INTRODUCTORY NUTRITION

INTRODUCTORY NUTRITION

Helen Andrews Guthrie, B.Sc., M.S., Ph.D.

Professor of Nutrition, The Pennsylvania State University,
University Park, Pennsylvania

FOURTH EDITION

with 233 illustrations

The C. V. Mosby Company

ST. LOUIS • LONDON • TORONTO 1979

FOURTH EDITION

Printed in the United States of America

The C. V. Mosby Company
11830 Westline Industrial Drive, St. Louis, Missouri 63141

Library of Congress Cataloging in Publication Data

Guthrie, Helen Andrews.
Introductory nutrition.

Bibliography: p.
Includes index.
1. Nutrition. I. Title.
TX354.G8 1979 641.1 78-16649
ISBN 0-8016-2001-5

TS/VH/VH 9 8 7 6 5 4 3 2 1 02/C/222

Preface

Since the publication of the first edition of this text in 1967, interest in nutrition has been increasing at a phenomenal rate. This has been evidenced in many ways—more health-food stores, more magazine articles and anecdotal accounts and testimony on the merits of certain nutritional practices, more government action on nutrition issues, more students enrolled in nutrition courses at the junior college, university, and adult levels, and increased funding for nutrition research and nutrition education activities. The number of college texts designed to teach the basic principles of nutrition and their applications has increased proportionately. Each, as this one, has its own merits and limitations. This text is based on the content of an introductory college course that has proved effective in teaching basic principles of nutrition for both students seeking a career in nutrition and those with a personal motivation for enrolling.

Experience has shown that the scope of this book is suited to the capabilities of most high school students who have had experience dealing with the concepts of the biological and physical sciences but no college training in science. It has also become evident that the level of presentation is equally valuable and suited to the needs of the student with a more sophisticated background. The primary purpose remains one of providing an in-depth introduction to the principles of nutrition for students at all levels of competence. It has been gratifying to know many have found this book meets their need.

A companion text, *Programmed Nutrition,* has been developed to help the student identify the concepts basic to an understanding of nutrition and utilize the principles of programmed instruction to reinforce an understanding of these concepts. In addition, to aid students, basic concepts from the related sciences are outlined in the first chapter, and a glossary and list of prefixes and suffixes with meanings are included in the appendices.

I hope that in mastering the material presented, students will become discerning consumers of nutrition information, with a comprehension of the basic principles adequate to enable them to discriminate the scientific from the pseudoscientific and fact from fallacy in the vast literature of both the lay and the scientific press. In addition to developing their own understanding of nutrition, students should be adequately prepared to interpret their knowledge of nutrition for the general public—a need that is becoming increasingly evident.

Another purpose of this book is to create awareness of the importance of nutrition in such a way that students will be motivated to apply this knowledge in establishing good eating habits. The extent to which this is achieved is more difficult to measure. It is also hoped that some students will be stimulated to continue the study of nutrition to acquire the level of competence needed to qualify them for the many challenging career opportunities in the field. The growing interest in the broad social and political implications of adequate nutrition has greatly expanded the horizons of the professional nutritionist.

An assessment of the advances in our knowledge of nutrition in the twelve years that have elapsed since the first edition indicates that nutritional biochemists, cell biologists, and physiologists have made significant contributions to our knowledge of metabolic processes. Many of their findings are beyond the scope of this presentation, but I have attempted to interpret those of greatest significance in the application of nutritional principles to the practical task of feeding people. For the most part, however, I have drawn on the studies of clinical nutritionists, who have focused on the questions of metabolism and nutrient needs of the total organism. Many of them have emphasized the role of social, economic, and psychological factors, as well as physiological and biochemical factors, involved in the availability and utilization of nutrients. Again, as in the previous editions, I have chosen to mention some of the more recent nutritional concepts and theories, with full recognition that they may have to be modified or deleted in subsequent editions.

The final chapter, dealing with the questions of hunger and malnutrition as national and international concerns, reflects a growing interest in the social implication of sound nutrition. Recognition of the effect that even moderate degrees of undernutrition may have on mental as well as physical health and development points to the availability and safety of the food supply as crucial factors in national planning. At the same time, a sizable portion of the population and certain of the readers of this book are being called on to cope with the equally complex problems of overnutrition.

Again, the revision was possible only through the help and encouragement of my husband, children, colleagues, and students. In addition to the innumerable people who gave valuable suggestions, Christine Lewis and Marian DeAngelo provided technical help, Joanne Green, a critical review of many chapters, and my two daughters, frank evaluation from a student perspective.

Helen Andrews Guthrie

Contents

PART ONE

Basic principles of nutrition

1

Overview of nutrition

Until five years ago nutrition was a topic that evoked little interest among either the public or legislators. Publicity of the relationship between diet and health performance or intelliegnce and questions to the effect of the changing food supply on our nutrient intake have kindled considerable interest in nutrition. Much of this interest is generated by persons questioning the adequacy of our food supply, some by those concerned with the safety of our changing food supply, and some by those who recognize the importance of a food intake derived from a variety of foods. At the same time that there is a growing interest in nutrition there is an ever-increasing opportunity for the spread of nutrition misinformation. This book is designed to provide the student with the core of information needed to make informed choices. This chapter provides a historical perspective on the growth of the science of nutrition.

The science of nutrition has been defined in many ways. Most simply it has been expressed as the science of nourishing the body properly or the analysis of the effect of food on the living organism. Yudkin chooses to define nutrition as the relationship between man and his food and implies the psychological and social as well as the physiological and biochemical aspects. Others propose defining it as a science devoted to the determination of the requirements of the body for food constituents both qualitatively and quantitatively and to the selection of food in kinds and in quantity to meet these requirements. The Council on Foods and Nutrition of the American Medical Association elaborates still further in declaring nutrition as "the science of food, the nutrients and other substances therein, their action, interaction, and balance in relation to health and disease and the processes by which the organism ingests, digests, absorbs, transports, utilizes and excretes food substances."

Regardless of the basic definition, persons studying nutrition agree that they are concerned with the changes that occur in food and the way in which the body uses it from the time food is ingested until it is eventually incorporated into the body tissues, participates in biological reactions, or is excreted from the body. This includes the study of digestion, absorption, and transportation of nutrients to the cells and their metabolism within the many types of body cells. In addition, nutritionists are becoming increasingly concerned with the factors that determine what a person chooses to eat and with monitoring the nutritive quality of the available food resources.

The nutrients in food with which nutrition is concerned are those chemical components of the food that perform one of three roles in the body: supply energy, regulate body processes, or promote the growth and repair of body tissue.

The science of nutrition is a relative youngster in the scientific community, having been recognized as a distinct discipline only in 1934 with the organization of the American Institute of Nutrition. As a science relying on the techniques of the chemist and biologist, nutrition developed only after development of these other branches of science. Nutrition, like other sciences, does not stand alone. It draws heavily on the basic findings of chemistry, biochemistry, microbiology, physiology, medicine, and, most recently, cellular biology. In turn, it also contributes to these fields of scientific investigation.

HISTORICAL BACKGROUND

Although the organized study of nutrition has been confined to the twentieth century, there is evidence of a long-standing curiosity about the subject. A few well-conceived nutritional experiments were performed earlier, but these stimulated little interest. Schneider has aptly divided the history of nutrition into three eras: the *naturalistic era* (400 BC-AD 1750), the *chemical-analytical era* (1750-1900), and the *biological era* (1900 to present). Running concurrently with the latter from 1955 to the present can be added the *cellular* or *molecular era,* in which emphasis has been directed to the study of nutrition within the highly organized individual cells. Although no attempt will be made to discuss all the findings of each era, a few highlights will be mentioned to give some picture of the extent of the knowledge of nutrition in each stage.

Naturalistic era. During the naturalistic era people had many vague ideas about food, most of which revolved around taboos, magical powers, or medicinal value. Just as millions do today, early man recognized that food was essential for survival and did not discriminate about the relative value of different foods. In Biblical times, however, Daniel observed that men who ate pulses and drank water thrived better than did those who ate the king's food and drank wine. Hippocrates, the father of medicine, in his discussion of food in health and disease in 400 BC considered food one universal nutrient. He believed that weight loss during starvation was caused by insensible perspiration. By the sixteenth century a doctrine of diet and longevity had been well established.

In the early seventeenth century an Italian physician, Sanctorius, curious about the fate of food in the body, weighed himself before and after each meal. His only explanation of his failure to gain weight commensurate with the amount of food taken in was that there must be weight loss in insensible perspiration. It was during this period that such men as Harvey and Spallanzani, with their interest in circulation and digestion, made observations that eventually facilitated the study of nutrition. At the end of this era the first controlled nutrition experiment was carried out in 1747 by a British physician, Lind, who attempted to find a cure for scurvy by treating twelve sailors ill with the disease with six different substances. He determined that either lemon or lime juice was effective, while the others, such as oil of vitriol, seawater, and vinegar, were ineffective in curing this scorbutic condition.

Chemical-analytical era. The chemical-analytical era in the study of nutrition was initiated in the eighteenth century by Lavoisier, who became known as the father of nutrition. His work involved the study of respiration, oxidation, and calorimetry—all concerned with the use of food energy. His work with guinea pigs on oxygen uptake, with and without food and during work, was the first investigation that showed the relationship between heat production and oxygen use in the body. Black and Priestley, also working in the eighteenth century, contributed to the growing knowledge of respiration and energy metabolism.

Early in the nineteenth century, methods for determining carbon, hydrogen, and nitrogen in organic compounds were developed. Analyses of foods for these elements led Liebig to suggest that the nutritive value of foods was a function of its nitrogen content. He also postulated that an adequate diet must provide plastic foods (protein) and fuel foods (carbohydrate and fat). Dumas, a French chemist, tested this hypothesis during a siege of Paris in 1871. His efforts to produce a synthetic milk of carbohydrate, fat, and protein in the proportions believed to be found in cow's milk proved unsuccessful, and the infants to whom he fed it died. Dumas logically concluded that milk must contain some unknown nutritive substance.

A similar conclusion was reached in 1881 by Lunin, who found that mice fed a diet of purified casein (a protein), milk sugar (a carbohydrate), milk fat, and the inorganic ash from milk died, while those who were fed milk thrived. Between then and 1906 there were reports of twelve experiments on the use of purified diets in the feeding of animals. All led to essentially the same conclusion that the addition of "astonishingly" small amounts of natural foods was necessary to promote growth and to maintain health in the animals. Obviously, food contained more than carbohydrate, fat, protein, and mineral ash, but the nature of the other substances remained a mystery. In spite of these findings the United States Department of Agriculture steadfastly maintained until 1910 that carbohydrate, fat, and protein were the only nutrients essential in the human diet.

By 1912 it had been well established that there was an additional dietary essential besides carbohydrate, fat, protein, and mineral ash. Funk, recognizing that this dietary component was essential to life *(vita)* and believing it to be *amine,* or nitrogen containing, introduced the term *vitamine* to describe this elusive dietary factor. Two independent studies showed that there were at least two vitamins—fat-soluble vitamin A and water-soluble vitamin B. McCollum's work at the University of Wisconsin showed that some fats such as butter contained an essential growth factor, whereas others such as lard did not. Eijkman observed that a water-soluble substance in rice bran prevented beriberi, a disease common in the Orient. By 1920 when it was established that all vitamins did not contain nitrogen, the final "e" was dropped to obtain the term *vitamin,* which persists to this day.

In spite of the relatively slow communication in this period, scientists in Europe, Asia, and North America made rapid progress in identifying essential dietary components. Many times discoveries were made almost simultaneously by scientists working independently and in widely separated laboratories. The concept that diseases such as beriberi, scurvy, rickets, and pellagra, previously considered to be caused by toxic substances or to be infectious in nature, were in reality the result of an absence of nutrients needed in very small amounts did much to stimulate the attempts to identify the nature of these dietary essentials.

Biological era. The early part of the biological era was characterized by the discovery of many factors with vitamin-like properties. It soon became clear that there were several components of both fat-soluble A and water-soluble B. By 1940 four fat-soluble and eight water-soluble vitamins had been identified as essential elements of the human diet, and several others had been identified for various species of animals. The chemical structure of each had been established, many had been synthesized, and knowledge of their biological roles was accumulating rapidly. Since 1940 only two essential vitamins, folic acid and vitamin B_{12}, have been identified. The emphasis in nutrition research has changed from a search for essential dietary components to a study of the interrelationships among nutrients, their precise biological roles, and the determination of human dietary requirements. More recently, interest has been directed toward the problems of nutrition education as the result of the widening gap between our theoretical knowledge of nutrition and its application in the improvement of nutritional status.

During this same period the noncombustible component, or mineral ash, of the diet was being studied, and it too proved to be a complex mixture of elements—twenty of which have been established as dietary essentials for humans. The essentiality of several others is still uncertain. Here again there was evidence of involved interrelationships among mineral elements; some were capable of replacing others, whereas a high intake of one could cause the excretion of another.*

Cellular or molecular era. Since 1955 the development of the electron microscope, the ultracentrifuge, microchemical techniques, the use of radioactive isotopes and immunoassays has made it possible to study the nutritional needs and metabolism of the individual cells and even the subcellular components, or organelles, of the cell. At the present time a vast body of information is accumulating, which is leading to a more complete understanding of the intricacies of cell structure and the complex and vital role that nutrients play in the growth, development, and maintenance of the cell. Nourishment of the cell is basic to the nourishment of the collection of cells known as tissue, and this in turn is basic to the nourishment of organs of the body and ultimately of the whole complex body.

It is now well established that lack of an essential nutrient results in a failure to form an essential enzyme or other cellular component or in an inability to use these components. This results in malfunctioning or death of the cell, which eventually shows up in a specific physical symptom of ill health.

PRESENT STATUS

We now find ourselves, more than a hundred years after the first studies that showed that more than carbohydrate, fat, and protein were necessary for normal growth and development, with a vast, complex, and rapidly expanding knowledge of over forty nutritional principles that must be supplied by food for normal body functioning. The absence of any one of these, regardless of the amount needed, can have a profound effect on the functioning of the whole body.

Although it is now over thirty years since the discovery of the last vitamin, nutrition remains a vital, exciting field in which new information is being accumulated at a phenomenal pace. The contributions of the nutritionist alone have been many and significant. When one integrates with these the related findings of the biochemist, physiologist, biologist, and physicist, one realizes that understanding the complexity of the process of nourishing the body is a challenging frontier of science that is only beginning to be explored.

The fact that scurvy, rickets, beriberi, pellagra, and kwashiorkor, all nutritional deficiency diseases representing but a small fraction of nutritional problems, can be found in affluent and developing countries alike is stark evidence of our failure to apply what nutrition information we do have. In attempts to eliminate this paradox, nutritionists are now turning to social scientists and communication specialists to assist them in effecting the kinds of behavioral changes that will result in improved nutritional health.

Many new approaches to the study of nutrition are emerging. The study of the cell has stimulated interest in the role that genetics may play in influencing the nutritional needs of the organism. The interaction between nutrition and genetics in the developmental process is providing an explanation for some congenital abnormalities and metabolic defects. The role of nutrition in brain development, behavior, resistance to infection, and stress and the role of environmental factors such as pollution and the use of drugs on nutrition are but some of the newer concepts being studied.

Recognition that nutritional factors are among those implicated in the development of cardiovascular disease, hypertension, diabetes, and cancer, all leading causes of death, has prompted extensive investigations of the possible roles of nutrition in the cause and prevention of these diseases. Unfortunately there are many unsubstantiated claims for the effectiveness of specific foods or specific nutrients in preventing or miraculously curing these degenerative diseases. The nutritionist is now as concerned about com-

*The serious student who is interested in reading some of the classic studies in nutrition is referred to a series being reprinted in *Nutrition Reviews* beginning in 1973 (Nutrition Foundation, Inc., New York).

batting misinformation as with delivering sound nutrition information.

As biochemists become more concerned with the intricacies of metabolism and less and less with the total organism, nutritionists are turning much of their attention to the integration of the theoretical knowledge from many fields of study and to the application of this to the maintenance of health and the prevention and treatment of disease.

Iatrogenic nutrition, which is concerned with nutritional disease resulting from the activities of a physician in treating a patient with drugs, surgery, or therapeutic diets, represents another area of interest.

The rate at which the time, effort, and money expended on nutrition research increased after the concept of vitamins was first postulated can be judged by the number of scientific publications in the field. In 1913 there were four publications, all by Casimir Funk; by 1920 the number had risen to 73; and in 1930, 724 articles appeared. In 1978 reviews of current literature on single nutrients routinely list from 200 to 500 references. At least ten scientific journals are devoted entirely to reporting findings of nutrition research and many more carry research that has either direct or indirect impact on nutritional policies and practices. In 1978 over 4000 papers dealing directly or indirectly with subjects of significance in nutrition were presented at a single scientific meeting. The large number of investigators who consider nutrition their major interest is obvious from the number of members in scientific organizations devoted to nutrition and from their attendance at professional meetings. The Institute of Nutrition, whose membership is restricted to scientists who have made significant contribution to the field, has over 1500 members. The Society for Nutrition Education was formed in 1971 in recognition of the need for a forum for professionals concerned with the application of nutrition knowledge in prevention as well as cure and understanding of malnutrition.

The year 1968 saw the beginning of a surge of public interest in nutrition in the United States. This was the result of the realization that hunger and malnutrition existed in the midst of plenty. The first White House Conference on Food, Nutrition, and Health, which convened in 1969, represented a concern on the part of the federal government that the problem be identified and that steps be taken to alleviate it. Since that time a number of federally supported nutrition activities have been initiated, including nutrition programs for the elderly, comprehensive nutrient labeling of all processed food products for which any nutritional claim is made, and nutrition education in elementary schools. Other programs such as school feeding and food stamps have been expanded. At the same time a nutrition-conscious nation has manifest its concern with increased expenditures on health foods and increased reliance on alternate food patterns. The effectiveness of the activity resulting from the 1969 conference was assessed at a follow-up conference in 1974.

The passage in 1977 of the Child Nutrition Bill mandating that each state establish a nutrition education program was designed to enhance nutritional awareness among a growing group of consumers. It should also provide the next generation of consumers with the knowledge base to allow them to function as nutritionally literate decision makers. Also, nutrition research and education have for the first time been pinpointed in various pieces of proposed legislation.

The controversial statement on Dietary Goals for the United States (p. 554) issued by the Senate Committee on Nutrition and Human Needs in early 1977 and revised in 1978 provided further evidence of increasing government interest in the nutritional health of the country. At the same time it raised the question as to whether the development of such guidelines should be the role of a legislative or scientific group.

On an international level the importance that political leaders attach to nutrition is best illustrated by the fact that the first

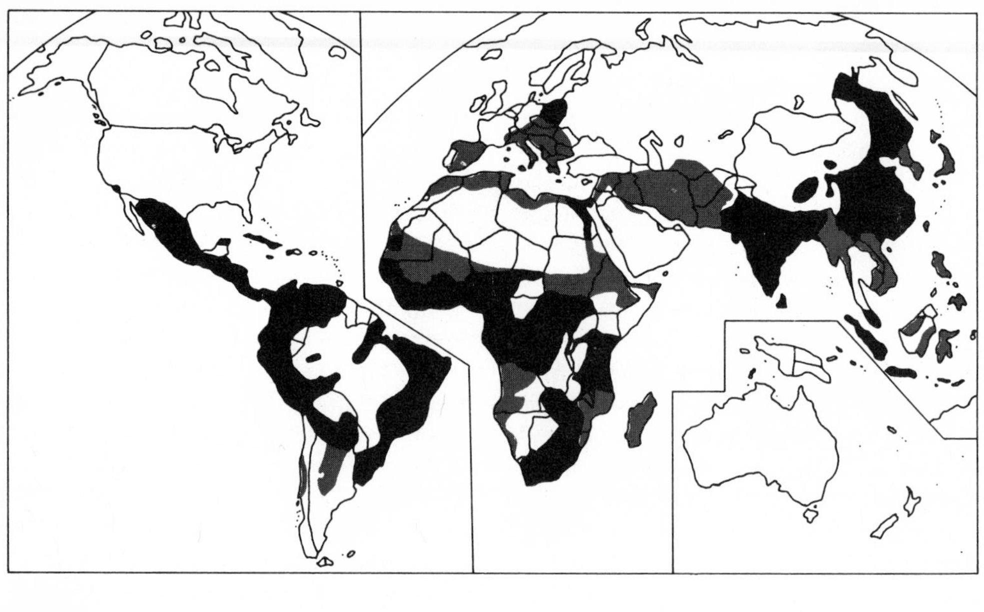

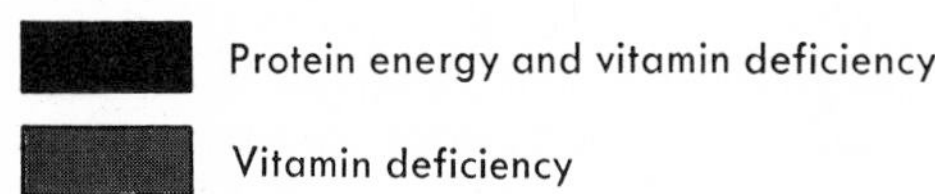

Fig. 1-1. Distribution of protein- and vitamin-deficiency diseases in the world.

agency authorized within the United Nations was the Food and Agricultural Organization, commonly known as FAO. In 1944 it was charged with the responsibility of devising ways to improve the nutritional status of the world's population as one of the major pathways to peace. Since then, interest in international nutrition problems has increased rapidly.

WHO (World Health Organization) allocates much of its resources toward the solution of nutrition problems, as do national groups such as the Agency for International Development. A large number of privately funded organizations and foundations also work actively to contribute to solutions for nutrition problems. Numerous conferences are devoted to discussion of efforts to improve the nutritional status of the expanding populations of developing countries. The necessity of making maximum use of indigenous food products to provide a level of nutrition capable of supporting health and promoting individual productivity is an ever-present challenge to nutritionists. The World Food Conference that convened in Rome in 1976 brought together a multinational group representing politicians, scientists, clinicians, educators, and the public concerned about the world food and nutrition policy and dedicated to finding ways to achieve more equitable food distribution and alleviate health problems associated with dietary inadequacies.

In spite of these efforts, malnutrition and undernutrition existing in conjunction with a rapidly expanding population and inadequate medical care remain the most important health problems in the world today. The worldwide incidence of nutritional deficiency diseases indicates the scope of the problem (Fig. 1-1).

IMPORTANCE OF GOOD NUTRITION

Before launching on an intensive study of the individual nutrients, the student of nutrition may legitimately ask, "What evidence is there that nutrition makes a difference?" The United States Department of Agriculture (USDA) has attempted to estimate the costs of malnutrition in the United States. It suggests that appropriate nutrition intervention activities can reduce morbidity and mortality from heart disease by 25%, from respiratory and infectious diseases by 20%, from cancer by 20%, and from diabetes by 50%. The preventable costs attributable to such conditions are estimated at billions of dollars annually. Good nutrition may indeed be one of our most valuable untapped resources.

Over the years several investigators have provided evidence that good nutrition does make a difference. Although a comprehensive review of studies in this area is well beyond the scope of this text, a few examples may serve to illustrate the point.

A change from the use of poorly refined brown rice to more highly refined white rice with its improved keeping qualities occurred in the Philippines and other rice-eating countries around the turn of the century. With this change there was a marked increase in the incidence of the disease beriberi, which first was believed to be caused by a toxic substance in rice and later was attributed to unsanitary milling conditions. By 1935, however, an antiberiberi factor in rice bran had been identified, establishing that beriberi was the result of a lack of a nutrient which was apparently removed in the milling process. This nutrient became known as thiamin. Once this vitamin had been synthesized and was available commercially, the Philippine government and the Williams Waterman Fund backed a study of rice enrichment to determine the effect of adding thiamin back to the rice. People on one half the island of Bataan ate rice enriched with thiamin, whereas those on the other half ate the unenriched milled white rice. After nine months 90% of the population on enriched rice who had previously shown mild or definite signs of the disease were improved and the death rate had dropped by two thirds. At the end of the second year there were *no* deaths from beriberi in the enriched-rice group, indicating clearly that the addition of the nutrient brought about a general improvement in the health of the population and a marked decrease in the incidence of beriberi.

In 1946 Burke, working with patients at the Boston Lying-In Hospital at Harvard, studied the relationship between the quality of the diet of the mother during pregnancy and the health of the infant at the time of birth. Of the infants born to mothers whose diet was rated good or excellent, 94% were judged in superior or good physical condition at the time of birth, and only 6% were rated in fair or poor condition. Conversely, when the diet was assessed as poor, only 8% of the infants received a superior or good rating, whereas 92% were judged in fair or poor condition. These observations are illustrated in Fig. 1-2. Since people change food habits slowly even under conditions of high motivation such as pregnancy, the dietary ratings undoubtedly reflected long-standing patterns of eating rather than those that prevailed only during pregnancy. Failure of subsequent studies to show such a clear-cut relationship may reflect an overall improvement of the diet of mothers as our knowledge of nutrition has increased.

The reduction in the incidence of simple goiter experienced in Michigan after an intensive educational campaign on the use of iodized salt is further evidence of the differences between poor and adequate nutrition in respect to one nutrient. In a thirty-year period there was a drop from 47.2% to 1.4% in the reported cases of simple goiter. Similarly, the addition of fluorine to drinking water has resulted in a 50% to 70% reduction in the incidence of tooth decay among children.

In Newfoundland a nutritional survey in 1945 revealed a high incidence of subclinical evidence of nutritional deficiency, such as rough dry skin, cracks in the corner of the lips, and soft bleeding gums. This was at-

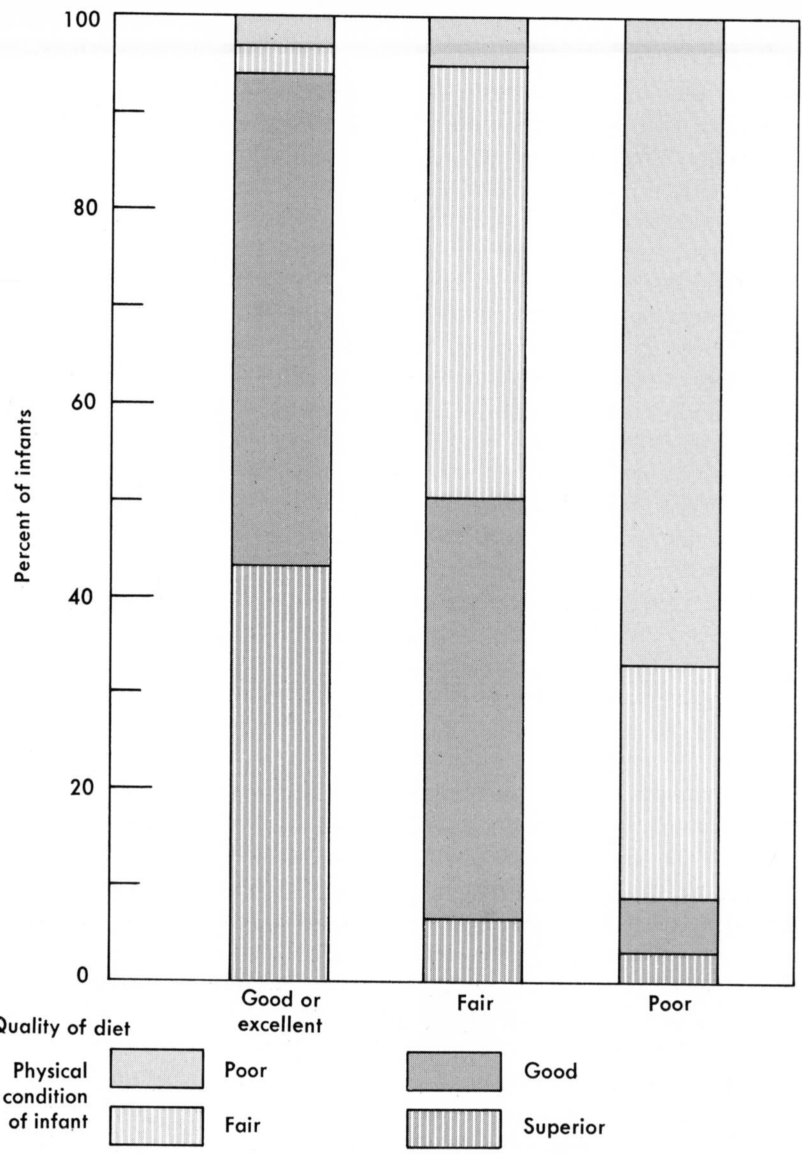

Fig. 1-2. Relationship between quality of mother's diet and condition of infant at birth. (Modified from Burke, B. S.: J. Nutr. **38**:453, 1949.)

tributed to suboptimal intakes of the B vitamins, vitamin A, and ascorbic acid. A program of enriching flour with thiamin, riboflavin, niacin, and iron and enriching margarine with vitamin A resulted in a marked reduction in these conditions.

The change in stature of children in the United States that has occurred in the past few decades has been in part attributed to improved nutrition. There is ample evidence that children are heavier and taller than their parents. For instance, Philadelphia schoolchildren in first through fifth grades in all socioeconomic groups averaged 5 cm (3 inches) taller and 1.35 kg (3 pounds) heavier in 1951 than in 1925. In 1880, 5% of the male college freshmen were over 1.8 m (6 feet) tall, whereas in 1955, 30% reached this stature. Nutrition has undoubtedly contributed to this gain, but one must also keep in mind advances in other areas of medicine that have reduced the incidence of infection and other deterrents to optimal growth at an early age. Adult heights have not shown a comparable increase. The question is now being raised as to how much of these increases in growth rate is desirable. Evidence from animal studies indicates a decrease in life-span among animals fed at a level to stimulate early and rapid growth. On the other hand, women over 1.63 m (5 feet 4 inches) tall, possibly the better nourished members of the population, were found to have fewer complications during pregnancy and easier deliveries than did those under 1.63 m (5 feet 4 inches) tall.

HOW THE BODY USES FOOD

Food fulfills many roles for the individual. Its psychological value, its social significance, and its satiety value are more likely determinants of when, how much, and what foods are consumed than are nutritional considerations.

The role of food to which our interests will be directed primarily, however, is that of nourishing the body. Food chosen wisely provides all the nutrients essential for the normal functioning of the body. If food is not properly chosen, there will be a deficiency of one or more of the essential nutrients. An essential nutrient is defined as one that must be provided to the organism by food because it cannot be synthesized by the body at a rate sufficient to meet its needs. Nutrients essential for one species may not be essential for another.

Although we have a rapidly expanding body of information on the biological role of and the need for specific nutrients, the long-established broad classification of the function of nutrients in the body is still valid. The major functions are to supply energy, promote growth and repair body tissues, and regulate body processes.

The nutrients that perform these functions may be divided into six main categories: carbohydrate, lipid, protein, minerals, vitamins, and water. A classification of the essential nutrients in each of these broad groupings follows.

Carbohydrate
- Glucose

Fat or lipid
- Linoleic acid

Protein
- Amino acids*
  - Leucine
  - Isoleucine
  - Lysine
  - Methionine
  - Phenylalanine
  - Threonine
  - Trytophan
  - Valine
  - Histidine
- Nonessential nitrogen

Minerals
- Calcium
- Phosphorus
- Sodium
- Potassium
- Sulfur
- Chlorine
- Magnesium
- Iron
- Selenium
- Zinc
- Manganese
- Copper
- Cobalt
- Molybdenum
- Iodine
- Chromium
- Fluorine
- Vanadium
- Tin
- Nickel
- Silicon

Vitamins*
- Fat-soluble vitamins
  - A (retinol)
  - D (cholecalciferol)
  - E (tocopherol)
  - K
- Water-soluble vitamins
  - Thiamin
  - Riboflavin
  - Niacin
  - Biotin
  - Folacin
  - Pyridoxine
  - Vitamin B_{12}
  - Pantothenic acid
  - Ascorbic acid

Water

The nutrients listed are absolutely essential to human growth and maintenance. Some nutrients are present in a wide variety of foods in nature and there is little likelihood of deficiency occurring. On the other hand, some are distributed in a limited number of foods and will be present in less than optimal amounts if the variety of foods in the diet is limited.

Differences in the extent to which various foods contribute these essential nutrients are illustrated in Table 1-1. From this table it is evident that the first four nutrients constitute 98% of the weight of food and that the vitamins and minerals constitute an extremely

*Chemical formulas are shown in Appendix L.

Table 1-1. Approximate composition of some representative foods

	Whole milk (%)	Bread (%)	Carrots (%)
Water	87.0	35.8	88.2
Carbohydrate	5.0	50.4	8.4
Lipid	3.5	3.2	0.2
Protein	3.7	8.7	1.1
Minerals	0.7	1.1	1.9
Vitamins	0.1	0.1	0.1

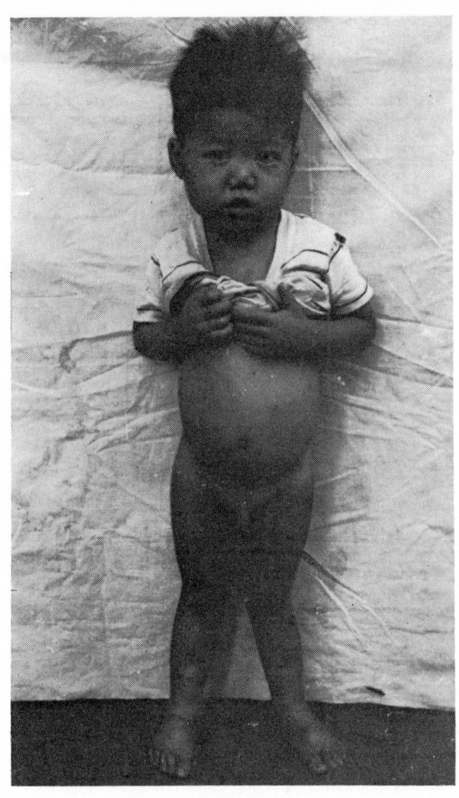

Fig. 1-3. Hidden hunger. This child, 4 years of age, looks plump enough. Closer inspection shows pitting edema of the legs caused by dietary protein deficiency and low serum albumin level. This is kwashiorkor (without dermatosis). The child is also dull, apathetic, potbellied, and has ophthalmic xerosis and Bitot's spots on the conjunctiva of both eyes. (Courtesy WHO Regional Office, Manila.)

small portion of food. These small amounts are, however, sufficient to make the difference between a healthy, well-functioning body and one with evidence of nutritional inadequacies.

It is clear from the following classification of nutrients according to functions that some, such as protein, perform all three functions, whereas some of the minerals are involved in two, and vitamins, directly, in only one. A nutrient that performs only one function is equally as essential as one involved in all three functions.

Source of energy
- Carbohydrate
- Lipid
- Protein
- Mineral elements*
- Vitamins*

Growth and maintenance of tissue
- Protein
- Mineral elements
- Vitamins*
- Water*

Regulation of body processes
- Protein
- Mineral elements
- Vitamins
- Water

The amount of each of the essential nutrients needed for normal body functions bears no relationship to its importance in the diet. In the adult male, needs vary from 3 μg (3/28,000,000 ounce) of cobalamin (vitamin B_{12}) to 46 g (1½ ounces) of protein to as much as 340 g (¾ pound) of carbohydrate depending on his energy needs. A deficiency of a nutrient needed in extremely small amounts may precipitate more severe symptoms more rapidly than a deficiency of one needed in much larger amounts. In addition, deficiencies can result from increased needs, decreased absorption, or depressed utilization of a nutrient. Fig. 1-3 shows the effects of a

*These play an indirect role, since they are necessary to catalyze the use of the three nutrients directly involved.

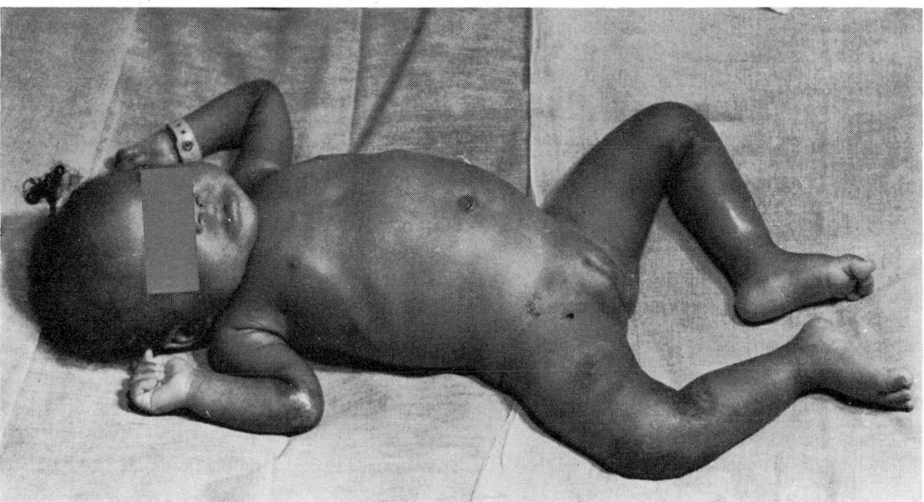

Fig. 1-4. Case of infantile scurvy caused by a lack of abscorbic acid (vitamin C). Note typical frog position, swelling of right thigh, and hyperpigmentation of skin. (From Ossofsky, H. J.: Amer. J. Dis. Child. **109:**173, 1965.)

severe or prolonged lack of a nutrient. Fig. 1-4 illustrates the effect of lack of a nutrient needed at one-thousandth the level of that producing the effect seen in Fig. 1-3. It was the search for a cause and cure of diseases such as these that stimulated much of the early research in nutrition.

One factor that influenced the ease with which nutritional factors were identified is the rapidity with which body reserves are depleted in times of dietary deficiency. Table 1-2 shows that the time varies from a few hours in the case of labile amino acids, which the body has virtually no capacity to store, to about sixty days for many water-soluble vitamins, to seven years for calcium. The major site of storage differs with the nutrient—liver for iron, vitamin A, and carbohydrate; the adrenal gland for vitamin C; and bone for calcium. For some nutrients there is no storage site. In these cases, deficiency symptoms will become evident once the individual cells have become depleted of the nutrient.

Table 1-2. Extent of body reserves of nutrients

Nutrient	Time required to deplete reserves
Amino acids	Few hours
Carbohydrate	13 hours
Sodium	2-3 days
Water	4 days
Fat	20-40 days
Thiamin	30-60 days
Ascorbic acid	60-120 days
Niacin	60-180 days
Riboflavin	60-180 days
Vitamin A	90-365 days
Iron	125 days (women) 750 days (men)
Iodine	1000 days
Calcium	2500 days

The elucidation of the role of individual nutrients was further complicated by the interrelationships and interdependence that exist among the nutrients. For instance, the need for thiamin (vitamin B_1) is a function of the amount and kind of carbohydrate in the diet, the absorption of calcium is dependent on a supply of vitamin D, vitamin E protects vitamin A, and the nature and amount of fat in the diet affects the vitamin E requirement. Current research is bringing forth further evidence of the complexity of these interrelationships. Manipulation of one dietary component may lead to changes in the utilization or need of many others.

In addition, nutrient needs and their use may be influenced by many nonnutritional factors such as the use of drugs, exposure to environmental contamination, or physical, emotional, or physiological stresses. Hence the evaluation of the results of manipulating one dietary factor depends on knowledge of the status of all other dietary factors as well as many nondietary influences.

BASIC CONCEPTS FROM RELATED SCIENTIFIC FIELDS

Although this treatment of introductory material basic to the understanding of nutrition does not presuppose any previous training in the related fields of biochemistry, physiology, and cellular biology, certain concepts from these fields will facilitate the understanding of the processes involved in nourishing the body. They are well within the grasp of any college student and will be presented here as an elementary review for those with previous instruction in these fields and as the bare fundamentals for those unfamiliar with the subject matter.

Role of enzymes, coenzymes, and hormones. The conversion of food into a form in which it can provide for the body's needs for growth, energy, and maintenance involves a series of biochemical changes. Some occur in the digestive tract, but the majority occur in the individual cells of the body. Many of these changes require the assistance of **enzymes,*** which are proteins produced by the cells of the body and either secreted into the body fluids or produced and used within the cells. Although most enzymes are composed of only protein, some contain a mineral as a part of their structure. Thus such an enzyme cannot be formed if either the material to form the protein or the mineral part of the enzyme is missing.

An enzyme performs a specific function and acts to facilitate one specific reaction. In some cases, such as digestion, the enzyme attaches itself to a specific spot in the complex substance and, either alone or with the help of another substance, causes the splitting of the large molecule into two or more smaller portions or the removal or change of some portion of the molecule. Conversely, enzymes may act to help build new substances from smaller units within the body. Many enzymes act to bring about the synthesis, or building, of body tissue, which occurs during growth, by making it possible for the two or more parts of a new substance to be joined together.

Some enzymes do not act by themselves but require the help of **coenzymes,** most of which are nonprotein organic compounds and all of which have a vitamin as part of their structure. Thus a reaction that requires both an enzyme and a coenzyme before it can take place requires that both the vitamin and the protein be available.

Hormones also play an important role in regulating biochemical changes within the body. In contrast to vitamins, which must be supplied in the food, and enzymes, which are produced in most body cells, hormones are produced in the glands and are transported through the blood to another part of the body where they exert their action. Often the action of a hormone is to stimulate the production of an enzyme, but a hormone may also influence the function of a tissue, such as the kidney.

Physiology. Before the cells, the smallest structural units of the body, can receive nourishment, the food taken into the body in a complex state must undergo many changes to reduce it to a form in which it can be transported to and used by the cells. These changes occur primarily in the digestive tract of the body (Fig. 1-5). The digestive tract is essentially a coiled tube about 9 meters long passing through the center of the body; until

*Terms that appear in boldface type are essential to the understanding of nutrition. They are either explained in the text or in the glossary (Appendix A).

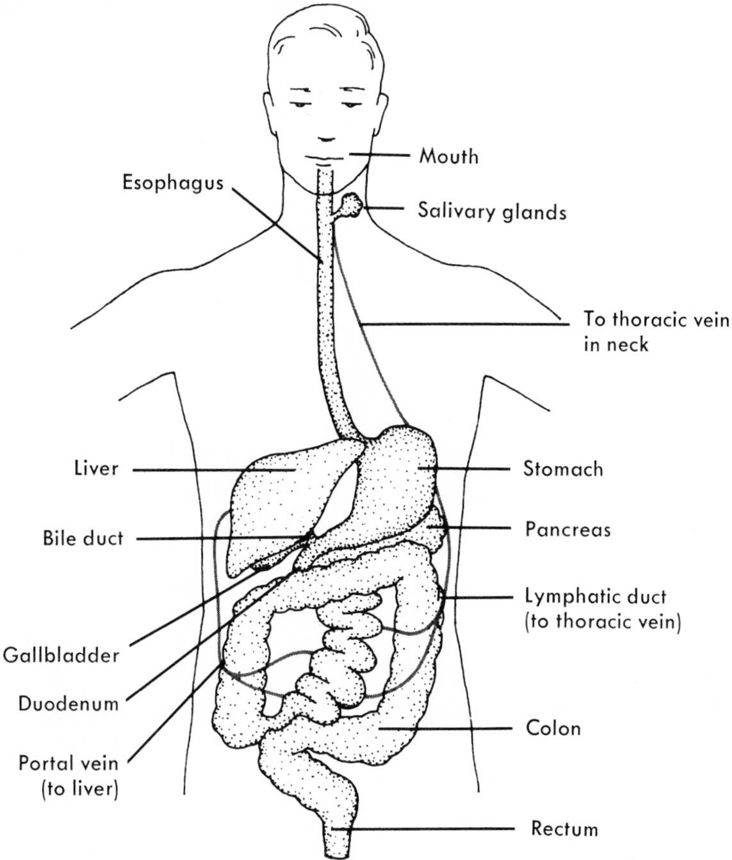

Fig. 1-5. Essential features of the human digestive system.

food passes through the walls of this tube, it is, from a physiological standpoint, still outside the body. The walls of the intestines regulate not only the form in which nutrients enter the body but also the amounts.

Digestion is accomplished by mechanical and chemical processes. Mechanically, food is broken down into small pieces by the action of chewing in the mouth. This increases the surface area on which the enzymes of the digestive juices can act. As the food mass passes down the digestive tract, **peristalsis,** the churning action resulting from the contraction and relaxation of the very muscular wall of the tract, reduces the size of food particles still further and mixes them thoroughly with digestive juices. The sites and nature of changes within the digestive tract are summarized in Table 1-3.

Chemically, the character of ingested food is changed by the action of digestive enzymes secreted in the salivary juice in the mouth, the gastric juice in the stomach, and the bile from the gallbladder, the pancreatic juice, and the intestinal juice secreted into the small intestine. In addition, some digestion, known as membrane digestion, occurs within the wall of the small intestine. Together these digestive juices provide all the enzymes necessary to prepare food to pass from the digestive to the circulatory system for use by the body.

Enzymes are specifically designed to act on each class of nutrient. Those which act on

Table 1-3. Summary of sites and nature of digestion

Site	Type of action	How accomplished
Mouth	Mechanical	Chewing
	Chemical	Salivary enzymes
Stomach	Mechanical	Peristalsis
	Chemical	Action of hydrochloric acid
		Gastric enzymes
Small intestine	Mechanical	Peristalsis
	Chemical	Pancreatic enzymes
		Intestinal enzymes
		Bile

carbohydrate are known as **amylases,** those on lipids as **lipases,** and those on proteins as **proteases.** Some digestive secretions contain enzymes that act on all three groups whereas others have enzymes for only one or two classes of nutrients.

Once the food has been changed chemically into the simple form in which the body can use it, it passes through the wall of the intestinal tract into the blood or lymph, by which it is carried to the body cells. Most absorption occurs through walls of the small intestine, but some also occurs in the stomach and large intestine, and extremely little in the mouth. For some nutrients the passage through the intestinal wall is by diffusion, for others by osmosis, and for many by **active transport,** a process that requires energy and often a special carrier. In any case, the nature and amount of food that enters the body from the digestive tract is regulated in the intestinal wall.

After the digested food has passed through the wall of the digestive tract, it is picked up by one of two circulatory systems of the body—the arteriovenous, or the blood system, or the **lymphatic** system. The relationship of these two systems is illustrated in Fig. 1-6. Nutrients that enter the arteriovenous system are carried by the portal vein to the liver, where they are released into the general circulatory system. In the circulatory system they are distributed through the arteries and very small blood vessels, the capillaries, and finally to the extracellular fluid bathing each individual cell of the body. Nutrients, primarily fats and fat-soluble nutrients that enter the lymphatic system (an auxiliary circulatory system serving primarily to collect body fluids), bypass the liver and enter the general arteriovenous circulation at a point in the neck just before the blood enters the heart. From this point they are distributed to the cells in the same way as nutrients that first passed through the liver. It is from the extracellular fluids bathing the cells that the cell obtains the nutrients it needs. In this case the cell membrane acts as a selective barrier to regulate the entrance of material into the cell.

The waste products of cellular metabolism are released into the extracellular fluid, enter the bloodstream, and are eventually excreted from the body, primarily through the lungs and kidneys.

The lungs serve as the main excretory organ for carbon dioxide and for 10% of the water. The kidneys, through which most of the water leaves the body, act as an efficient and selective filtering system for the bloodstream. They are capable of concentrating in the urine waste products of metabolism, such as creatinine and urea, and excreting them. They will also allow excesses of such nutrients as water-soluble vitamins to leave the body. However, for nutrients such as glucose, which the body needs to conserve, the kidneys will resorb practically all that is present in the blood filtered through them. In the case of some other nutrients, such as sodium, they will resorb the amounts needed to maintain normal blood and tissue levels and will release the rest. They are extremely sensitive to the needs of the body and will regulate the nature and amount of the metabolites excreted in response to the many regulatory forces, such as hormones, that influence

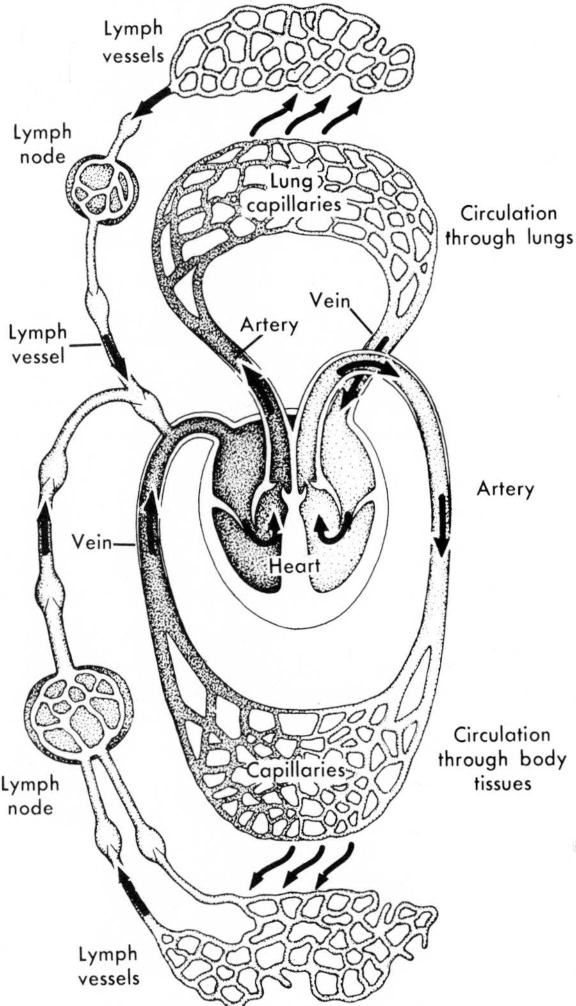

Fig. 1-6. This schematic diagram shows the relationship between the arterial and venous systems and the lymphatic system. Blood is pumped by the heart through a network of capillaries in the lung. The oxygenated blood returns to the heart, where it is then pumped out to supply the various parts of the body with oxygen and nutrients. After passing through the tissues the blood returns to the heart to again be pumped to the lungs. However, in both the lung circulation and body tissue circulation some of the fluid leaves the blood capillaries and enters spaces within the tissues. This fluid is picked up by the lymph capillaries and returned to the bloodstream. Lymph nodes are important in the removal of foreign particles and in the production of antibodies. (From Berry, J. W., Osgood, D. W., and St. John, P. A.: Chemical villains: a biology of pollution, St. Louis, 1974, The C. V. Mosby Co.)

them. Some nutrients are also lost from the body through the skin—either in perspiration or in the sloughing of epithelial cells or the loss of hair and nails. Cells lining the intestinal tract are completely replaced every three to four days, and the old ones are excreted in the feces. Fecal excretions may also contain nutrients that are part of the digestive juices, which are not reabsorbed. A determination of the kinds and amounts of nutrients lost from the body through any or all of these pathways sheds much light on the need for various nutrients and the way in which they are changed in the body.

Biochemistry. The nature of the nutrients and the chemical changes that occur in them from the time they are taken into the body until they are built into body tissue, are used, or are excreted is part of the subject matter of biochemistry—the chemistry of living material. All biological compounds contain the elements carbon and hydrogen, practically all contain oxygen, and they may have nitrogen, sulfur, or other inorganic elements.

Basic to any understanding of biochemistry is knowledge of the chemistry of carbon compounds. Carbon, an element capable of reacting with negatively charged elements, *always* has a valence of 4, which means that there are four places (bonds) on a carbon atom to which some other element is attached:

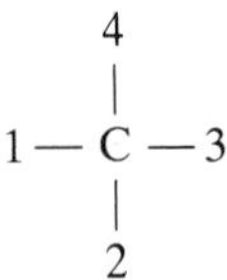

If two adjacent carbon atoms are unsaturated (do not have anything to attach to their carbon bonds), they will join together, forming what is known as a double bond:

```
     4    4
     |    |
1 —  C =  C — 3
```

This is a relatively reactive bond easily broken to two single bonds if some elements become available to attach to the bonds. Compounds that contain double carbon bonds are active chemically, since they are receptive to the addition of other elements.

In general, however, carbon compounds are relatively inert, reacting slowly with each other, with water, and with oxygen.

About 30% of the body is made up of biological material whose basic chemical structure involves carbon compounds. These range from simple 2-carbon compounds, such as acetate, to the extremely large molecules of hormones and enzymes containing several hundred carbon atoms linked together in a straight chain, a branched arrangement, or a multidimensional molecule.

Some compounds are biologically active, undergoing constant and sometimes rapid change, whereas others are relatively inert, changing slowly. A portion of the study of nutrition involves studying the nature and extent of the changes and the way in which various nutrients are involved in these changes. The biological material enters the body as carbohydrate, fat, protein, or vitamins and eventually is excreted through the lungs as carbon dioxide and water and in the urine as a variety of substances. The time elapsing between these two extremes may be a matter of seconds or a matter of years. In the interval they may be subjected to a few minor biochemical changes or a series of very complex biochemical actions and interactions. Thus, when we refer to changes involving a single carbon unit, such as a methyl group (CH_3), we are speaking of one small molecule or a small portion of a molecule; when we talk of a long-chain carbon unit, such as peptide chain or a fatty acid, we may be referring to a large portion of a biological compound.

Biochemical compounds are subject to the same fundamental reactions that inorganic compounds undergo. Thus biochemical substances such as carbohydrate may unite with oxygen in a process called **oxidation** or combustion. The removal of a hydrogen atom (**dehydrogenation**) has the same effect and is another way in which oxidation can occur. On the other hand, if hydrogen is incorporated, the substance is said to have been reduced or to have undergone **hydrogenation.** The removal of oxygen is also a reducing reaction. A compound that has been either reduced or oxidized will have physical, chemical, or biological properties that differ from the original compound. Nutritionally, the value of a nutrient may be completely destroyed or reduced by either oxidation or hydrogenation; in some cases the biological value of a nutrient is unaffected and in others it is enhanced.

In biochemical compounds the presence of an OH, or hydroxyl group, in a terminal position identifies the compound as an alcohol (comparable to hydroxide in inorganic compounds). When this is oxidized, it forms an aldehyde, —CHO, which can be further oxidized to an acid in which the terminal group is —COOH. This conversion of alcohol to aldehyde to acid by oxidation may be reversed by reduction reactions.

Other biochemical reactions that a nutrient may undergo are **deamination,** the removal of the amino group (NH_2) from a compound; **transamination,** the transfer of NH_2 from one compound to another; and **transmethylation,** the transfer of a methyl group (CH_3).

Cellular biology. The smallest unit of body structure is the cell, which occurs in many sizes and shapes in the body. Fig. 1-7 shows various types of cells that have specific characteristics, depending on the particular tissues of which they are a part. Development of the electron microscope has allowed scientists to determine a definite structure within individual cells, indicating a high degree of organization of subcellular particles, or **organelles.** The use of the ultracentrifuge and various microchemical techniques has made possible the determination of the biochemical makeup of these organelles and has indicated definite biochemical specialization in these small subcellular units. Even the cell membrane is a highly structured, complex, and functional unit of the cell.

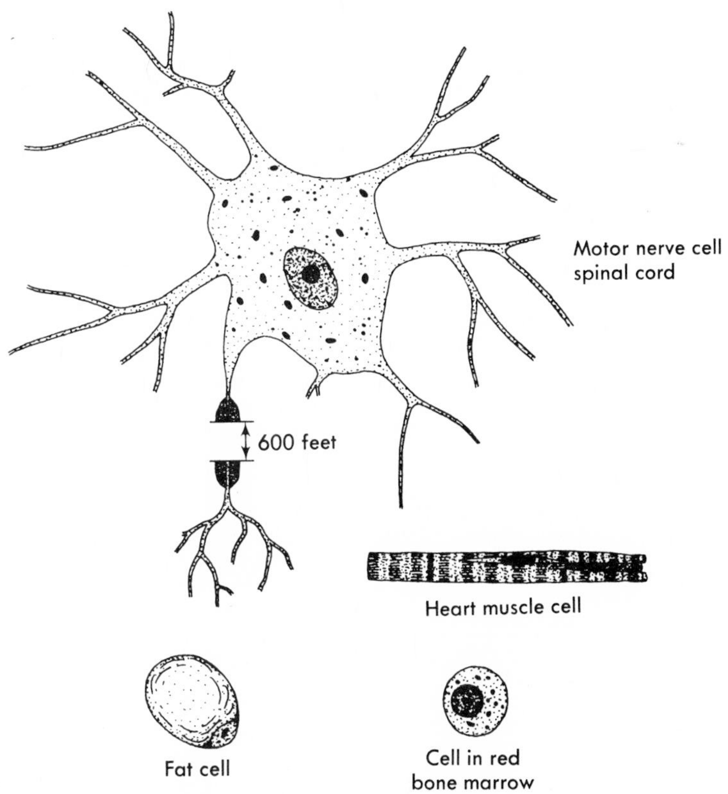

Fig. 1-7. Some typical mammalian cells.

Since many of the advances in nutrition are the result of the study of cellular nutrition and since popular publications are using these findings with increasing frequency, a familiarity with cell structure seems desirable for a student of nutrition. Just as there is no typical human, there is no typical cell. Each varies according to its function. Fig. 1-8 however, is a representation of the essential features of most cells.

Among the main organelles, or functional units, of the cell is the **cell membrane,** composed of protein and lipid, which regulates the uptake of material from the external environment of the cell, the extracellular fluid. It also governs the release of material, either newly synthesized material or waste products from the cell. In a sense, it is the "doorkeeper" of the cell. Within the cell is a mass of material, the **cytoplasmic matrix,** in which there are several highly organized areas.

The **mitochondrion,** another double-membraned structure within the cell, contains upward of 500 enzymes involved in the release of energy from energy-yielding nutrients. Its vital role in energy metabolism has led to its designation as the "powerhouse" of the cell. The number of mitochondria within a cell varies, depending on the function of the cell, but in extremely active cells, such as those of liver or heart muscle, there may be as many as 1000.

Lysosomes contain the digestive enzymes of the cell and serve to digest particles that may enter the cell in a form which must be changed before they can be used. Lysosomes are capable of digesting complex substances in the cytoplasm of the cell and releasing them as their simple components into the cytoplasm again. If released from their membranes, the enzymes of the lysosomes are capable of digesting the cell itself. This occurs at the death of the cell.

Throughout the cytoplasm is a network of canals, some of which are lined with small granules. The canals are known as **endoplasmic reticulum** and serve as communication channels within the cell and between cells. The small granules are **microsomes** in which the synthesis of protein within the cell occurs. Canals with ribosomes attached are identified as rough endoplasmic reticulum, whereas those without the protein-synthesizing mechanism are known as the smooth endoplasmic reticulum. The latter may be involved in hormone synthesis.

Within the cell, separated from the cytoplasm by a membrane, is the **nucleus.** The

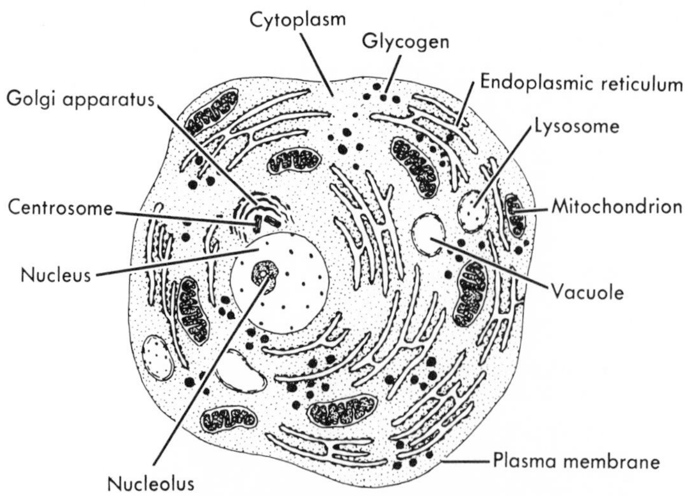

Fig. 1-8. Diagrammatic representation of a typical cell.

nucleus contains the genetic information that allows the cell to reproduce in the pattern of the parent cell. The code contained in the genetic material, deoxyribonucleic acid (DNA), is transmitted through the nuclear membrane to the ribosomes by another nucleic acid, messenger ribonucleic acid (RNA), produced in the nucleus.

CURRENT ISSUES IN NUTRITION

While physiologists, biochemists, cell biologists, food scientists, and nutrition scientists are continuing to unravel the mysteries of what goes on within the cell and its subcellular components, there is a growing concern and interest in the relationship of our changing food supply and dietary practices to health. The issues change from time to time, reflecting the balance between our scientific knowledge and nutritional practices. Some of the applied aspects of nutrition receiving attention currently, and which will be discussed throughout the text, are outlined here.

Iatrogenic malnutrition. This is a state of malnutrition that may be the result of the medical treatment of another condition. For instance, the use of oral contraceptives has resulted in changes in the need for certain nutrients so that amounts considered adequate before the use of these drugs are no longer sufficient to meet the body's needs. Similarly, some antibiotics interfere with the activity of intestinal bacteria that synthesize certain nutrients. Anticonvulsant drugs have a marked effect on the need for vitamin D. An operation that involves shortening the gastrointestinal tract reduces the absorption of nutrients and may lead to a relative nutrient deficiency.

Nutrition in space. The challenge of maintaining men in prolonged space flights has opened a whole new area of nutritional investigation. Not only is there the question of how to prepare food in a way it can be ingested without undue hazard, but variations in nutritional needs, metabolism, and taste sensations and problems of dehydration and electrolyte balance must be considered as well.

Relation of nutrition to degenerative diseases. There is a growing belief that the course of many conditions such as cardiovascular disease, hypertension, diabetes, and possibly cancer is influenced by dietary factors. As a result, considerable effort is being directed at determining the kind of dietary practices throughout life that will reduce the likelihood of these developing.

Megavitamin therapy. Suggestions that the use of nutrients, expecially vitamins, in amounts far in excess of accepted standards or what could reasonably be obtained from food will prevent or cure such conditions as schizophrenia, the common cold, and aging have led to widespread use of large (mega) doses of nutrients. Information on the benefits of their use is limited as is knowledge of any adverse effects from what must be considered pharmacological dosages.

Nutrition and national policy. It is now becoming evident that the nutritional status of a population is determined to a large extent by governmental policies on issues such as agricultural price and wage supports, import tariffs, and public works projects (roads and credit policies). Since all these concerns and many more reflect directly or indirectly on the availability of food, there is increasing interest in encouraging policy makers to consider the nutritional implications of their decisions.

Safety of food supply. In addition to being concerned about the nutritional quality of the diet, nutritionists have recently been joining food scientists in directing their attention to the safety of the food supply. The importance of both intentional and incidental additives, environmental contaminants such as herbicides and pesticides, the use of hormones in animal feeds, and naturally occurring toxicants are but a few of the issues that are of concern to the public and about which a nutritionist must be knowledgeable.

BIBLIOGRAPHY

Alcantara, E. N., and Speckmann, E. W.: Diet, nutrition and cancer, Am. J. Clin. Nutr. **29:**1035, 1976.

Barnes, R. H.: Dual role of environmental deprivation

and malnutrition in retarding intellectual development, Am. J. Clin. Nutr. **29**:912, 1976.
Brozek, J.: Malnutrition and behavior, J. Am. Diet Assoc. **72**:1, 1978.
Committee on International Nutrition Programs: The relationship of nutrition to brain development and behavior, Nutr. Today **9**:12, 1974.
Chichester, C. O., and Darby, W. J.: The historical relationship between food science and nutrition, Food Tech. **28**:38, 1974.
Crane, R. K.: A perspective of digestive-absorptive function. Am. J. Clin. Nutr. **22**:242, 1969.
Darby, W. J.: Nutrition science: an overview of American genius, Nutr. Rev. **34**:1, 1976.
Goldblith, S. A., and Joslyn, M. A., editors: Milestones in nutrition, Westport, Conn., 1964, AVI Publishing Co.
Goldsmith, G. A.: Nutrition and world health, J. Am. Diet. Assoc. **63**:513, 1973.
Gori, G. B.: Diet and cancer. an overview for perspective, J. Am. Diet. Assoc. **71**:375, 1977.
Griffith, W. H.: Food as a regulator of metabolism, Am. J. Clin. Nutr. **17**:391, 1965.
Hartshorn, E. A.: Food and drug interactions, J. Am. Diet. Assoc. **70**:15, 1977.
Hathcock, J. N.: Nutrition: toxicology and pharmacology, Nutr. Rev. **34**:65, 1977.
Hegsted, D. M.: Nutritional requirements in disease, J. Am. Diet. Assoc. **56**:303, 1970.
Hurley, L. S.: Nutrients and genes: interactions and development, Nutr. Rev. **27**:3, 1969.
King, C. G.: Notes on the history of nutrition in America, J. Am. Diet. Assoc. **56**:188, 1970.
Lowenberg, M. E., and Lucas, B. L.: Feeding families and children—1776 and 1976. A Bicentennial study, J. Am. Diet. Assoc. **68**:207, 1976.
McCollum, E. V.: A history of nutrition, Boston, 1957, Houghton Mifflin Co.
Ross, M. L.: The long view, J. Am. Diet. Assoc. **56**:295, 1970.
Schneider, H.: What has happened to nutrition? In Ingle, D. J., editor: Life and disease, New York, 1963, Basic Books, Inc., Publishers.
Sebrell, W. H.: Changing concepts of malnutrition, Am. J. Clin. Nutr. **20**:653, 1969.
Snook, J. T.: Adaptive and non-adaptive changes in digestive enzyme capacity influencing digestive function, Fed. Proc. **33**:88, 1974.
Todhunter, E. N.: Development of knowledge in nutrition. I. Animal experiments. II. Human experiments, J. Am. Diet. Assoc. **41**:328, 335, 1962.
Todhunter, E. N.: Some classics of nutrition and dietetics, J. Am. Diet. Assoc. **44**:100, 1964.
Todhunter, E. N.: The evolution of nutrition concepts, J. Am. Diet. Assoc. **46**:120, 1965.
Todhunter, E. N.: Chronology of some events in the development and application of the science of nutrition, Nutr. Rev. **34**:353, 1976.
Weininger, J., and Briggs, G. M.: Nutrition update, 1976, J. Nutr. Ed. **8**:172, 1976.
Weininger, J., and Briggs, G. M.: Nutrition update, 1977, J. Nutr. Ed. **9**:173, 1977.
Weir, C. E.: Benefits from human nutrition research, Human Nutrition, Report No. 2, U.S. Department of Agriculture, Washington, D.C., 1971.
Wynder, E. L.: The dietary environment and cancer, J. Am. Diet. Assoc. **71**:385, 1977.
Youmans, J. B.: Changing face of nutritional diseases in America, J.A.M.A. **189**:672, 1964.
Yudkin, J.: Disagreement, Nutr. Today **3**(3):25, 1969.

2

Carbohydrate

Carbohydrates, which are generally recognized as starches and sugars, the form in which plants store energy, are the major source of energy for most populations, providing from 45% to 80% of the caloric intake in various cultures. Only recently has it been recognized that carbohydrate is an essential nutrient and that the kind and proportion of carbohydrate in the diet may have a major determining role in the development of conditions such as coronary heart disease, diabetes, hyperlipidemia, cancer, and dental caries. In general, it is recommended that the current trend toward an increasing amount of simple sugars in the diet be reversed to favor the inclusion of more complex carbohydrates and fiber.

Carbohydrate, an energy-yielding nutrient, is the largest single component, aside from water, of most diets. About 300 g (⅔ pound) of carbohydrate is present in a 2400-kilocalorie (kcal) diet consumed by a typical adult. Carbohydrates are recognized by most people as starches and sugars. They provide slightly less than half the calories in the typical American diet. Carbohydrates account for about three fourths of the energy in the plant world on which animal life depends for food. In the last sixty-five years the total consumption of carbohydrate in the United States has declined by at least 25% and that of starches over 40%. At the same time, the consumption of sugar, after dropping to 39.2 kg (87 pounds) during World War II, has now risen to 46.8 kg (104 pounds) per capita per year. These data indicate the proportion of sugar has increased even though actual amounts per capita have only recently reached the level of 1920. Data on sugar use show that a decreasing amount is being consumed directly in the home and that two thirds is now being used by the food industry. The largest amount is included in beverages, followed by cereals and baked goods.

The health implications of the trends in consumption of simple and complex carbohydrate has been the subject of much speculation and some research. These trends are depicted in Fig. 2-1.

Since carbohydrate foods are easy to grow, can be stored at room temperature with a minimum of deterioration, and have a high energy yield per unit of land, they are relatively inexpensive sources of energy. As a result, when the amount of money available for food is restricted and where plant life is abundant, the proportion of carbohydrate foods in the diet increases. Although refined carbohydrates contribute little other than calories to the diet, the less refined products may make substantial contributions of other nutrients. The amount varies inversely with the degree of refinement.

Although carbohydrate was one of the first nutrients to be chemically identified, only now is evidence appearing to indicate that it is essential in human nutrition. It is a compound composed of the three elements carbon, hydrogen, and oxygen. The ratio of hydrogen to oxygen in all carbohydrates is 2:1, the same ratio found in water (hydro); hence

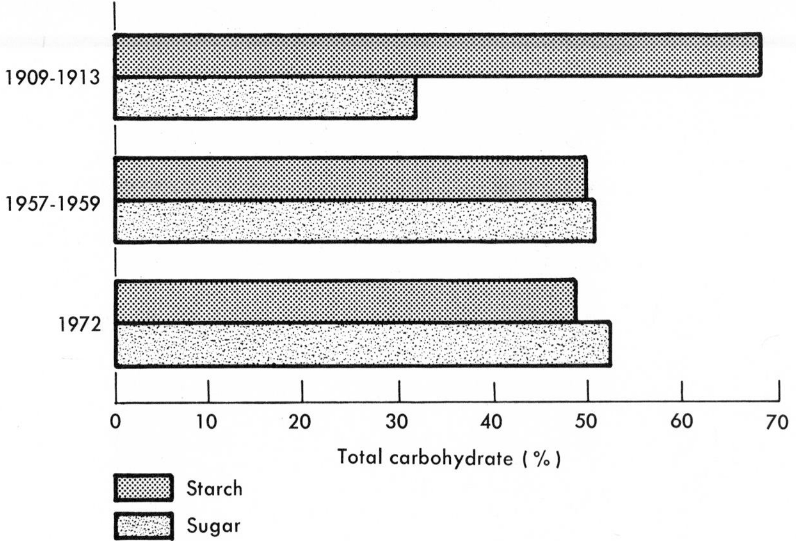

Fig. 2-1. Changes in patterns of carbohydrate intake.

the term *carbohydrate.* In simple carbohydrates there are equal numbers of carbon atoms and water molecules ($C_n[H_2O]_n$); for complexes of two or more simple carbohydrates there is one less water equivalent than carbon atoms ($C_n[H_2O]_{n-1}$). It is as these carbohydrates that green plants store the energy they derive from the sun.

SYNTHESIS

Plants with green leaves are able to trap the radiant energy of the sun and through a process known as **photosynthesis** store it as chemical energy in carbohydrates. This process is essential for the continuation of life. As shown in Fig. 2-2, the carbon dioxide of the atmosphere and water from the soil are picked up by the plant and combined in the presence of chlorophyll, the magnesium-containing pigments of plants, to form an energy-rich carbohydrate stored as starch or sugar. In some plants, such as potatoes, wheat, and rice, the carbohydrate is in the form of starch; in others, such as sweet peas, bananas, cherries, and sugar beets, it is in the form of sugar. In peas and corn, carbohydrate is stored initially as sugar and is changed to starch as the seed matures. The

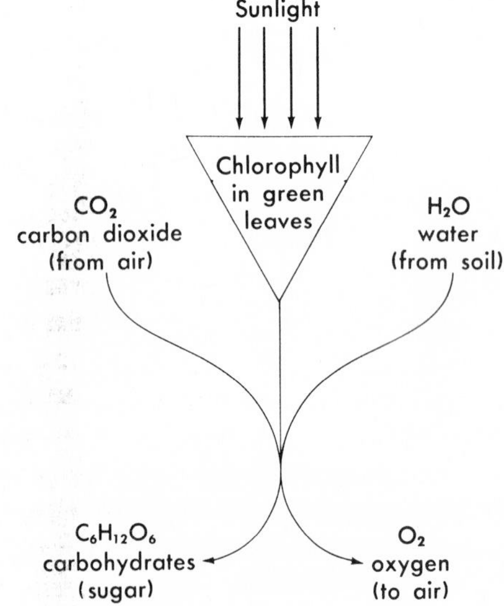

Fig. 2-2. Process of photosynthesis.

sweetness of carrots also declines when the sugar in the root is converted to starch as the carrot is stored. On the other hand, starch in immature fruits such as bananas, apples, and pears is converted to sugar during the ripening process. On further ripening, this sugar ferments to either acid or alcohol, as found in

Glucose	Fructose	Galactose	Mannose
O	H	O	O
‖	|	‖	‖
C—H	H—C—OH	C—H	C—H
H—C—OH	C=O	H—C—OH	HO—C—H
HO—C—H	HO—C—H	HO—C—H	HO—C—H
H—C—OH	H—C—OH	HO—C—H	H—C—OH
H—C—OH	H—C—OH	H—C—OH	H—C—OH
H—C—OH	H—C—OH	H—C—OH	H—C—OH
H	H	H	H

(Boxed areas are where structure differs from glucose.)

overripe fruits. Regardless of the form in which it is stored or whether it is stored in the root, leaf, seed, or fruit of the plant, carbohydrate represents the reserve of energy for the plant.

CLASSIFICATION

Monosaccharides. The simplest structural unit of carbohydrates is a **monosaccharide,** one sugar unit. This is the chemical building block or unit from which all more complex carbohydrates are built. Most of the monosaccharides are also known as hexoses, since they are composed of a 6-carbon chain or ring to which hydrogen and oxygen atoms are attached as hydrogen and hydroxyl (OH) groups. There are three monosaccharides of importance in nutrition—*glucose, fructose,* and *galactose.* A fourth, *mannose,* has limited significance in human nutrition, since it is found in foods in only poorly digested complexes. All hexoses contain the same number and kinds of atoms—6 carbon atoms, 12 hydrogen atoms, and 6 oxygen atoms ($C_6H_{12}O_6$). They differ from one another only in the way in which the hydrogen and oxygen atoms are arranged around the chain of carbon atoms. The differences in monosaccharides can be observed from the formulas at the top of the page.

These different arrangements of atoms within the carbohydrate molecule account for the variation in sweetening power, solubility, and other properties of the different monosaccharides. One method of identifying sugars involves passing a beam of polarized light through a solution of the sugar. On the basis of its effect of polarized light, glucose, which causes the light to rotate to the right, has been named **dextrose.** A fructose solution, on the other hand, causes polarized light to rotate to the left. Hence fructose is known as **levulose.**

Monosaccharides occur in fruits and in some vegetables, accounting for 1% to 16% of their weight. The monosaccharides glucose and fructose, which account for approximately 10% of dietary carbohydrate, occur in varying amounts in fruits and vegetables as shown in Table 2-1. The remaining monosaccharides that are used in the body are derived from the digestion or breakdown of more complex carbohydrates rather than being provided as such by food.

Glucose is found in fruits, vegetables, and honey, which together provide about 16 g per

Table 2-1. Distribution of sugars in selected foods*

Food	Glucose	Fructose	Sucrose
	g/100 g food		
Cabbage	1.6	1.2	0.2
Carrot	0.9	0.9	4.2
Onion	2.1	1.1	0.9
Potato	1.0	1.2	1.7
Squash	1.0	1.2	1.6
Tomato	1.1	1.3	0
Melon	2.6	2.6	5.9
Apple	1.2	6.0	3.8
Blueberries	3.8	3.8	0.2
Grapes	5.4	5.3	1.3
Peach	0.9	1.1	6.9
Cherry	4.3	3.3	0.4
Strawberries	2.1	2.14	1.0

*From Schallenberger, R. S.: Occurrence of various sugars in foods. In Sipple, H. L., and McNutt, K. W., editors: Sugars in nutrition, New York, 1974, Academic Press.

capita per day. It is frequently referred to as blood sugar, since it is the primary carbohydrate found in the general circulation of the body, where it occurs in both the blood plasma and the red blood cells. It is the primary source of energy used by the central nervous system. The total amount of glucose in blood and extracellular tissue is estimated at 17 g in an adult male. Normal fasting blood glucose levels are about 100 mg/dl (100 ml) of blood. The level usually rises following a meal and falls gradually until it hits the fasting level, associated with the onset of hunger. When levels rise above 160 mg/dl, the condition is known as **hyperglycemia.** This usually occurs only in diabetes, where a lack of the hormone insulin results in a decreased uptake of glucose from the blood by the cells. Under these conditions blood glucose levels get so high that the kidneys, which normally prevent the loss of sugar from the body, cannot resorb it, and sugar appears in the urine. The process of excreting sugar necessitates an increase in urine volume; thus additional early symptoms of diabetes are frequency of urination and thirst.

Blood glucose levels below 60 mg/dl are characteristic of a condition known as **hypoglycemia.** These low blood sugar levels are generally associated with changes in neuromuscular coordination, convulsions, stupor, unconsciousness, and even death. Recently there has been a tendency to attribute feelings of fatigue, malaise, "uptight feelings," irritability, and a host of other symptoms to hypoglycemia and the resulting decrease in the supply of glucose to the brain. In most cases these symptoms can be attributed to mental or health problems rather than to dietary problems. Since the disorders of the nervous or endocrine system, such as excess insulin secretion, which are the cause of hypoglycemia are rare, it is unlikely that true hypoglycemia is as widespread a problem as popular diagnoses would suggest.

Glucose can be reduced to an alcohol sugar, sorbitol. Sorbitol, with a sweetening power equivalent to glucose and one half that of sucrose, has been used in some weight-reducing aids on the theory that the body cannot utilize it. It now appears that the body can use it without the help of insulin. Because of the slow rate at which it is absorbed, it permits blood sugar levels to remain high after a meal and delays the onset of hunger sensations; in some persons, however, flatulence and diarrhea result. It has been found in many fruits and vegetables.

Fructose, which is also known as fruit sugar, occurs naturally in many fruits and berries. It constitutes half the sugar in honey and is responsible for its sweetness. Recently it has been possible through the use of enzymes to produce a low-cost crystalline fructose from the glucose derived from cornstarch or from sucrose. High-fructose corn syrups (42% fructose) are also available. Since fructose has a sweetening power 70% greater than sucrose, it is possible to achieve the same degree of sweetness with less fructose and hence fewer calories than would be required with sucrose. Fructose is also less

$$\underset{\textit{Monosaccharide}}{C_6H_{12}O_6} + \underset{\textit{Monosaccharide}}{C_6H_{12}O_6} \underset{\text{Hydrolysis}}{\overset{\text{Synthesis}}{\rightleftarrows}} \underset{\textit{Disaccharide}}{C_{12}H_{22}O_{11}} + \underset{\textit{Water}}{H_2O}$$

likely to contribute to the formation of the plaque involved in the development of dental caries. Although it appears to have none of the undesirable characteristics of artificial sweeteners, the possibility that an increased use of fructose may pose difficulties for those individuals who are unable to metabolize or use fructose is leading to research to determine if there is indeed a problem. Unlike glucose, fructose, which is absorbed more slowly and evenly, may be used in amounts up to 1.5 g/kg of body weight by diabetics who lack the hormone insulin. Most fructose is changed to glucose in the liver. Fructose may not, however, be used to raise blood sugar levels. It has also been observed that fructose serves to alleviate the symptoms of alcoholism by speeding up the metabolism of alcohol. Physiologically, fructose appears in fetal blood and the cerebrospinal fluid.

Mannose is found in limited amounts in apples, peaches, and oranges and then only in poorly digested complexes.

Mannitol, another alcohol sugar used as a drying agent in some foods, has a sweetening power similar to glucose, but because only partially metabolized, it yields only half as many calories per gram as other carbohydrates. It is found in pineapple, olives, asparagus, carrots, and sweet potatoes.

So far no food has been found that contains free galactose. It does occur as a component of the more complex carbohydrates in milk and the seed coat of legumes.

Some 5-carbon sugars, pentoses, are found occasionally in plants but do not represent an appreciable source of dietary carbohydrate. Ribose, arabinose, and xylose are the most common. In the body, ribose is part of some vital body compounds, such as the riboflavin- or vitamin B_2–containing enzymes, and nucleic acids, the genetic material in the nucleus and cytoplasm of the cell. The body can produce ribose from glucose and therefore does not depend on a dietary source of 5-carbon sugars to form the essential nucleic acids.

Xylose, a 5-carbon sugar, is the second most abundant sugar in nature. Xylitol, a 5-carbon alcohol sugar, derived from xylose in birch trees, plant shells, and straw, is being promoted as a sweetening agent, since it does not have the usual adverse effect of sugar on teeth. It will not support the growth of microorganisms that must occur if carbohydrate is to contribute to dental decay. It may prove useful in confectionary products. Xylitol enters the cell without the help of insulin and thus has proved useful for diabetics and patients on intravenous feedings (total parenteral nutrition). It has been shown to be safe up to 90 g/day, although recently there was concern that it might be carcinogenic as it occurs in sugarless gum. About 900 metric tons (1000 tons) per year are produced.

Disaccharides. The **disaccharides,** each composed of two monosaccharide units, account for 35% of dietary carbohydrate. When two monosaccharides are joined to form a disaccharide, one molecule of water is split off. Conversely, when a disaccharide is broken into its two component monosaccharide units, as occurs in digestion, a molecule of water must be added in a process known as hydrolysis. Thus we have a reversible reaction as seen at top of page.

The most common disaccharide, *sucrose,* which is obtained from both sugarcane and sugar beets, is a combination of glucose and fructose. Granulated sugar has traditionally been 100% sucrose, but with increasing costs of raw sugar, a combination of fructose and glucose formed from the hydrolysis and enzyme treatment of less expensive cornstarch is appearing on the market. Brown sugar, the slightly less refined, more flavorful product made by adding some molasses to either beet or cane sugar, is 97% sucrose. The world consumes 74 million metric tons of sucrose a year, two thirds of it coming from sugarcane and one third from sugar beets. Both cane and beet sugar yield far more calories per acre of land than any other crop. The consumption of sucrose in the American diet has hit a plateau at approximately 128 g/day. There is concern that it may be a contributing factor to the high incidence of tooth decay and possibly heart disease.

Of the 9 million metric tons of sugar marketed in the United States each year approximately 32% is sold directly for home use, 63% is employed in the food industry, and 5% is sold to other industrial users. Within the food industry 25% is used in beverages, 24% in cereal, and 22% in baked goods—almost a 50% increase from the amount utilized in 1960. The average amount of sugar added to foods ranges from 3% in baby-processed vegetables and 5% in snack foods to 12% in processed fruit juices and drinks, 13% in beverages, 26% in cereals, 32% in jams and jellies, and 42% in chewing gum.

Almost all sucrose is digested to glucose and fructose in the cells lining the intestinal tract, but at high levels of intake some may be absorbed unchanged to be excreted unchanged in the urine.

Lactose, which accounts for 25 g of the total dietary carbohydrate, is a combination of glucose and galactose. It is found only in milk, where it makes up half the total solids. Sometimes known as milk sugar, it was first identified in 1633 and is the source of the monosaccharide galactose. In the intestine certain microorganisms cause the production of lactic acid from any unabsorbed lactose. This increased acidity in the lower intestinal

Table 2-2. Comparison of physical properties of carbohydrates (relative values)

Monosaccharides	Sweetening power	Soluble	Rate of absorption
Hexoses			
Fructose	173	Yes	30
Glucose	74	Yes	100
Galactose	32	Yes	110
Mannose			10
Alcohol sugars			
Sorbitol	60	Yes	
Mannitol	50	Slightly	
Pentoses			
Ribose	—	Yes	
Xylose	40	Yes	15
Arabinose	—	Yes	9
Disaccharides			
Sucrose	100	Yes	
Maltose	32	Yes	
Lactose	16	Yes	
Polysaccharides			
Dextrin		Slightly	
Starch		No	
Glycogen		No	
Cellulose		No	

tract creates a medium in which the organism *Lactobacillus bifidus* grows to produce the *bifidus factor* believed to be beneficial to very young infants in preventing the growth of the less desirable bacteria that cause intestinal putrefaction. This factor is found primarily in the intestines of breast-fed infants, and its presence has been identified as one of the advantages of breast-feeding over bottle-feeding.

There is evidence that a relatively soluble calcium-lactose complex increases the extent to which calcium is absorbed or that lactose increases the permeability of the intestinal membrane to ions such as calcium. Whatever the mechanism, it is interesting to note that the best source of lactose and of calcium in the diet is the same food—milk.

Maltose, the third disaccharide, is found in germinating cereals. It is composed of two molecules of glucose and makes a negligible contribution to the diet, accounting for less than 3% of dietary carbohydrate.

All members of the monosaccharide group and disaccharide group are considered sugars, as indicated by the suffix *-ose.*

Sugars differ in their sweetening power, as shown in Table 2-2. The sweetening power of sugar parallels its solubility. Fructose, with the greatest sweetening power, is most soluble and therefore difficult to crystallize from a solution and to obtain in crystalline form. This makes it useful in syrups but also means that because it is so difficult to keep in crystalline form, the small amount of crystalline fructose available is expensive. Lactose, which is relatively insoluble, is difficult to incorporate in a solution and hence is not practical as a sweetening agent for liquids. The contribution of individual sugars to total sugar consumption in the United States is shown in Table 2-3.

Table 2-3. Percent contribution of individual sugars to total sugars provided by United States diet*

	1909-1913	1947-1949	1972
Total sugar (g/day)	156	192	201
Sucrose	64.8	62.0	61.8
Lactose	13.6	14.5	12.5
Fructose	4.0	2.6	1.7
Glucose	3.5	5.6	6.4
Maltose	1.1	1.7	2.7
Other	2.1	2.4	3.2

*From Page, L., and Friend, B.: Level of use of sugars in the United States. In Sipple, H. L., and McNutt, K. W., editors: Sugars in nutrition, New York, 1974, Academic Press.

Polysaccharides. The third group of carbohydrates, the **polysaccharides,** are much more complex and are considered starches rather than sugars. Starches represent about half the dietary carbohydrate. They are composed solely of glucose units linked together in long chains. A polysaccharide may contain as many as 2000 glucose units, which may be in one long chain (an amylose) or in a branched arrangement (an amylopectin), as illustrated:

$$G - G - G - G - G - G - G - G - G_n$$

Amylose

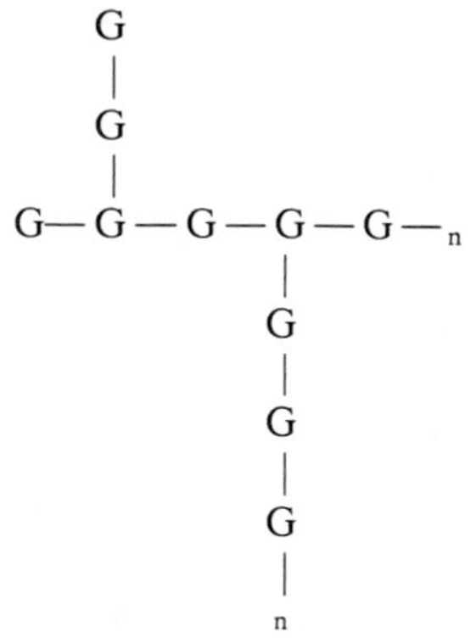

```
   G
   |
   G
   |
G— G — G — G — G —n
           |
           G
           |
           G
           |
           G
           |
           n
```

Amylopectin

The number of glucose units and their arrangement within the molecule determine the characteristics of the starch. Each plant deposits a starch characteristic of its species. Granules of potato starch can thus be distinguished from granules of rice, wheat, cassava, corn, or any other starch by microscopic examination of the shape and size of the granule. In addition, each of these starches has unique properties in regard to solubility, thickening power, and flavor. Nutritionally, the body does not discriminate among starches but is able to break all cooked starches into their component glucose units for absorption and utilization by the body cells.

The animal stores a limited amount of carbohydrate as the polysaccharide *glycogen.* It is stored primarily in liver and muscle, the only two animal tissues aside from milk and blood that contain carbohydrate. The adult human stores only about 340 g of glycogen—a third as liver glycogen and two thirds as muscle glycogen. The energy thus stored represents only enough energy to last an adult human about half a day.

The capacity of the liver and muscles to store glycogen may be increased 100% by manipulating the diet in association with exercise. This procedure, known as **carbohydrate loading,** is frequently used by athletes such as soccer players or long distance runners who need a large amount of energy derived from muscle glycogen over a period of 30 minutes or more. Under these circumstances, an athlete depletes his muscle reserves of glycogen by exercising for several days while on a diet low in carbohydrate. Two or three days before the contest, the diet is switched to one in which carbohydrate is the major source of energy. This results in the accumulation of larger than normal amounts of glycogen in the muscles, where it is available when needed. This procedure also causes an increase in liver glycogen reserves, which can be easily converted into glucose for use by the central nervous system and to prevent hypoglycemia. For short periods of less sustained exercise little glycogen is required for energy.

When used as food, animal liver or muscle contains no glycogen, since most is converted into lactic acid at the time of slaughtering.

Dextrin, another nutritionally important polysaccharide, is the slightly soluble product resulting from the initial breakdown of a starch when the very long glucose chains are split into shorter chains by the orderly removal of maltose units. This may be accomplished by enzymes, as occurs during digestion, or by action of dry heat on starch, as in toasting bread or browning flour. In either case the resulting dextrin is sweeter and more soluble than the original starch. A starch hydrolysate, dextromaltose, is often used in infant feeding, since it helps to prevent the formation of a heavy curd in the infant's stomach and does not ferment readily. Completely dextrinized breads such as zwiebach are well suited to the digestive capacities of the infant.

Cellulose, which is also composed of many glucose units linked in a slightly different manner from starch units, is an important dietary constituent. It accounts for 50% of all carbon in vegetables and is the most abundant organic compound in the world. Cellulose is the structural framework of plant tissue, and the human body lacks the enzyme necessary to break its monosaccharide linkages. This indigestible residue contributes bulk to the diet and is important in maintaining intestinal motility.

Ruminants have a bacterial enzyme system capable of fermenting cellulose linkages, which explains their ability to exist on grasses and forage crops composed largely of cellulose, whereas humans cannot. This fermentation produces short-chain fatty acids used for energy and a useless gas, methane.

The data on fiber recorded in tables of food composition have traditionally been for crude fiber or the portion of the plant that resists destruction by strong acid or alkali. From a nutritional standpoint, however, data on dietary fiber are needed. This term includes all plant fibers that are not affected by digestive enzymes and includes, in addition to crude fiber or cellulose, a group of related carbohydrates known as pectins, lignins, and hemicelluloses. It has been suggested that this component of food, which has also been referred to as bulk or roughage, be called "plantix." Values for dietary fiber in Table 2-4 tend to be considerably higher in most foods than those for crude fiber. Dietary fiber is found only in foods of plant origin such as legumes, nuts, whole-grain cereals, and fruits and vegetables.

Interest in the role of fiber as a dietary essential has been stimulated by the observation that groups of people consuming diets with 25 to 30 g of fiber compared to the 2 to 3 g in the American diet had a very low incidence of cancer of the colon and diverticulitis. In diverticulitis, a weakening of the wall of the large intestine caused by the pressure created by extremely hard stools, is usually accompanied by infection.

The relationship between lack of dietary fiber and cancer of the colon has been attributed to accompanying changes in the microorganisms in the gastrointestinal tract. It is postulated that either these microorganisms favor the formation of cancer-producing substances or they prevent or limit the breakdown of carcinogens, which are normally destroyed when the fiber content of the diet is higher. It is also possible that fiber exerts its beneficial effect by speeding the passage of the feces through the large intestine so that carcinogens are in contact with the intestinal wall for a shorter period of time or by providing sufficient bulk to dilute any carcinogens. The ability of fiber to reduce problems from constipation and diverticulitis can be attributed to its tendency to absorb water and maintain a bulky, moist stool, which passes through the colon rapidly.

Table 2-4. Total dietary fiber in 100 g of selected foods*

Bran	48.0
Whole wheat flour	11.7
Brown flour (90% extraction)	8.7
Peas	7.7
Carrots	3.7
White flour (72% extraction)	3.4
Cabbage	2.9
Pear	2.4
Strawberries	2.1
Banana	1.8
Plum	1.5
Apple	1.4
Tomatoes	1.4

*From Southgate, D. A. T.: The definition and analysis of dietary fiber, Nutr. Rev. **35**:31, 1977.

The possibility that diets high in fiber provide some protection against coronary heart disease can be explained by the decreased intake of lipid, protein, and simple carbohydrates which are generally recognized as risk factors and are usually high on a low-fiber diet. Some fibers, especially pectins, tend to bind cholesterol and reduce its absorption or resorption from the intestinal tract. Fiber may also favor the growth of microorganisms responsible for the breakdown of bile acids, which release cholesterol that is usually reabsorbed.

Because of the limited data available on the dietary fiber content of foods, it is difficult to recommend a desirable intake. Currently the best estimates are that 6 to 8 g/day will afford more protection than the 2 to 4 g believed to represent the intake associated with the typical American diet. The recommendation will undoubtedly vary with the source of the fiber, since the type and amount of the separate fiber components vary greatly from one food to another.

Related carbohydrates. Mucopolysaccharides and mucoproteins are a group of compounds that are extremely important body constituents; they occur in the body but are not found in food. Mucopolysaccharides are complex combinations of two or more compounds, one of which is a carbohydrate. Many consist of loose combinations of amino sugars with protein. Some of the common mucopolysaccharides are hyaluronic acid, present in the fluid lubricating the joints and in the vitreous humor of the eyeball; chondroitin sulfate in cartilage, skin, and bone; heparin, an anticoagulant; and keratosulfate, found in hard structures such as nails. Mucoproteins such as the protein in eggs and some hormones are more tightly bound polysaccharides and proteins.

DIGESTION

Before carbohydrate can fulfill its established roles in the body, it must be converted into sufficiently small units to pass through the walls of the intestine into the bloodstream. The monosaccharides are the only units that normally cross the intestinal membrane. The process by which complex carbohydrates are reduced to their component monosaccharide units is one aspect of digestion. Virtually all the changes involved are brought about by starch-splitting enzymes called **amylases** and specific disaccharide-splitting enzymes, sucrase, lactase and maltase.

The amylases are present in two digestive juices—the saliva in the mouth and the pancreatic juice in the small intestine, and disaccharidases are in the intestinal juice or wall of the intestine. The salivary amylase of the saliva, which mixes with the food in the mouth, acts on the starch in a slightly alkaline medium to convert it to simpler carbohydrates, usually dextrins. If it remains in contact with the saliva sufficiently long before being acidified by the hydrochloric acid secreted in the

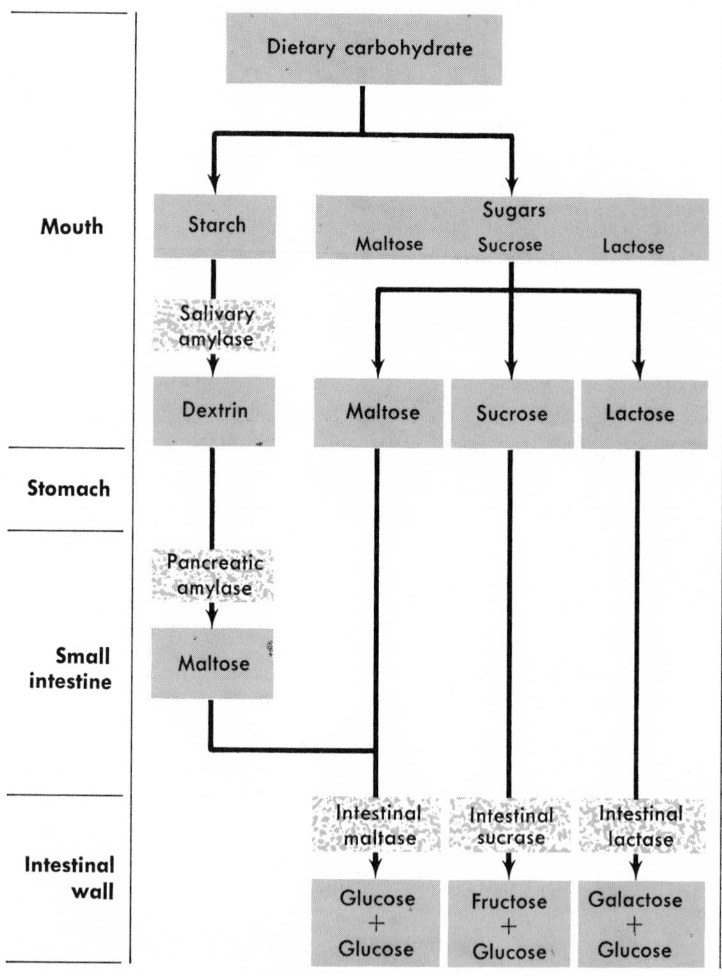

Fig. 2-3. Summary of digestion of carbohydrate.

stomach, the starch may be split as far as the disaccharide maltose. As much as 75% of potato starch may be digested by salivary amylase before it is inactivated by gastric acidity.

Virtually no digestion of starch occurs in the stomach, which possesses no starch-splitting enzyme. Some sucrose, in the presence of hydrochloric acid secreted in the stomach, may undergo acid hydrolysis to glucose and fructose. From the stomach the digestive mass passes to the small intestine, where alkaline secretions neutralize the hydrochloric acid and create the slightly alkaline medium necessary for the action of the starch-splitting enzymes secreted into the small intestine. Pancreatic amylase attacks complex carbohydrates and converts them into the disaccharide maltose.

The final conversion of sucrose to fructose and glucose is accomplished by intestinal sucrase. A further change of 26% to 70% of fructose to glucose may occur at the same time in the intestinal wall. Maltose is converted to two glucose molecules by intestinal maltase, and lactose is converted to glucose and galactose by intestinal lactase. The longstanding belief that these enzymes act within the intestinal lumen or tract is now being questioned. Evidence indicates that these enzymes are not secreted into the intestinal cavity but remain in the membrane of the cells lining the intestinal cavity, where they accomplish the ultimate conversion of the disaccharides to the monosaccharides.

The digestibility of carbohydrates varies with the source but ranges from 90% to 98% for most foods. The digestion of carbohydrate is summarized in Fig. 2-3.

ABSORPTION AND TRANSPORTATION

During absorption, monosaccharides pass freely across the walls of the villi, the small fingerlike projections lining the intestinal tract, but the rate varies with the type of sugar. Galactose is absorbed slightly faster than glucose, whereas fructose is absorbed at less than half the rate of glucose. The rate of absorption tends to decrease with time; it increases with an increase in concentration of the carbohydrate solution, and in the presence of the hormones insulin, secreted by the pancreas, and thyroxin, secreted by the thyroid glands.

From the intestinal wall the monosaccharides accumulate in the small blood vessels that eventually carry them to the portal vein. This large blood vessel carries the absorbed monosaccharides to the liver, where two paths may be followed by the monosaccharides glucose, fructose, and galactose. They may all be converted into glycogen up to the capacity of the liver to store glycogen, or the galactose and fructose may be converted to glucose and, along with the absorbed glucose, may be released to the bloodstream to be carried to various cells in the body. In muscle cells some glucose may be stored as muscle glycogen. Most glucose, however, will be used as an immediate source of energy for the cells. The nerve and lung cells depend entirely on glucose as a source of energy, since they are unable to utilize other energy-yielding nutrients.

METABOLISM

The liver releases carbohydrate as glucose to the bloodstream at a rate to maintain a minimal level of 80 mg of glucose/dl of blood. After a meal, the level of glucose may rise considerably above this but will drop again as it is withdrawn by the cells. One theory of regulation of appetite proposes that the difference between blood sugar levels in arterial and venous blood, Δ-glucose, influences the appetite-regulating mechanism, the hypothalamus of the brain. A small difference, representing depletion of blood glucose reserves, triggers the appetite. A large difference, showing an available supply of blood sugar, leads to a depressed appetite.

Glucose released from the liver is carried by the bloodstream to all tissues of the body. Here the individual cells take up the glucose through a process involving energy, an exchange of sodium, and a carrier system in the cell membrane. Once within the cell, the glucose is oxidized to pyruvic acid. Then in the

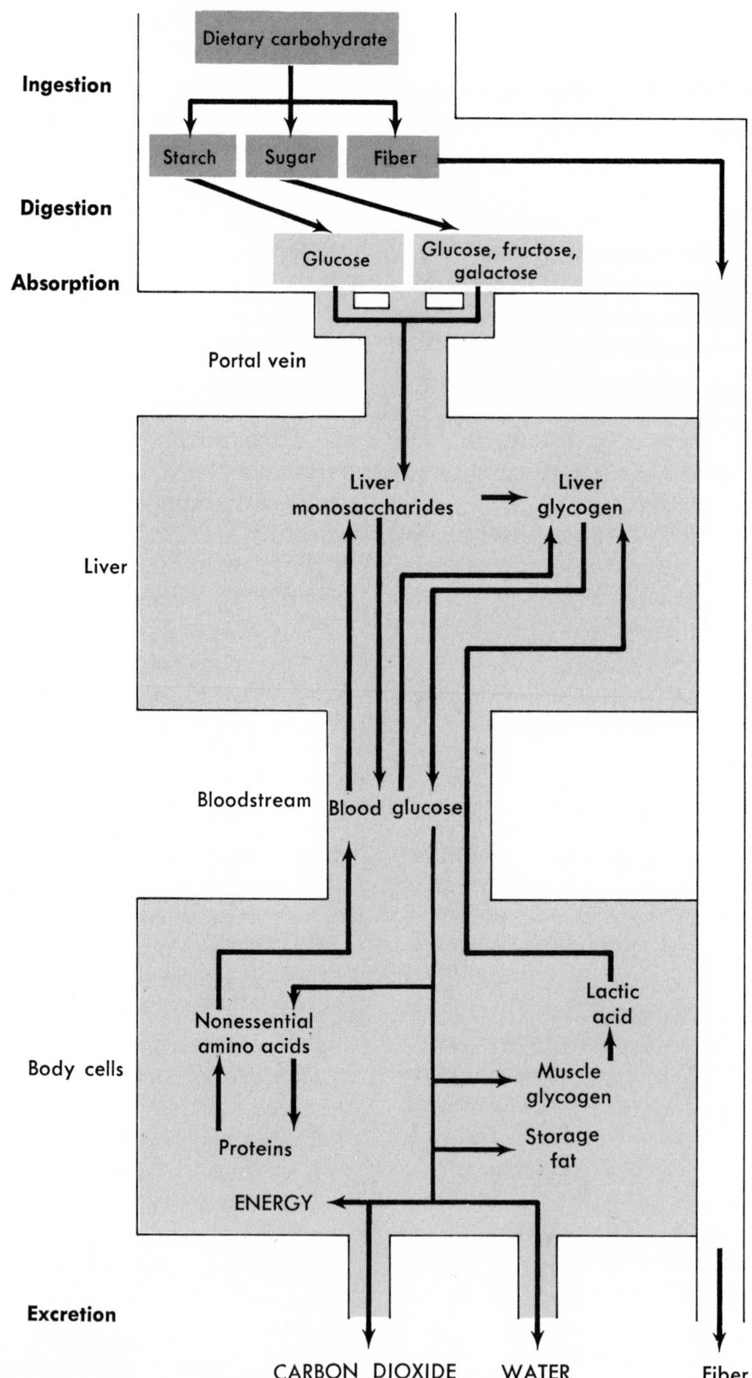

Fig. 2-4. Summary of carbohydrate digestion and metabolism. Items in capital letters are end products of metabolism.

mitochondrion the energy stored in the carbohydrate is released to supply energy for the many needs of the body, such as heat, muscle contraction, synthesis of essential compounds, and conduction of nerve impulses. Within the mitochondrion are concentrated the many enzymes necessary for the orderly and slow release of energy from glucose in the form of adenosine triphosphate (ATP). Once the energy of glucose has been released, the other end products of carbohydrate metabolism, carbon dioxide and water, are released from the cell and eventually excreted from the body.

STORAGE

When carbohydrate is supplied in the diet and monosaccharides are absorbed beyond the body's immediate needs for energy and its capacity to store glycogen, they cannot be excreted but must be converted into a form for storage in the body. The body has an unlimited capacity to store fat. It also has the ability to convert extra carbohydrate into fat. This conversion of glucose to fatty acids occurs primarily in the microsomes of the liver, although it can occur in all tissues. The glucose molecule is broken down from 6-carbon into 2-carbon fragments that are then synthesized into fatty acids. These are transported in the bloodstream to the adipose tissue cells, where they combine with a 3-carbon compound, glycerol, also derived from glucose, to form fat.

The digestion and metabolism of carbohydrate is summarized schematically in Fig. 2-4. It is clear that carbohydrate in food is used primarily in one of three ways in the body, depending on metabolic needs:

1. Metabolized or oxidized immediately as a source of energy
2. Converted into glycogen and stored as liver glycogen or muscle glycogen when carbohydrate intake exceeds the amount needed immediately for energy
3. Converted into fat and stored as a reserve of energy in regular cells or in special adipose cells when the carbohydrate intake exceeds the amount needed immediately for energy and when the limited glycogen reserves are saturated

The eventual end products of carbohydrate metabolism are carbon dioxide, water, and energy. The period of time elapsing between the intake of carbohydrate and its excretion as carbon dioxide and water may range from a few minutes to a few hours to several months.

FUNCTIONS

Source of energy. The major function of carbohydrate is as a source of energy. Although this function is not unique to carbohydrate, carbohydrate is the least expensive source of energy. Nervous tissue and lung tissue can use only glucose as a source of fuel, but since glucose can be produced from part of the fat molecule and from some amino acids in the process called **gluconeogenesis**, even these tissues can get along without dietary carbohydrates. When blood glucose levels fall below normal, the brain is deprived of glucose, its only source of energy, and it reacts by firing off uncontrolled and uncoordinated impulses that produce the symptoms of convulsions. Although glucose is the preferred source of energy for muscles, it can be replaced by fatty acids, which are utilized 4% to 5% less efficiently.

The amount of energy provided by carbohydrate is almost constant for all forms. One gram of carbohydrate provides 4 kcal of energy regardless of the source—starch, sugar, monosaccharides, or disaccharides. In the typical American diet in 1972 carbohydrate provided slightly less than 50% of the total calories. The proportion of total carbohydrate from starches has declined from 68% to 53% and that from sugar has increased from 31% to 53% between 1913 and 1972 (Fig. 2-1).

The amount of carbohydrate in the diet tends to increase with a decrease in the amount of money available to spend on food, since it is a much less expensive source of calories than are protein and fat. In some countries, such as Japan and Indonesia, where rice or cassava is the staple in the diet, as much as 80% to 85% of the calories come from carbohydrate. At the other extreme, carbohydrate provides only 8% of the energy in the high-fat diet of Eskimos living where available plant life is limited.

Since the caloric value of carbohydrate is the same from all sources, when a sauce can be thickened with half as much cornstarch as wheat starch, it will have half the calories from starch. Similarly, a sugar with high sweetening power will contribute the same degree of sweetness with less sugar and fewer calories than one of low sweetening power. Conversely, the use of a starch with a low thickening power and a sugar with a low sweetening power may help increase the caloric value of a diet without appreciably changing its character.

Dietary essential—an unexplained role. Although carbohydrate can be replaced by fat and protein as a source of energy, recent evidence indicates that a diet devoid of carbohydrate produces many indesirable symptoms. Persons on a diet of only protein and fat may rapidly develop the same symptoms as persons on a starvation regimen. They lose very large amounts of sodium, are unable to prevent the breakdown of body protein except at very high levels of protein intake, and develop ketosis from the accumulation in the blood and urine of abnormal products of fat metabolism by the second day of a carbohydrate-free diet. The subjects all experience dehydration, fatigue, and loss of energy. All these undesirable results of a lack of carbohydrate in the diet are reversed by the addition of carbohydrate, which would indicate that carbohydrate is a dietary essential.

No evidence has been compiled to indicate whether the need is for any carbohydrate, specifically for one group such as monosaccharides, disaccharides, or polysaccharides, or for a specific carbohydrate. Persons on a diet lacking in carbohydrate experience the same rapid loss of weight as do persons subjected to total starvation. It should be pointed out, however, that diets are seldom totally devoid of carbohydrate and that intakes as low as 60 g will prevent these undesirable symptoms. The hazards associated with low-carbohydrate diets suggest that they should be used only under strict medical supervision.

Carbohydrates or products derived from them also serve as precursors of vital body compounds, such as nucleic acids and connective tissue matrix.

FOOD SOURCES

Carbohydrate is found almost exclusively in foods of plant origin. Milk, with its high lactose content, is the only important source of animal carbohydrate. Human milk contains considerably more lactose (7%) than cow's milk (4.8%). Eggs contain a very small amount, and scallops and oysters are the only other animal tissues that contain carbohydrate. The small amount in the liver is almost all converted to pyruvic and lactic acids during the slaughtering process.

Table 2-5 shows some typical sources of carbohydrate. The figures for total carbohydrate include the utilizable sugars and starches and the nondigestible cellulose, or fibers. The values for fiber content represent crude fiber and the best currently available values for dietary fiber but may be low. When tables of food composition are used to determine the utilizable carbohydrate in the diet, the values for fiber should be subtracted from those for total carbohydrate.

Some foods, such as sugar and cornstarch, are over 80% carbohydrate. Others, such as the potato and rice, commonly considered carbohydrate foods, are about 20% carbohydrate. Most of the caloric content of the foods listed in Table 2-5 is derived from carbohydrates with some from protein but little from fat.

The range in the amount of carbohydrate in fruits and vegetables is evident. Persons who must regulate the carbohydrate content of their diets are well aware of the classification of fruits and vegetables into exchange lists based on the carbohydrate content. The amounts of the different foods with equiva-

Table 2-5. Carbohydrate content of foods*

Food	Total carbohydrate	Crude fiber	Dietary fiber
	g/100 g food		
Sugar, granulated	99.5	0	
Sugar, brown	96.4	0	
Cornstarch	87.6	0.1	
Raisins	77.4	0.9	
All-purpose flour (72% extraction)	76.1	0.3	3.4
Macaroni, dry	75.2	0.3	
Chocolate fudge	75.0	0.2	
Maple syrup	65.0	—	
Enriched white bread	50.5	0.2	
Whole wheat bread	47.7	1.6	
Muffins	42.3	0.1	
Rice, coated	24.2	0.1	
Macaroni, cooked	23.0	0.1	
Potatoes, baked	21.1	0.6	
Bananas	22.2	0.5	1.8
Ice cream	20.6	0.8	
Lima beans, cooked	19.8	1.8	
Corn, cooked	18.8	0.7	
Grapes	15.7	0.6	
Apples, not pared	14.5	1.0	1.4
Ginger ale	8.0	—	
Beans, green	7.1	1.0	
Cabbage	5.4	0.8	2.8
Beef liver	5.3	0	
Whole milk	4.9	0	
Oysters, raw	3.4	0	
Pears, cooked	2.0	0.6	2.4

*Based on Watt, B. K., and Merrill, A. L.: Composition of foods—raw, processed and prepared, Handbook No. 8, Washington, D.C., 1963, U.S. Department of Agriculture; and Southgate, D. A. T.: The definition and analysis of dietary fiber, Nutr. Rev. **35**:31, 1977.

lent amounts of carbohydrate are included in these lists to facilitate making substitutions (Appendix I).

Carrageenin, or Irish moss, is a polysaccharide that cannot be utilized by the human. Because of its ability to absorb water, it is a useful ingredient for several synthetic foods such as imitation milk. Methyl cellulose, a synthetic product, is used in low-calorie cookies, mayonnaise, and candy.

MILLING OF CEREALS

Since cereals are a major source of calories, there is considerable interest in the effect of milling on the nutritive value of cereals. The structure of a typical cereal grain is shown in Fig. 2-5. Starch is the major constituent of the endosperm in the center of the seed where energy is stored. Although some other nutrients are provided in the endosperm, many occur in higher amounts in the

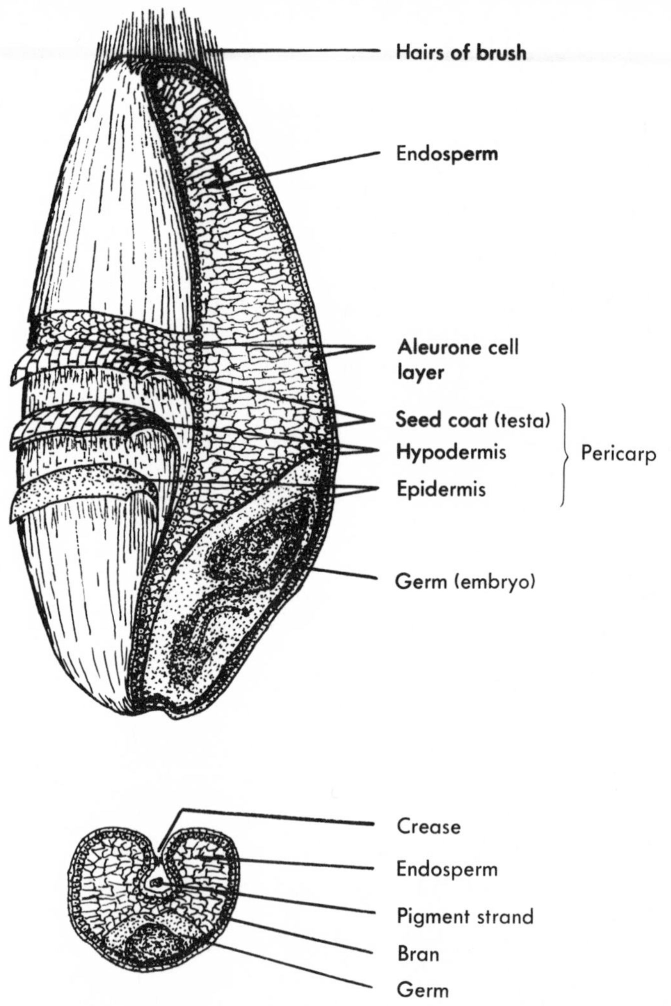

Fig. 2-5. Diagrammatic representation of cereal grain in longitudinal and cross section.

Table 2-6. Distribution of nutrients in cereal grain (percent of total content)

	Protein	Total mineral	Thiamin	Riboflavin	Niacin	Pyridoxine	Pantothenic acid
Endosperm	72	20	3	32	12	6	43
Pericarp	4	7	1	5	4	12	9
Aleurone	15	61	32	37	82	61	41
Germ (embryo)	3	4	2	12	1	8	3
Scutellum	5	8	62	14	1	12	4

bran and the germ, as shown in Table 2-6. Thus the nutritive value of cereals depends, to a large extent, on the amount of the bran that is retained when a cereal is milled. The higher the extraction (percentage of wheat remaining after milling), the more bran retained and the higher the amount of the other nutrients. The wheat germ contains a large proportion of the thiamin and vitamin E in the seed and is usually removed in milled cereals because it has a high content of oil, which becomes rancid quickly and results in spoilage.

DIETARY REQUIREMENTS

Since the body can function with considerably less carbohydrate than is present in most diets, it has been impossible to establish a dietary standard for carbohydrate. Diets low in or devoid of carbohydrate are so unpalatable that there is little likelihood of their being consumed for any appreciable length of time. In addition, the fact that carbohydrate is the most economical source of calories leads to its use in sufficent quantities to ensure at least a minimum intake. The Food and Nutrition Board of the National Research Council recommends an intake of 100 g of carbohydrate a day to prevent the undesirable consequences of a lower intake, such as ketosis, excessive breakdown of protein, and other undesirable metabolic responses. Most diets provide over 200 g.

ABNORMALITIES OF METABOLISM

There are several pathological conditions that cause difficulty in utilization of carbohydrate. The most common is diabetes, in which there is a relative lack of the hormone insulin necessary for uptake of glucose by the cell. Whether this is because of decreased production of insulin by the pancreas or an excess of an insulin inhibitor in the blood, the cell cannot pick up and utilize carbohydrate from the bloodstream at a normal rate.

Another condition is caused by the lack of the enzyme necessary to convert galactose to glucose in the liver. Galactose then appears as an abnormal constituent of the blood and the condition is known as galactosemia. This may also occur when the intake of galactose is extremely high. Weight loss, vomiting, and mental retardation are some of the consequences of galactosemia.

The lack of the enzyme needed to release stored glycogen from the liver leads to glycogen storage disease.

Lactose intolerance. In the past few years evidence has accumulated showing that practically all adults, but especially those of Oriental or Negro ancestry, suffer from a deficiency of the enzyme lactase, which is needed to convert lactose to glucose and galactose so that it can be absorbed. As a result, these adults are unable to tolerate any appreciable amount of lactose and thus develop gastrointestinal symptoms following the ingestion of more than a limited amount of milk. They are, however, able to consume fermented milks and cheese in which the lactose has been changed to lactic acid by the action of microorganisms. Symptoms of lactase insufficiency or lactose intolerance include diarrhea, flatulence, abdominal cramps, and bloating caused by either the osmotic effect of the undigested lactose in the lower gastrointestinal tract or the production of organic acids and carbon dioxide in the fermentation of lactose by gastrointestinal organisms.

Two theories have been advanced to explain the condition. One suggests that the enzyme deficiency is an adaptive one in which the child who does not receive milk after weaning no longer has any use for the enzyme and therefore fails to produce it. Similarly, this theory suggests that the ability of some adults to tolerate lactose is a result of their ability to induce or "turn on" the gene that synthesizes lactase when milk is regularly consumed. The second theory maintains that in populations that do not normally consume milk after weaning, lactase deficiency is a normal, genetically transmitted trait and that the milk-drinking populations have had to develop a gene to promote lactase production.

In general, symptoms of lactose intolerance do not appear until adolescence and there is some evidence that those who are intolerant may be able to adapt to a diet in which milk is fed in small quantities. This may be the result of the production of the enzyme to digest lactose, of the ability of lactose to prevent the degradation of lactase, or of a change in the intestinal flora that allows new bacteria to digest lactose and thus prevent fermentation, which leads to the characteristic symptoms.

Observations that black children who may have the defect consume less milk than white children, presumably because of the discomfort associated with the ingestion of milk, raise questions about the relevance of milk in school feeding programs for black children. Similarly, others have questioned the use of milk in international feeding programs for population groups who are likely to be lactase deficient. However, since milk is the major dietary source of calcium and often of protein and since it is possible to alleviate symptoms by slowly increasing the amount given over a period of time, it seems desirable to determine the degree of lactose intolerance before recommending complete elimination of milk. Milk intolerance and lactose intolerance may not be the same thing.

Research is being directed toward the development of low-lactose milk. Lactases from yeasts and molds are introduced during processing to split lactose to glucose and galactose. There is also evidence to suggest that tolerance to whole milk is greater than to nonfat milk or to lactose alone.

CARBOHYDRATE AND ATHEROSCLEROSIS

Research to identify a dietary factor involved in atherosclerosis, now a leading cause of death in the United States, has suggested that both the kind and amount of carbohydrate in the diet may be important factors. Epidemiological data show that a high intake of sugar is among the dietary risk factors associated with coronary heart disease. Data from animal studies have failed to confirm this with results that vary, depending on age, species, and sex of the animal, length of the experiment, and amount of dietary cholesterol. Data from human studies are confusing and often contradictory, undoubtedly because of difficulty in manipulating only one dietary factor. In general, it is impossible to conclude that when sucrose represents from 20% to 30% of the calories consumed, it has any undesirable effect or as great an effect as the type and amount of dietary lipid on blood lipids, atherosclerosis, or coronary heart disease. The addition of sucrose to the diet may, however, exaggerate the effect of dietary fats on blood lipids. On the other, hand, we have no evidence of undesirable effects from a reduced sugar intake. In summary, at this time no evidence of a firm association between sugar consumption and coronary artery disease exists.

CARBOHYDRATE AND DENTAL HEALTH

Carbohydrate is often implicated as one of many factors in the cause of dental caries. In the preeruptive stage when the tooth is forming and is being nourished through the bloodstream, carbohydrate has little direct effect on tooth quality. However, if carbohydrate in the diet replaces protective foods that carry nutrients such as calcium, vitamin D, and vitamin C, which are necessary for normal tooth formation, they indirectly have an adverse effect on the health of the tooth before eruption.

In the posteruptive stage when the tooth is exposed to the oral environment and has only limited systemic connection, carbohydrate, especially sucrose, assumes importance. It has been established that before tooth decay occurs, there must be present both microorganisms and food for the microorganisms-carbohydrate. Complex carbohydrates or carbohydrates in solution that do not adhere to the tooth surface cause relatively little harm. However, a sucrose-rich food, such as toffee, or caramel, that tends to adhere to the tooth surface provides the food needed by the bacteria to form polysaccharides called dextrans or polyglucans, which adhere to the tooth to form plaques. These in turn are acted on by other bacteria to form the acid that ultimately facilitates the solution of tooth enamel, with resultant decay of the caries-susceptible tooth. In dental health the form of the carbohydrate is equally as important as the amount.

A high incidence of dental caries in children who are given a bottle at bedtime and allowed to fall asleep with it in their mouths has been described as the "nursing bottle syndrome." These conditions are conducive to the growth of organisms and the formation of dental caries, especially in the upper teeth.

Carbohydrate has less detrimental effect on tooth health if it is followed by liquids or other detergent foods, such as apples, that tend to remove the carbohydrate from the tooth surface or when consumed as part of a meal rather than at between-meal feedings.

SUGAR SUBSTITUTES

Since a large segment of the population, especially the obese and diabetic, is concerned with calorie control and yet wishes to enjoy the pleasure associated with eating sweet foods, there is a constant search to identify a safe, low-calorie sweetening agent. Some, such as fructose, Monellin, Naringin, and aspartame, a dipeptide, achieve a high degree of sweetening with very few calories, either by contributing a sweet taste or by acting directly on the taste buds to increase their sensitivity to the natural sweetness. Other nonnutritive sweeteners such as saccharin or cyclamates contribute a sweet taste without calories. Before any nonnutritive substance can be introduced on the market, the Delaney Amendment requires convincing evidence that there is no possibility of carcinogenic effects. As a result, aspartame and sodium and calcium cyclamates, which had been widely used (5.85 million kg in 1967), have been banned in 1974 and 1970, respectively, from use in food products as possible carcinogens. The safety of saccharin, which has been used since 1879, is under review. Monellin, or Serendip, which is a protein, is unstable when heated and of no value in cooked products. Thus, at the present time fructose is the only approved sweetening agent whose safety has not been ques-

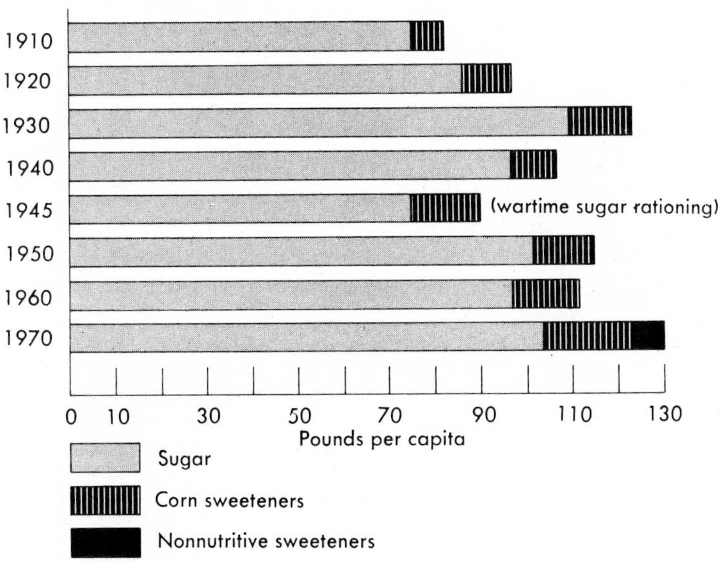

Fig. 2-6. Trends in consumption of sugar and other sweeteners.

tioned. However, it is almost twice as expensive for the same sweetening effect and still has half the calories of sucrose. Naringin, which is bitter tasting, is a naturally occurring substance found in the rind of grapefruit. It can be converted into a substance that has a sweetening power 1500 times that of sugar and three times that of saccharin. It is being considered as a substitute for nonnutritive synthetic sweetening agents. Since it is totally excreted in either the urine or feces within 24 hours, it is unlikely to prove toxic. It has the advantage of being stable over a wide range of temperatures. Aspartame, a dipeptide of aspartic acid and phenylalanine, both of which are amino acids, is 160 times as sweet as sugar but has been found unsafe. The amino acid tryptophan is thirty times as sweet as sucrose. Xylitol, a 5-carbon sugar, has been used as a sweetener in diabetic diets, but it contributes an appreciable number of calories, since from 49% to 95% of the sugar is absorbed.

Three additional chemicals derived from the rind or oranges and grapefruit and belonging to a group of substances known as bioflavonoids also show promise as acceptable sweeteners without caloric value. Trends in the use of sugar and sweeteners are shown in Fig. 2-6.

ALCOHOL (ETHANOL)

Ethyl alcohol, produced from the fermentation of glucose in the presence of enzymes in yeast and in the absence of oxygen, statistically accounts for an average energy intake of 76 kcal per capita per day. However, since about two thirds of the population do not use alcohol, the contribution of this nutrient to the energy intake of those who do may reach as high as 10% of the total caloric intake. Thus it is appropriate that a student of nutrition have an understanding of its metabolism.

Absorption and metabolism

Ethanol is a small, neutral, water-soluble molecule that does not require digestion. It is absorbed by diffusion throughout the length of the gastrointestinal tract. As much as 80% of the intake is absorbed in the small intestine immediately after leaving the stomach. There is no upper limit on the rate of absorption, and the absorbed alcohol, being water soluble, immediately disperses throughout the body fluids. Its concentration in any one tissue parallels the water concentration of the tissue. Thus a large amount of absorbed alcohol is found in the blood and relatively little in adipose tissue and bone. Little alcohol is excreted. Less than 5% is lost through the kidneys and lungs. However, since the amount in the expired air and in the urine is in equilibrium with that in the blood, it is possible to use a measure of alcohol content of these as a legally valid measure of alcohol content of the blood. A blood concentration of 0.1% is considered a maximum, and a level of 0.15% is evidence of intoxication. A level of 0.4% causes respiratory arrest.

The metabolism of alcohol begins in the liver and kidney, which contain the enzyme alcohol dehydrogenase and two other enzyme systems necessary to oxidize or convert the alcohol to the form in which it can be used in the same way that carbohydrate and fatty acids are used as a source of energy. Since skeletal muscles lack this enzyme, the metabolism of alcohol cannot be initiated there, but once the intermediate has been formed, muscle tissue as well as all other tissues can use it as an energy source. It is possible that alcohol could be converted to fat and stored, but in general it is metabolized immediately to carbon dioxide, water, and energy in preference to fatty acids and glucose. By sparing these energy sources, ethanol can contribute to positive caloric balance. The brain also contains some alcohol dehydrogenase, which allows it to metabolize sufficient alcohol to make local adjustments to control the neural effects of alcohol that would result otherwise.

Alcohol contributes 7 kcal of energy/g or 5.6 kcal/ml. Thus 29.6 ml (1 fluid ounce) of 100-proof alcohol (50% alcohol) contains 12 g of alcohol, which contribute 84 kcal of energy. Similarly, 355 ml (12 oz) of beer with an alcohol content of 3% or 118 ml (4 oz) of wine with a 12% alcohol content contribute 80 kcal to the energy pool. Evidence that alcohol use stimulates energy expenditure suggests that the net result of alcohol ingestion may be less than 7 kcal/g, with the remainder being dissipated as heat. Individuals vary greatly in the rate at which they metabolize alcohol, but for most people it ranges between 100 and 200 mg/kg of body weight/hr. This is equivalent to one fifth of a gallon of 100-proof whiskey a day for a 70 kg man.

The absorption of alcohol can be modified by interaction with other drugs. Once absorbed, the rate of metabolism is speeded up by both injected and dietary fructose. It is unaffected by physical exercise, vitamin supplements, thyroid hormones, and caffeine.

The consumption of alcohol in excessive amounts can lead to severe liver damage and the accumulation of fat in liver tissue. By inhibiting glycolysis (the conversion of glycogen to glucose) and gluconeogenesis (the formation of glucose from amino acids and glycerol) and stimulating the production of NADPH (a lipid precursor), alcohol consumption often results in a low blood sugar level, fatty liver, and the accumulation of ketones or intermediates of fat metabolism in the liver. In cases in which alcohol consumption does not lead to a decreased intake of other nutrients, the liver is generally protected against damage.

The caloric value is some commonly used alcoholic beverages is presented in Table 2-7.

Table 2-7. Caloric content of alcoholic beverages

Beverage	Amount	Calories
Beer	8 oz	110
Ale	8 oz	150
Gin		
80 proof	1 oz	65
86 proof	1 oz	78
Rum	1 oz	70
Whiskey	1 oz	80
Wine		
Red	3 oz	145
Dry	3 oz	90
Vermouth, sweet	1 oz	50
Manhattan	3 oz	165
Martini	3 oz	140
Old Fashioned	3 oz	180

BIBLIOGRAPHY

Ahrens, R. A.: Sucrose, hypertension, and heart disease: an historical perspective, Am. J. Clin. Nutr. **27**:403, 1974.

Bayless, T. M., and Huang, S.: Inadequate intestinal digestion of lactose, Am. J. Clin. Nutr. **22**:250, 1969.

Bing, F. C.: Dietary fiber—in historical perspective, J. Am. Diet. Assoc. **69**:498, 1976.

Brown, A. T.: The role of dietary carbohydrates in plaque formation and oral disease, Nutr. Rev. **33**:353, 1975.

Burkitt, D. P., Walker, A. R. P., and Painter, N. S.: Dietary fiber and disease, J.A.M.A. **229**:1068, 1974.

Committee on Alcoholism and Drug Dependence: Alcohol and society, J.A.M.A. **216**:1011, 1971.

Council on Foods and Nutrition, American Medical Association: A critique of low carbohydrate ketogenic weight reduction regimens. A review of Dr. Atkin's Diet Revolution, J.A.M.A. **224**:1415, 1973.

Danouski, T. S., Nolan S., and Stephen, T.: Hypoglycemia, World Rev. Nutr. Diet. **22**:288, 1975.

Federation of American Societies for Experimental Biology: Evaluation of health aspects of sucrose as a food ingredient, SCOGS-69, Washington, D.C., 1976.

Goodhart, R. S.: Cyclamate sweeteners in the human diet—a scientific evaluation, North Chicago, 1968, Abbott Laboratories.

Gray, G. M.: Carbohydrate digestion and absorption: role of the small intestine, N. Engl. J. Med. **292**:1225, 1975.

Hardinge, M. G., Swarner, J. B., and Crooks, H.: Carbohydrates in foods, J. Am. Diet. Assoc. **46**:197, 1965.

Harper, A. E.: Carbohydrates. In Food yearbook of agriculture, Washington D.C., 1959, U.S. Department of Agriculture.

Hegsted, D. M.: Food and fibre: evidence from experimental animals, Nutr. Rev. **35**:45, 1977.

Inglett, G. E.: A history of sweeteners—natural and synthetic, J. Toxicol. Environ. Health **2**:207, 1976.

Johnson, H. L., and Consolazio, C. F.: Dietary carbohydrate and work capacity, Am. J. Clin. Nutr. **25**:85, 1972.

Kelsay, J. L.: A review of research on effects of fiber intake on man. Am. J. Clin. Nutr. **31**:142, 1978.

Kretchmer, N.: Lactose and lactase, Sci. Am. **227:**70, 1972.

Kritchevsky, D., Tepper, S. A., and Story, J. A.: Nonnutritive fiber and lipid metabolism, J. Food Sci. **40:**8, 1975.

McDonald, J. T., and Margen, S.: Wine versus ethanol in human nutrition. I. Nitrogen and calorie balance, Am. J. Clin. Nutr. **29:**1093, 1976.

McMichael, H.: Intestinal absorption of carbohydrate in man, Proc. Nutr. Soc. **30:**248, 1971.

McNutt, K.: Perspective. Fiber, J. Nutr. Educ. **8:**150, 1976.

Mazur, R. H.: Aspartame—a sweet surprise, J. Toxicol. Environ. Health **2:**243, 1976.

Mendeloff, A. I.: Dietary fibre, Nutr. Rev. **33:**321, 1975.

Moore, K. K.: Xylitol: Uncut gem among sweeteners, Food Prod. Dev. **11:**66, 1977.

National Academy of Sciences: Sweeteners, issues and uncertainties, Washington, D.C., 1975.

Nutrition Foundation, Marabou Symposium on Food and Fibre, Nutr. Rev. **35:**1, 1977.

Painter, N. S.: Unprocessed bran in the treatment of diverticular disease of the colon, Br. Med. J. **2:**137, 1972.

Southgate, D. A. T.: The definition and analysis of dietary fibre, Nutr. Rev. **35:**31, 1977.

Southgate, D. A. T., Bailey, G., Collinson, E., and Walker, A. F.: A guide to calculating intakes of dietary fiber. J. Hum. Nutr. **30:**303, 1976.

Spiller, G. A., and Shipley, E. A.: Perspectives on dietary fiber in human nutrition, World Rev. Nutr. Diet. **27:**106, 1977.

Stare, F. J., Editor: Sugar in the diet of man, World Rev. Nutr. Diet. **22:**236, 1975.

Stevens, H. A., and Ohlson, M. A.: Estimated intake of simple and complex carbohydrates, J. Am. Diet. Assoc. **48:**294, 1966.

Symposium on Alcohol in Nutrition, Proc. Nutr. Soc. **31:**77, 1972.

Trowell, J.: Definition of dietary fiber and hypotheses that it is a protective factor in certain diseases, Am. J. Clin. Nutr. **29:**417, 1976.

Van Soest, P. J.: What is fibre and fibre in food? Nutr. Rev. **35:**12, 1977.

Victor, M.: Alcohol and nutritional diseases of the nervous system, J.A.M.A. **167:**65, 1958.

Westerfeld, W. W., and Schulman, M. P.: Metabolism and the caloric value of alcohol, J.A.M.A. **170:**197, 1959.

Wightman, N.: Saccharin—are there alternatives? J. Nutr. Educ. **9:**106, 1977.

Woodruff, C. W.: Milk intolerances, Nutr. Rev. **34:**33, 1976.

Yudkin, J.: Sugar and disease, Nature **239:**197, 1972.

3

Fat or lipid

Fats or lipids are clearly identifiable components of many foods that have been accounting for an increasing proportion of the energy in the American diet. Because of a possible relationship between dietary fat and the incidence of several degenerative diseases, the public is concerned not only about how much fat is consumed but also about the source and composition of the fat. While nutritionists are seeking to learn the role of dietary lipid in the development of coronary heart disease, cancer, and obesity, food technologists are developing ways to modify the amount and kind of fat in the American diet. As a concentrated source of energy, lipid, when taken in excess of caloric needs, is implicated in the obesity problem in the United States.

Next to water and carbohydrate, the predominant nutrient in the American diet is **lipid** or fat. Some of the dietary sources of this nutrient are readily identified as visible fats and oils such as butter, margarine, salad oil, and the fat surrounding meat. These food sources, however, account for only 40% of the lipid in the diet. The remaining 60% is invisible fat, including that marbled throughout meat fibers, in finely divided form either emulsified in egg yolk or homogenized in whole milk, or found as a constituent of whole-grain cereals and nuts. Currently about 60% of our dietary fat comes from animal sources and the remainder from vegetable sources, primarily vegetable oils. (See Fig. 3-1.)

As seen in Fig. 3-2, the lipid content of the American diet increased steadily from 125 g/day, which provided 32% of the calories in 1910, to 159 g/day, providing 41% of the energy of the diet in 1972. By then the average person was consuming 57.7 kg/yr. Data for 1976, indicating an intake of 157 g/day, suggest that this upward trend is being reversed. While the amount of fat consumed has been changing, there has been a marked shift in the proportions coming from animal and vegetable sources. The widespread use of margarine instead of butter, cooking oils rather than lard, and nondairy creamers to replace cream has resulted in a decline from 84% to 60% in the proportion of fat from animal sources and a concurrent increase in the amount of vegetable fat consumed. Soybean oil accounts for about three fourths of the vegetable oil used in the United States with cottonseed, corn, and coconut oil accounting for 8%, 5%, and 4% of the consumption, respectively. There has been an increase from 25% to 41% in the contribution of beef to the fat from the meat group and a decrease from 60% to 36% in the contribution of pork.

The nature and amount of fat in a diet is influenced as much by social, cultural, geographical, and economic factors as by nutritional concerns. For instance, the Japanese diet is traditionally low in fat, whereas the Italians have a high-fat intake, emphasizing the use of olive oil. The type of fat included in many processed foods is determined by economic considerations.

Although on the one hand there are concerns about adverse effects from an increased use of dietary fat, on the other hand

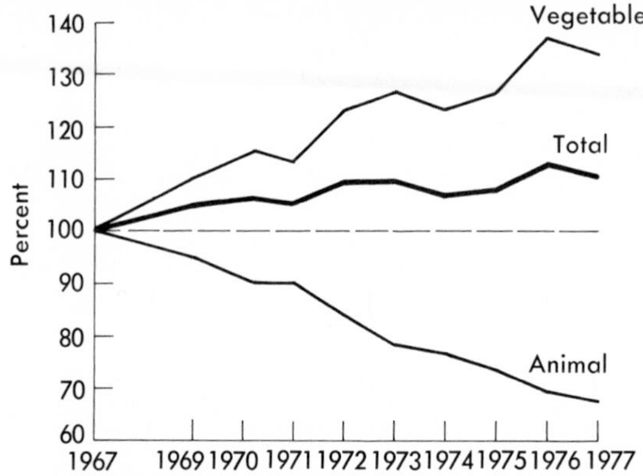

Fig. 3-1. Sources of fat in diet. (From Fat in the diet, Washington, D.C., 1977, U.S. Department of Agriculture.)

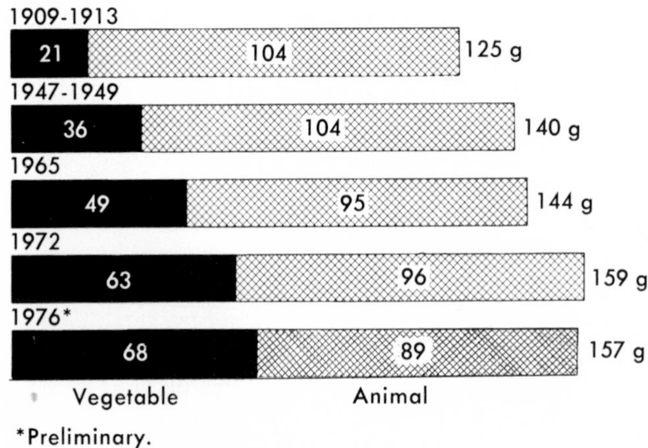

Fig. 3-2. Trends in the consumption of animal and vegetable fat in American diet. (Based on data from National food situation NFS-161, Washington, D.C., 1977, Economic Research Service.)

it is important to recognize that fat is an essential dietary component both from a nutritional and a palatability standpoint.

CHEMICAL COMPOSITION

Like carbohydrate, lipid is composed of the three elements carbon, hydrogen, and oxygen. It differs from carbohydrate, however, in that the ratio of oxygen to carbon and hydrogen is much lower, being 1:2 in simple carbohydrates and from 1:7 to 1:30 in simple fats. This lower amount of oxygen in relation to the other two elements accounts for the fact that fat is a more concentrated source of energy than is carbohydrate.

Most of the energy from dietary fat is provided by the class of lipids called triglycerides. Biochemically, these lipids have two major components—*glycerol* and *fatty acids*. The glycerol portion, a 3-carbon alcohol, is common to practically all dietary lipids. The fatty acid portion varies from one fat to another.

$$\begin{array}{ccc} & \mathrm{H} & \\ & | & \\ \mathrm{H}- & \mathrm{C} & -\mathrm{OH} \\ & | & \\ \mathrm{H}- & \mathrm{C} & -\mathrm{OH} \\ & | & \\ \mathrm{H}- & \mathrm{C} & -\mathrm{OH} \\ & | & \\ & \mathrm{H} & \end{array}$$

As constituents of dietary lipids, fatty acids are composed of an even-numbered carbon chain, 4 to 22 carbon atoms in length. In addition, fatty acids differ from one another, depending on the number of hydrogen atoms attached to the carbon chain. In a saturated fatty acid, 2 hydrogen atoms, the maximum possible, are attached to each carbon atom other than the first carbon, which has 3 hydrogens (CH_3) and the last, which is known as a carboxyl group (COOH). In contrast, unsaturated fatty acids have fewer than the maximum number of hydrogen atoms attached to the carbon chain. In a monounsaturated fatty acid, 1 hydrogen atom is missing from each of 2 adjacent carbons. To compensate for the loss of hydrogen atoms, the 2 carbons form an additional chemical bond, introducing a double bond (=) in the carbon chain. Thus instead of having this form

$$\begin{array}{ccccccccc} & & & \mathrm{H} & & \mathrm{H} & & & \\ & | & & | & & | & & | & \\ - & \mathrm{C} & - & \mathrm{C} & - & \mathrm{C} & - & \mathrm{C} & - \\ & | & & | & & | & & | & \\ & & & \mathrm{H} & & \mathrm{H} & & & \end{array}$$

the chain looks like this:

$$\begin{array}{ccccccccc} & | & & & & & & | & \\ - & \mathrm{C} & - & \mathrm{C} & = & \mathrm{C} & - & \mathrm{C} & - \\ & | & & | & & | & & | & \\ & & & \mathrm{H} & & \mathrm{H} & & & \end{array}$$

In some long-chain fatty acids, double bonds appear in two or more places, and these fatty acids are known as **polyunsaturated** fatty acids (PUFA). The chain may look like this:

$$\begin{array}{cccccccccccc} & | & & & & & & | & & & & \\ - & \mathrm{C} & - & \mathrm{C} & = & \mathrm{C} & - & \mathrm{C} & - & \mathrm{C} & = & \mathrm{C} \\ & | & & | & & | & & | & & | & & | \end{array}$$

Fatty acids are classified on the basis of the number of carbons in their carbon chains. Short-chain fatty acids with 2 to 6 carbons are relatively rare; medium-chain fatty acids with 8 to 12 carbons are more common, constituting 4% to 10% of fatty acids in food, whereas long-chain fatty acids with 16 or 18 carbons predominate in natural fats. The nature and source of the common fatty acids are shown in Table 3-1.

Fats as they occur in food and in the body represent a combination of one to three fatty acids with a glycerol molecule. A fat may contain only one fatty acid; it is then known as a **monoglyceride. Diglycerides** have two fatty acids attached to the glycerol molecule and triglycerides have three. The most common lipids are **triglycerides,** accounting for 95% of fat in food. If the fatty acids are all the same, the fat is referred to as a simple triglyceride, whereas if they differ from one another, the fat is called a mixed triglyceride.

The general formula for glycerides may be written as follows (FA represents a fatty acid):

$$\begin{array}{ccc} & \mathrm{H} & \\ & | & \\ \mathrm{H}- & \mathrm{C} & -\mathrm{OH} \\ & | & \\ \mathrm{H}- & \mathrm{C} & -\mathrm{OH} \\ & | & \\ \mathrm{H}- & \mathrm{C} & -\mathrm{O}-\mathrm{FA_1} \\ & | & \\ & \mathrm{H} & \end{array}$$

Monoglyceride

$$\begin{array}{ccc} & \mathrm{H} & \\ & | & \\ \mathrm{H}- & \mathrm{C} & -\mathrm{OH} \\ & | & \\ \mathrm{H}- & \mathrm{C} & -\mathrm{O}-\mathrm{FA_1} \\ & | & \\ \mathrm{H}- & \mathrm{C} & -\mathrm{O}-\mathrm{FA_2} \\ & | & \\ & \mathrm{H} & \end{array}$$

Diglyceride

$$\begin{array}{ccc} & \mathrm{H} & \\ & | & \\ \mathrm{H}- & \mathrm{C} & -\mathrm{O}-\mathrm{FA_1} \\ & | & \\ \mathrm{H}- & \mathrm{C} & -\mathrm{O}-\mathrm{FA_2} \\ & | & \\ \mathrm{H}- & \mathrm{C} & -\mathrm{O}-\mathrm{FA_3} \\ & | & \\ & \mathrm{H} & \end{array}$$

Mixed triglyceride

Table 3-1. Composition and sources of fatty acids most commonly found in food

Name	General formula $CH_3—(CH_2)_n—COOH$	Length of carbon chain	Position of double bond	Common source
Saturated				
Butyric	$CH_3—CH_2—CH_2—COOH$	4		Butter
Caproic	$CH_3(CH_2)_4COOH$	6		Butter
Caprylic	$CH_3(CH_2)_6COOH$	8		Coconut oil
Capric	$CH_3(CH_2)_8COOH$	10		Palm oil
Lauric	$CH_3(CH_2)_{10}COOH$	12		Coconut oil
Myristic	$CH_3(CH_2)_{12}COOH$	14		Butterfat Nutmeg Coconut oil
Palmitic	$CH_3(CH_2)_{14}COOH$	16		Animal and vegetable
Stearic	$CH_3(CH_2)_{16}COOH$	18		Animal and vegetable
Arachidic	$CH_3(CH_2)_{18}COOH$	20		Peanut oil and lard
Unsaturated				
Palmitoleic	$CH_3(CH_2)_2—CH{=}CH—(CH_2)_7COOH$	16	9-10	Butter and seed oils
Oleic	$CH_3(CH_2)_7—CH{=}CH—(CH_2)_7COOH$	18	9-10	Most fats and oils
Linoleic	$CH_3(CH_2)_4CH{=}CH—CH_2—CH{=}$ $CH—(CH_2)_7COOH$	18	9-10 12-13	Seed fats
Linolenic	$CH_3CH_2CH{=}CH—CH_2—CH{=}$ $CH—CH_2CH{=}CH(CH_2)_7COOH$	18	9-10 12-13 15-16	Soybean oil
Arachidonic	$CH_3(CH_2)_4CH{=}CH—CH_2CH{=}CH—CH_2CH{=}$ $CH—CH_2CH{=}CH(CH_2)_3COOH$	20	5-6 8-9 11-12 14-15	

When the fatty acids are attached to the glycerol molecule, the carboyxl end of the fatty acid joins the hydroxyl (OH) portion of the glycerol molecule with the release of 1 molecule of water. The chemical bond that holds them together is called an ester bond.

Since glycerol is common to all triglycerides, differences are due to the number and kind of fatty acids and the order or place in which they are attached to the glycerol core. The characteristics of the fat reflect the nature of the fatty acids in the molecule and their arrangement on the glycerol base. Most food fats contain glycerides with eight to ten fatty acids—a mixture of saturated and unsaturated. Unsaturated fatty acids produce a fat that is liquid at room temperature with a low melting point, whereas fats with saturated fatty acids predominating will have a high melting point and be solid at room temperature. The proportion of unsaturated to saturated fatty acids in a fat is called the P/S ratio. The higher the ratio, the more unsaturated fatty acids are present in the fat and the more likely it is to be liquid (oil). A P/S ratio is often used in advertising and food labelling to help consumers know what kind of fat they are buying. In general, animal fats are high in saturated fatty acids and vegetable fats are low. Exceptions are chicken fat and fish, which have a high P/S ratio. Coconut oil has a low P/S ratio but is liquid because of the large proportion of short-chain fatty acids.

Table 3-2. Iodine values of common fats and oils*

Oil	Iodine number
Linseed oil	177-209
Corn oil	115-124
Soybean oil	130-138
Cottonseed oil	105-115
Peanut oil	85-100
Olive oil	79-90
Lard	50-65
Butter	26-38

*The higher the value the more unsaturated the fat.

Fatty acids in fats will combine with iodine in proportion to the number of double bonds they contain. This property of fatty acids is the basis of a test to determine the degree of saturation of a fat. The iodine number for a fat will be high if it contains many unsaturated fatty acids and low if it contains few. Iodine values of some common fats and oils are shown in Table 3-2.

The double bonds in fatty acids also make unsaturated fatty acids vulnerable to deterioration as the result of oxidation. The double bond reacts with atmospheric oxygen to produce peroxides, which are responsible for the rancidity and "off" flavors in some fats. It is often necessary to add antioxidants to unsaturated oils if they must be kept for long periods without deterioration.

Monounsaturated fatty acids constitute about 40% of dietary fat, polyunsaturated 12%, and saturated 37%. Although hydrogen cannot be removed to make unsaturated fatty acids from saturated, it is possible to chemically convert unsaturated fatty acids to saturated by the addition of hydrogen. This process of **hydrogenation** is used commercially to convert less expensive oils such as cottonseed and soybean oil into fats with the physical characteristics of more expensive animal fats. For instance, margarine and shortening are produced by the hydrogenation of vegetable oils. By manipulating the process, it is possible to retain many of the unsaturated fatty acids and still have a fat with the desired characteristics. The extent to which hydrogenated fats are used is evident by the fact that over 1.35 billion kg are consumed in the United States each year.

Although each animal tends to produce a fat characteristic of its own species, it is possible to change the nature of animal fat by modifying the diet of the animal. Livestock producers take advantage of this phenomenon to market a product with the type of fat that consumers want. For instance, in some areas the softer fat produced by feeding pigs peanuts is more acceptable than the harder fat that results when corn is fed. Ruminants normally change the character of fat by saturating fatty acids in the rumen. Cattlemen have now learned they can bypass this step and produce beef with more unsaturated fat by feeding the cattle oil in a capsule that is not released until it reaches the intestine, where the animal can no longer change it to a saturated fat.

The physical form of lipid varies among foods. In foods such as egg yolk the fat is in finely divided particles surrounded by a thin layer of a phospholipid-protein complex that keeps them from joining together, or coalescing, to form visible fat globules. These fats are known as emulsified fats and because the fat is in fine particles, it has a much larger surface area than an unemulsified fat. Homogenized milk is whole milk with the fat globules broken up mechanically and dispersed so that they no longer rise to form a layer of cream. Similarly, the oil in mayonnaise is mechanically emulsified and stabilized by a layer of egg protein.

RELATED LIPIDS

In addition to the monoglycerides, diglycerides, and triglycerides, foods also contain a small amount of a related group of substances known as **phospholipids.** In these lipids, one of the fatty acids is replaced by a phosphate (PO_4) group and either a nitrogen-containing or a carbohydrate-like substance. Since these groups are water soluble, phospholipids serve to increase the solubility of the lipid and to keep fats in a finely divided emulsified form. The best known of the phospholipids is **lecithin,** in which the chemical choline is the nitrogen-containing portion of the molecule. It serves as the natural **emulsifier** in eggs and is present in cell membranes within the body. In spite of the popular use of lecithin as a dietary supplement, there is no evidence that it is absorbed unchanged or that it must be provided in the diet.

Cholesterol, an alcohol lipid or sterol, is present in all animal fats. It is necessary for the formation of many essential substances such as steroid hormones and bile salts; it is an integral part of all membranes of the body including myelin, which forms a protective sheath around nerve fibers. Cholesterol can be synthesized in the body, primarily in the liver and small intestine. The amount synthesized is regulated, depending on the quantity needed and available in the diet.

Phytosterols are a group of related lipids found in plants. One of these, sitosterol, apparently competes with cholesterol for absorption, thus causing a decreased absorption of cholesterol. Another, ergosterol, found in yeast, is a precursor of vitamin D.

ESSENTIAL FATTY ACIDS

The term **essential fatty acids** has traditionally been used to refer to linoleic, linolenic, and arachidonic acids. Originally, essential fatty acids (EFA) were considered those known to cure dermatitis and restore the growth of young animals fed a diet devoid of or very low in fat. Newer techniques for analysis have resulted in a reevaluation of the essentiality of certain fatty acids and findings are still inconclusive.

Linoleic acid, an 18-carbon fatty acid with two double bonds, cannot be produced by the body and has been clearly demonstrated to both restore growth and prevent dermatitis. For this reason linoleic acid has been designated an EFA and must be provided preformed in the diet.

Arachidonic acid is a 20-carbon polyunsaturated fatty acid with four double bonds found in some animal fat. Since the body can convert linoleic acid to arachidonic acid, it is not strictly speaking an essential fatty acid even though it performs some of the same functions as linoleic acid. Arachidonic acid is said to have partial EFA activity.

Evidence indicates that linolenic acid, an 18-carbon fatty acid with three double bonds, cannot be synthesized by mammals. This acid has no antidermatitis effect. Although there are a number of discrepancies in information concerning the essentiality of linolenic acid, present knowledge suggests that since it does not fulfill all the known functions of an EFA, it cannot be considered essential. It may, however, be required for

Table 3-3. Interrelationship of fatty acids

Fatty acid	Structure	Biological role	Sources
Linoleic ↓	18 carbons 2 double bonds	Growth factor Antidermatitis factor	Vegetable Seed oils
Arachidonic	20 carbons 4 double bonds	Antidermatitis factor	Animal fat
Linolenic	18 carbons 3 double bonds	Growth factor	Soybean oil

some function as yet unknown. The relationship among these fatty acids is shown in Table 3-3.

PHYSICAL PROPERTIES

Fat is insoluble in water but soluble in solvents such as ether, chloroform, and benzene. Fats are less dense than water; therefore they will rise to the surface of any aqueous mixture. In emulsified fats the fat particles are in finely divided form and are kept separated from one another by an emulsifying agent; thus they are prevented from coalescing or fusing together to form large globules. The dispersed fat in homogenized milk is an example of a fat emulsified by mechanical means; egg yolk fat is a naturally emulsified fat.

Fat is not affected by temperatures normally used in food preparation; however, heating at high temperatures leads to the decomposition of fatty acids and the production of acrolein from glycerol. Acrolein has a very pungent acrid fume extremely irritating to the nasal passages and the gastrointestinal tract. Fats are also subject to oxidation. Natural fats containing unsaturated fatty acids are extremely susceptible to oxidation, especially in the presence of catalysts such as iron. When they are low in antioxidants, which retard oxidation, they become rancid because of the production of peroxides of fatty acids, a major cause of spoilage in fats. Fats may also become unpalatable because of their tendency to absorb odors and flavors.

DIGESTION

Before fat can be absorbed across the intestinal wall to enter the circulatory system for transport to the various tissues, it must be broken down chemically into units small enough to be taken up by the cells lining the intestinal tract. Although some of the dietary triglycerides are changed to fatty acids and glycerol, the majority are split into monoglycerides and fatty acids.

A limited amount of digestion of fats, primarily those with short-chain fatty acids, occurs in the stomach, where the emulsified dietary fat is changed to fatty acids and glycerol by the action of gastric lipase, a fat-splitting enzyme secreted in the gastric juice from the stomach wall. Some of the fatty acids and glycerol liberated here recombine immediately to form new triglycerides, resulting in a fat with different characteristics than that consumed. Long-chain fatty acids are less likely to be attacked by gastric lipase or reincorporated into fat than are short-chain fatty acids.

Most of the digestion of fat takes place in the intestine. There, bile salts formed in the liver but stored in and secreted from the gallbladder arrange themselves on the surface of unemulsified triglycerides to break them into very small particles. These small particles with a larger surface area and smaller diameter can be more readily altered by digestive enzymes. Once the lipid is in this finely divided form, the pancreatic lipase secreted into the intestine from the pancreas can attack each triglyceride molecule and release the fatty acids attached to carbons 1 and 3 at either end of the 3-carbon glycerol core. This releases two fatty acids and leaves a monoglyceride with a fatty acid attached in the middle, or number 2, position. Sometimes this fatty acid is eventually split off. The release of a fatty acid is a hydrolytic reaction requiring the addition of 1 molecule of water for each fatty acid released. The digestion of fat is summarized in Fig. 3-3.

Absorption. After the monoglycerides, often referred to as monoacylglycerol, and fatty acids are formed, they combine with bile salts to form water-soluble complexes known as micelles, in which the diameter of each fat-containing particle is about 1/100 of that of the emulsified fat and the surface area 10,000 times greater.

These micelles enter the minute spaces between the small projections on the intestinal wall to come in close contact with the cells lining the intestinal tract. The fatty acids and monoglycerides enter the mucosal cells; the bile salts remain in the lumen of the intestine, incorporating more lipid into micelles to be transported to the absorbing cells.

Once the fatty acids, glycerol, and monoglycerides have entered the mucosal cells,

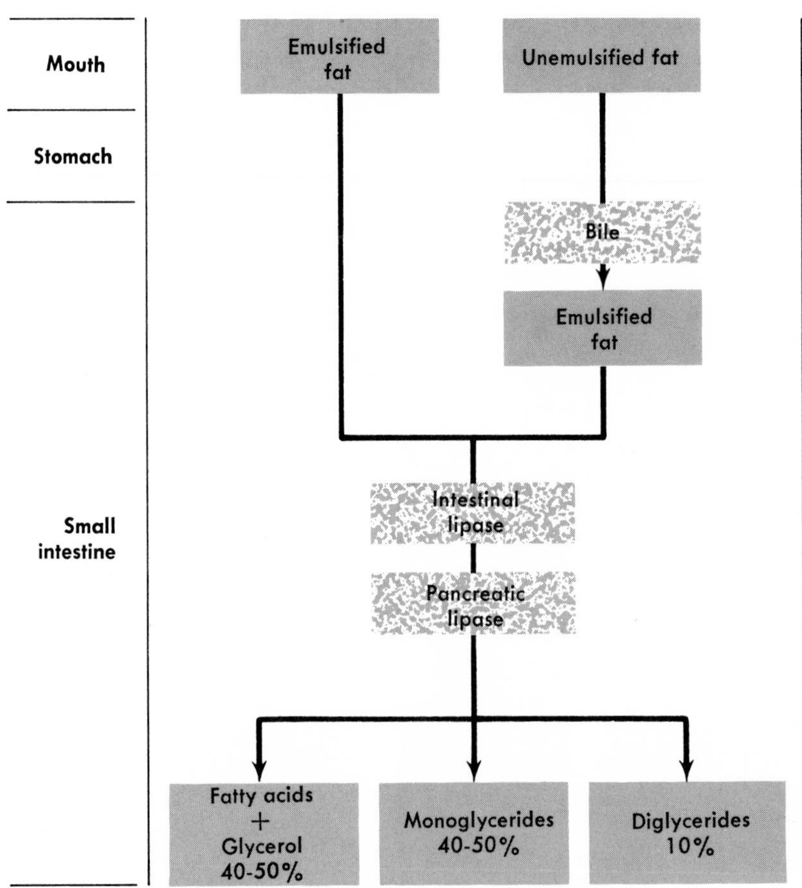

Fig. 3-3. Summary of fat digestion.

the longer-chain fatty acids are immediately recombined with the monoglycerides to form triglycerides. This process requires energy. About 70% of the absorbed fatty acids recombine to form triglycerides, whereas the 30% less than 12 carbons in length do not reform triglycerides. Each type of lipid enters the bloodstream in a different way.

To enter the bloodstream, the resynthesized triglycerides must be packaged in a water-soluble form that will enable them to be transported by the blood and other aqueous fluids of the body. This is accomplished by the formation of complexes of lipids with proteins known as **lipoproteins.** These water-soluble mixtures serve to transport lipid throughout the body. Lipoproteins differ from very low-density substances consisting of 99% lipid and 1% protein to high-density complexes with only 55% lipid and 45% protein.

The triglycerides formed within the intestinal wall can be packaged into two specific water-soluble lipoproteins—chylomicrons and very low-density lipoproteins (VLDLS). These leave the intestinal cells by reverse pinocytosis—the large molecules are more or less "spit out" of the cells. They are then picked up by the lacteals, the fat-collecting ducts for the lymphatic system. The lymphatic system gathers body fluids, including those containing the lipoproteins from the intestine, and returns them to the general circulation through the thoracic duct, which enters in the neck region just above the heart (Fig. 1-6). From there the lipid-rich particles, which contribute a turbid milky appearance to the blood, are transported to all tissues of the body. Most of the 100 g of lipid transported this way each day are removed by the adipose, or fat-storing, tissue.

The glycerol portion of the fat, representing 22% of the absorbed lipid, is transported unchanged across the intestinal wall and appears in the portal vein, to be carried to the liver. Medium- and short-chain fatty acids that are not reesterified combine with albumin, a protein carrier, and are transported in the portal system. Fats such as co-

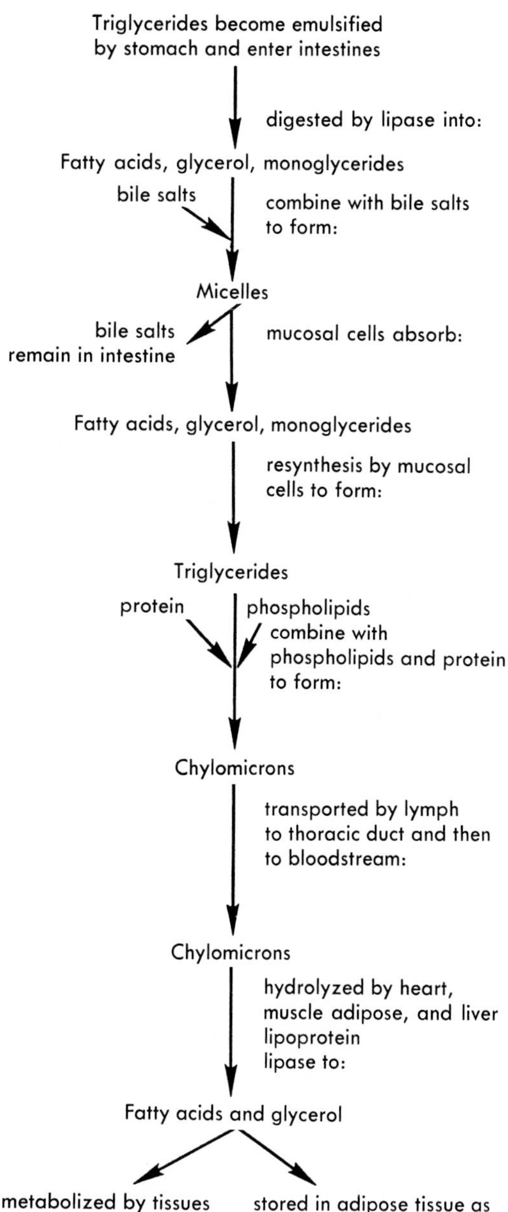

Fig. 3-4. Summary of the absorption of fat. (From Fat: nutritional perspectives, No. 2, Evansville, Ind., 1976, Mead Johnson Laboratories.)

conut oil contain triglycerides with fatty acids of medium-chain lengths and are absorbed more efficiently than fats with long-chain fatty acids, especially by low–birth weight infants and those who have absorption problems. The absorption of lipid is summarized in Fig. 3-4.

METABOLISM

Once the chylomicrons are delivered to the adipose or other tissue cells, lipoprotein lipases are released, which separate triglycerides from the carrier proteins. The lipids are removed from the chylomicrons in a matter of minutes and from the VLDLS in a few hours. The released triglycerides are then split by other specific lipases into fatty acids and glycerol. The fatty acids may enter the cells, and the water-soluble glycerol portion is transported in the general circulation. As the VLDL loses its triglyceride, it becomes a cholesterol-rich low-density lipoprotein (LDL). These carriers, with a protein content of about one fourth, are responsible for transporting about two thirds of the total circulating cholesterol.

Once the fatty acids are taken up by the cells, they may be used in several ways. Some may be oxidized or burned immediately as a source of energy. This involves a complex series of biochemical changes that ultimately results in the production of carbon dioxide, water, and energy. Fatty acids are the only energy source used by the heart muscle. Others may form triglycerides and be stored in the cells. Others make up the lipid portion of cell walls, whereas some may be used as precursors in the synthesis of essential compounds such as prostaglandins. In the mammary gland, fatty acids are incorporated into milk fat, which varies according to the types of fatty acids available. In the liver, some of the glycerol and fatty acids are reassembled as triglycerides and released into the circulation as components of VLDLS.

Certain specialized cells, known as adipose cells, function as storage sites for fat. When the body has need for its energy reserves, the fat stored in these cells is hydrolyzed or split by special lipases within the cells to form fatty acids and glycerol. As the fatty acids leave the cells, they become attached to the protein albumin in the blood and are carried to the tissues requiring energy. These complexes are usually 1% fatty acids and 99% protein. Because they have not recombined (esterified) with glycerol, they are known as nonesterified fatty acids (NEFA). Since the adipose cells do not have adequate amounts of the enzyme necessary to use glycerol to reform fats, glycerol diffuses into the plasma and is removed by the liver or kidneys, which do possess the enzymes needed to use it.

The digestion and metabolism of lipid is shown in Fig. 3-5. In general, lipid made available to cells as fatty acids and glycerol follows one of four pathways during metabolism:

1. It is used immediately as a source of energy.
2. It is stored in adipose or other cells as an energy reserve.
3. It is incorporated into the structure of cells.
4. It is used in the synthesis of essential compounds.

Cholesterol metabolism

Cholesterol, a lipid-related substance present in all mammalian cells, is metabolized in a different way. In addition to being provided preformed in food of animal origin, it is synthesized in all cells (especially the liver and small intestine) from precursors provided by both lipid and carbohydrate.

Cholesterol is present in food as a free alcohol or attached to long-chain fatty acids from which it can be released by enzymes in the intestinal mucosa. From 24% to 50% of ingested cholesterol appears to be absorbed into the lympatic system, depending on the amount available. In addition, cholesterol secreted in the bile and intestinal cells or resulting from the loss of intestinal cells is reabsorbed. Absorption takes place in the same way as that of fatty acids from micelles, but the amount absorbed is controlled by the in-

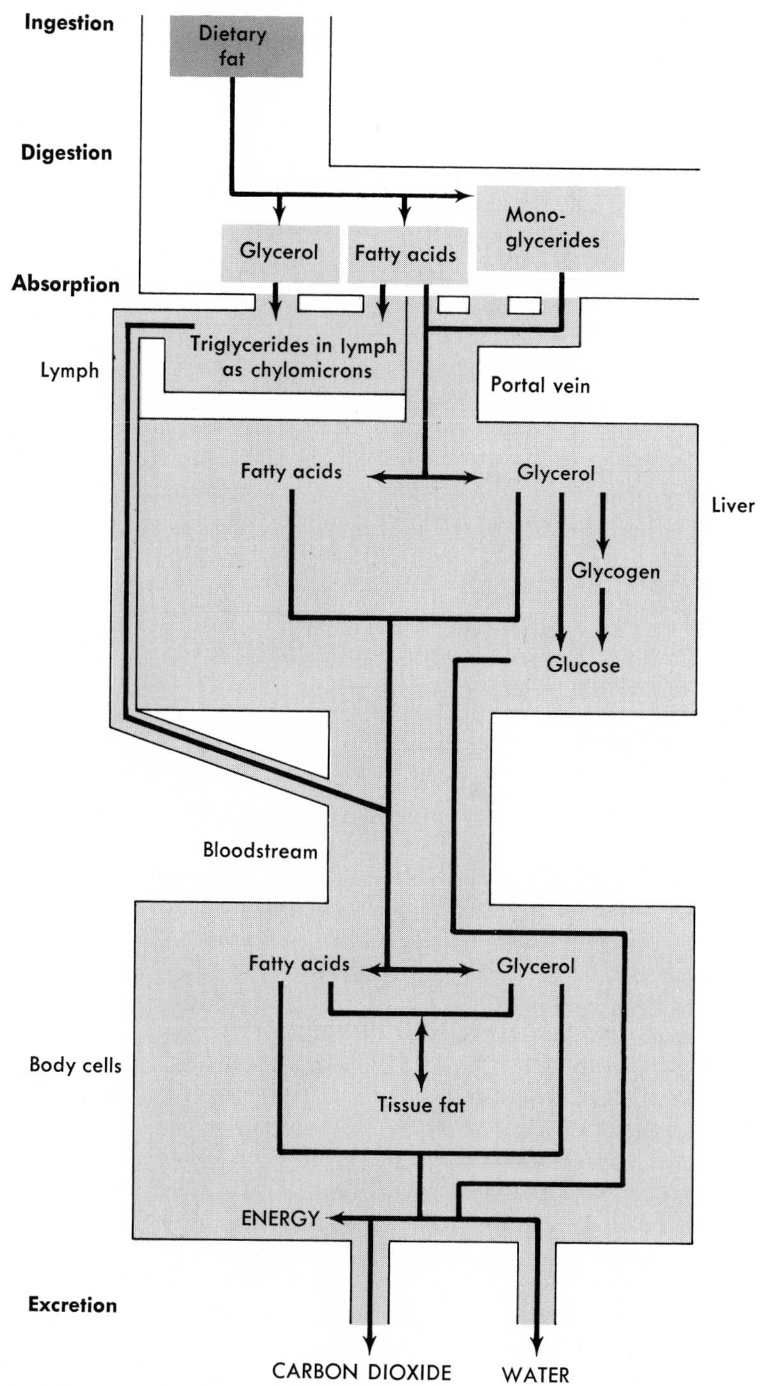

Fig. 3-5. Summary of fat digestion and metabolism. Terms in capital letters are end products of metabolism.

testinal mucosa. Once absorbed, cholesterol is released to the blood as part of the chylomicrons and VLDLS. After the triglycerides are removed by various tissues, the chylomicrons become proportionately richer in cholesterol. It is eventually removed by the liver.

The amount of circulating cholesterol (approximately 11 g) is a function of three factors—the amount synthesized in the liver, the amount absorbed by the intestine, and the amount of cholesterol secreted in the bile, which is not resorbed but excreted in the feces. There is an elaborate interplay between these factors with the amount synthesized reflecting the amount present in the blood.

FUNCTIONS IN DIET

Source of energy. Fat serves as a concentrated source of energy. Each gram of fat, whether animal or vegetable, liquid or solid, provides 9 kcal—2¼ times as much energy as an equal weight of either carbohydrate or protein. Fat represents the form in which the animal stores excess energy; thus the amount of fat in an animal product is determined by the energy balance of the animal. Practically all animal foods contain some fat. Even relatively lean steak has 28% fat, which contributes 70% of its energy.

In processing foods in which it is desirable to maintain the characteristics contributed by fat but to reduce the number of calories, polymers of triglycerides, known as polyglycerol esters, with 6.5 to 8.5 instead of 9 kcal/g have been used.

Satiety value. Fat tends to leave the stomach relatively slowly, being released approximately 3½ hours after ingestion. This delay in the emptying time of the stomach helps to delay the onset of hunger pangs and contributes to a feeling of satiety after a meal. Because of its high caloric value, fat is frequently reduced and visible fats virtually eliminated from diets suggested for weight control. Current research shows that the inclusion of some fat—whole milk, butter on vegetables and bread, or oil on salads—increases the satiety value of low-calorie diets so that they are more easily adhered to. This more than compensates for the concentrated caloric content of the fat. Currently, moderate-fat reducing diets are considered more successful than low-fat diets.

Carrier of fat-soluble vitamins. Among the dietary essentials are four fat-soluble vitamins—A, D, E, and K. Dietary fat serves as a carrier for these nutrients or their precursors. Thus the elimination of fat from the diet leads to a reduced intake of these nturients. Fat at a level of at least 10% of the energy intake also appears necessary for the absorption of vitamin A precursors from nonfat sources such as carrots. Similarly, anything that interferes with the absorption or utilization of fat, such as an obstruction of the bile duct or rancidity of fat, depresses the availability of the fat-soluble vitamins.

Source of essential fatty acids. Among the fatty acids is a polyunsaturated fatty acid, linoleic acid, which is effective in curing the dermatitis and restoring the growth of young animals fed a diet devoid of or very low in fat. Because it cannot be produced by the body, linoleic acid is considered an essential fatty acid (EFA).

Saturated fatty acids have no EFA activity and may increase the need for EFA. Young animals need more EFA than older animals, males more than females, and diabetics and persons with hypothyroidism more than those with no metabolic abnormality. Need also increases in pyridoxine deficiency. The need for essential fatty acids is usually met when 2% of the total calories are provided by linoleic acid. Linoleic acid is present in highest concentrations in vegetable oils, with some, such as corn oil, sunflower, and safflower oil, containing over 50% linoleic acid. Lesser and variable amounts are present in hydrogenated fats or spreads made from these oils. Most diets provide many times the minimum EFA requirements. The fatty acid composition of some representative fats is given in Table 3-4. EFA deficiency occurs most frequently in infants fed a nonfat milk formula. It is practically unknown among adults. The essential fatty acid requirement of infants has been set at 3% of the total calories. This is easily met by breast milk, in

Table 3-4. Fat content and major fatty acid composition of selected foods (in decreasing order of linoleic acid content within each group of similar foods)*

Food	Total fat (%)	Fatty acids[1] Saturated[2] (%)	Unsaturated Oleic (%)	Unsaturated Linoleic (%)
Salad and cooking oils	100	10	13	74
Safflower	100	11	14	70
Sunflower	100	13	26	55
Corn	100	23	17	54
Cottonseed	100	14	25	50
Soybean[3]	100	14	38	42
Sesame	100	11	29	31
Soybean, specially processed	100	18	47	29
Peanut	100	5	68	17
Rapeseed	100	11	76	7
Olive	100	80	5	1
Coconut	100	23	23	6-23
Vegetable fats—shortening				
Margarine, first ingredient on label[4,5]	80	11	18	48
Safflower oil (liquid)—tub	80	14	26	38
Corn oil (liquid)—tub	80	15	31	33
Soybean oil (liquid)—tub[6]	80	15	33	29
Corn oil (liquid)—stick[6]	80	15	40	25
Cottonseed or soybean oil, partially hydrogenated—tub[6]	80	16	52	13
Butter	81	46	27	2
Animal fats				
Poultry	100	30	40	20
Beef, lamb, pork	100	45	44	2-6
Fish, raw[6]				
Salmon	9	2	2	4
Mackerel	13	5	3	4
Herring, Pacific	13	4	2	2
Tuna	5	2	1	1
Nut				
Walnuts, English	64	4	10	40
Walnuts, black	60	4	21	28
Brazil	67	13	32	17
Peanuts or peanut butter	51	9	25	14
Pecan	65	4-6	33-48	9-24
Egg yolk	31	10	13	2
Avocado	16	3	7	2

*From Fats in food and diet, Agricultural Information Bulletin No. 361, 1974, Washington, D.C., U.S. Department of Agriculture.

[1]Total is not expected to equal total fat.

[2]Includes fatty acids with chains from 8 through 18 carbon atoms.

[3]Suitable as salad oil.

[4]Mean values of selected samples and may vary with brand name and date of manufacture.

[5]Includes small amounts of monounsaturated and diunsaturated fatty acids that are not oleic or linoleic.

[6]Linoleic acid includes higher polyunsaturated fatty acids.

which 6% to 9% of the calories come from linoleic acid.

With the greater use of vegetable oils rather than animal fats in the American diet the amount of EFA is increasing.

Precursors of prostaglandins. In 1962 a group of substances capable of stimulating the contraction of smooth muscles in the walls of blood vessels were identified as **prostaglandins.** Further study of these has shown that there are at least four forms and all are synthesized from 20-carbon fatty acids. They perform many important and varied functions, ranging from promoting conception and inducing labor and abortions to regulating transmissions of nerve impulses, inhibiting lipolysis and gastric secretion, and regulating blood pressure. It appears that prostaglandins are synthesized and used locally in a tissue rather than being transported to act on other tissues. As a result they have become known as local hormones.

Palatability. The role of fat in contributing to the palatability of food is appreciated best by those forced to exist on a low-fat diet. The use of fat for frying food, as a spread, as a base for salad dressing, and as a flavor adjunct for vegetables does much to improve the taste appeal of meals. Many substances responsible for the flavors and aromas of food are fat soluble. It has also been suggested that fat in the diet stimulates the flow of digestive juices.

ROLE IN THE BODY

Energy reserve. Body fat represents the primary form in which energy is stored in the body. Since it is an essential constituent of the cell membrane, all tissues contain some fat. In addition, the body has a group of specialized cells, called adipose cells, whose main function is the storage of fat. Although the size of the cells may increase in the adult in response to a need for more storage sites for fat, there is considerable evidence that the number of adipose cells in many parts of the body is determined within the first few years of life and again during adolescence. The amount of fat stored will reflect the extent to which the adipose cells are saturated with fat rather than of the rate increase in number of cells. Once fat has been formed and deposited in the adipose tissues, the body has no way of excreting it. Thus body fat can be reduced only by oxidizing, or burning, it as a source of energy when caloric intake is less than caloric expenditure. A certain amount of body fat, about 18% to 20% of body weight for women and 15% for men, is considered normal and desirable. Reserves of fat in excess of this represent, at first, overweight and, in extreme cases, obesity with all the associated physical, physiological, and aesthetic disadvantages.

Body regulator. As an essential constituent of the membrane of each individual cell, fat helps to regulate the uptake and excretion of nutrients by the cell.

Insulation. Deposits of fat beneath the skin (subcutaneous fat) serve as insulating material for the body, protecting it against shock from changes in environmental temperature. Here, again, a certain minimum layer is desirable to prevent excessive heat loss from the body, but too thick a layer slows down the rate of heat loss during hot weather, with resultant discomfort to the individual. Thick subcutaneous fat layers impede physical movement and present many aesthetic problems.

Protection of vital body organs. The fat deposits that surround certain vital organs serve to hold them in position and shield them from physical shock. The kidneys and heart are protected in this way. These are the last deposits to be reduced when there is a caloric deficit.

FOOD SOURCES

The amount of fat in representative foods is shown in Table 3-4, which also indicates the amount present as saturated and unsaturated fatty acids. Some advertisers are making use of a P/S ratio to identify the nature of the fat in their product. They assume that a high P/S ratio is desirable because of some evidence that polyunsaturated fatty acids reduce serum cholesterol levels more than do other fatty acids. Special margarines now on the market have a P/S ratio of 1.0 to 2.4 compared with 0.2 to 0.5 for regular margarines. In the hydrogenation of polyunsaturated fatty acids, essential fatty acids may be converted into monounsaturated acids, that lack the effectiveness of the essential fatty acids. In addition, the double bond sometimes shifts so that the common *cis* form is changed to the less well utilized *trans* form of the acid. These may constitute up to 35% of the fatty acids in margarines, with smaller amounts found in soft margarines. At present it is difficult to assess or to predict the effect of these on metabolism and on cell membranes.

In studying the linoleic acid content of vegetable oils, it is obvious that coconut oil, chocolate, and palm kernel oils contain virtually no EFA. On the other hand, wheat germ oil and walnut oil contain 57% and 73% linoleic acid, respectively. Poultry and game are good sources of EFA.

It is difficult to present precise data on the fatty acid composition of animal fats because of the differences resulting from variation in the diet of the animal. The method of food processing and storage may also have an effect on the fatty acid composition of the food as it is consumed.

The percentage of calories contributed by fat tends to be relatively high in most animal foods. In whole milk with 3.2% fat, 53% of the calories come from fat; in cheese with 32% fat, 68%; in beef with 28% fat, 72%; and in frankfurters containing 27% fat, 70%.

Vegetable foods contain less fat. Whole-grain cereals have from 2% to 9% fat, mainly in the germ. The fat in seeds ranges from 4% in corn to 17% in soybeans. Peanuts have 48% fat, and pecans have 41%. Avocado with 16% and ripe olives with 30% are the only fruits with any appreciable fat.

Based on its nutrient composition, bacon is correctly designated as a fat food rather than a protein food. It contains 69% fat in raw form and 52% fat when cooked, although the latter figure varies with the extent of cooking.

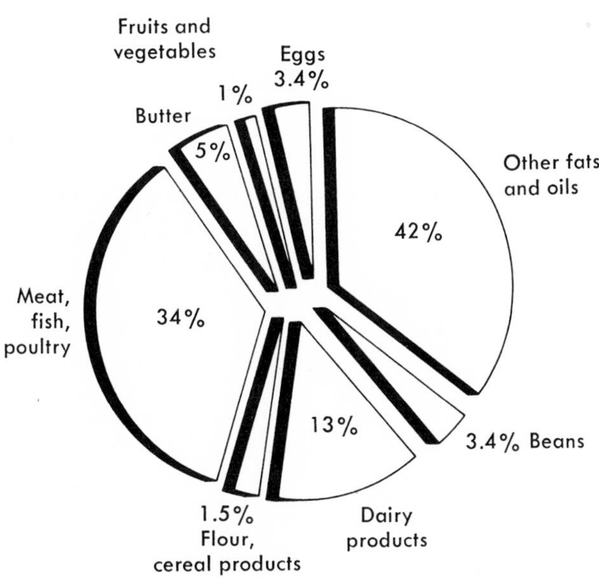

Fig. 3-6. Contribution of various food groups to total fat in American food supply. (Based on Contribution of major food groups to nutrient supplies available for civilian consumption, National Food Review NFR-1, Washington, D.C., 1978, Economic Research Service.)

Fig. 3-6 shows the contribution of various food groups to the total fat in the American food supply.

Because of the frequent suggestion in popular literature that mineral oil be substituted for vegetable oils in salad dressings, it is appropriate to mention it although mineral oil has no nutritional value. It is hydrocarbon, a by-product of the oil-refining process. The body possesses no enzymes capable of digesting it; therefore it passes through the digestive tract unchanged, acting as a lubricant and contributing no calories to the body's energy pool. Unfortunately, however, it acts as a solvent for the fat-soluble vitamins, which are then excreted along with the mineral oil. Since the low-calorie homemade mineral oil salad dressings are generally used on vegetable greens, one of the best sources of vitamin A, its use in the diet should be discouraged.

DIETARY REQUIREMENTS

Aside from the need for a dietary source of linoleic acid, the human does not require fat in the diet. A diet providing 2% of its calories from linoleic acid meets this requirement. However, as a concentrated source of energy, fat is important in allowing us to meet our energy requirements without eating large quantities of food. The current practice of obtaining as much as 40% of the calories from fat is being questioned because of the prevalence of excessive calorie intake and the possibility of an adverse effect of high-fat diets in cardiovascular diseases. Nutritionists suggest that an intake of fat providing 25% to 30% of the calories is more compatible with good health. This amount usually provides essential fatty acids and facilitates the absorption of fat-soluble vitamins.

Modification of dietary fat intake may be desirable in several conditions. In gallbladder disease, the amount of bile secreted is limited, and it may be necessary to restrict the total to as little as 10% of the calories from fat or to substitute emulsified fats for nonemulsified ones. Medium- and short-chain fatty acids can be absorbed in the absence of bile. In addition, they are transported through the portal vein to the liver, where they are usually metabolized as a source of energy, instead of being incorporated into tissue lipid. As a result, they can be used in the treatment of steatorrhea without requiring reduction in the total amount of fat in the diet. Some disorders of absorption, such as sprue or ileitis (inflammation of the ileum), inhibit the absorption of fat, and the usual manifestation of this is the appearance of as much as 60 g of fat in the stools daily compared to normal levels of 2 to 5 g. Until the cause of the problem can be corrected, the person is given as much fat as he can absorb, since a restriction limits both caloric intake and the absorption of fat-soluble vitamins. Hyperlipidemia, in which levels of certain fat constituents of the blood are elevated, may call for a restriction in either the kind or amount of dietary fat. Some types of hyperlipidemia do not respond to dietary changes and can be treated only with drugs.

The necessity of restricting fat intake in such conditions as hepatitis, cirrhosis, and jaundice is now questioned.

RELATIONSHIP TO HEART DISEASE

The necessity of a discussion on the relationship of dietary fat and artherosclerosis in an elementary text can be legitimately questioned. However, since the topic is being widely discussed in popular literature, it seems appropriate to include a statement of the current interpretation of the question. This is done with the full recognition that scientific thinking on the topic can change within short periods of time.

Interest in a possible relationship between dietary factors and the incidence of heart disease was triggered by the observation that persons who suffered heart attacks almost always had above-normal levels of blood cholesterol. Cholesterol, a fat-related compound present in many animal foods that the body can also synthesize, was shown to be a major constituent of the atherosclerotic plaques, or precipitates, that form on the inside of some blood vessels. These plaques eventually narrow the passage to the point that if a clot forms, it closes the vessel entirely. It was also noted that the incidence of heart disease is greater in populations deriving a higher percentage of their calories from saturated fat than it is in populations consuming less saturated and more unsaturated fats.

Efforts to lower blood cholesterol levels by dietary manipulation were made after studies on rabbits showed that a restriction of dietary cholesterol resulted in lower levels of cholesterol in the blood. In humans, however, control of dietary cholesterol by restricting the amount of cholesterol-containing foods such as eggs, meat, and liver did not consistently result in lowering of blood cholesterol levels or a reduction in heart disease. The reason became clear when it was learned that the body can synthesize in the liver as much as 2 g of cholesterol from fat, carbohydrate, and protein whenever the amount of these in the diet exceeds the body's need for energy. This is considerably more than the 0.5 g provided from a normal diet. Since a certain amount of cholesterol is vital for the synthesis of sex hormones, for the transport of essential fatty acids, and as a component of all cell membranes, it must be considered a normal body constituent.

Attention was next focused on the nature of fat in the diet with the observation that persons who consumed liquid fats or oils rather than solid fats had lower blood cholesterol levels than those who ate more solid animal fats. Since liquid fats differ from solid fats primarily in the proportion of PUFA they contain, emphasis in dietary treatment shifted toward an increased use of vegetable oils high in PUFA. This dietary modification, when PUFA provided about half the dietary fat, did indeed lead to a reduction in blood cholesterol levels but not to concurrent reduction in heart disease. Among the unsaturated fatty acids those with 10 to 16 carbon atoms have the greatest effect in lowering blood cholesterol. Vast research has shown that dietary patterns may be reflected in blood cholesterol levels, depending on the initial levels.

Interest shifted to a search for another fat-related component of the blood associated with a tendency toward atherosclerosis. It was found that heart disease occurred most often in persons who had a high blood cholesterol level coupled with a high blood triglyceride level. Triglycerides appear in the blood after a meal high in fat, but their presence also reflects the synthesis of fat from excess carbohydrate, primarily in the liver but with some occurring in the intestinal wall. Carbohydrate in the form of sugar rather than the complex starches is more likely to stimulate triglyceride synthesis. This situation generally occurs when caloric intake exceeds outgo and carbohydrate intake is high. It would appear, then, that modifying the diet to limit simple carbohydrates and substituting polyunsaturated fats for saturated fats would be most favorable for a reduction of the triglyceride and cholesterol content of the blood—especially if accompanied by a control of caloric intake and the maintenance of optimum body weight. Such a regimen is not universally effective, however.

Knowledge of the dietary factors involved and the balance that exists among these factors in the development of atherosclerosis is at present far from conclusive. It is believed that any drastic modification of the American diet on the basis of current information is unnecessary. However, high-risk, overweight, middle-aged men with high blood cholesterol and triglyceride levels, those with a family history of heart disease, and individuals who are working under emotional tension—the type of person most likely to suffer from atherosclerosis—should adhere to a prudent diet. Additionally, there would be no harm and possibly there would be benefits for most persons (1) if the amount of fat in the diet were reduced from the present level of 40% of total calories to less than 35% of calorie intake, (2) if the amount of dietary cholesterol were restricted to less than 300 mg, (3) if polyunsaturated fat were substituted for some of the saturated fat in the diet, (4) if saturated fat were limited to 15% of total calorie intake, and (5) if energy intake was adjusted to maintain desirable body weight. There is evidence that the nature of the American diet is shifting in these directions; at the same time there is a reduction in mortality from coronary heart disease.

Techniques for identifying those persons in whom dietary restrictions are most likely to result in change in blood lipids are now available. Data on the cholesterol content of representative foods are shown in Table 3-5.

LIPID AND CANCER

Epidemiological data showing greater cancer incidence in populations with a higher proportion of fat in the diet has directed attention to the possibility that dietary fat plays

Table 3-5. Cholesterol content of common measures of selected foods (in ascending order)*

Food	Amount	Cholesterol (mg)
Milk, skim, fluid or reconstituted dry	1 cup	5
Cottage cheese, uncreamed	½ cup	7
Lard	1 tablespoon	12
Cream, light table	1 fl oz	20
Cottage cheese, creamed	½ cup	24
Cream, half and half	¼ cup	26
Ice cream, regular, approximately 10% fat	½ cup	27
Cheese, cheddar	1 oz	28
Milk, whole	1 cup	34
Butter	1 tablespoon	35
Oysters, salmon	3 oz cooked	40
Clams, halibut, tuna	3 oz cooked	55
Chicken, turkey, light meat	3 oz cooked	67
Beef, pork, lobster, chicken, turkey, dark meat	3 oz cooked	75
Lamb, veal, crab	3 oz cooked	85
Shrimp	3 oz cooked	130
Heart, beef	3 oz cooked	230
Egg	1 yolk or 1 egg	250
Liver, beef, calf, hog, lamb	3 oz cooked	370
Kidney	3 oz cooked	680
Brains	3 oz raw	More than 1700

*From Fats in food and diet, Agricultural Information Bulletin No. 361, 1974, Washington, D.C., U.S. Department of Agriculture.

a role. It has been suggested that a high-fat content in the feces encourages the growth of bacteria, which produce carcinogens from the increased bile acids resulting from a high-fat diet.

BIBLIOGRAPHY

Albrink, M.: Triglyceridemia, J. Am. Diet. Assoc. **62:**626, 1973.

Alfin-Slater, R. B.: Fats, essential fatty acids, and ascorbic acid, J. Am. Diet. Assoc. **64:**168, 1974.

Atherosclerosis: the cholesterol connection, Science **194:**711, 1976.

Food and Nutrition Board and Council of Foods and Nutrition, American Medical Association: Diet and coronary heart disease, Washington, D.C., 1972, National Academy of Sciences.

Food and Nutrition Board: Dietary fat and human health, Publication No. 1147, Washington, D.C., 1966, National Academy of Sciences–National Research Council.

Fristrom, G. A., and Weikraug, G. L.: Comprehensive evaluation of fatty acids in foods, J. Am. Diet. Assoc. **69:**517, 1976.

Gatto, A. M., and Scott, L.: Dietary aspects of hyperlipidemia, J. Am. Diet. Assoc. **62:**617, 1973.

Glueck, C.J., and Conner, W.E.: Diet—coronary heart disease relationships reconnoitered, Am. J. Clin. Nutr. **31:**727, 1978.

Holt, P.R.: Dietary triglyceride composition related to intestinal fat absorption, Am. J. Clin. Nutr. **22:**279, 1969.

Keys, A., Grande, F., and Anderson, J. T.: Bias and misrepresentation revisited. Perspective on saturated fat, Am. J. Clin. Nutr. **27:**188, 1974.

Kolata, G. B.: Atherosclerotic plaques: competing theories guide research, Science **194:**592, 1976.

Kritchevsky, K., Tepper, S. A., and Story, J. A.: Nonnutritive fiber and lipid metabolism, J. Food Sci. **40:**8, 1975.

Kritchevsky, D.: Diet and atherosclerosis, Am. J. Pathol. **84:**615, 1976.

Kritchevsky, D.: Diet and cholesteremia, Lipids **12:**49, 1977.

Kummerow, F. A., Kim, Y., Hull, J., Pollard, J., Ilinov, P., Dorossiev, D. L., and Valek, J: The influence of egg consumption on the serum cholesterol level in human subjects, Am. J. Clin. Nutr. **30:**664, 1977.

Long term effects of diets prescribed in coronary prevention programs, Nutr. Rev. **35:**140, 1977.

Mann, G. V.: Diet-heart: end of an era, N. Engl. J. Med. **297:**644, 1977.

Metzner, H. L., Lamphiear, D. E., Wheeler, N. C., and Larkin, F. A.: The relationship between frequency of eating and adiposity in adult men and women in the Tecumseh Community Health Study, Am. J. Clin. Nutr. **30:**712, 1977.

Mueller, J. F.: Dietary approach to coronary artery disease, J. Am. Diet. Assoc. **62:**613, 1973.

Nichols, A. B., Ravenscroft, C., Lamphiear, D. E., and Ostrander, L. D.: Daily nutritional intake and serum lipid levels. The Tecumseh study, Am. J. Clin. Nutr. **29:**1384, 1976.

Report Working Party of Royal College of Physicians of London and British Cardiac Society: Prevention of coronary heart disease, Nutr. Rev. **34:**220, 1977.

Reiser, R.: Oversimplification of diet: coronary heart disease relationship and exaggerated diet recommendations, Am. J. Clin. Nutr. **31:**865, 1978.

Reiser, R.: Saturated fat in the diet and serum cholesterol concentration: a critical examination of the literature, Am. J. Clin. Nutr. **26:**524, 1973.

Saudek, C. D. , and Felig, P.: The metabolic events of starvation, Am. J. Med. **60:**117, 1976.

Sheig, R.: Absorption of dietary fat: use of medium-chain triglycerides in malabsorption, Am. J. Clin. Nutr. **21:**3000, 1968.

Scheig, R.: What is dietary fat? Am. J. Clin. Nutr. **22:**651, 1969.

Slater, G., Mead, J., Dhopeshwarkar, G., Robinson, S., and Alfin-Slater, R. B.: Plasma cholesterol and triglycerides in men with added eggs in the diet, Nutr. Rep. Int. **14:**249, 1976.

Subbiah, M. T. R.: Dietary plant sterols: current status in man and animal sterol metabolism, Am. J. Clin. Nutr. **26:**219, 1973.

Truswell, A. S.: Diet and plasma lipids—a reappraisal, Am. J. Clin. Nutr. **31:**977, 1978.

Vergroesen, A. J.: Role of fats in human nutrition, London, 1975, Academic Press, Inc.

Vergroesen, A. J.: Physiological effects of dietary linoleic acid, Nutr. Rev. **35:**1, 1977.

Walker, A. R. P.: Colon cancer and diet, with special reference to intakes of fat and fiber, Am. J. Clin. Nutr. **29:**1410, 1976.

Whyte, H. M., and Hevenstein, N.: A perspective view of dieting to lower the blood cholesterol, Am. J. Clin. Nutr. **29:**784, 1976.

4

Protein

Protein, first recognized as a dietary essential over fifty years ago, is vital for the growth and maintenance of body tissue. The fact that it is a part of thousands of hormones and enzymes regulating almost all body processes accounts for the long-standing interest in this nutrient and the vast amount of information we have of its role. However, there are still many mysteries about the function of protein. Traditionally we have relied on foods of animal origin to meet our protein needs, but concern over the ability of the world to provide adequate animal protein such as meat, fish, eggs, and milk has led to interest in the use of mixtures of vegetable proteins such as cereals and legumes in meeting our protein needs.

The term *protein*, meaning, "to take first place," was introduced by Mulder, a Dutch chemist, in 1838. He attributed it to a nitrogen-containing constituent of food that he believed to be of prime importance in the functioning of the body and without which life was impossible. Although it is now difficult to maintain that protein is more important than other nutrients, it is unlikely that Mulder had any conception of the extremely important roles this group of compounds plays in the body or of the number or complexity of the protein components of the body and of food. We now have evidence that protein is a constituent of every living cell. Half the dry weight and 20% of the total weight of an adult is protein. Almost half is in muscle, a fifth in bone and cartilage, a tenth in skin, and the rest in other tissues and body fluids. All enzymes are protein in nature. Many hormones are either protein or protein derivatives. Viruses are proteins. The nucleic acids in the cell nucleus responsible for the transmission of genetic information in cell reproduction often occur in combination with protein as nucleoproteins. The only body constituents that normally contain no protein are urine and bile.

In the absence of dietary protein there is a failure in body growth, followed by a loss of already established body tissue . Proteins, as part of every enzyme and many hormones, are vital in the regulation of body processes. If the energy intake is adequate, after the needs for growth and repair of tissue have been met, any remaining protein is used as a source of energy.

Early in the twentieth century, with the availability of methods of analyzing for protein by determining the nitrogen content in food and tissues, there was widespread interest in protein nutrition and especially in qualitative differences in proteins. The most significant work was done by Folin, who differentiated between **endogenous** and **exogenous** protein metabolism. He showed that endogenous metabolism (the metabolism of body proteins) is reflected in the excretion of a nitrogen-containing substance, creatinine, a fairly constant indicator of body mass and basal energy expenditure. On the other hand, the metabolism of the exogenous dietary protein results in the excretion of urea, which fluctuates with dietary intake in relation to body needs.

With the discovery of vitamins in the

period between World Wars I and II, emphasis in nutrition research shifted toward a clarification of their role and structure. Again, however, in the early 1950s interest in protein was revived. Several factors were responsible for this:

1. Recognition of a widespread protein deficiency disease, kwashiorkor, which plagues a large segment of the world's population, especially young children in developing countries
2. Availability of radioactive isotopes, broadening the scope of investigations beyond that previously possible
3. Recognition of blood and plasma transfusions as means of saving lives

Current interest in protein nutrition is evident from the vast literature on the subject in scientific journals and books.

Table 4-1. Amino acids in food and body tissue*

Classification	Amino acid
Naturally occurring amino acids	
Essential for all humans	Isoleucine
	Leucine
	Lysine
	Methionine
	Phenylalanine
	Threonine
	Tryptophan
	Valine
	Histidine
Nonessential	Glycine†
	Glutamic acid
	Arginine‡
	Aspartic acid
	Proline
	Alanine
	Serine
	Tyrosine
	Cysteine
	Asparagine
	Glutamine
Related compounds sometimes classified as amino acids	Hydroxyglutamic acid
	Hydroxylysine
	Hydroxyproline
	Thyroxin
	Norleucine
	Cystine

*Chemical formulas are shown in Appendix L.
† Essential for chicks.
‡ Essential for birds and rats.

CHEMICAL COMPOSITION

Proteins are extremely complex substances made up of many amino acids, the structural units of protein. These are the basic units from which protein is synthesized and into which it is converted in the course of digestion or catabolism, the breakdown of body tissue. The twenty different naturally occurring amino acids that have been identified as the building blocks for body protein are listed in Table 4-1. Chemically, the amino acids are composed of a carboxyl group (COOH), a hydrogen atom (H), an amino group (NH_2), and an amino acid radical (R) attached to a carbon atom as shown below:

```
      COOH
       \
    H—C—R
       /
     NH2
```

The nitrogen of the amino group is characteristic of protein and is not found in any other nutrients. On the average, it represents 16% of the amino acid molecule. It ranges from 15% in milk protein to 16% in meats, 17% in cereals, and 18% in nuts. Because of this constancy of nitrogen in protein, most studies of protein metabolism are based on nitrogen determinations. The carboxyl group, the amino group, and the hydrogen atom are common to all amino acids. It is the nature of the *R group* that distinguishes one amino acid from another. *R* varies from a single hydrogen (H) atom as found in glycine, the simplest amino acid, to longer carbon chains of 1 to 7 carbon atoms. Those in which the carbon atoms are arranged in a hexagon (benzene ring) rather than a straight

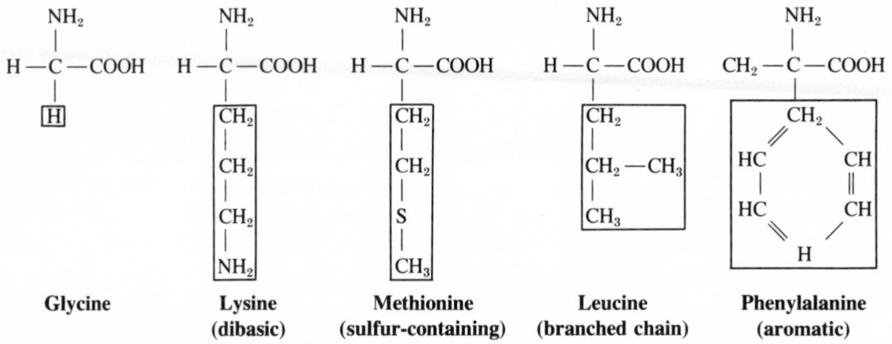

Fig. 4-1. Representative formulas for classes of amino acids. *Boxed portion* is unique to the specific amino acid.

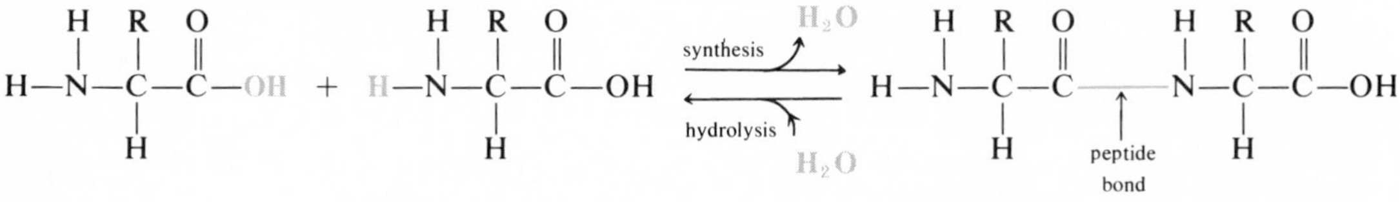

Fig. 4-2. Synthesis and hydrolysis of a dipeptide.

line are called aromatic amino acids. Tyrosine and phenylalanine are examples. Others, such as cysteine and methionine, also contain sulfur. Lysine, arginine, histidine, and tryptophan contain a second nitrogen atom and are thus called dibasic amino acids. Examples of classes of amino acids are given in Fig. 4-1.

SYNTHESIS

Proteins can by synthesized by both plant and animal cells. Plants obtain the essential nitrogen through the soil either from that provided by chemical fertilizers or released from nitrogen-containing organic fertilizers by the action of bacteria. In addition, some plants such as legumes have small nodules of bacteria on their roots that are capable of fixing, or trapping, nitrogen from the atmosphere. Animals obtain most of their nitrogen as amino acids from either plant or animal sources but do have a limited capacity to synthesize amino acids in their gastrointestinal tract.

In both plants and animals the synthesis of protein involves the formation of long chains of amino acids called peptide chains. These chains are so named because the chemical bond that holds two amino acids together is called a **peptide bond.** In forming the chain an amino group of one amino acid joins with a carboxyl group of the next with the release of 1 molecule of water. Conversely, when the peptide linkage is broken, as in digestion, water must be added before the amino acids can be split apart by either acid or enzyme hydrolysis. This is illustrated in Fig. 4-2.

Proteins, as found in nature, consist of many amino acids linked together. The characteristics of a particular protein are determined not only by the types of amino acids that are used and the number of times they are repeated but also by the order in which they are joined together. Since each amino acid may be used any number of times in any relation to other amino acids, the possibility for the formation of different proteins becomes enormous. It is analogous to the number of combinations of fifty or more letters that could be made from an alphabet of twenty letters with practically no limitations on the order in which they may be joined. In addition, the spatial arrangement of the amino acid chain, whether coiled, folded, or straight and whether or not there are additional cross linkages, influences manyfold the properties of the resulting protein and the possibilities of the number of proteins.

It is unlikely that anywhere near the theoretical number of proteins exists in nature, but we have evidence that a great many do. The human body contains hundreds of different proteins, some containing as many as 200 amino acids. It is estimated that a liver cell alone contains a thousand different enzymes, each being a protein. In addition, every species builds proteins characteristic of itself. Thus, although the hemoglobin protein of a horse resembles that of a duck or a dog or a human, the proteins differ sufficiently that they cannot be interchanged with one another. In fact, the protein of one species is frequently toxic to another if introduced before being hydrolyzed or digested into its constituent amino acids. This, of course, makes transfusion of blood from one species to another impossible. These slight differences in hemoglobin from one species to another can be used as a basis for identifying the source of a blood sample, an invaluable tool in criminal investigations.

Only in the last twenty-five years have analytical techniques enabled scientists to determine the amino acid composition of a protein. It was even more recently that they could establish the order in which amino acids occur in a peptide chain. Now further advances have allowed scientists to determine the spatial relationship of the amino acids in a protein molecule. **Myoglobin,** consisting of 150 amino acid units representing nineteen different amino acids, is considered a simple protein and was the first for which the complete composition and structure was known. It was elucidated in 1961. Since then, rapid progress has been made in determining the amino acid composition and sequence in many of the proteins that had previously been isolated from natural sources.

Once the composition of a protein was known, it was relatively simple to synthesize it in the laboratory. As a result, in 1969 two groups of scientists almost simultaneously announced the synthesis of the enzyme ribonuclease. The complex structure of this enzyme is depicted in Fig. 4-3. The investigators used different methods and produced slightly different forms of the same enzyme. They accomplished after fifty years of work what the ribosome responsible for protein synthesis within the cell accomplishes in 1 to 3 minutes. Since then, the synthesis of other enzymes has followed rapidly, opening up a new approach to nutritional investigations.

One of the long-term goals of biologists, nutritionists, and biochemists has been to determine how the cell "knows" which protein to build, that is, the kind and order and number of amino acids to incorporate when building new protein. This goal was reached in 1962 when Watson and Crick showed that the pattern for protein synthesis was present, or encoded, in the substance **DNA (deoxyribonucleic acid),** the genetic material in the nucleus of the cell. The pattern is transferred to the **ribosomes,** the protein-synthesizing organelle in the cytoplasm of the cell by another nucleic acid **RNA (ribonucleic acid),** known as messenger RNA. The ribosome is able to pick up, in the proper order, the required amino acids carried to it by yet another form of RNA, called transfer RNA, and to incorporate them in a protein molecule in a prescribed order dictated indirectly from DNA through messenger RNA. Proteins that are used within a cell are synthesized by clusters of ribosomes called polyribosomes within the cytoplasm of the cell. Those which are to be secreted from the cell are synthesized by similar clusters of ribosomes located on the surface of channels leading to the outside of the cell. In the case of viruses the pattern for protein synthesis may be passed from RNA to DNA.

The code or codes for specific amino acids have been identified. They consist of a triplet

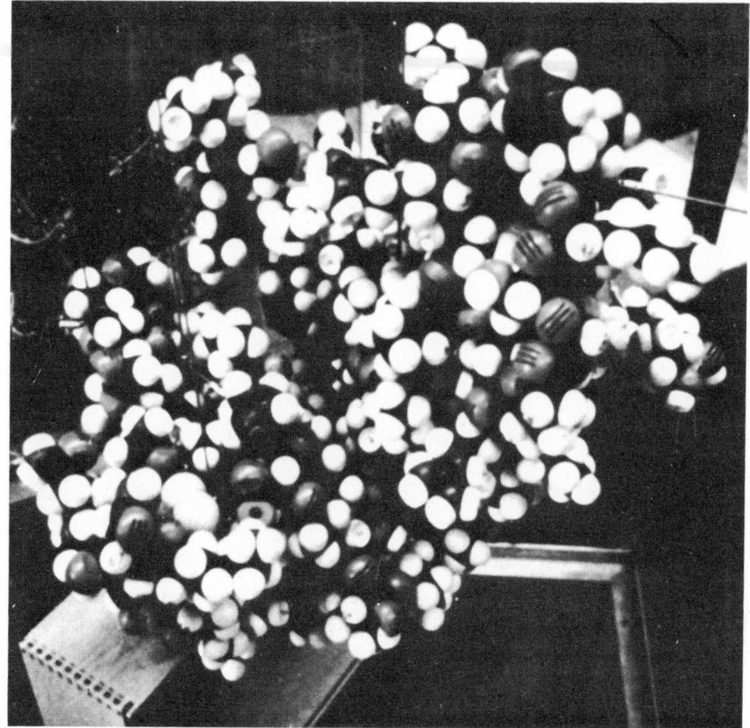

Fig. 4-3. Ribonuclease—three-dimensional structure. (Courtesy Dr. H. W. Wyckoff; from Denkewalter, R. G., and Hirschmann, R.: Am. Sci. **57:**389, 1969.)

(combination of three) of the four substances purines or pyrimidines present in the DNA molecule—adenine (A), guanine (G), cytosine (C), and thymine (T). Thus, when DNA gives the code GAG, the ribosome gets a message through messenger RNA to incorporate the amino acid glutamic acid, which will be brought to it from the amino acid pool within the cell by transfer RNA. After glutamic acid has been attached to the growing amino acid chain, the ribosome will read the next triplet code, perhaps ACG, telling it to add 1 molecule of the amino acid threonine. This process continues until all the amino acids of a particular protein have been joined together in a prescribed order.

If a particular amino acid is not available or cannot be produced immediately within the cell, the synthesis of the protein ceases. In addition, that part of the protein already formed will be broken down into its component amino acids, since it cannot be stored as a partially complete protein until the missing amino acid is available.

The mechanisms determining that messenger RNA will carry a message to the ribosome to call for the synthesis of a new protein are equally complex, and although they are relatively well understood, a discussion of them is beyond the scope of this book. However, with the level of understanding we now have about the control of protein synthesis, geneticists have available to them the information to change the message and hence the resultant protein. This offers much promise in the control of genetic defects that result in the production of a defective protein, usually an essential enzyme. In addition, it opens the possibility for genetic engineering to produce a protein or a living organism such as a virus with either specific or unknown characteristics. The awesome implications of this have led to heated debates and a moratorium on so-called "recombinant research" involving the production of new genetic material to direct the synthesis of previously unknown proteins.

FOOD AS A SOURCE OF AMINO ACIDS

The ultimate value of a food protein lies in its amino acid composition, since the amino acids rather than the protein are the essential nutrients. Many foods commonly designated as proteins are more accurately called protein-rich foods, and their nutritive value lies in the amino acid composition of their various proteins. Some foods, such as gelatin, contain only one protein, but almost all others have more. For example, hemoglobin, myoglobin, elastin, and collagen are all found in meat, casein and lactalbumin in milk and gliadin and glutenin in wheat.

CLASSIFICATION

Amino acids. From a functional nutritional standpoint, amino acids are classified into two groups—essential (indispensable) and nonessential (dispensable). An indispensable amino acid is one that cannot be synthesized by the body *at a rate* sufficient to meet the needs for growth and maintenance. In the classification in Table 4-1 it is seen that nine of the twenty amino acids are essential and must be provided by the diet. Until recently, histidine was considered essential for infants but not adults. It is now believed that adults are not capable of producing enough histidine to meet their needs over a long period of time and must rely on food. If sufficient nitrogen is available, humans can synthesize the other eleven amino acids needed to build body proteins. Other species may require different amino acids.The nitrogen used in the synthesis of nonessential acids may come from other nonessential amino acids or an excess of essential amino acids. In addition, there is some evidence that the human, like many animals, can make use of a limited portion of nitrogen provided by nonprotein nitrogen, such as urea, for the synthesis of nonessential amino acids. Amino acids from food that serve as a source of nitrogen for the synthesis of other amino acids undergo a process called *transamination,* in which the amino group is transferred to another substance, often a carbohydrate derivative, to form the required amino acid. Since the body must obtain this nitrogen from food, dispensable nitrogen is now considered a dietary essential.

Protein. Proteins in food are classified on the basis of their amino acid content. Although there is an overlap in the classification, it provides a simple basis on which to evaluate protein quality. Proteins that contain all essential amino acids in proportions capable of promoting growth when they are the sole source of protein in the diet are described as complete proteins, good-quality proteins, or proteins of high biological value. They contain about 33% essential and 66% nonessential amino acids. All animal proteins except gelatin which is limited in both tryptophan and lysine, are complete proteins.

The pattern of amino acids in these proteins is able to meet human needs best because it closely resembles the pattern of human amino acid requirement. Thus, if they are used as the sole source of protein in an amount to meet human nitrogen needs, they provide enough of all the essential amino acids. Extra amounts of essential amino acids would be used to synthesize nonessential amino acids to supplement those already present in the protein. Fig. 4-4 compares the amino acid profile of a high-quality protein (protein A) to the adult requirement.

However, all animal proteins are not equally good in meeting growth requirements, although none of them is totally lacking in essential amino acids. Incomplete proteins, poor-quality proteins, or proteins of low biological value are those which lack one or more essential amino acids. They have about 25% essential amino acids. In contrast to complete proteins, if these low-quality proteins (protein B) are used as the sole source of protein in the diet, they could not provide all the essential amino acids necessary for the synthesis of body proteins.

Some proteins that contain all essential amino acids but a relatively small amount of one have sufficient amino acids to repair body tissue if they are the sole source of dietary protein, but they do not have enough to promote growth. They are designated as partially complete proteins. The amino acid present in the smallest amount relative to the amount required is called the *limiting amino acid.* Arginine is the limiting amino acid in casein, as is methionine in fish and eggs. Ly-

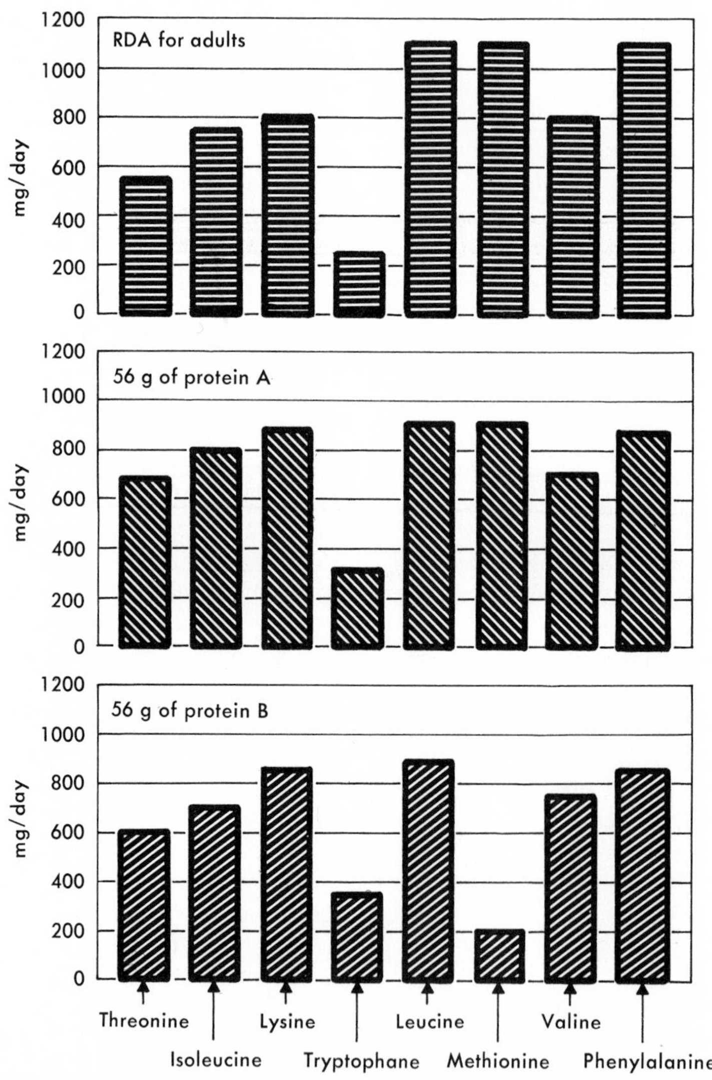

Fig. 4-4. Comparison of amino acid pattern of good-quality protein A and poor-quality protein B with pattern of protein requirement of adult male. Methionine is limiting amino acid in protein B. (Courtesy Dr. Barbara Shannon, Pennsylvania State University.)

sine is the amino acid most often lacking in cereal protein and methionine the most limiting in legumes, although it does vary from one protein to another. A complete protein functions as a partially complete protein when it constitutes a small portion of the diet.

Fig. 4-5 shows the results of feeding complete, partially complete, and incomplete proteins to rats. Fig. 4-6 shows 9-week-old littermates raised on a 3% and an 18% protein diet, respectively, since birth.

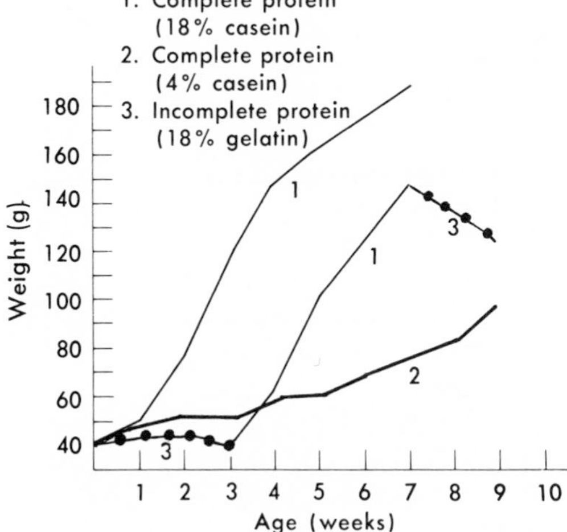

Fig. 4-5. Effect of complete, partially complete, and incomplete protein on growth of weanling rats.

There is also wide variation among vegetable protein in the pattern of amino acids they contain. Both soy protein and nuts contain some of all the essential amino acids but are sufficiently limited in one or more that they are less effective than most animal proteins in meeting needs for growth. Other vegetable proteins are so deficient in one or more amino acids that they can neither repair tissue nor support growth.

Supplementary value of proteins. It is possible to simulate a complete protein by supplying simultaneously two vegetable proteins that complement one another or to supplement an incomplete protein with a small amount of animal protein. For instance, a combination of wheat lacking in lysine, but plentiful in methionine and soybeans limiting in methionine but containing lysine would provide a mixture containing all essential amino acids. Similarly, a small amount of milk taken with a wheat cereal would provide the missing amino acid lysine and would enhance the biological value of the wheat protein.

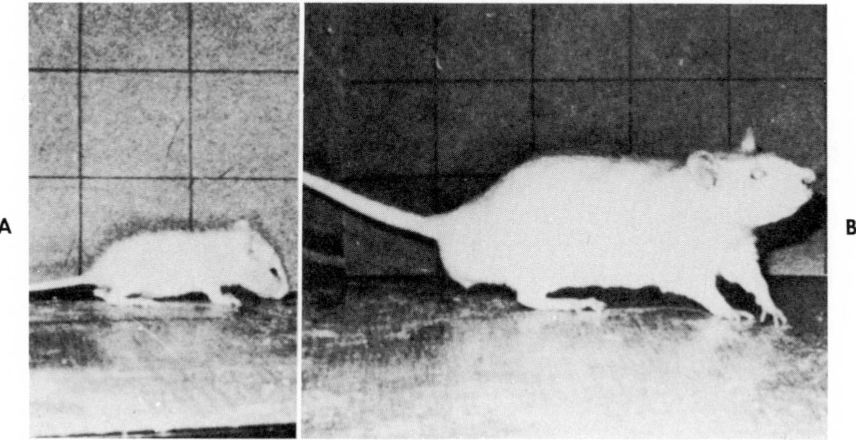

Fig. 4-6. Nine-week-old weanling rats. **A,** Rat raised in litter of 16 was fed a diet with 3% casein after weaning and weighed 19 g. **B,** Rat raised in litter of 8 was fed diet with 18% casein after weaning and weighed 311 g.

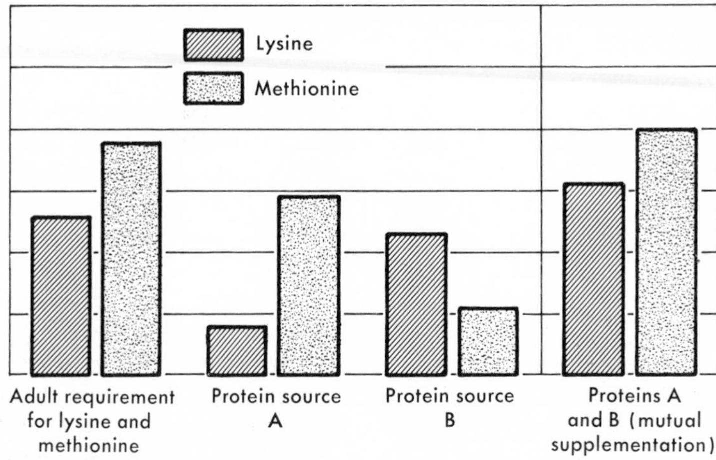

Fig. 4-7. Mutual supplementation of low-quality proteins lacking in lysine (A) and lacking in methionine (B). They complement one another to provide a high-quality protein. (Courtesy Dr. Barbara Shannon, Pennsylvania State University.)

Fig. 4-7 illustrates how two proteins, each of which alone is unable to support growth, are able to complement each other and, if eaten together, be as effective as a high-quality protein in meeting nutritional needs.

EXTENDING HIGH-QUALITY PROTEIN

The essential amino acids are generally present in animal protein in such amounts that small quantities of animal products will make up the essential amino acid deficits of the plant proteins. When this method of providing dietary protein is used, it is wise to rely on the more concentrated sources of plant proteins such as dried beans, peas, or grain products such as noodles so the total quantity of food which must be consumed is reasonable. Examples of protein extension are chicken and rice, chili con carne, tuna and noodle casserole, wheat cereal with milk, and macaroni and cheese. Use of protein extension provides high-quality protein less expensively than relying totally on animal sources for protein needs.

FUNCTIONS

Although we must rely on protein-rich foods as a source of amino acids, it is the essential amino acids that are the ultimate nutrients for the body. The type and amounts of amino acids provided by the dietary protein determine how effectively the body can perform the functions for which amino acids are needed. The needs for amino acids fall in six broad categories:

1. *Essential for growth and maintenance of tissue.* Before cells can synthesize any new protein, they must have available simultaneously all the essential amino acids, plus sufficient nitrogen to incorporate with other materials to form the nonessential amino acids. Growth or increase in body mass is impossible in the absence of the proper mixture of amino acids. Moreover, for growth to occur, amino acids must be present in amounts over and above those needed for maintenance. The growth of some tissues calls for specific amino acids such as the sulfur-containing amino acids characteristic of hair, skin, and nails.

Gain in body weight per se is not an adequate criterion of protein nutrition. Pups fed a diet with a wheat protein, gluten, as the source of protein gained as much weight as a group receiving egg protein. However, they were obese and inactive and had delayed skeletal development, whereas the egg-fed pups were lean and active and had gained three times as much body protein.

On the other hand, rather than store fat if the dietary amino acid pattern does not lead to protein synthesis, some animals reduce their food intake.

In addition to cell division and growth, which are dependent on protein, synthesis of much of the structural material of the body requires protein. The matrix for bones and teeth, in which calcium and phosphorus are deposited, is protein. Collagen is the basic protein in tendons and ligaments and serves as the intercellular material that binds the cells together. Myosin, which is the material responsible for muscle contractions, and fibril filaments, which contribute to muscle mass, are other structural proteins.

Most protein tissue in the body is in a dynamic state, being alternatively broken down and resynthesized. The rate of breakdown and subsequent repair varies greatly from one tissue to another with a total of 300 g or 3% of the 10 kg of body protein being replaced each day. About 75 g of muscle are replaced each day and the wall of the intestine, the most active tissue, is regenerated every four to six days, requiring the synthesis of as much as 70 g of protein a day. Failure to replace these results in a loss of body weight.

2. *Formation of essential body compounds.* Hormones such as insulin, epinephrine, and thyroxin have been identified as protein substances. Every body cell contains many different enzymes, each catalyzing a specific reaction. All enzymes so far identified are protein. However, coenzymes necessary for the action of enzymes have a nonprotein structure usually associated with a specific vitamin.

Hemoglobin, the substance in blood responsible for its oxygen and carbon dioxide-carrying properties so vital in respiration, is a protein complex. Most of the many substances in the blood responsible for clotting are protein in nature, as are the substances in the eye responsible for vision.

The amino acid tryptophan acts as a precursor to niacin, itself having a regulatory function as a vitamin. In the brain, trytophan serves as a precursor for serotonin and tyrosine for norephinephrine, both essential **neurotransmitters** responsible for the transmission of nerve impulses.

The formation and replacement of these vital compounds have high priority within the body and will suffer only in severe protein deprivation. Some tissue enzymes may be reduced 10% to 20% during protein depletion, those of brain being resistant to change and those of kidneys, skeletal muscle, and spleen showing some reduction.

3. *Regulation of water balance.* Fluid in the body is separated into three components: that (1) within the cells **(intracellular fluid),** (2) between the cells **(extracellular** or **intercellular fluid),** and (3) in the blood vessels **(intravascular fluid).** It is important that the distribution of fluid on either side of a cell membrane within each of these systems be maintained at a fairly constant level. The balance from one area to another is regulated by electrolytes, such as sodium, which exert osmotic pressure to draw the fluid in or out of the cells, and proteins in the blood, which exert oncotic pressure and draw fluid into the vascular system. As blood is pumped through the body to the capillaries, the hydrostatic pressure, which builds up as the blood flows into increasingly smaller blood vessels, finally forces fluid into the intercellular spaces to nourish the cells. Protein present in the blood does not pass out of the capillaries and thus exerts oncotic pressure, attracting the fluid back into the blood vessels. When the level of plasma protein is low, such as occurs in a protein deficiency, the water is not drawn back into the circulatory system completely and accumulates in the intercellular spaces, making the tissue spongy and waterlogged or edematous. This condition, known as **edema,** is an early sign of a protein deficiency.

4. *Maintenance of body neutrality.* Proteins are considered amphoteric substances, or buffers, capable of reacting with either acids or bases to neutralize them. Their presence in the blood helps to prevent the accumulation of too much acid or base, either of

which would interfere with normal body functioning. When an excess of base occurs, the protein acts as an acid by combining with the base to neutralize it and prevent it from contributing to the alkalinity of the blood. Conversely, when excess acid appears in the body fluids, the proteins of the blood act as a base to neutralize it. Thus plasma protein performs an important function in helping to maintain body neutrality essential to normal cellular metabolism.

5. *Stimulation of antibody formation.* The antibodies responsible for the body's ability to combat infection are protein substances. Since a specific antibody is produced in response to a particular infective agent or allergenic substances, the need for protein in this role may be quite extensive. The increased susceptibility to infection noted in persons on a low-protein diet is attributed to a lower level of antibodies capable of combating the infective agents.

The ability to detoxify poisonous material in the body is controlled by enzymes that are protein in nature, located primarily in the liver. In protein depletion the ability to counteract the toxic effect of chemicals is reduced, rendering persons more susceptible to certain poisons or drugs.

6. *Transportation of nutrients.* Protein plays an essential role in the transport of nutrients from the intestine across the intestinal wall to the blood, from the blood to the tissues, and across the cell membrane into the cell. Most substances that carry nutrients are proteins. They may be specific to one nutrient such as transferrin, which carries only iron; they may be able to carry several different nutrients that compete with each other to be carried; or they may carry a whole group of substances such as lipid carried as lipoproteins. If there is a lack of protein, less carrier will be synthesized and either the absorption or transportation of some nutrients will be reduced.

DIGESTION

All dietary proteins consisting of complex units of amino acids joined together are too large to pass through the intestinal wall. They must be broken down in the digestive tract to simple units of one or two amino acids so that they can pass into the bloodstream and be carried to the tissues. Digestion is accomplished by the action of specific protein-splitting enzymes known as proteases, which are available in the stomach, small intestine, and the intestinal wall. Digestion involves breaking the peptide linkages joining the amino acids.

There are no protein-splitting enzymes in the saliva, and so the first attack on the peptide or amide linkages of a complex protein is made in the stomach. Here in the acid medium of the gastric contents, gastric protease (pepsin—the protein-splitting enzyme of the gastric juice) attacks specific linkages in the peptide chain involving the amino acids phenylalanine and tyrosine. Breaking these linkages, which are remote from the ends of the chain, results in shorter units of amino acids, known as polypeptides, proteoses, and peptones. From the stomach the polypeptides or shorter chains of partially digested proteins pass into the small intestine, where the acid is neutralized and the mixture becomes slightly alkaline. The digestive secretion from the pancreas contains two protein-splitting enzymes, pancreatic protease and chymotrypsin. Pancreatic protease, or trypsin, attacks specific protein linkages—those involving carboxyl groups of lysine and arginine, while chymotrypsin breaks peptide linkages involving the carboxyl group of tyrosine, phenylalanine, tryptophan, and methionine. About 30% of the protein is released as amino acids and absorbed directly. The remaining shorter fragments, representing 70% of ingested protein, may contain two amino acids (dipeptides) or three (tripeptides) but may also be more complex. One enzyme capable of breaking the short protein fragments into their component amino acids is carboxypeptidase, which attacks the linkage next to the carboxyl end. Another enzyme, an aminopeptidase, secreted by the intestine, attacks the amino end, releasing amino acids until only two remain joined as dipeptides. These two-unit peptides enter the brush border lining the intestinal wall, where another enzyme, intestinal dipeptidase, completes protein digestion by breaking them into two separate amino acid units.

Most of the digestion of dietary protein occurs in the upper half of the intestine. In the lower half these same protein-splitting enzymes digest the 50 to 70 g of endogenous protein that results from the loss of intestinal cells. These proteins resist digestion longer than dietary protein because they are not changed in shape or denatured by the acid in the stomach.

All the protein-splitting enzymes are hydrolytic in that they require water to free the amino acids. This is a reversal of the process of synthesis, in which the amino acids are joined together with the release of 1 molecule of water for each linkage formed. Protein digestion is summarized in Fig. 4-8.

The apparent digestibility of protein based on differences between dietary nitrogen and fecal nitrogen averages about 92%, but the fact that a variable amount of fecal nitrogen comes from intestinal cells and digestive enzymes makes true digestibility difficult to determine.

Coefficients (percentage) of digestibility for protein range from 78% for legumes and nuts to 75% and 80% for most cereals (except whole grain). 85% for fruits, 74% for vegetables, and 97% for meats and eggs. In some foods amino acids are bound in a way that resists the action of gastrointestinal en-

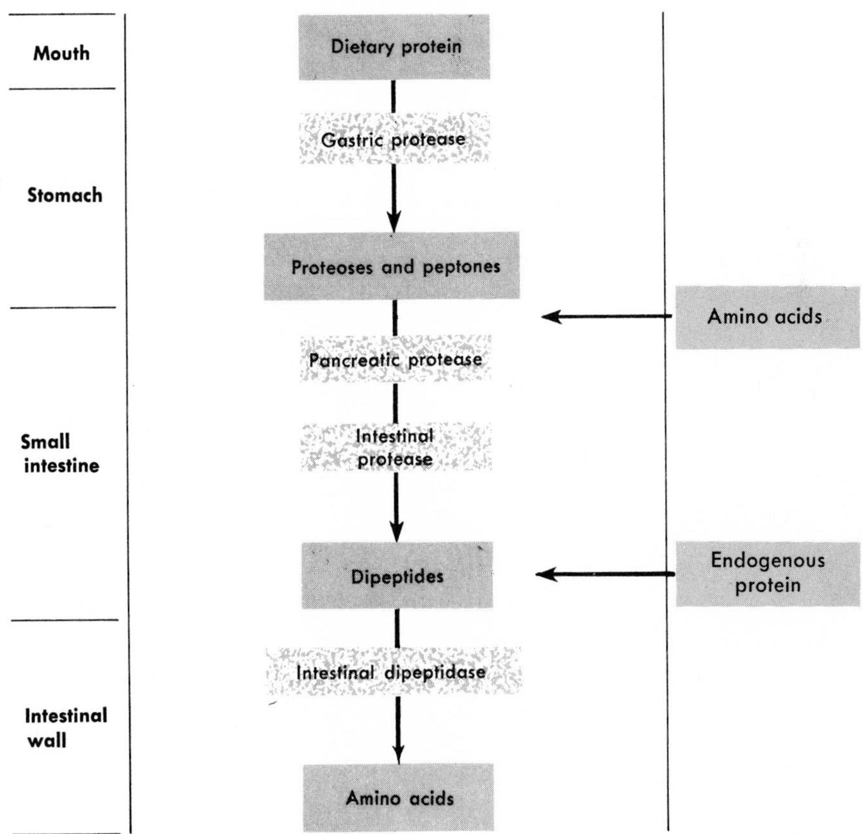

Fig. 4-8. Summary of protein digestion.

zymes. The digestibility can often be improved if the foods have been heated with strong acids or alkalies in processing.

ABSORPTION

The amino acids formed in the process of digestion are in sufficiently simple form chemically to pass from the wall of the intestinal tract into the bloodstream either by diffusion or by the energy-requiring process of active transport. Apparently some competition exists among amino acids for the carrier to transport them across the intestinal wall, which accounts for the effect of an excess of one amino acid on the absorption of another. About 11% of the free amino acids are absorbed in the stomach, 60% in the small intestine, and 28% in the colon. From the intestine they are carried by the portal vein to the liver, where they are released into the general circulation and carried to the various tissues and cells. Amino acids from vegetable proteins are less well absorbed than those from animal proteins, a difference that is only partially explained by the high fiber content of vegetables.

A few fragments containing several amino acids or complete proteins may also be absorbed. Except for dipeptides containing glycine or proline, they cannot be utilized for protein synthesis and may be responsible for the sensitization, or allergic reaction, to specific proteins.

METABOLISM

Absorbed amino acids are released from the intestinal wall into the portal vein and carried directly to the liver. The level of amino acids in the portal vein fluctuates and immediately following a meal may be several times higher than in the general circulation, depending on need. If amino acids are not needed, they will be degraded or deaminated to produce urea, which is then excreted in the urine. Some are synthesized into plasma proteins by the liver, and the remainder are released into the general circulation. From the blood the amino acids are taken up by the individual cells that use them in the synthesis of a specific protein. If the cell is to synthesize a protein, all the essential amino acids needed for the enzymes or structural proteins must be provided simultaneously. If they are not available, the cell will release the other essential amino acids, to be taken up by the other cells or used for energy, and no protein will be formed. In addition to the essential amino acids that the cell cannot manufacture, many nonessential amino acids are provided from the bloodstream. The cell will pick up at the same time any of the nonessential amino acids needed or, if they are not available in the amino acid pool, will synthesize them, using the nitrogen of other amino acids. It is conceivable that every cell is not capable of synthesizing all of the dispensable amino acids but may rely on those synthesized by other cells and released into the amino acid pool of the bloodstream. For some particular cells, then, there may be additional essential amino acids. Although very complex, the whole process of protein synthesis is extremely rapid, sometimes taking only minutes.

Amino acids not needed by any of the body cells for building new protein will be used for other purposes. The extra branched amino acids (leucine, valine, isoleucine) not needed for protein synthesis are taken up by muscle cells, especially if insulin levels are high. There they are converted to the amino acid alanine; glutamine is derived from another amino acid, glutamic acid. These are returned to the liver along with the other extra amino acids, where the nitrogenous group (NH_2) is removed in a process called *deamination* (a reaction requiring vitamin B_6). The nonnitrogenous residue enters the metabolic cycle for carbohydrates and fats and will either be oxidized to provide energy or will be converted into fat and stored as energy reserve. (See Appendix to Part One.) The nitrogen portion undergoes a series of chemical changes and is converted into urea by the liver and excreted by the kidneys in the urine. Since the kidneys are called on to excrete this urea as metabolic waste, a high protein intake in excess of needs for building body tissue and essential body compounds may tax the capacity of the kidneys to excrete waste, especially when intake of fluid to produce urine is low.

An amino acid that, after deamination, is metabolized as a carbohydrate is described as a *glucogenic* amino acid. One that is metabolized as a fatty acid is a *ketogenic* amino acid.

Early concepts of protein metabolism maintained that body proteins were relatively static. However, once radioactive isotopes became available, it was soon demonstrated that body proteins are in a state of dynamic equilibrium with a constant interchange of nitrogen from one tissue to another and between newly absorbed and older amino acids. Tissue proteins are continually being broken down and resynthesized—contributing to and taking away from the metabolic pools of amino acids to which dietary proteins also contribute. Although there is no major storage site for extra protein, the liver will increase in size when protein is available, and some tissue proteins, such as plasma albumin, represent small labile protein reserves. In a deficiency of either quantity or quality of dietary protein, storage protein is broken down to provide amino acids for more vital uses in the body. Plasma globulin (the other major protein in blood) levels, however, are maintained in periods of protein depletion at the time albumin levels are being depleted. Liver, gastric mucosa, pancreatic, muscle, and skin proteins can be used as labile reserves of amino acids, but the protein of the brain is resistant to change. The labile protein reserves, which can be reversibly depleted and repleted, comprise up to 25% of total body protein, and the amino acid pool represents about 0.5 g of nitrogen/kg of body weight.

The total amount of protein in the body does not change as long as the body is in nitrogen equilibrium, but the rate of turnover of body protein varies from tissue to tissue. Some, such as the gut, pancreas, and liver, exhibit a very rapid amino acid turnover, whereas muscle and collagen with a half-life of several hundred days, turn over their amino acids more slowly. The rate of turnover in all tissues tends to decrease when dietary protein is limited. The half-life of total body protein is estimated at eighty days, and the rate of synthesis of protein in the adult male is estimated at 0.3 g/kg of body weight/day.

The digestion and metabolism of protein is summarized diagrammatically in Fig. 4-9. It is clear that dietary protein available to the cells as amino acids may be used in several ways.

1. If the caloric intake is adequate, amino acids are used for synthesis of protein as far as is needed.

2. If caloric intake is insufficient to meet energy needs *or* if more amino acids are available than are needed for synthesis of protein *or* if all the essential amino acids are not present simultaneously, amino acids are deaminated, with the amino group being excreted as urea and the nonnitrogenous fraction being used as a source of energy.

3. If glucogenic amino acids (capable of forming glucose), such as alanine, cystine, and methionine, are deaminated, they are converted into glucose and then are metabolized as glucose, that is, used as an immediate source of energy, stored as glycogen, or stored as fat.

4. If ketogenic amino acids (capable of forming fatty acids directly), such as leucine, isoleucine, phenylalanine, and tyrosine, are deaminated, they are converted into fatty acids and either are used directly as a source of energy or are converted into triglycerides and stored as fat.

The end products of protein metabolism are carbon dioxide, water, energy, and nitrogenous products in the urine. As with carbohydrates, the time elapsing between ingestion and excretion may vary from a few minutes to several months, depending on the intermediary steps involved and the stability of the protein in the body.

FACTORS AFFECTING PROTEIN UTILIZATION

Amino acid balance. Equally important as the presence of all essential amino acids for growth is the balance of amino acids available to the cell. The pattern, or balance, of

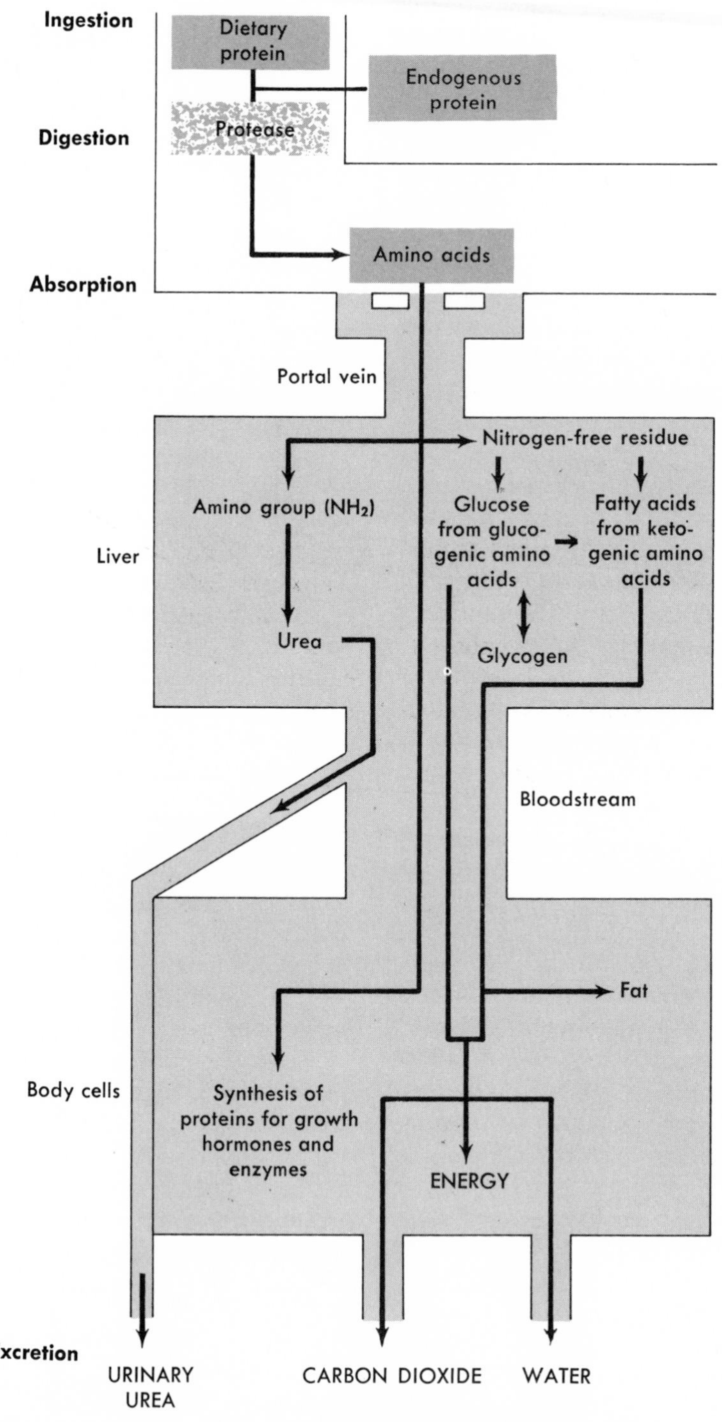

Fig. 4-9. Summary of protein digestion and metabolism. Terms in capital letters are end products.

amino acids in egg protein and lactalbumin in milk is considered excellent for growth. Deviations from such a balance of amino acids results in less efficient growth response. It has been suggested that the limiting factor in the biological value of a protein is as frequently the pattern as the quantity of the essential amino acids. One of the hazards of supplementing a low-protein diet with a single amino acid is that an imbalance would occur in the amino acid pattern of the total diet. If too much of one amino acid were added relative to the others present, growth might be depressed rather than improved. Such growth depression is not present when a high-protein diet is supplemented.

Caloric intake. The protein content of the diet cannot be adequately evaluated without a consideration of the caloric content. As the caloric value of the diet drops below a certain critical point, the retention of nitrogen drops, indicating that part of the protein was deaminated and used for energy purposes. If the caloric level is adequate, the level of protein utilization depends on the protein needs and the quality of the protein.

Immobility. The ability to synthesize protein is influenced by activity. It has been observed that bedridden patients, especially older people, experience a negative nitrogen balance even when dietary protein seems adequate. A healthy individual in bed at rest loses nitrogen at a rate of 12 to 18 g/day. Protein tissue lost in febrile illness (fever) is regained at a slower rate than that at which it is lost.

Injury. Increase in nitrogen excretion after injury is well documented. It may reach as high as 20 g/day of nitrogen on a normal food intake. High protein intakes immediately after injury neither prevents nor reverses the nitrogen loss. The losses are recovered once healing begins.

Emotional stability. Emotional stresses such as fear, anxiety, or anger increase the secretion of epinephrine, which in turn causes a series of changes that result in loss of nitrogen. Students lose nitrogen under the stress of examinations, as do persons experiencing severe pain, those whose work requires them to reverse normal night and day patterns, and those experiencing personal anxieties. Stress of a cold also increases nitrogen excretion.

NITROGEN BALANCE

Since practically all proteins have a constant and equal percentage of nitrogen, scientists have been able to use the relatively simple Kjeldahl determination of nitrogen as indicative of protein. Nitrogen accounts for 16% of the protein molecule, therefore values for nitrogen can be multiplied by 6.25 (100/16) to give protein values. Thus studies of nitrogen metabolism have become the basis for assessing protein metabolism. The few vitamins and the nucleic acids that contain any nitrogen have so little that the results are not appreciably affected.

Nitrogen balance studies involve a determination of the nitrogen content of all food intake compared to the amount of nitrogen excreted. They have provided us with basic information on the overall gain or loss of body protein; however, they do not give information on changes among tissues. Most nitrogen is excreted either in the urine or feces. Urinary nitrogen represents both endogenous nitrogen from the breakdown of body tissue and exogenous nitrogen, which represents that from digested and absorbed amino acids in excess of the body's need to build or repair body tissue from vital body compounds. In both cases the nitrogen has been removed from the absorbed amino acids so that the rest of the protein molecule can be used as a source of energy. Exogenous nitrogen will appear in the urine when protein intake exceeds the body's need for protein, when caloric intake is insufficient to meet needs of the body, or when the protein does not contain enough of the essential amino acids to allow the body to synthesize protein to replace that lost through the breakdown of body tissue. The small and fairly constant percentage of ingested nitrogen that appears in the feces and represents undigested protein amounts to about 8% of the total intake, although this varies with the source of protein as reflected in Table 4-2.

In addition to the urinary and fecal losses, which average 37 mg/kg and 12 mg/kg of body weight respectively, small losses of 5 mg/kg occur through the sloughing of skin, perspiration, saliva, shedding of hair, and expiration. Because these losses are difficult to measure, typical nitrogen balance studies frequently underestimate excretion.

When nitrogen intake equals nitrogen excretion, the individual is said to be in nitrogen equilibrium. This indicates that the protein intake is sufficient to replace and repair body tissue but that no growth or increase in body tissue is occurring. This condition should prevail in any adult who is receiving at least the minimum protein needed. It also occurs at any level above minimum where no growth is occurring.

When nitrogen intake exceeds nitrogen excretion, positive nitrogen balance prevails. Under these conditions growth can occur. Tissue or vital body compounds are being built faster than they are being destroyed. Positive nitrogen balance should prevail throughout the period of childhood and adolescence and during pregnancy and lactation (if protein in milk is considered). It will also occur in recovery from an illness in which protein has been lost.

Nitrogen excretion in excess of intake (negative nitrogen balance) indicates that body tissue is wearing out or breaking down at a rate faster than it is being repaired. It occurs not only when protein is low but also when calories are restricted. This is an undesirable situation, reflecting wasting of body tissue and loss of body protein. Low levels of intake produce a negative balance when fed after a higher intake has been established. However, there is some evidence that individuals adapt to low protein intakes. Eventually, these levels may be sufficient to establish nitrogen equilibrium as the body adjusts toward more efficient use of the amount available.

Fig. 4-10 shows the amount of nitrogen needed to maintain body tissue and meet requirements for growth with increasing age. In infants almost equal amounts are needed for growth and maintenance, but in older children the proportion needed for maintenance increases and that for growth de-

Table 4-2. Coefficient of digestibility of representative proteins

Food	Coefficient of digestibility
Eggs	97
Meat, fish	97
Milk	97
Wheat (70% to 74% extraction)	89
Fruits	85
Rice	84
Wheat cereals	79
Legumes (peas, beans, etc.)	78
Oatmeal	76
Root vegetables	74
Other vegetables	65

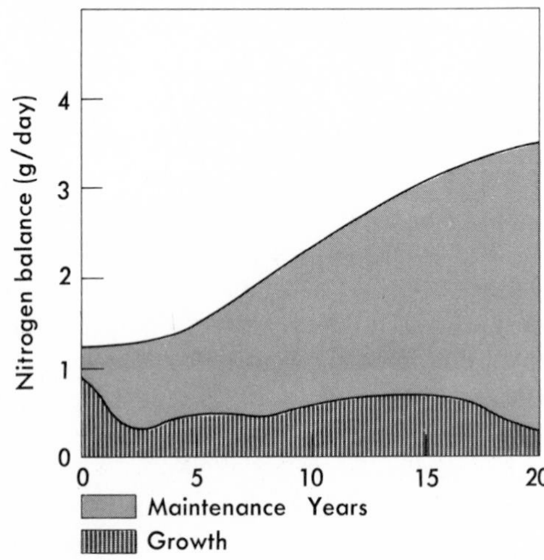

Fig. 4-10. Amounts of nitrogen needed for maintenance and growth of boys at various ages. (Modified from Allison, J. B.: Trans. N. Y. Acad. Sci. **25**:293, 1963.)

creases until adulthood, when virtually none is used for growth. An unexplained retention of nitrogen above that needed for repair of tissue has been observed in many adults. It has been designated as nitrogen needed for adult growth, although the nature of the need remains obscure.

Nitrogen balance studies yield information only on total protein mass and give no indication if a shift in body proteins from one tissue to another is occurring. For instance, plasma albumin levels may drop in an individual in nitrogen equilibrium, indicating that this labile nitrogen pool has been depleted to meet needs of another tissue. Thus it is possible for a suboptimal level of protein nutrition to prevail before it is manifest in negative nitrogen balance.

The significance of nitrogen balance data is illustrated in Fig. 4-11.

DETERMINATION OF MINIMAL NEEDS

Nitrogen balance studies have been used to determine both minimum total protein and essential amino acid needs. In this technique the subject is fed progressively lower levels of nitrogen in successive balance periods, usually of three to seven days' duration during which energy intake is adequate and all intake and excreta are collected and analyzed. As long as the individual is in nitrogen equilibrium, he is getting enough total protein, or if one amino acid is being tested, he is getting a sufficient amount of that amino acid. The point at which his nitrogen balance becomes negative is that at which his needs exceed his intake. His minimal protein need falls between the lowest point at which he was in equilibrium and the level at which his balance is negative. It is possible to arrive at a more precise figure by gradually increasing the protein in successive balance periods until the individual is again in equilibrium. By using this technique, it has been established that the requirements for the essential amino acids are surprisingly low. It is also evident that there are wide individual differences in needs for amino acids, as for other nutrients. There is still much controversy over proposed values. In addition to the minimum amounts proposed for these amino acids, sufficient nonessential nitrogen must be allowed for the synthesis of nonessential amino acids. With the recognition that the body needs

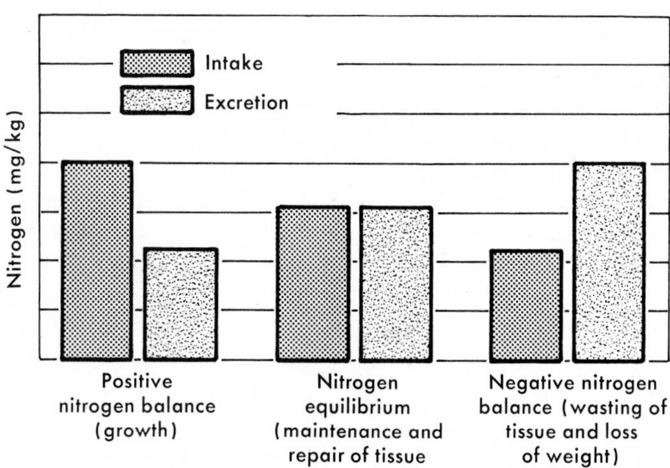

Fig. 4-11. Diagrammatic representation of nitrogen balance.

amino acids, nitrogen, and organic acids rather than protein as such for protein synthesis, the term *protein requirement* is becoming outmoded. However, in the following discussion of requirements the amount of protein necessary to provide the amino acids and nitrogen by age and sex will be considered.

DIETARY REQUIREMENTS

Estimates of desirable protein intakes may be obtained in two ways. They may be based on observations of the minimum amount of protein that will promote growth in children and maintain nitrogen balance in adults. Alternatively, they may be based on calculations of the losses of nitrogen that occur through the urine and feces on a protein-free diet, allowing for the obligatory losses through the skin, sweat, and sloughing of cells. Amounts needed to allow the increase in body mass during growth as assessed by changes in body composition must also be considered. Because of the lack of uniformity in the available data, recommendations for desirable levels of intake have been based on considerations of both types of data. For instance, there are considerable experimental data on nitrogen balance in adult males, some in adult females and infants, but only meager data for other groups. Similarly, data on obligatory nitrogen losses are available for infants and children but not for adults.

In 1973 both the Food and Agriculture Organization (FAO) and the Food and Nutrition Board of the National Research Council (NRC) published recommended dietary allowances for protein. Although for most other nutrients the former proposes a practical allowance and the latter an allowance to meet the physiological needs of essentially all healthy individuals, their recommendations for protein are essentially the same for all age and sex categories except for pregnant women. The values reflect a safe level of intake or one adequate for maintenance of good nutrition. Since there is no evidence of adverse effects from intakes above minimal requirements and since the effects of inadequate intakes are well documented, both groups have set their recommended levels at 2 standard deviations above the minimal requirement. This, they believe, will meet the needs of nearly all healthy persons and exceed those of the majority of the population.

From a comparison of the two standards in Table 4-3, it is evident that when the FAO recommendation for intake of a protein of high quality is compared to the NRC recommended allowances, the latter is slightly lower in some categories and the same in others. For pregnant women, however, the Food and Nutrition Board recommends an intake 30 g above nonpregnant needs whereas FAO recommends an increase of only 9 g.

In calculating the protein requirements, the Food and Nutrition Board estimates that in the adult male, losses of nitrogen through urine amount to 1.35 mg/kcal of basal energy needs. Losses in feces, varying with amount of food consumed, its fiber content, and its digestibility, were estimated at 0.9 g/day. In addition, obligatory losses through sweat, hair, nails, sloughed skin, and various body secretions and excretions, although small, represent a nitrogen loss of 300 mg/day. These losses amount to 3.7 g of nitrogen or 23 g of protein for a 70 kg man. A more realistic estimate of 33 g or 0.47 g/kg is based on data from low-protein diets. Since most proteins are utilized at 75% efficiency, the NRC recommends an additional 33% to take into account variability in protein quality. After considering that an additional 30% must be added to account for variation from one individual to another, NRC suggests that an intake of 0.8 g of protein/kg of body weight will provide the protein needed by most healthy persons. This is essentially the same recommendation as made by FAO.

Since these protein allowances are relatively low, they represent only 10% of the energy needs. This is considerably lower than the 15% recommended for adolescents and the percentage usually found in the American diet. Although it is less costly to obtain energy from carbohydrate and fat, it is

Table 4-3. Comparison of protein standards for selected age groups (in grams)

Age group	NRC recommended dietary allowances*		Nutrient allowances, United Kingdom†	Canadian dietary standards‡	FAO/WHO safe intake	
	Per person	Per kilogram			Per person	Per kilogram
	←g/day→		←g/day→	←g/day→	←g/day→	
Infants						
0-0.5 yr		2.2	20	2.2/kg		—
0.5-1 yr		2.0	20	1.4/kg	14	1.53
Children						
1-3 yr	23	1.8	30-35	22	16	1.19
4-6 yr	30	1.5	40	27	20	1.01
7-10 yr	36	1.2	53	33	25	0.88
Males						
11-14 yr	44	1.0		52	30	0.81
15-18 yr	54	0.9	75	54	38	0.60
19-22 yr	54	0.8				
23-50 yr	56	0.8	75	56	37	0.57
51+ yr	56	0.8				
Females						
11-14 yr	44	1.0			29	0.76
15-18 yr	48	0.9	58	43	31	0.63
19-22 yr	46	0.8				
23-50 yr	46	0.8	55	41	29	0.52
51+ yr	46	0.8				
Pregnant	+30	1.3	60	+20	+ 9	—
Lactating	+20		68	+24	+17	—

*Food and Nutrition Board: Recommended dietary allowances, ed. 8, Washington, D.C., 1974, National Academy of Sciences—National Research Council.
†Department Health and Social Security, Recommended intakes of nutrients for the United Kingdom, Reports on Public Health and Medical Subjects No. 120, London, 1969, Her Majesty's Stationary Office.
‡Dietary standards for Canada, Canadian Bulletin on Nutrition, vol. 6, No. 1, March, 1964, Rev. 1975.
§Joint FAO/WHO Expert Group: Protein requirements, FAO Nutrition Meeting Report Series No. 52, Rome, 1973.

possible that by restricting protein to 10% of the calories, it will be difficult to obtain adequate amounts of other nutrients during periods of high nutrient needs.

In calculating the needs during growth, the Food and Nutrition Board assumed that an increase in body weight was 18% protein and proposed an appropriate figure based on observations of growth rate.

For infants and children experiencing a rapid increase in body weight, much of which is bone and muscle growth, the recommended levels of protein intake are considerably higher per unit of body weight. Intakes of 2.2 g/kg of body weight are proposed for the first 5 months, and 2 g from 6 to 12 months of age.

Minimum protein level needed by infants

will usually be reached when protein provides 6% of the caloric intake. For breast-fed infants this amounts to 1.5 to 2.5 g/kg.

In children from 1½ to 3 years of age, increase in muscle accounts for half the weight gain. The amount needed to ensure normal growth is again a function of the biological value of the protein in the diet as well as the individual characteristics of the child but approximates 1.8 g/kg of body weight, or about 30 g.

In children up to 9 years of age the skeleton grows faster than the body as a whole; therefore protein needs are proportionately higher. As legs grow in length and the center of gravity becomes farther from the floor, more muscles must be developed to maintain posture and to permit activity.

For adolescents one recommendation is that 15% of the calories be provided by protein. Since protein has a physiological fuel value of 4 kcal/g, a person needing 3000 kcal should receive 450 kcal from protein, or 112 g of protein. This is in considerable excess of the RDA of 54 g.

During pregnancy the NRC suggests intakes 30 g above those of nonpregnant women. This is necessary not only for the growth of the fetus but also for the growth of the uterus, placenta, and mammary glands. A 3 kg baby has 0.5 kg of protein, acquired primarily in the last half of pregnancy. This growth calls for 4 to 6 g of protein/day above maintenance requirements. Restriction of protein in the mother's diet leads to the birth of shorter, lighter infants. Two thirds of the protein in the diet of pregnant women should be of high biological value. In lactation the requirement is raised by 20 g. The production of 850 ml of mature human milk with a protein content of 1.2% involves the synthesis of 10 g of milk protein, mostly lactalbumin.

One adverse effect of a high-protein diet has been identified in relation to calcium retention. An intake of 2 g/kg of body weight in men results in loss of body calcium, or negative calcium balance.

Amino acids. In the determination of the requirements of essential amino acids based on nitrogen balance studies, amino acids must be provided in purified form and the level of all amino acids as well as that of nonessential nitrogen must be carefully con-

Table 4-4. Minimal amino acid requirements*

Amino acid	Infants (mg/kg)	Adult female (mg/day)	Adult male (mg/day)
Isoleucine	70	550	700
Leucine	161	730	1100
Lysine	103	545	800
Methionine (+ cystine)	58	700	1100
Phenylalanine (+ tyrosine)	125	700	1100
Threonine	87	375	500
Tryptophan	17	168	250
Valine	93	622	800
Histidine	34	—	—
(Suggested adult protein intake is 0.55 g/kg/day.)			

*Energy and protein requirements, FAO Nutrition meetings Report Series No. 52, Rome, 1973.

trolled. The technique is costly and time consuming. The results of experiments to assess the amino acid needs of infants, adult men, and adult women have not been accepted uncritically. The currently accepted standards are given in Table 4-4, although it is recognized that further work will undoubtedly lead to modifications.

FOOD SOURCES

Some of the major food sources of protein and their contribution to the total protein requirement are shown graphically in Fig. 4-12. Values are expressed in terms of 100 g of the food and 100 kcal. It must be remembered that the ultimate value of a protein-rich food to the diet is determined by its amino acid pattern. Generally, proteins of animal origin have a better distribution of amino acids than do those of vegetable origin, but within each group there is a wide range in biological values. Table 4-5 gives the index of nutrient quality (INQ) for protein representation for some food items.

The effect of heat on the utilization of dietary protein has been the subject of much research. The results of such studies have not been conclusive, however. The peak level of amino acids in the blood after the ingestion of overheated pork was not reached for 5 hours, indicating slow digestion of the protein. Weight gain was reduced 22% on overheated pork. When soybeans were fed, moderate heating of the beans increased plasma amino acid levels, whereas overheating reduced them. The beneficial effects of heating were believed to be caused by greater ease in the release of the limiting amino acid methionine. On the other hand, the protein of wheat and oats is adversely affected by heat, as is that of nine out of seventeen types of legume seeds tested. Heat used in the preparation of evaporated and dried milks seems to improve the digestibility and utilization of the protein. When heat decreases the nutritive value of proteins, the effect seems to be caused by a reduction in hydrolysis of heated proteins by digestive enzymes, indicating that heating has produced complexes resistant to the action of digestive enzymes. If heating affects the *rate* of release of amino acids from a protein, it could affect the nutritive value that is dependent on the release of all amino acids simultaneously.

Some protein-rich foods such as peanuts and soybeans cannot be eaten raw because they contain either toxic substances or enzymes that must be destroyed before they are of value to the human body. Some are susceptible to the growth of toxic molds known as aflatoxins.

Since protein-rich foods are one of the most expensive items in the average diet, it is helpful to have information on the cost of similar amounts of protein from various sources. Such information is provided in Fig. 4-13, which shows the cost of 15 g or one third of a day's allowance of protein for the adult male. In interpreting these data, it must

Table 4-5. INQ* for selected sources of protein providing at least 15% of the U.S. RDA per serving

Broiled chicken	6.2
Fish and shellfish (tuna)	5.0
Cottage cheese	4.5
Hamburger (ground beef)	4.4
Veal	4.4
Lamb, leg of	3.3
2% milk	2.4
Pork	2.4
Beefsteak	2.1
Spaghetti (meatballs and tomato sauce)	2.0
Chili con carne	2.0
Peanuts	1.6
Whole wheat bread	1.5

*INQ (index of nutrient quality) =

$$\frac{\text{\% U.S. RDA of nutrient}}{\text{\% requirement of energy}} = \frac{\text{Amount in food (g of protein)}}{\text{U.S. RDA (protein)}} \div \frac{\text{Energy in food (kcal)}}{\text{Energy requirement (2300 kcal)}}$$

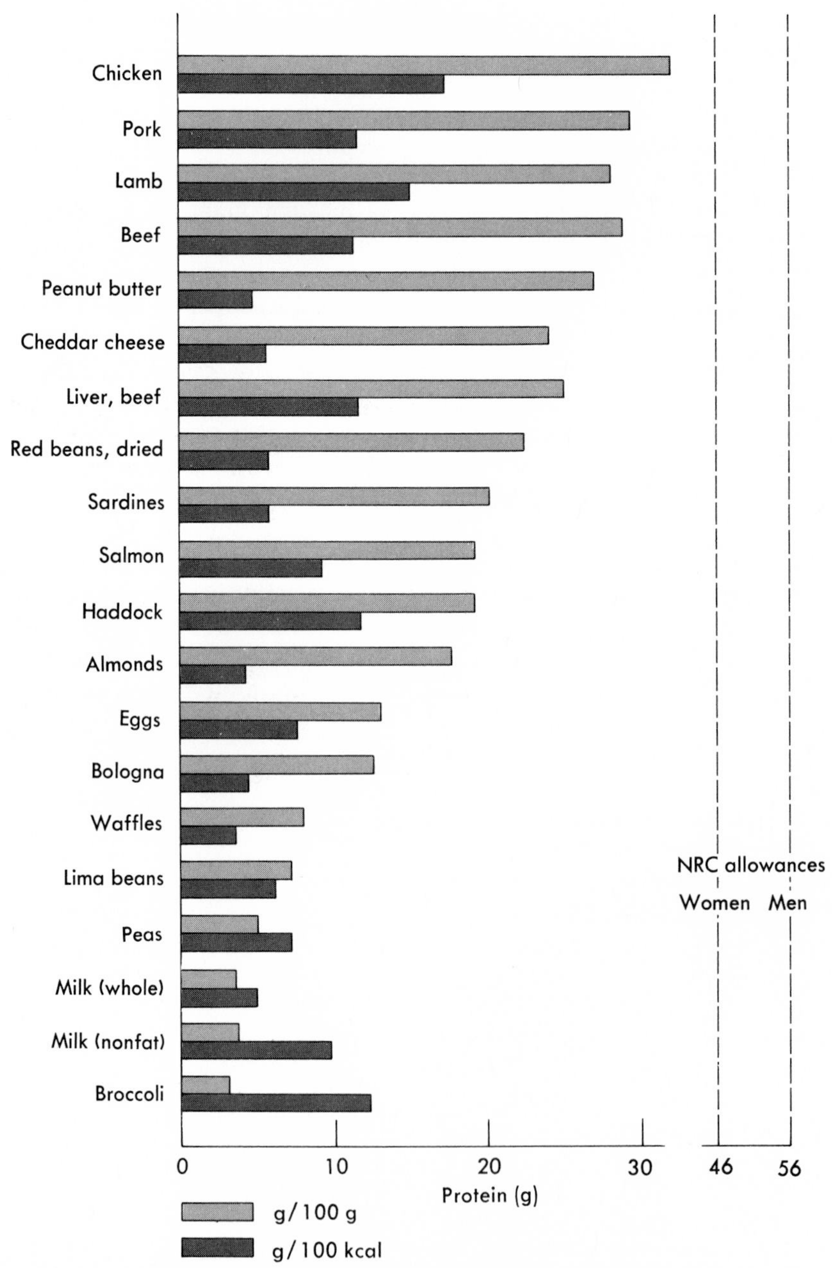

Fig. 4-12. Protein contribution of 100 g and 100 kcal portions of some representative foods. (Based on Watt, B. K., and Merrill, A. L.: Composition of foods—raw, processed and prepared, Handbook No. 8, Washington, D.C., 1963, U.S. Department of Agriculture.)

be kept in mind that they are based on average prices in 1977 and may not be accurate at any specific date in the future, especially in the light of seasonal variations in costs of products such as eggs and pork. They are presented only to give some concept of relative costs. Many of the foods represented make significant contributions of other nutrients as well.

In assessing the value of a day's diet, it is important to look at the distribution of dietary protein throughout the day's meals. Generally, it is recommended that at least one third of the protein be from animal sources of high biological value. The typical American diet is more likely to contain 60% to 80% animal protein. But if this is not distributed so that the amino acid composition of each meal is adequate through some complete protein or a mixture of vegetable proteins that supplement one another, the body will be unable to use protein as a body builder and will be forced to deaminate it for use as a source of energy. Traditionally, complete protein supplements incomplete protein in the diet. The serving of milk with cereal, cheese with macaroni, meat with rice, and peanut butter with bread are examples of these complementary relationships. The increasing use of dried milk solids in commercially baked bread has a supplementary effect on the amino acid pattern of the wheat protein and improves the biological value of the bread protein. Any baked flour product such as muffins or waffles will have the protein quality of the flour enhanced by the egg protein.

Seeds such as sunflower, pumpkin, and sesame have a relatievely high-protein content but are not practical source, since 28 g will provide 14 g of fat and only 7 or 8 g of protein at a cost of about 20 cents. The high-fiber content (10% to 12%) may also prove irritating to many persons.

With the increasing cost of food and concern over inefficiency in using natural resources for the production of animal foods, many persons are looking for alternatives to relatively costly animal proteins. Increasing numbers are turning to vegetarianism. The ovolacto-vegetarian who consumes milk, eggs, and cheese in addition to legumes and cereals should have no difficulty in achieving an adequate intake of good quality protein. The true vegetarian who relies exclusively on vegetable protein, by carefully selecting

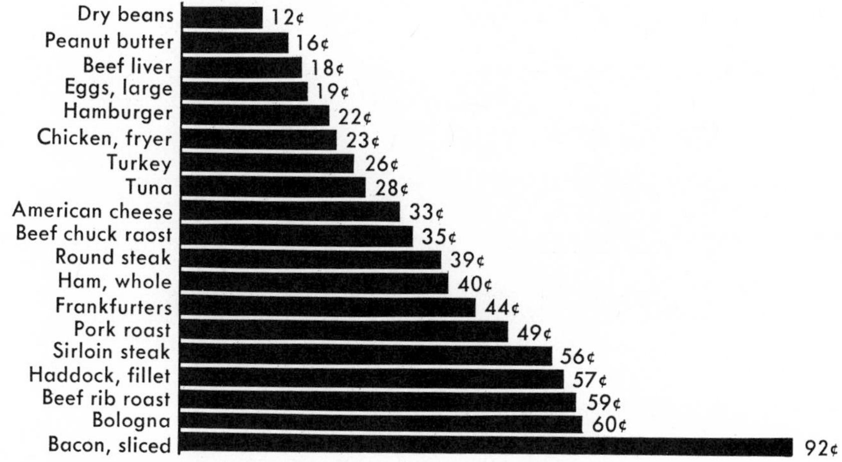

Fig. 4-13. Costs of one third of Recommended Daily Allowance for protein for 20-year-old man. Bureau of Labor Statistics average prices for United States cities. (From Meats and meat alternates, Washington, D.C. 1977, U.S. Department of Agriculture.)

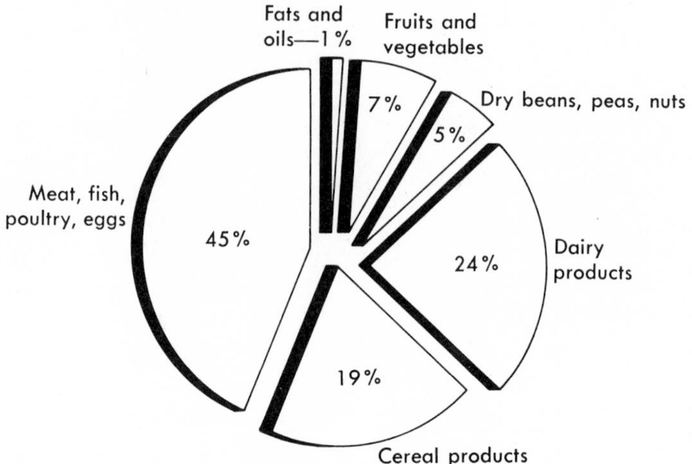

Fig. 4-14. Contribution of food groups to protein content of the American food supply. (Based on Contribution of major food groups to nutrient supplies available for civilian consumption, National Food Review NFR-1, Washington, D.C., 1978, Economic Research Service.)

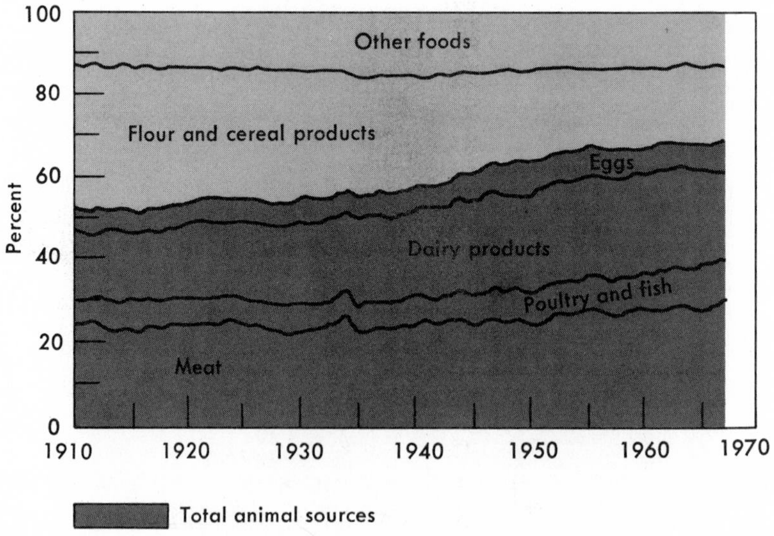

Fig. 4-15. Trends in contribution of various food groups to protein content of American diet from 1910 to 1968. (Data from 1968 preliminary data, Agricultural Research Service, U.S. Department of Agriculture, 1969.)

foods, can also obtain the recommended level of protein of a sufficiently high biological value to maintain body tissue. It is more difficult but not impossible to meet the relatively high needs for growth in a young child or during pregnancy. The most important consideration is to include simultaneously, rather than at successive meals, a combination of foods whose amino acid compositions provide all the essential amino acids. Examples of such combinations are wheat low in lysine and beans low in methionine or corn and rice. The use of nuts, with a biological value of 60, is also recommended. In general, it is advisable to choose two vegetable proteins from different classes of food to supplement one another; for example, a cereal and a legume, a legume and a nut, or a root crop such as yams with a legume.

The efforts of some commercial interests to promote the addition of lysine to bread and flour and methionine to vegetable pro-

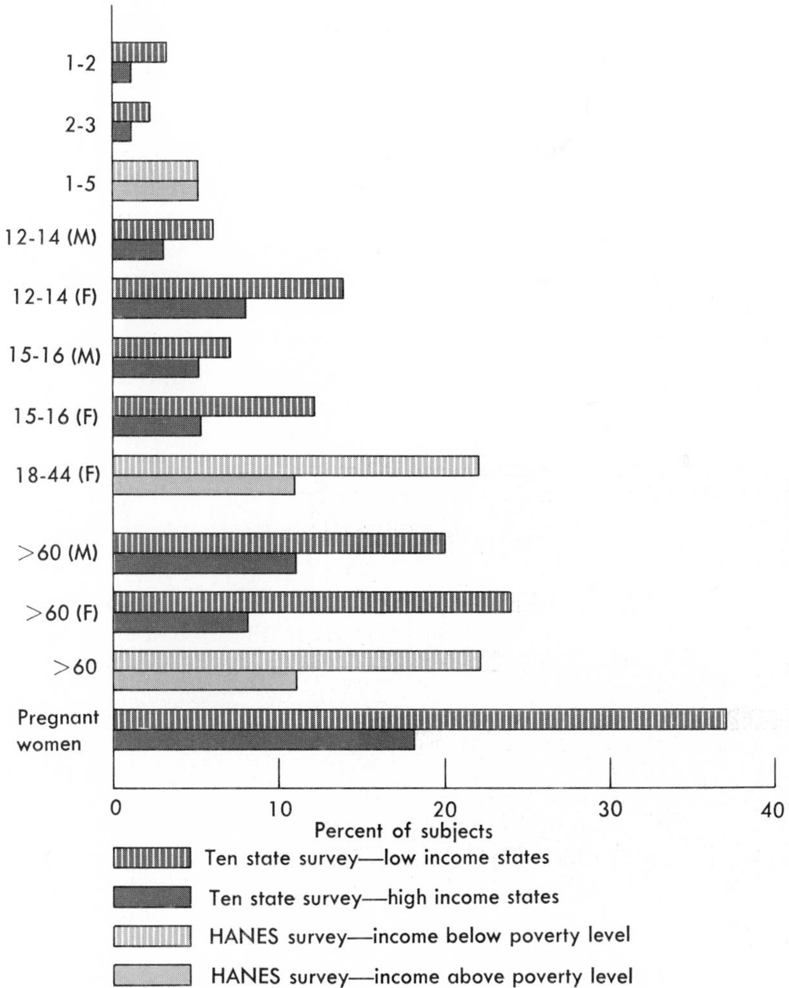

Fig. 4-16. Percentage of persons with dietary protein intake below two-thirds Recommended Dietary Allowances by age, sex, and income level. Data based on results of Ten-State Nutrition Survey (1968-1970) and preliminary findings of First Health and Nutrition Examination Survey (HANES) (1971-1972).

teins in the United States are likely not justified, since there is no evidence of a lysine deficiency in the American diet. In addition, studies suggest that protein quality may be depressed rather than increased if the level of one amino acid is increased out of proportion to the others. Amino acid supplementation of a low-quality protein may be justified when it is a staple item in a total diet of low biological value, but not when protein quality is high or when vegetable proteins that can supplement one another are available.

The relative contribution of various food groups to the protein in the American diet is shown in Fig. 4-14 and trends in the contribution of various food groups to total protein intake in Fig. 4-15. The extent of diets inadequate in protein in the United States is depicted in Fig. 4-16. From this it is evident that a relatively small number of individuals have been identified with dietary intakes below established standards.

EVALUATION OF PROTEIN QUALITY

Since the amino acid content of a protein as well as the total amount of the nutrient in the diet determines its value for growth or maintenance, the problem of measuring the relative value of various proteins as dietary constituents is complex. Both biological and chemical methods of evaluating protein quality have been tried.

A widely used index is the **biological value** (BV). This is a measure of the relationship of protein retention to protein absorption on the assumption that more will be retained when the essential amino acids are present in sufficient quantity to meet the need for growth. The biological value is assessed by determining the amount of nitrogen in the food intake and in the urinary and fecal excretions of both a test diet and on a protein-free diet. Urinary nitrogen includes that from absorbed amino acids that have been deaminated. Fecal nitrogen represents that which was unabsorbed, plus nitrogen from any cells sloughed off the lining of the digestive tract or from digestive enzymes that have not been digested and reabsorbed. The formula for determining biological value becomes

$$\text{BV} = \frac{\text{Dietary N} - (\text{Urinary N} - \text{U}_0)(\text{Fecal N} - \text{F}_0)}{\text{Dietary N} - (\text{Fecal N} - \text{F}_0)} \times 100$$

(where U_0 and F_0 represent excretion on a protein-free diet). A protein with a biological value of 70 or more (that is, 70% of the intake of nitrogen is retained) is considered capable of supporting growth, assuming that the caloric value of the diet is adequate. Diets with a biological value of less than 70 are less capable of supporting growth through the use of more of that protein. This index may be applied to single proteins, single foods, or combinations of protein in foods. The biological value of representative proteins is given in Table 4-6. Testing for the biological value of a protein is usually done with rats. It is necessary to feed the protein at the level needed for maintenance or slightly below so that it will be used with maximum efficiency.

Since the BV is based only on the amount of nitrogen absorbed, it does not take into account differences in digestibility from one protein to another. The measurement of protein quality by an index known as *net protein utilization* (NPU) has been introduced to express in a single measurement both the digestibility of the protein and the biological value of the amino acid mixture absorbed from the intestine. NPU = N retained/N intake and can be represented by BV × coefficient of digestibility. NPU represents the percentage of dietary protein retained. It is essentially the same as another test, the NPR-net protein ratio.

Determination of BV and NPU values for humans is costly in terms of both time and money and is of limited usefulness during periods of growth where ethical considerations preclude limiting the protein intake. Data from rat studies, however, are not necessarily applicable to humans.

The protein efficiency ratio (PER) is the simplest method of determining protein quality, since it requires no chemical analy-

Table 4-6. Biological value of representative proteins

Food	Biological value
Egg	100
Milk	93
Rice	86
Fish	75
Beef	75
Casein	75
Corn	72
Cottonseed flour	60
Peanut flour	56
Wheat gluten	44

ses. It merely requires calculating the weight gain of a growing animal in relation to its protein intake when calories are ample and the protein source is fed at an adequate level (9% protein) for a sufficiently long period of time (four weeks) to assess the protein in comparison to casein with a known PER of 2.5. It is based on the assumption (which may be in error) that weight gain of a growing animal is in proportion to gain in body protein. A variation of the PER in which several levels of protein are fed and the slope of the line joining the PER values interpreted is known as the RNV (relative nutritive value). This new technique involving the PER at various levels of protein intake is more precise but also much more complex.

In addition to the biological methods of evaluating protein quality, there are several chemical methods based on the determination of the amino acid pattern of a particular food and a comparison of this to a reference protein. In 1957 the FAO proposed a reference protein based on the amino acid requirements of humans but in 1965 decided to abandon its use in favor of an amino acid pattern of whole egg or human milk as a standard. In 1973 the FAO introduced still another scoring pattern. Chemical scores based on these standards are in closer agreement with the biological indices of protein quality (Table 4-7). To obtain a chemical score, the

Table 4-7. Chemical score and net protein utilization values of common foods*

Protein	Chemical score	Net protein utilization†
Whole egg	100	
Human milk	100	95
Cow's milk	95	81
Soybean milk	74	75
Sesame	50	54
Ground nut (peanut)	65	57
Cottonseed	81	41
Maize	49	36‡
Rice	67	63‡
Whole wheat	53	49‡

*From Food and Agriculture Organization: Energy and protein requirements, FAO Nutrition Meeting Series No. 52, Rome, 1973.
†Based on values for children 3 to 7 years old receiving 6.7% of energy from protein.
‡Based on values for children 8 to 12 years.

amount of each essential amino acid is expressed as a ratio of total essential amino acids in the reference protein.

The amino acid score of a protein or a mixture of proteins is calculated by the following formula:

$$\text{Amino acid score} = \frac{\text{mg of amino acid in 1 g test protein}}{\text{mg of amino acid in reference protein}} \times 100$$

This yields a score that reflects the extent of the deviation of the most limiting amino acid, which approximates the probable efficiency of utilization of the test protein. This score may underestimate the quality of protein for adults whose essential amino acid needs are lower. Since lysine, sulfur-containing amino acids, and tryptophan have been found to be the most limiting amino acids, for practical purposes these are the only scores that need to be calculated.

Chemical scores do not take into consideration imbalances in amino acid patterns or differences in absorption of amino acids.

Both these factors could account for discrepancies between results from biological and chemical evaluation of protein quality. In addition, the adequacy of the energy intake, the availability of the amino acid (which is dependent on digestion and absorption), the treatment of protein in processing may influence the value of a food as a source of dietary protein. Chemical scores of representative proteins are shown in Table 4-7.

The fact that so many standards for evaluating protein quality have been and are being proposed is evidence that we lack any single satisfactory standard. Many based on biological assays are more costly and time consuming than chemical analyses of amino acid composition. However, protein metabolism is apparently so complex that a determination of chemical makeup of a protein gives only limited information on the manner in which the animal may utilize it. Similarly, proteins that can effectively repair body tissue may have limitations as a source of growth protein. A comparison of various estimates of protein quality appears in Table 4-8.

KWASHIORKOR

The importance of protein in world nutrition has been emphasized in the last thirty-five years with the identification of the condition *kwashiorkor* as a protein-deficiency disease. This condition occurs primarily among children between the ages of 2 and 5 years, when they are weaned from mother's milk to a diet of starchy cereal pastes practically devoid of protein. Fig. 1-3 shows a child with kwashiorkor. This term, applied by the Ga tribe in Ghana to a sickness of a weanling child, means literally "first-second." It was appropriate because the first child developed the condition within three or four months after being abruptly weaned from the breast on the arrival of the second child. This corresponds to the time when milk, the child's only source of good-quality protein, is removed. Kwashiorkor is considered the major nutrition problem in the world today; many infants are dying as a result of it, and untold numbers are suffering from subclinical symptoms of the disease and increased susceptibility to infection. In kwashiorkor there is a deficiency both in quality and quantity of

Table 4-8. Comparison of estimates of protein quality on the basis of several measures

	BV	NPU	PER	Chemical score
Polished rice	64	57	2.18	57
Egg	94	94	3.92	100
Fish	76	80	3.55	71
Cow's milk	85	82	3.09	60
Brewer's yeast	67	56	2.24	57
Beef	74	67	2.30	69
Sesame seeds	62	53	1.77	42
Soybeans	73	61	2.32	47
Peas	64	47	1.57	37
Peanuts	55	43	1.65	55
Whole wheat	65	40	1.53	43
Oats	65	66	2.19	57

dietary protein in the presence of adequate calories. *Marasmus* is the term applied to the condition resulting from a caloric deficit that is usually accompanied by a protein deficiency. The terms protein calorie malnutrition and protein energy malnutrition are now being replaced by energy protein malnutrition (EPM) and energy protein deficits (EPD), which recognize more recent thinking that energy rather than protein may be the most limiting nutrient, but that both are involved. Fig. 4-17 shows a child with characteristic EPM on admission and discharge four weeks later.

The main clinical symptoms of kwashiorkor are as follows:

1. Failure to grow in both weight and length, with weak, thin, and wasting muscles
2. Behavioral changes manifest as irritability in kwashiorkor and apathy in marasmus
3. Edema—the accumulation of fluid in the tissues, causing them to be soft and

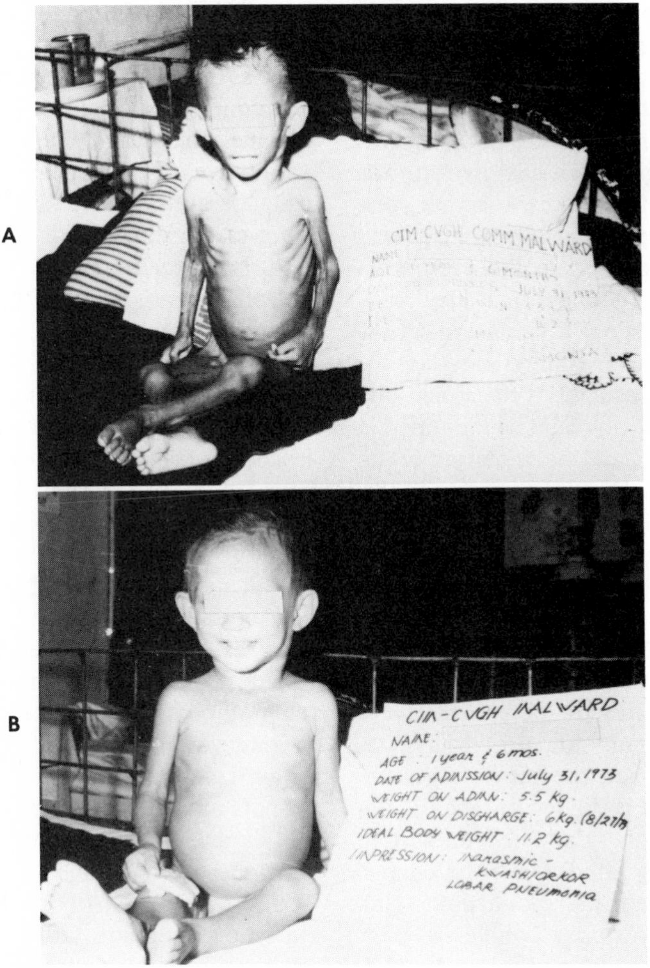

Fig. 4-17. Child with marasmic-kwashiorkor on admission to hospital, **A,** and on discharge one month later, **B.** (Courtesy Dr. Florentino Solon, Cebu Institute of Medicine, Philippines.)

spongy, especially in the lower half of the body
4. Skin changes, especially in the lower part of the body, including abnormal color in some areas, lack of color in others, and drying and peeling of the skin resulting in the formation of ulcers
5. Changes in hair, which becomes sparse and loses its pigmentation or takes on a characteristic reddish color
6. Loss of appetite, vomiting, and diarrhea
7. Enlargement of the liver
8. Anemia

The ability of the child to combat infection is very low and death is usually attirbuted to an infection, such as measles or pneumonia, that would not normally be fatal in a more adequately nourished child.

Unfortunately, many children with kwashiorkor are never given medical help or are brought in for treatment only when the condition is well advanced, usually when a concurrent infection has led to high temperatures and obvious debilitation. The most helpful diagnostic sign is a change in serum albumin levels, but this change does not occur in the very early stages of the condition. Prekwashiorkor, which could be identified if the growth of the child were plotted regularly, can be treated simply by improving the amount and quality of protein in the diet. The treatment must also take into account the anorexia, or loss of appetite, that is common, complicating recovery because of the difficulty in getting the child to eat. In more advanced cases, extreme care must be taken to compensate for the low potassium levels that usually accompany low protein intake. Nonfat milk has been the most successful therapeutic food. It is diluted at first and increased in strength gradually until full strength can be tolerated. Once the edema has been eliminated and blood potassium levels have been restored, whole milk or nonfat milk with coconut and corn oil added are necessary to provide sufficient calories to stimulate growth.

Since infection is a complicating and often precipitating factor in kwashiorkor, any dietary treatment should be accompanied by efforts to improve environmental sanitation. This may be even more important as a means of protecting subsequent children than it is for the affected child.

The most promising attack on the problem of kwashiorkor is prevention, which implies the maintenance of a diet adequate in good-quality protein and calories. Most attempts to provide sufficient animal protein are impractical where there is limited land available and the cost of animal protein is economically unfeasible for most of the population. The situation will become progressively worse as population pressures increase. The one inexpensive source of animal protein that has promise is fish, but problems of preservation in tropical climates limit the extent to which this is exploited.

Efforts are being encouraged to provide a palatable low-cost food with an adequate balance of amino acids that can be made from indigenous plant substances for use in the postweaning diet of infants to supplement the basic cereal diet. Since no one plant protein provides a desirable balance for mammalian needs, a search for such a mixture of plant proteins has been the incentive for much research. One promising effort has been that of the Institute of Nutrition in Central America and Panama, commonly referred to as INCAP. They have succeeded in producing a mixture of 58% ground maize and sorghum, 36% cottonseed flour, 3% torula yeast, 1% $CaCO_3$ and vitamin A. It is sold under the name of Incaparina and is being promoted for use as a relatively low-bulk beverage or gruel at a cost of less than 4 cents a day. This mixture provides the critical pattern of amino acids required for child growth and at the same time corrects the nutrient deficiencies that usually accompany kwashiorkor—vitamin A, riboflavin, calcium, niacin, and potassium. Other combinations of leaf protein and legumes available in regions such as Lebanon and India have been developed and show promising results.

Some efforts have been made to enrich or to fortify cereals with the limiting amino acids, such as adding lysine to wheat, lysine and threonine to rice, and lysine, threonine, and methionine to barley. This has not proved practical, as it is feasible only where cereals are milled in a central facility. It only improves the quality of the protein and does not solve the problem of low protein and low calorie intake. In addition, only methionine and lysine are sufficiently low in cost to be economically feasible. The possibility of creating an imbalance in the amino acid pattern by the addition of too much of the limiting amino acid is another reason for caution.

A third approach has been to supplement basic cereal diets with small amounts of animal protein. The addition of 20% nonfat milk powder or 10% fish flour to a maize and pea mixture or a mixture of corn, soy, and milk produces a protein equal to milk in nutritive value. The development of protein concentrates that can be incorporated into basic cereal products has been encouraging. Fish flour, with a protein content of 85% and produced from small fish that normally have no commercial value, is acceptable when it has been defatted and deodorized. Concentrates from coconut seed press cakes, other seed kernels, and cottonseed by-products, which are often discarded, are inexpensive and promising as a partial solution to the problems of protein malnutrition. Care must be taken, however, to exclude any toxic substances that are naturally present or that develop during processing.

Plant geneticists have succeeded in developing Opaque II corn with a protein of greatly improved nutritive value. The "miracle rice," a high-yield variety with a short growing period and a high resistance to disease, shows great promise in increasing the amount of rice available in Southeast Asia. Many commercial companies are investigating the potential of soybean-based beverages for increasing protein consumption in developing countries. The possibilities of using chlorella, a microscopic plankton that abounds in the sea, or a single-celled protein produced when bacteria grow on petroleum, manure, and other energy sources also are being studied experimentally.

In addition to having a protein content of high biological value, any food that will provide any hope for meeting the nutritional needs in developing countries must meet certain other criteria. (1) It must be locally available or capable of being produced locally, (2) it must be acceptable within the culture, (3) it must be within economic reach of the segment of the population needing it, (4) it must have long storage life under hot, humid conditions, (5) it must be easily transported, and (6) it must have acceptable characteristics of taste, odor, and physical properties. On the other hand, if it is too popular, it may become a prestige food in the culture and be consumed by the ranking adult males rather than by children and pregnant women whose needs are greatest. The food must be free from toxic and deleterious effects in the form proposed and must not be currently used to a maximum as human food. Many foods or combination of foods have been suggested, but at present, in addition to fish flour, the most promising appear to be soy products with a protein value of 25%, peanut flour, sesame flour, cottonseed flour, oil seed cakes, and coconut protein. Algae and yeast, although theoretically good sources, have not proved sufficiently palatable for human use. Others have been eliminated because of their unknown nutritive value, the uneconomical aspects of their production, a limited production of the raw material, or the presence of a toxic substance.

The provision of dietary protein is ineffective unless the diet includes adequate calories simultaneously. In fact, in many instances prevention of EPM requires only increasing the quantity of food without changing the composition of the diet.

ABNORMALITIES IN AMINO ACID METABOLISM

Some infants are born with an inability to produce the enzymes necessary for phenylalanine metabolism. These children need a small amount of this essential amino acid for protein synthesis but have no ability to metabolize the rest, with the result that phenylalanine and some of its partially oxidized derivatives accumulate in the blood and urine. They have an adverse effect on nervous tissue and the resulting condition, known as phenylketonuria (PKU), is characterized by mental retardation. Early diagnosis is crucial to successful treatment and prevention of mental retardation. A diet very low in phenylalanine is indicated.

A similar failure to metabolize leucine and valine is reflected as maple sugar urine disease, so named because of the characteristic odor of the urine. Failure to metabolize histidine appears related to speech defects. Up to 250 other inborn errors of metabolism involving other enzyme defects have been reported.

BIBLIOGRAPHY

Allison, J. B., and Wannemacher, R. W., Jr.: The concept and significance of labile and over-all protein reserves of the body, Am. J. Clin. Nutr. **16:**445, 1965.

Broquist, H. P.: Amino acid metabolism, Nutr. Rev. **34:**289, 1977.

Committee Report: Assessment of protein nutritional status, Am. J. Clin. Nutr. **23:**807, 1970.

Chapra, J. G., Forbes, A. L., and Habicht, J. P.: Protein in the U.S. diet, J. Am. Diet. Assoc. **72:**253, 1978.

el Lozy, M., and Hegsted, D. M.: Calculation of the amino acid requirements of children at different ages by the factorial method, Am. J. Clin. Nutr. **28:**1052, 1975.

Food and Agriculture Organization: Amino acid content of foods and biological data on proteins, FAO Nutrition Studies, No. 24, Rome, 1973.

Food and Agriculture Organization: Energy and protein requirements, FAO Nutrition Meeting Report Series, No. 52, Rome, 1973.

Food and Nutrition Board: Evaluation of protein quality, Publication No. 1100, Washington, D.C., 1963, National Academy of Sciences–National Research Council.

Food and Nutrition Board: Improvement of protein nutriture, Washington, D.C., 1974, National Academy of Sciences–National Research Council.

Garza, C., Scrimshaw, N. S., and Young, V. R.: Human protein requirements: the effect of variations in energy intake within the maintenance range, Am. J. Clin. Nutr. **29:**280, 1976.

Harper, A. E.: Some implications of amino acid supplementation, Am. J. Clin. Nutr. **9:**533, 1961.

Harper, A. E., Payne, P. R., and Waterlow, J. C.: Assessment of human protein needs, Am. J. Clin. Nutr. **26:**1168, 1973.

Hegsted, D. M.: Amino acid fortification and the protein problem, Am. J. Clin. Nutr. **21:**688, 1968.

Hegsted, D. M.: Minimum protein requirements of adults, Am. J. Clin. Nutr. **21:**352, 1968.

Holt, L. E., Jr., Halac, E., Jr., and Kadji, C. N.: The concept of protein stores and its implication in the diet, J.A.M.A. **181:**699, 1962.

Irwin, M. I., and Hegsted, D. M.: A conspectus of research on amino acid requirements of man, J. Nutr. **101:**539, 1971.

Joint FAO/WHO Expert Group: Protein requirements, WHO Techn. Rep. Ser. 301, 1965.

Korslund, M. K., Leung, E. Y., Meiners, C. R., Crews, M. G., Taper, J., Abernathy, R. P., and Ritchey, S. J.: The effects of sweat nitrogen losses in evaluating protein utilization by preadolescent children, Am. J. Clin. Nutr. **29:**600, 1976.

Miller, D. S., and Payne, P. R.: The assessment of protein requirements by nitrogen balance, Proc. Nutr. Soc. **28:**225, 1969.

Payne, P. R.: Safe protein-calorie ratios in diets. The relative importance of protein and energy intake as causal factors in malnutrition, Am. J. Clin. Nutr. **28:**281, 1975.

Schrimshaw, N. S.: Nature of protein requirements: ways they can be met in tomorrow's world, J. Am. Diet. Assoc. **54:**94, 1969.

Spencer, R. P.: Intestinal absorption of amino acids. Current concepts, Am. J. Clin. Nutr. **22:**292, 1969.

Stifel, F. B., and Herman, R. H.: Is histidine an essential amino acid in man? Am. J. Clin. Nutr. **25:**182, 1972.

Vauy, R., Schrimshaw, N. S., and Young, V. R.: Human protein requirements: obligatory urinary and fecal nitrogen losses and factorial estimation of protein needs in elderly males, J. Nutr. **108:**97, 1978.

5

Energy balance

Energy balance is a topic freely discussed by the general public but widely misunderstood. While research scientists are attempting to understand the mechanisms controlling appetite, many individuals and groups are capitalizing on the fears of a large segment of the population that they either are or are likely to become obese. They provide diet and exercise plans and panaceas that require neither calorie restriction nor increased activity but give no long-range help. This chapter emphasizes that energy intake and expenditure are both measured in units of heat known as kilocalories, which the body can use or store as fat. This energy can neither be destroyed nor excreted.

ENERGY SOURCES

The energy value of the diet is provided entirely by its carbohydrate, fat, protein, and alcohol components. These may make up from 4% of foods such as lettuce to 100% of foods such as sugar, salad oil, and dry gelatin. The remaining portion of the food consists of water, cellulose, minerals, and vitamins, none of which yields energy. In the typical American diet, carbohydrate provides from 50% to 60% of the energy; protein, from 10% to 15%, and fat, from 35% to 45%. The source of energy in diets varies with many factors—agricultural, cultural, social, and economic. For instance, in rice-eating countries, carbohydrate makes a large contribution to the energy intake; in countries with emphasis on dairying, protein assumes greater importance. Italians, with the extensive use of cooking oil, derive more energy from fats. In America the trend has been toward greater use of protein and a decrease in complex carbohydrate consumption with an increase in the amount of money available for food. More recently, however, with a growing concern about the potential of the world food supply to meet the needs of an expanding population, many persons are reducing their intake of animal protein and substituting cereal grains.

Unit of measurement

The energy value of a food is currently expressed in terms of a unit of heat, a **kilocalorie** (kcal).* This represents the amount of heat required to raise the temperature of 1 kg (slightly over 1 quart) of water 1° C. Although this unit is correctly designated as a kilocalorie to distinguish it from the smaller unit, a calorie (0.001 kcal), used in most physical and chemical measurements, many nutrition sources still refer to it as the Calorie or calorie, assuming that it is a sufficiently standardized term in nutrition that no distinction need be made.

There is a growing interest in using the terms *joule* and *kilojoule* to express the energy potential of food or the energy cost of activity. One kilojoule represents the energy involved in physically moving a 1 kg (2.2 lb)

*A proposal that the *joule* (1 kcal = 4.18 kilojoules [kJ]) be adopted as the unit of energy in nutrition has been endorsed by many organizations concerned with nutrition.

weight 1 m (39 inches) by the force of 1 Newton (a unit of force). If the kilojoule is ever universally adopted, to make the transition, it will be necessary to multiply all values currently given in kilocalories by 4.2 (1 kcal equals 4.18 kJ). Any discussion of energy will then involve much larger numbers. It will undoubtedly be some time before the term *calorie,* as used in popular literature, will be replaced by the more correct *kilocalorie,* and even longer before the concept of the joule as the unit of measurement of energy receives popular endorsement.

An appreciation of the amount of energy or heat available from foods may be obtained by noting that 2 tablespoons of sugar provide 100 kcal, enough heat to raise the temperature of slightly over 4 cups of water from 0° C (freezing) to 100° C (boiling), assuming the availability of oxygen and a high degree of efficiency in the conversion of energy. Five teaspoons of fat or 4½ cups of shredded cabbage have a similar energy potential. In humans, about 20% of the energy obtained from food is converted into mechanical, osmotic, and chemical energy and 80% into heat.

The ability of animals to release energy from food sources depends not only on the presence of oxygen but also on the availability of minerals, vitamins, and enzymes, which catalyze the many and complex chemical changes involved in converting the energy in the simple energy-yielding nutrients, glucose and fatty acids, into ATP (adenosine triphosphate), a high-energy compound. Energy is trapped in this form and is released in slowly regulated amounts for use within the cell. The final steps in transfer of energy to ATP take place almost exclusively in the mitochondrion of the cell. ATP is used, however, in virtually all organelles of the cell for the synthesis of complex substances from simple nutrients and for all physical changes and metabolic reactions that require energy. When 1 molecule of phosphate splits off, the needed energy is released and ADP remains.

DETERMINATION OF ENERGY VALUES

Direct calorimetry

Much of our information on the energy value of foods is obtained by **direct calorimetry** or the direct measurement of heat. The instrument used for this is the *bomb calorimeter,* a highly insulated, compact, boxlike container about 1 cubic foot in size. The essential features of a bomb calorimeter are shown in Fig. 5-1. A dried sample of food is

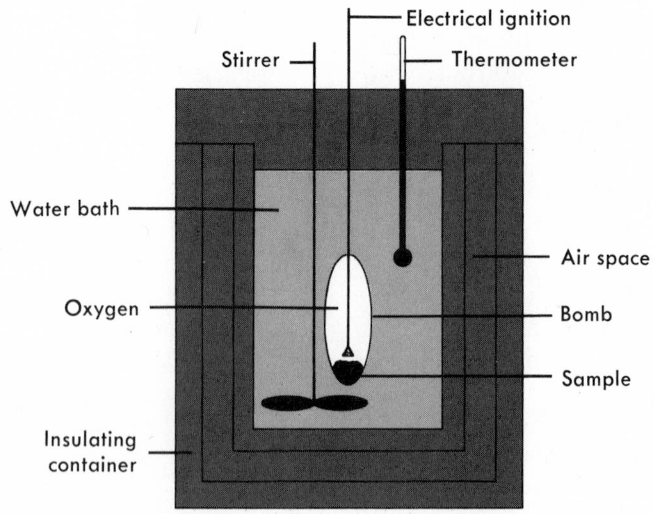

Fig. 5-1. Cross section of a bomb calorimeter showing essential features.

completely burned in the oxygen-rich environment within the container, and all the heat produced is absorbed by a weighed amount of water surrounding the combustion chamber. The change in temperature of this fluid is measured. Since a kilocalorie is defined as the amount of heat required to change the temperature of a certain volume of water, the amount of heat required for the observed change in a known amount of water can be readily calculated. Because the bomb is sufficiently insulated so that no heat exchange takes place with the environment, the heat necessary for the increase in water temperature must be derived from the dried sample of food, which is completely burned to release all its energy. A single bomb calorimeter determination takes about 20 minutes but must be preceded by the time-consuming processes of precise weighing and careful drying of the sample.

Heat of combustion

The energy value of a sample of food determined in a bomb calorimeter is known as the **heat of combustion,** the maximum amount of energy, measured as heat, that the sample is capable of yielding under conditions providing for complete burning or oxidation.

When purified samples of carbohydrate, fat, and protein are burned in the bomb calorimeter, the amount of heat produced will vary slightly with the source and chemical composition of the nutrient. However, values of 4.1 kcal/g of carbohydrate, 9.45 kcal/g of fat, and 5.65 kcal/g of protein are generally considered representative for the American diet.

The heat of combustion represents the energy produced by the oxidation of the carbon molecule to carbon dioxide, the hydrogen to water, and the nitrogen of protein to nitrous oxide. The body is capable of releasing the energy potential of carbon by the process of *decarboxylation,* or removal of carbon dioxide, and of hydrogen through a series of reactions referred to as *coupled oxidative phosphorylation.* It cannot, however, release or utilize the energy potential of nitrogen. Thus the heat measured in the bomb calorimeter from the oxidation of nitrogen is not available when protein is utilized in the body for energy. It is necessary then to subtract the amount of heat representing the oxidation of nitrogen from the total heat of combustion of protein in estimating the amount available to the body. The oxidation of nitrogen accounts for 1.3 kcal of the 5.65 kcal/g of protein, leaving a potential of only 4.3 kcal/g of protein available to the body.

Coefficient of digestibility

Since the body is not 100% efficient in digesting (preparing food for absorption), absorbing, or metabolizing nutrients, in determining the amount of energy available to the body from an energy-yielding nutrient, it is necessary to take into account the availability of the ingested nutrient to the cells where energy is ultimately released. The extent of digestion varies from one nutrient to another and is also influenced by the nature of the food in which it is found. However, to calculate the potential energy from carbohydrate, fat, and protein, representative *coefficients of digestibility* expressing the percentage of the nutrient ultimately available are used. For carbohydrate, which is 98% digested, fat, 95% digested, and protein, 92% digested, the coefficients of digestibility are 0.98, 0.95, and 0.92, respectively. Although nutritionists are well aware that these factors may not be accurate for any one food, they do represent the best currently available factors to apply to the energy-yielding nutrients in the American diet for calculating the *physiological fuel value,* or the amount of potential energy available from a diet. It has been observed that other factors would be more appropriate for use in other countries where the composition of the diet and its digestibility may be different.

Physiological fuel value

The calculation of the physiological fuel value of the three energy-yielding groups is summarized in Table 5-1.

Table 5-1. Calculation of physiological fuel value of nutrients

	Carbohydrate	Fat	Protein
	kcal/g		
Heat of combustion	4.15	9.45	5.65
Energy from combustion of nitrogen unavailable to the body	—	—	1.3
Net heat of combustion	4.15	9.45	4.35
Coefficient of digestibility	0.98	0.95	0.92
Physiological fuel value	4.0	9.0	4.0

The factors 4, 9, and 4, representing the amount of energy available to the body per gram of carbohydrate, fat, and protein in the diet, are widely used in nutrition and dietetics. Although they may be influenced by many variables and their use may lead to some small inaccuracies, they represent a useful tool in calculations involving energy values of diets.

Indirect calorimetry, or oxycalorimetry

The energy value of a substance may also be determined by indirect calorimetry, in which the oxygen used in burning the samples and the carbon dioxide produced are measured. Although results obtained in the *oxycalorimeter* correspond closely to those from the bomb calorimeter, oxycalorimetry is seldom used.

ENERGY VALUE OF FOODS

A determination of the fuel value of a food may be made in two ways: by calorimetry or by calculation based on its carbohydrate, fat, and protein content.

Direct calorimetry

The bomb calorimeter is used in determining the caloric value of a food by direct calorimetry. A weighed sample of food or mixture of foods is dried to a constant weight and burned in the bomb calorimeter, and the amount of heat given off is measured directly. The values obtained in this way represent the heat of combustion of the food and not its physiological fuel value. The values are from 7% to 10% higher than the actual fuel values, depending on the percentage of calories from protein. The more protein, the greater the error.

Proximate composition

For most foods we now have analytical data for *proximate composition*—the percentage of carbohydrate, fat, protein, and water found in a typical sample of the food. If very precise data on the energy value of a food are not needed, this method is quicker and less costly than the use of the bomb calorimeter. For example, from tables of food composition we may learn that a particular food contains 9.2% fat, 21.4% utilizable carbohydrate, and 5.5% protein—the only energy-yielding nutrients in food. The value for fat in a food can be assessed directly by extracting the lipid chemically. Protein is estimated from an analysis for nitrogen and water by drying the food. Carbohydrate is determined by the difference between the total weight of the food and that accounted for by lipid, water, protein, and crude fiber. Since carbohydrate values include some nonutilizable dietary fiber, they may be overestimated and hence less accurate than the values for lipid and protein. Calculation of the energy value of 100 g of food is shown in Table 5-2.

From the information that this food sam-

Table 5-2. Calculation of energy value of a food from proximate analysis

Nutrient	Percent in food	Amount in 100 g (g)	Energy value/g (kcal)	Energy value of 100 g (kcal)
Carbohydrate	21.4	21.4	4	85.6
Fat	9.2	9.2	9	82.8
Protein	5.5	5.5	4	22.0
TOTAL ENERGY				190.4

Table 5-3. Size and caloric value of an average serving of food and the amount of food needed to provide 100 kcal

Food	Average serving	Kcal /serving	Amount to provide 100 kcal
Lettuce	¼ head	6	4 heads
Cabbage	½ cup	10	5 cups, shredded
Asparagus	6 spears	15	40 spears
Carrots	1 medium	30	3½ medium
Sugar	1 tablespoon	50	2 tablespoons
Bread	1 slice	70	1½ slices
Apple	1 medium	80	1¼ apples (7 cm in diameter)
Egg	1 large	80	1¼ large
Potato	1 medium	75	1 large
Banana	1 medium	76	1⅓ medium
Nonfat milk	1 cup	90	1 cup +
Pear	1 medium	100	1
Dates	4	100	4
Butter	1 tablespoon	100	1 tablespoon
Mayonnaise	1 tablespoon	100	1 tablespoon
Salad oil	1 tablespoon	120	⅚ tablespoon
Whole milk	1 cup	150	⅔ cup
Chicken breast	1	160	1.7 oz
Pork chop	1	305	0.9 oz

*From Nutritive value of foods, Home and Garden Bulletin No. 72, Agriculture Research Service, Washington, D.C. 1977, U.S. Department of Agriculture.

ple provided, 190.4 kcal/100 g or 1.9 kcal/g one can readily calculate the energy value of a food sample of any size. By knowing the total carbohydrate, fat, or protein content of the diet, one can determine the percentage of total calories contributed by any one nutrient group. In fact, by knowing the sample size and any three of the four variables—carbohydrate, fat, protein, and total energy—one can calculate the unknown factor.

Variation in energy value

The energy value of a particular food is a function of its carbohydrate, fat, and protein composition in relation to cellulose and water. Foods with a high percentage of fat are concentrated sources of calories, as are foods with a low water content. Since small amounts of them are required to yield a relatively large number of calories, they are often erroneously considered "fattening" foods. Although it is easier to eat excess calories from foods low in water or high in fat content, the foods themselves are not to be condemned as fattening. Only the total diet can be described as fattening and only then when its energy value exceeds the need of the individual for energy.

Table 5-3 presents the amounts of various foods required to provide 100 kcal and also the size and caloric value of an average serving. It is evident from the bulk of food required that if one wishes to increase his caloric intake, foods from the bottom of the list should be chosen. Conversely, if one wishes to restrict caloric intake, more satisfaction in terms of bulk in the stomach and the amount of chewing required will be obtained from using foods from the top of the list. Items with concentrated calories, such as sugar, flour, butter, and cheese, are often used to enhance the palatability of foods relatively low in calories. Examples of the effect of methods of food preparation on the caloric value of a food are shown in Table 5-4.

The relationship between the weight of a food and its caloric value is evident in Table 5-5. Foods low in water and high in fat have a high caloric density, and those low in fat but high in water and cellulose are lower in calories.

Exchange lists

Since diabetics must regulate their caloric intake, the American Dietetic Association has developed an exchange list to relieve these persons of the need to constantly calcu-

Table 5-4. Effect of method of preparation on energy value of an average serving of a single food

Food	kcal
Apple	70
Applesauce	185
Baked apple	225
Apple Betty	350
Apple pie	330
Apple pie a la mode	440
Potato (1 medium)	
Boiled	90
Mashed with 1 teaspoon butter	120
Baked (served with 1 pat butter)	140
French fried	155
Creamed	200

Table 5-5. Caloric value of 100 g (3.5 oz) portions of food*

Food	Caloric value/ 100 g
Lettuce (½ head)	14
Asparagus (6 spears)	20
Cabbage (1½ cups shredded)	24
Carrots (2)	31
Nonfat milk or buttermilk (⅖ cup)	36
Milk (3.7% fat; ⅖ cup)	66
Peas (⅝ cup)	68
Potato (1 small)	76
Lamb (1 serving)	197
Chicken (1 serving)	208
Pork (1 serving)	236
Bread (4 slices)	250
Dates (10)	274
Sugar (½ cup)	400
Butter (7 tablespoons)	716
Mayonnaise (7 tablespoons)	718
Salad oil (7 tablespoons)	884

*From Watt, B. K., and Merrill, A. L.: Composition of foods—raw, processed and prepared, Handbook No. 8, Washington, D.C., 1963, U.S. Department of Agriculture.

late their intake of energy. This exchange system is equally applicable to nondiabetics who wish to regulate their energy intake or know the approximate amount of carbohydrate, lipid, or protein in their diets. Exchanges are presented in six food groupings, and foods categorized in one group are similar in carbohydrate lipid, protein, and energy content. The approximate content of each group is shown in Table 5-6 and the complete exchange lists in Appendix I. Carbohydrates such as sugar that do not appear on these lists provide approximately 5 g of carbohydrate per teaspoon.

BODY'S NEED FOR ENERGY

An individual's need for energy is a function of several factors, each of which can be estimated and will be discussed separately—basal metabolism, activity, and the effect of food. All of these, in turn, are a function either directly or indirectly of a person's size; a larger person always has higher requirements than a smaller person.

ENERGY EXPENDITURE

Basal metabolism

Basal metabolism represents the minimum amount of energy for internal work needed to carry on the vital body processes. It is an expression of the energy needs during physical, emotional, and digestive rest. These processes, without which life is impossible, include respiration, circulation, glandular activity, cellular metabolism, and maintenance of muscle tonus and body temperature. It is well known that the rate of respiration increases during strenuous exercise or in the absence of sufficient oxygen, as occurs at high altitudes. These changes are a response to a need for oxygen in the cells. On the other hand, a certain minimum respiratory rate is necessary to provide sufficient oxygen to maintain life at a minimum level of cellular respiration, a rate that differs from one individual to another.

The assessment of basal metabolic energy needs includes the amount of energy necessary to carry on this minimum rate of respiration. Similarly, a minimum rate of circulation must be maintained to carry oxygen and nutrients to the cells and waste products away from the cells. The energy required for this minimum rate of circulation compatible with life is included in a basal metabolism determination. As long as life continues, glands, such as the thyroid, the adrenals, the pancreas, and the pituitary, produce and secrete hormones that control the level and nature of cellular metabolic activity. The synthesis and secretion of these substances into the bloodstream require energy. No matter how relaxed the person may be, there is still a state of muscular contraction or muscular elasticity. If not, the body would become a shapeless mass of protoplasm. The

Table 5-6. Proximate analysis of diabetic food exchange groups

Exchange	Carbohydrate (g)	Protein (g)	Lipid (g)	Energy (kcal)
Nonfat milk	12	8	0	80
Vegetables	5	2	0	25
Fruit	10	0	0	40
Bread	15	2	0	70
Lean meat	0	7	3	55
Fat	0	0	5	45

energy required to maintain this muscle tonus is also measured when basal metabolic needs are assessed. In addition, metabolic processes, such as the uptake of nutrients, the synthesis of new compounds, the excretion of waste, and the maintenance of internal environment of the cells, are constantly going on as long as the cell is living. The minimum amount of energy to maintain this cellular activity is also included in basal metabolism, as is energy needed to maintain the nervous system.

Measurement of basal metabolism

Basal metabolism can be measured in two ways—by direct or indirect calorimetry. A third test, a clinical evaluation of the protein-bound iodine (PBI) in a blood sample, will give relative but not exact energy costs.

Direct calorimetry. Direct calorimetry involves the measurement of the heat given off by the body in a respiration chamber, a small insulated room that operates on the same principle as the bomb calorimeter. By measuring the change of temperature of a known volume of water circulating in pipes in the top and walls of the chamber, it is possible to determine the amount of heat produced by a subject inside it. In addition, a measurement is often made of the exchange of carbon dioxide and oxygen that takes place. This allows the calculation of a respiratory quotient (RQ), as follows:

$$\frac{CO_2 \text{ expired}}{O_2 \text{ consumed}}$$

From this, one can determine whether carbohydrate, fat, or protein was burned. This is a useful piece of information in certain clinical situations. If carbohydrate is the sole source of fuel, the RQ is 1, indicating that one volume of carbon dioxide is produced from every volume of oxygen used in respiration. Fat has an RQ of 0.7, protein, approximately 0.8, depending on the amino acid mixture, and mixtures of carbohydrate, fat, and protein have intermediate values. Under basal conditions the RQ is usually 0.82. If the test is conducted under basal metabolic conditions,

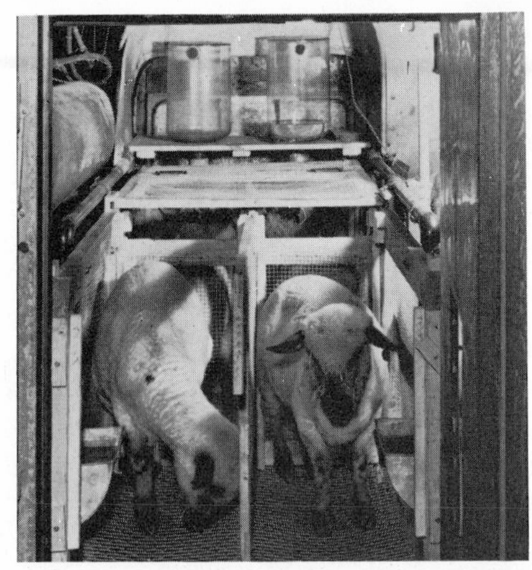

A

B

Fig. 5-2. A, Sheep in the Armsby calorimeter participating in a metabolism experiment in animal nutrition for which the chamber was originally designed. **B,** Two men entering the same calorimeter to participate in a 72-hour metabolism study, after its conversion for use with human subjects in the 1950s. In both photos note the thickness of the walls with intervening air spaces. (Photographs by R. Beese; courtesy Dr. G. Barron, The Pennsylvania State University.)

the heat produced represents the minimum energy need of the individual. Since the cost of operating a respiration calorimeter is high and there are few available, it is used only under carefully controlled experimental conditions. Fig. 5-2, *B,* shows subjects entering one of the few respiration calorimeters in the world. This one is located at The Pennsylvania State University.

A modification of the respiration chamber, the metabolic chamber, measures the heat given off by the subject with thermocouples and heat-exchange disks attached to the skin. Any changes in temperature are re-

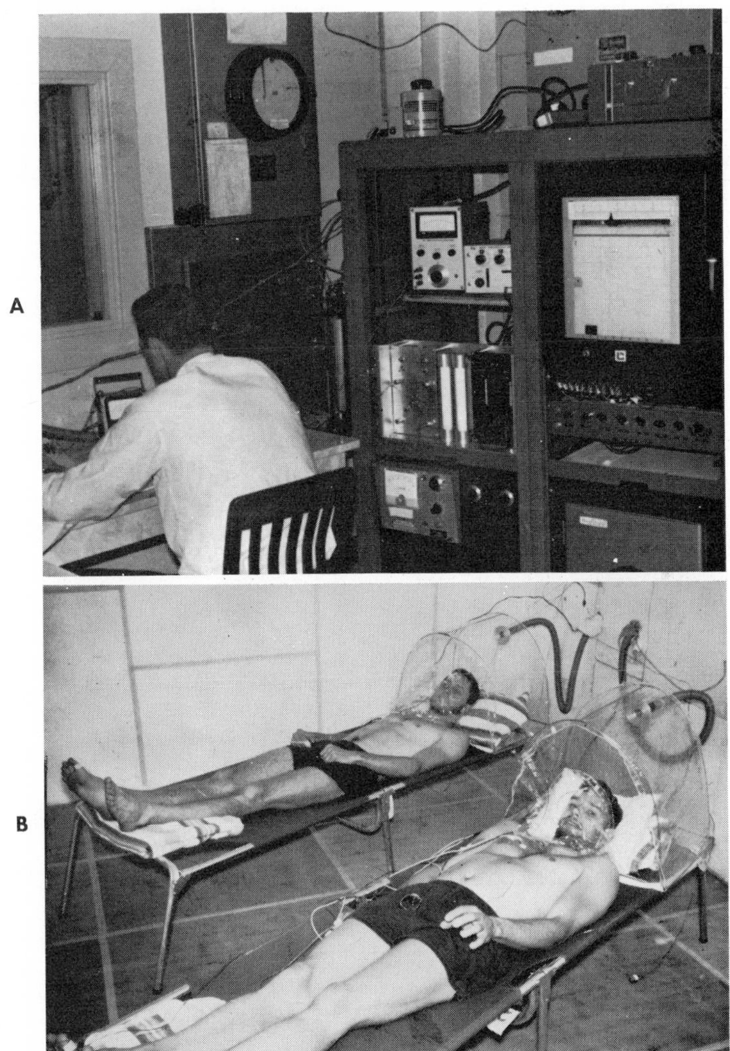

Fig. 5-3. A, Technician at control panel outside metabolic chamber at the Human Performance Laboratory at The Pennsylvania State University, monitoring the oxygen consumption, carbon dioxide excretion, and changes in surface temperature of subject in chamber behind glass. **B,** Subjects in metabolic chamber in which the effect of environmental temperature changes on oxygen consumption and skin temperature are being determined. (Courtesy Public Relations Department, The Pennsylvania State University.)

corded on instruments outside the chamber. Both chambers can be used for determinations of basal energy needs, and they also permit the assessment of energy costs of activities that can be performed in a limited space. Fig. 5-3 illustrates the use of one type of metabolic chamber.

Indirect calorimetry. Indirect calorimetry is a much simpler method; the basal metabolic energy needs are determined by measuring oxygen consumption. For many years the Benedict Roth respiration apparatus was the standard machine used for this purpose. It is a closed-circuit system in which the subject receives oxygen only from a measured source of pure oxygen and exhales into a container in which the carbon dioxide and water are removed and the remaining oxygen recirculated. By measuring the difference in the oxygen level in the container before and after the standard 6-minute test, the amount of oxygen consumed can be readily calculated. Since the use of 1 liter of oxygen represents 4.82 kcal when the RQ is 0.82, it is possible to calculate the caloric equivalent of a known volume of oxygen.

It has been shown that open-circuit indirect calorimetry is equally valid. It involves the use of room air and a determination of the amount of oxygen removed from it during a test period. A measured amount of atmospheric air is breathed from a closed container and the exhalations are passed over soda lime, removing the carbon dioxide. The amount of carbon dioxide removed from the exhaled air is readily measured by weighing

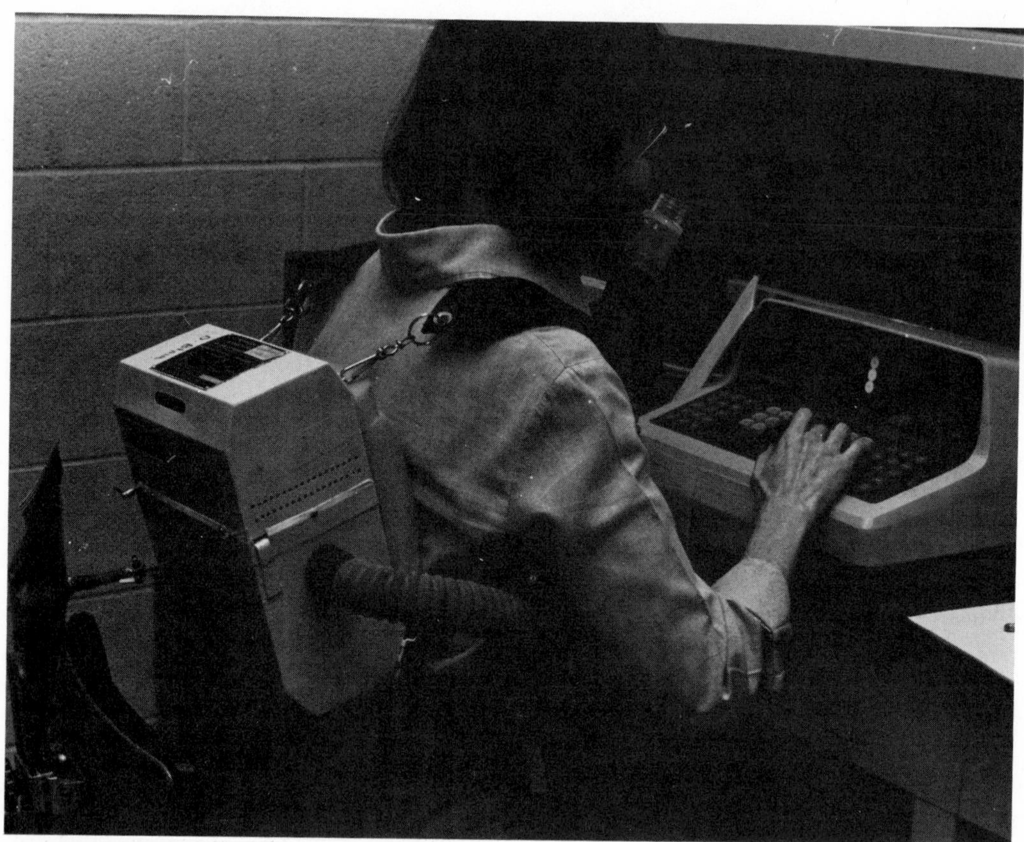

Fig. 5-4. Open-circuit respirometer used to measure energy expenditure. (Courtesy Dr. E. R. Buskirk, Noll Human Performance Laboratory, University Park, Pa.)

the soda lime container before and after the test. These values can be used along with oxygen figures as a basis for standardized calculations of the energy used during that period. The open-circuit method is less costly and reduces the possibility of stimulation in metabolism from the use of pure oxygen. A typical instrument used in this test is shown in Fig. 5-4.

A determination of the energy required for basal metabolism must be made when the subject is using a minimum amount of energy for respiration, circulation, glandular activity, and maintenance of musculе tonus. Virtually no energy should be expended for nonvital functions such as digestion and absorption or increased muscle tonus arising from fear, anger, or other emotional states, from an uncomfortable physical environment, or from physical exertion. To achieve these conditions, the subject must be lying down, preferably immediately after a night's sleep, awake, in an environment of a comfortable temperature and humidity, in a postabsorptive state (at least 12 hours since the last meal), and at a normal body temperature. Since cellular respiration in skeletal muscle accounts for the greatest part of the oxygen consumption, it is especially important that the subject's muscles be relaxed. In some tests drugs have been used to reduce mental and muscular tension to a minimum.

The protein-bound iodine test is discussed in Chapter 8.

Estimation of basal energy needs

Basal metabolic tests have yielded sufficient data so that it is now possible to predict basal energy needs from body measurements of height and weight. For persons of average body build an estimate based on body weight—1 kcal/kg of body weight/hr—gives a value that corresponds well to those obtained on actual basal metabolic tests. But when this formula is applied to persons whose body build deviates from standards either in the direction of obesity or leanness, it becomes increasingly less satisfactory, apparently because the simple measurement of body weight does not reflect body composition.

Estimates of heat production, or basal energy needs, based on body surface area have been considered more reliable than those based on body weight, since they reflect differences in body composition, a function of weight in relation to height. For instance, an individual who is 1.8 m tall and weighs 67 kg will have a greater surface area, higher proportion of muscle than fat, and a larger amount of more active tissue, than will a 67 kg person who is 1.5 m tall. Surface area can be determined by use of nomograms, or charts from which surface area is determined by the point that a line drawn from height to weight on vertical columns intersects one with the corresponding surface area measurement. Tables indicating energy costs per square meter of surface area per hour in relation to age and sex are available.

The best estimates of basal metabolism, however, can be obtained by using the metabolic, or fat-free, size of the body, sometimes called biological body weight or metabolic body size. It is obtained by calculating the body weight in kilograms to the 0.75 or ¾ power. This metabolic body size for different body weights is given in Table 5-7. Basal energy needs are then calculated as 70 × (weight in $kg^{3/4}$), a value that applies not only to persons of quite different body builds but to almost all animals as well. This amounts to about 1.3 kcal/kg of fat-free weight/hr.

For most individuals actual basal metabolic needs fall with ±10% of the predicted values. When deviations occur, they are expressed as a percentage of predicted values, such as −12 or 12% below. Deviations may be attributed to one or more of the factors discussed subsequently. The resting metabolic rate (RMR) is now being used in estimating total energy requirements. It is generally about 10% above basal energy requirements, since it includes needs for all functions except external work, and represents the minimum energy needs during sleep and for the other periods when there is no exercise and no exposure to cold. It also

Table 5-7. Body weights in pounds, kilograms (kg), and kg$^{3/4}$*

	Lb	kg	kg$^{3/4}$
Infants	8.8	4	2.8
	15.4	7	4.3
	19.8	9	5.2
Children	26.4	12	6.1
	30.8	14	7.2
	35.2	16	8.0
	41.8	19	9.1
	50.6	23	10.5
	61.6	28	12.2
Males	77	35	14.4
	94.6	43	16.8
	129.8	59	21.3
	147.4	67	23.4
	154	70	24.2
Females	96.8	44	17.1
	104.4	52	19.4
	118.0	54	19.9
	127.6	58	21.0

*From Food and Nutrition Board: Recommended dietary allowances, ed. 7, Publication No. 1694, Washington, D.C., 1968, National Academy of Sciences–National Research Council.

includes energy costs from the specific dynamic effects of meals.

Factors affecting basal energy needs

Body composition. Although all body tissue is metabolically active, undergoing constant breakdown and repair and participating in vital functions, some tissues experience these changes much more rapidly than others. Muscle, brain, glands, and organs such as the liver are relatively active, consuming large amounts of oxygen per unit of weight in their normal functioning. On the other hand, bones and adipose tissue, although far from static, are relatively inactive tissues and require less oxygen per unit of weight to maintain normal metabolic activity.

If we compare two men each weighing 67 kg, one 1.5 m tall and the other 1.8 m tall, we are comparing a short stocky person with less muscle and more fat to a tall thin person whose weight is composed or relatively less fat and more muscle. The taller person would have a higher basal metabolic energy need, since the muscle tissue requires more oxygen than the adipose tissue per unit of weight. The difference in body composition is reflected in body surface area measurements or in the measurement of metabolic body size—weight in kg$^{3/4}$.

Body condition. A person in good physical condition usually has developed more muscle tissue than one who has not had as much exercise. If we compare two men both 81 kg in weight and both 1.7 m tall, one of whom is an accountant in an essentially sedentary occupation and the other a stockman in an occupation calling for physical activity, we would find that the weight of the sedentary individual represents less muscle and more fat than that of the physically active person. The former's basal metabolic needs would be lower.

Sex. Differences in body composition between a male and a female of the same age, height, and weight have been documented. Women characteristically develop more adipose tissue and less musculature than men. This is reflected in a basal metabolic rate for women 5% lower than that for men.

Hormone secretions. The secretions of the ductless glands, the thyroid and the adrenals, have more influence on basal energy needs than any single factor. In fact, any marked deviation from predicted basal energy needs is usually attributed to oversecretion or undersecretion of the thyroid gland, although this is not the only possible cause. **Hypothyroidism,** with a below-normal secretion of thyroxin, the iodine-containing hormone of the thyroid gland, may be reflected in a basal metabolic rate depressed as much as 30%. This means that the energy required for vital body functions is 30% below that for a person with normal thyroid activity. This depressed secretion can be counteracted by the careful use of thyroxin available only under medical supervision. Conversely, hyperthyroidism, characterized by an above-normal thyroxin secretion, may elevate basal metabolism as much as 50% to 75%. Under such conditions a person would have an energy requirement for basal needs alone 50% to 75% above predicted levels. Hyperthyroidism is more difficult to correct. Drugs that interfere with the production of thyroxin or the uptake of iodine, an essential part of the thyroxin hormone, are very difficult to control. Partial thyroidectomy (removal of part of the thyroid gland) or a limitation in iodine intake to reduce the amount of raw material available for thyroxin synthesis are alternative approaches to treatment. Deviations in basal metabolism from predicted levels in excess of 20% are almost always indicative of disturbed thyroid function. The very high basal metabolic rate due to excess thyroxin production is characteristic of **exophthalmic goiter** or **hyperthyroidism.**

The secretion of the adrenal gland, epinephrine, is produced in response to intense emotional stimuli, such as anger or fear. The stimulation in metabolism resulting as more epinephrine is produced is intense but of short duration, with metabolic activity returning to normal levels in 2 or 3 hours.

Sleep. Measurements and estimates of basal metabolism are made assuming the individual is awake but muscularly and emotionally relaxed. During basal metabolic tests involving the use of special breathing apparatus, it is essential that the subject be awake. During sleep an individual achieves a greater degree of muscular and emotional relaxation, which causes a further drop in energy needs to 10% below waking levels. However, the energy savings due to relaxation in sleep may be counteracted by the energy expended in motion during sleep so that the values obtained from basal metabolism may well be applicable over a 24-hour period.

Age. The basal metabolic rate per unit of body surface changes with age. The rate is high at birth, increases up to 2 years of age, and then declines gradually except for a rise at puberty. In males it varies from 53 kcal/m^2/hr at 6 years to 41 kcal at 20 years to 34 kcal at 60 years of age. There is a similar gradual decline in basal energy needs for females except during pregnancy and lactation. The decline in energy needs between ages 25 and 35 amounts to only 35 kcal/day for a 60 kg person, but between ages 25 and 55 it amounts to a more significant decline of 145 kcal. A person who fails to adjust his caloric intake to reflect this reduced basal energy need will experience a slow and insidious gain in weight.

Pregnancy. During the last trimester of pregnancy there is an increase in basal metabolism of 20% above normal values. This may represent either the high metabolic activity of the fetus and placenta associated with growth or an increase in metabolic activity in maternal tissues.

Previous nutritional status. Basal energy studies in persons who have been subjected to prolonged caloric undernutrition yield values up to 20% below predicted levels. This apparently reflects the body's efforts to conserve energy when calories are restricted. Although the effect of starvation is not a significant factor among Americans, it may explain the ability of persons in areas of chronic undernutrition to maintain their body weight on caloric intakes that are lower than predicted needs.

Body temperature. Since heat acts as a catalyst to almost all chemical reactions, it is not surprising to find that basal metabolism increases with an increase in body temperature. A rise of 1° F in body temperature leads to an average increase of 7% in basal metabolism (13% per 1° C), although increases as high as 15% have been observed. It is obvious then that a person with a fever has a greater need for energy than normal.

Environmental temperature. Lowest basal metabolism readings are obtained at an environmental temperature of 26° C or 78° F with higher readings being reported at both higher and lower environmental temperatures. A temporary decrease in environmental temperature, not compensated for by additional clothing, will cause shivering and a temporary increase in basal metabolic needs as the body attempts to produce more heat to counteract the effect of low temperatures.

In summary, then, although many factors, such as body composition, hormonal secretions, sleep, and previous nutritional status, may influence basal metabolism, for most persons an accurate estimate of needs can be made on the basis of body surface area or metabolic body size. For many individuals,

Table 5-8. Energy cost of activities exclusive of basal metabolism and influence of food*

Activity	kcal/kg/hr	Activity	kcal/kg/hr
Bicycling (century run)	7.6	Piano playing (Liszt's "Tarantella")	2.0
Bicycling (moderate speed)	2.5	Reading aloud	0.4
Bookbinding	0.8	Rowing in race	16.0
Boxing	11.4	Running	7.0
Carpentry (heavy)	2.3	Sawing wood	5.7
Cello playing	1.3	Sewing, hand	0.4
Crocheting	0.4	Sewing, foot-driven machine	0.6
Dancing, foxtrot	3.8	Sewing, motor-driven machine	0.4
Dancing, waltz	3.0	Shoemaking	1.0
Dishwashing	1.0	Singing in a loud voice	0.8
Dressing and undressing	0.7	Sitting quietly	0.4
Driving automobile	0.9	Skating	3.5
Eating	0.4	Standing at attention	0.6
Fencing	7.3	Standing relaxed	0.5
Horseback riding, walk	1.4	Stone masonry	4.7
Horseback riding, trot	4.3	Sweeping with broom, bare floor	1.4
Horseback riding, gallop	6.7	Sweeping with carpet sweeper	1.6
Ironing (5-pound iron)	1.0	Sweeping with vacuum sweeper	2.7
Knitting sweater	0.7	Swimming (2 mph)	7.9
Laundry, light	1.3	Tailoring	0.9
Lying still, awake	0.1	Typewriting rapidly	1.0
Organ playing (30% to 40% of energy hand work)	1.5	Violin playing	0.6
Painting furniture	1.5	Walking (3 mph)	2.0
Paring potatoes	0.6	Walking rapidly (4 mph)	3.4
Playing ping-pong	4.4	Walking at high speed (5.3 mph)	9.3
Piano playing (Mendelssohn's songs)	0.8	Walking downstairs	†
Piano playing (Beethoven's "Apassionata")	1.4	Walking upstairs	‡
		Washing floors	1.2
		Writing	0.4

*From Taylor, C. M., and McLeod, G.: Rose's laboratory handbook for dietetics, ed. 5, New York, 1949, The Macmillan Co., p. 18.

†Allow 0.012 kcal/kg for an ordinary staircase with 15 steps without regard to time.

‡Allow 0.036 kcal/kg for an ordinary staircase with 15 steps without regard to time.

especially those engaged in sedentary or moderate activity, basal energy needs account for 50% to 70% of their total caloric requirements.

Activity

Energy costs of activities have been determined by measuring consumption of oxygen from an air bag carried on the back while a subject performs a specific activity (Fig. 5-4). Recently small transistorized units carried in the pocket have been used to record heart rate during various activities. These heart rates have been found to vary directly with oxygen consumption. This technique represents a greatly simplified approach to measuring energy costs of activity.

The energy required for physical activity above the needs for basal metabolism is a function of the type of activity, the duration of activity, and the size of the individual performing it. Since 75% of the energy expended in most activities is involved in moving the body, it has become common practice to base estimates of energy needs for activity on body weight. As a result, tables such as Table 5-8, giving the energy costs of various activities per unit of body weight, have traditionally been used in estimating energy costs. Although some workers have published tables of energy costs of activity based on the type of activity irrespective of the size of the individual (Table 5-9), most workers continue to base estimates on body weights (Table 5-8). Tables of energy costs represent our best available estimates, but before consulting them, one should be aware of the limitations in their usefulness.

First, individuals differ in the efficiency with which they perform a particular activity, either through training or innate ability, so that the actual costs may vary considerably from estimates. Calculations show that a 90 kg person will use 50% more energy in performing the same task for the same length of time than will a 60 kg person. The former's needs would be calculated to be same as a 60 kg person carrying a 30 kg (66-pound) load on his back. In neither case would the differences be this great because of efficiencies affected by the distribution of the weight over the whole body.

Second, while many activities that involve moving the body, such as walking, swimming, or bicycling, require an energy expenditure proportional to body size, others, such as knitting, writing, and piano playing, will likely not vary with body size but rather will require about the same amount of energy for all persons.

Third, since many of the values were based on a very few determinations or were extrapolated from data on similar activities, they should not be considered precise. For that reason the student is cautioned against attributing too much precision to calculations based on them. It should also be recognized that the energy expenditure attributable to the activity itself may represent a very small portion of the total energy used during the time, since a much larger portion may be used for basal metabolism. For instance, the energy cost for eating is 0.4 kcal while that for basal needs at the same time is 1.0 kcal/kg/hr. Energy costs of an activity such as swimming will be estimated accurately only if the person is swimming, not just in the water, for the entire time period.

Once the limitations are recognized, tables of energy costs can be useful tools in nutrition studies.

Many persons are dismayed to find the relatively small amount of energy expended in performing various activities. For instance, the energy cost of walking 3 miles in 1 hour is only 2 kcal/kg of body weight above maintenance requirements. Thus a 60 kg person will expend only an additional 120 kcal over basal needs or 96 kcal more than when sitting. Even 1 hour of skating will involve only 210 kcal for this same person, while bicycling requires 150 kcal over basal. The Canadian dietary standard suggests that light work, such as cooking, typing, or golfing, involves an average expenditure of 1.1 kcal/min, while moderately heavy work, such as gardening, carpentry, and swimming, costs 2.6 kcal/min. Heavy work, such as farm chores,

Table 5-9. Energy expenditure in specified activities, including basal energy and the effect of food*

	kcal/min	kJ/min
Man (65 kg)		
In bed asleep or resting	1.08	4.52
Sitting quietly	1.39	5.82
Standing quietly	1.75	7.32
Walking 3 miles/hr (4.9 km/hr)	3.7	15.5
Walking 3 miles/hr (4.9 km/hr) with a 10 kg load	4.0	16.7
Office work (sedentary)	1.8	7.5
Domestic work		
Cooking	2.1	8.8
Light cleaning	3.1	13.0
Moderate cleaning (polishing, window cleaning, chopping firewood, etc.)	4.3	18.0
Light industry		
Printing	2.3	9.6
Tailoring	2.9	12.1
Shoemaking	3.0	12.6
Garage work (repairs)	4.1	17.2
Carpentry	4.0	16.7
Electrical industry	3.6	15.1
Machine tool industry	3.6	15.1
Chemical industry	4.0	16.7
Laboratory work	2.3	9.6
Transport		
Driving lorry	1.6	6.7
Building industry		
Labouring	6.0	25.1
Bricklaying	3.8	15.9
Joinery	3.7	15.5
Decorating	3.2	13.4
Farming (European, mechanized)		
Driving tractor	2.4	10.0
Forking	7.8	32.6
Loading sacks	5.4	22.6
Feeding animals	4.1	17.2
Repairing fences	5.7	23.8
Forestry		
In nursery	4.1	17.2
Planting	4.7	19.7
Felling with axe	8.6	36.0
Trimming	8.4	35.1
Sawing—hand saw	8.6	36.0
power saw	4.8	20.1
Mining		
Working with pick	6.9	28.9
Shoveling	6.5	27.2
Erecting roof supports	5.6	23.4

*From Durnin, J. V. G. A., and Passmore, R.: Energy, work and leisure, London, 1967, as reported in Energy and protein requirements, FAO/WHO Technical Report No. 522, 1973.

Table 5-9. Energy expenditure in specified activities, including basal energy and effect of food—cont'd

	kcal/min	kJ/min
Man—cont'd		
Armed services		
Cleaning kit	2.7	11.3
Drill	3.7	15.5
Route marching	5.1	21.3
Assault course	5.8	24.3
Jungle march	6.5	27.2
Jungle patrol	4.0	16.7
Recreations		
Sedentary	2.5	10.5
Light (billiards, bowls, cricket, golf, sailing, etc.)	2.5-5.0	10.5-21.0
Moderate (canoeing, dancing, horse-riding, swimming, tennis, etc.)	5.0-7.5	21.0-31.5
Heavy (athletics, football, rowing, etc.)	7.5+	31.5
Woman (55 kg)		
In bed asleep or resting	0.90	3.77
Sitting quietly	1.15	4.82
Standing quietly	1.37	5.73
Walking 3 miles/hr (4.9 km/hr)	3.0	12.6
Walking 3 miles/hr (4.9 km/hr) with 10 kg load	3.4	14.2
Office work (sedentary)	1.6	6.7
Domestic work		
Cooking	1.7	7.1
Light cleaning	2.5	10.5
Moderate cleaning (polishing, window cleaning, chopping firewood, etc.)	3.5	14.6
Light industry		
Bakery work	2.3	9.6
Brewery work	2.7	10.0
Chemical industry	2.7	11.3
Electrical industry	1.9	7.9
Furnishing industry	3.1	13.0
Laundry work	3.2	13.4
Machine tool industry	2.5	10.5
Farming		
Threshing (Europe)	3.8-5.5	15.9-23.0
Binding sheaves (Europe)	3.0-4.9	12.6-20.5
Hoeing (Africa)	4.8-6.8	20.1-28.4
Recreations		
Sedentary	2.0	8.3
Light (billiards, bowls, cricket, golf, sailing, etc.)	2.0-4.0	8.3-16.7
Moderate (canoeing, dancing, horse-riding, swimming, tennis, etc.)	4.0-6.0	16.7-25.1
Heavy (athletics, football, rowing, etc.)	6.0+	25+

lumbering, or mountain climbing, costs 2.8 kcal/min and very strenuous work, 5.1 kcal. These are proposed in addition to the needs for basal metabolism independent of body size.

Disillusioning as it may be, it has been established that mental effort causes virtually no increase in energy requirements. The brain, however, even in the resting state uses up 20% of basal energy calories. The 3% to 4% increase sometimes recorded during mental work has been attributed to the increase in muscle tension rather than to brain cell activity.

The decline in caloric requirements for activity that occurs with aging is proportionately greater than the decline in basal energy requirements. It is estimated to decrease at 3%, 6%, 13.5%, 21%, and 31% of that at age 25 with each succeeding decade but obviously will vary with the individual and can be attributed to changing life-styles.

To estimate the caloric needs of an individual for activity, it is necessary to keep an accurate record of all activity for a specified period of not less than 24 hours. Activities are then grouped to determine the total time spent in a particular activity such as those given in Table 5-8. If a particular activity is not listed, a reasonable estimate can be made by classifying it with one involving a similar degree of muscular exertion. With the energy cost factors from Table 5-8 and the record of the time involved, caloric costs per kilogram for each activity can be calculated. The day's energy requirement for all activity is obtained by multiplying the total by the body weight in kilograms. The number of kilocalories needed for a day's activity vary greatly from one individual to another, but for a sedentary or moderately active person usually amount to 30% to 50% of basal energy needs. For active and extremely active persons, the needs for activity may equal or exceed basal energy needs.

The Canadian dietary standards use the values 23 kcal per unit of metabolic body size to estimate the energy cost of activity for a sedentary person, with an additional 23 kcal for light activity, 55 for moderate activity, such as gardening or making furniture, 80 for heavy activity, such as farm chores, lumbering, or active participation in competitive sports, and 107 for extremely heavy activity. These values are over and above the needs for basal metabolism. The Food and Nutrition Board suggests energy costs of 1.5, 2.9, 4.3, and 8.4 kcal/kg/hr for very light, light, moderate, and heavy activity for men. Comparable values for women are 1.3, 2.6, 4.1, and 8.0.

Effect of food

It has been recognized for some time that the ingestion of food causes an increase in energy needs not only for the digestion, absorption, and transportation of the nutrients but also as a result of a general stimulation in metabolism that follows the ingestion of food. This effect has been referred to as the *specific dynamic effect* of food, the calorigenic effect, and more recently as *dietary thermogenesis*. Experiments designed to determine the exact magnitude of this effect have produced no conclusive results. It is still generally believed that the effect of food amounts to about 10% of the total energy needed for basal metabolism and activity.

In some cases in which protein provides almost all of the calories, this stimulation in metabolism is even higher. The stimulating effect of the high-protein diet has been attributed to the action of some amino acids, the heat resulting from the deamination of protein, the synthesis and excretion of urea, or to the higher energy cost of releasing ATP from protein compared to glucose or fatty acids.

Since the effect of food represents an increase in energy expenditure, it must be added to the basal and activity needs in calculating the total energy requirements. If this factor were not considered, a diet providing only sufficient calories for basal and activity needs would lead to an inadequate caloric intake with subsequent weight loss.

Estimation of total energy needs

The method used to estimate total caloric needs depends on the degree of accuracy desired. Energy cost of activity can be measured by both direct and indirect calorimetry. The former is too costly to be practical and would permit study only of activities that can be performed in a limited amount of space. Indirect calorimetry also has limited usefulness. The subject must wear a mask and breathe from a monitored source of air in an apparatus worn on his back. More recently, the continuous monitoring of heart rate by a small electronic device has provided a method of assessing energy expenditure that does not interfere with the usual level of activity. The relationship between heart rate and oxygen consumption must first be determined for each subject.

Factorial method. More easily used and less expensive, but also less precise, is the *factorial method* of estimating caloric needs. It involves estimating basal metabolism from body weight or metabolic body size, activity needs from accurate activity records, and an additional factor for the effect of food. The factorial method for estimating caloric needs is outlined in Table 5-10 using either body

Table 5-10. Factorial estimation of total energy needs

Subject: Male Weight: 60 kg Height: 1.73 m Age: 35

Basal metabolism: 1 kcal/kg/hr

$1 \text{ kcal} \times 60 \times 24 = 1440 \text{ kcal}$

or

$70^* (\text{Wt}_{\text{kg}})^{3/4} = 70 \times 60^{3/4} = 70 \times 22 = 1540 \text{ kcal}$

Activity needs

Activity	Time (hr)	Energy cost: kcal/kg/hr	Energy cost: kcal/kg
Dressing	1.5	0.7	1.05
Sitting	6.0	0.4	2.4
Skating	0.5	3.5	1.7
Walking (3 mph)	2.0	2.0	4.0
Standing relaxed	1.0	0.5	0.5
Typing	4.0	1.0	4.0
Sleeping	8.0	—	—
Playing piano	0.5	2.0	1.0
Walking upstairs	4 flights	0.036†	0.14
Walking downstairs	4 flights	0.012†	0.04
			14.83

Energy cost of activity = 14.83 kcal × 60	889
Total energy cost for basal metabolism and activity	2329 or 2429
Specific dynamic effect (10%)	232 or 242
Total energy requirement	2561 or 2671

*70 is the caloric cost for basal metabolism per unit of metabolic size.

†Allowance per kilogram for ordinary staircase (15 steps) regardless of time.

weight or metabolic body size for estimating basal needs.

Rule of thumb. For a quick estimate of energy needs the U.S. Department of Agriculture suggests multiplying body weight in pounds by a factor determined by the type of physical activity in which the individual is engaged. These factors for women are 14 for sedentary, 18 for moderately active, and 22 for very active. For men, values of 16, 21, and 26 are used. The limitation in this method lies in the subjective judgment of the nature of a person's physical activity. The most common error is to confuse the terms *busy* and *active.* A typical college student may be very busy but very sedentary at the same time. A busy but sedentary person needs fewer calories than a physically active individual.

Canadian and FAO dietary standards. The Canadian dietary standards estimate total energy needs on the basis of metabolic body size. Their formula is 116 (weight in $kg^{3/4}$). The Food and Agricultural Organization of the United Nations (FAO) has also developed a formula from which they believe one can arrive at a figure representing the energy requirement for moderately active adults, ages 20 to 39. For men they use weight in kilograms × 46, and for women weight in kilograms × 40. They recommend adjusting these values by an index of 0.9 for light activity, 1.17 for very active persons, and 1.34 for exceptionally high activity. To account for age, factors of 0.95 for 44 to 49 years, 0.9 for 50 to 59 years, 0.8 for 60 to 69 years, and 0.7 for persons over 70 years are suggested.

Other methods. Durnin and Passmore have proposed a table of values for estimating energy expenditure of adults based solely on the activity and the time, exclusive of rest periods, involved without reference to body weight. They recognize that weight as well as training and efficiency of movement contribute to individual variability but feel that the use of this table (Table 5-9) provides reasonable estimates of energy costs.

NRC recommended allowances. The Food and Nutrition Board of the National Research Council has established the caloric allowances they believe provide sufficient energy to maintain body weight or rate of growth at levels most conducive to well-being for practically all healthy individuals. Recognizing the many factors that influence caloric requirements, they have expressed their recommendations for a reference man or woman and have then indicated a basis for making adjustments.*

As reference individuals they chose 22-year-old persons living in a temperate zone with a mean environmental temperature of 20° C (68° F), who are engaged in occupations requiring moderate physical activity. For the reference woman weighing 58 kg (128 pounds) allowance is set at 2100 kcal and for the 70 kg (154-pound) man at 2700 kcal, but values are planned primarily for assessing needs of groups rather than individuals.

Adjustment for age. Increasing age is accompanied by decreased caloric expenditures because of the progressive reduction in basal metabolic rate and the usual decline in physical activity. Although there may be wide individual differences in the extent to which needs for activity are reduced with age, a decrease in total caloric needs of 5% between 22 and 35, 3% per decade between ages 35 and 55, 5% per decade from ages 55 to 75, and 7% after age 75 is proposed as typical. Thus, at age 85 requirements are approximately 70% of those at age 20.

Adjustment for body size. A basic principle in physics states that the amount of work required to move a mass is proportional to the size of the mass. In assessing human energy requirements it is assumed that 75% of the energy expenditure is directly proportional to body size and 25% is independent of body weight. On this basis, formulas for caloric needs of RMR† + 13 (weight in kilograms) for men and RMR + 7 (weight in kilograms) for women 22 years of age have been developed

*Because of individual differences in need, energy allowances may be eliminated from 1979 RDA.

†Resting metabolic rate is basal metabolic rate plus 10%.

6

Mineral elements

At the turn of the century it was recognized that the noncombustible portion of food—the mineral ash—was essential for life. It was several decades, however, before the complexity of this small but important component was recognized. With increasingly sophisticated and sensitive analytical techniques, scientists are still finding new elements that appear to be essential in human nutrition. There is also growing recognition that the balance among the mineral elements of this ash is an important factor in human health.

It had been demonstrated by the middle of the nineteenth century that a mixture of the known constituents of food—the proximate principles, carbohydrate, fat, protein, and water—was not capable of supporting growth. Scientists then looked to the noncombustible fraction, or the mineral ash, of food for a clue to the growth-promoting properties of natural food absent in the synthetic mixtures. Because the mineral residue, when added to a synthetic diet, did not by itself stimulate growth or prevent death in animals, it did not arouse much interest at that time. Since the 1880s, however, the ash has been shown to be composed of many mineral elements that play vital roles in human nutrition. Research on the roles of these elements is commanding the attention of a large and growing number of scientists.

DISTRIBUTION

Ninety-six percent of body weight is made up of the elements carbon, hydrogen, and oxygen (the components of carbohydrate, fat, and protein), nitrogen of protein, and water. The remaining 4%, about 2.7 kg in the adult male, is made up of as many as sixty different mineral elements. Approximately twenty-one of these have been proved essential in human nutrition. However, an analysis of mineral ash reveals an additional twenty or thirty that may be present because of contamination from the environment or because they have an unestablished but essential role.

ESSENTIAL ELEMENTS

An essential mineral is one that must be provided in the diet and performs functions vital to life, growth, and reproduction. Its absence results in impaired cellular and physiological function and often causes illness. A mineral is considered essential if (1) there is a demonstrable improvement in the health and growth of an animal on addition of the mineral to a purified diet, (2) the removal of the element from a diet containing adequate but not toxic amounts of all other dietary essentials results in clear-cut evidence of deficiency symptoms, and (3) a low intake can be correlated with subnormal levels of the element in blood or other tissues. Even when it is determined that an element is a part of an essential enzyme system, it must still be established that the reaction cannot be catalyzed by some other means. The presence of a reserve, or pool, of the element that is influenced by hormones or other substances is considered further evidence of a biological role, as is its presence in fetal tissue.

The list of essential elements continues to

Table 6-1. Classification of mineral elements

Classification	Elements	Percent of body weight
Macronutrient elements essential for human nutrition (> 0.005% body weight or 50 ppm)	Calcium	1.5-2.2
	Phosphorus	0.8-1.2
	Potassium	0.35
	Sulfur	0.25
	Sodium	0.15
	Chlorine	0.15
	Magnesium	0.05
Micronutrient elements essential for human nutrition (< 0.005% body weight)	Iron (17th century)*	0.004
	Zinc (1934)	0.002
	Selenium (1957)	0.0003
	Manganese (1931)	0.0002
	Copper (1928)	0.00015
	Iodine (1850)	0.00004
	Molybdenum (1953)	
	Cobalt (1935)	
	Chromium (1959)	
	Fluorine (1972)	
	Silicon (1972)	
	Vanadium (1971)	
	Nickel (1971)	
	Tin (1970)	
Elements for which essentiality has not yet been established, although there is evidence of their participation in certain biological reactions	Barium	
	Arsenic	
	Bromine	
	Strontium	
	Cadmium	
Elements found in the body but for which no metabolic role has been elucidated	Gold	
	Silver	
	Aluminum	
	Mercury	
	Bismuth	
	Gallium	
	Lead	
	Antimony	
	Boron	
	Lithium	
	+20 others	

*Dates in parentheses identify year in which essentiality was established.

grow with the development of sensitive techniques for studying the metabolism of these elements. For instance, chromium and silicon, which were considered contaminants several years ago, are now known to perform essential functions.

The body has mechanisms for controlling the absorption of essential elements and can also regulate the amount retained by excreting them in the urine, bile, and other intestinal secretions. There appears to be no comparable mechanism for controlling the absorption and excretion of nonessential elements. Thus, at the same time that nutritionists want food processing methods to be controlled so that essential elements are not removed from the food supply, they want to ensure that these processes do not result in excessively high amounts of other elements. For some elements the body can tolerate a wide range of intakes; for others, such as iron, copper, selenium, cobalt, and zinc, the intake must be kept within a very narrow range to prevent diseases due to either a deficiency or an excess of the element.

Minerals occur in the body in several forms—in combination with organic compounds, such as the iron in hemoglobin, with other inorganic ions, such as the calcium phosphate of bone, or as free ionized ions, such as the calcium in the intercellular fluids.

Progressive refinement in the analytical techniques used to study mineral metabolism—atomic absorption spectroscopy, neutron activation, colorimetry, the use of radioactive isotopes, and flame photometry—has made possible studies of progressively smaller concentrations of minerals to as little as 1 ppb (part per billion) or nanogram amounts in biological tissue. This has helped elucidate roles for mineral elements that have established their essential nature.

CLASSIFICATION

The essential mineral elements are often grouped as macronutrient and micronutrient elements. Macronutrient elements are present in relatively high amounts in animal tissue; micronutrient elements, or trace elements, are present as less than 0.005% (50 ppm) of the body weight (Table 6-1). It is entirely possible that with the increasingly sensitive analytical techniques available, biological roles will be discovered for at least some of the elements now considered either contaminants or toxic in relatively small amounts.

Although certain elements listed are also vital for plant growth, some, such as cobalt, sodium, and iodine, are not essential. They do, however, occur in foods of plant origin, which become a major source of these elements in the human diet. The amount of a mineral element in an animal tissue reflects the amount present in the plants it eats, and this in turn is a function of the amount of the element present in the soil and the extent to which the plant is able to concentrate it.

Foods of animal origin, in which minerals are present in a higher concentration and in a form more readily absorbed, may be superior to plants as sources of minerals. In plants, trace elements are found in the highest concentration in the outer layers and the germ, both of which are removed with extensive milling. Since the phytic acid and fiber in the outer husk tends to interfere with absorption, the loss is not as great as would be expected when the whole grain is not consumed.

GENERAL FUNCTIONS OF MINERAL ELEMENTS

The complex interrelationships that exist among the mineral elements as they function in the body necessitate a discussion of the general functions of minerals. Some elements have been studied extensively and will be discussed individually. The ones on which the most information has been acquired are those most likely to be lacking in the diet and for which specific deficiency conditions have been recognized. This does not minimize the role of the other mineral elements; they are equally important in maintaining normal body function.

Maintenance of acid-base balance. The tremendous number of biological reactions that take place within the cell can occur only in a very specific internal environment. Just as the enzymes of the digestive juices require a certain acidity or alkalinity, the enzymes that work within the cells can perform their task only when the fluid in the cells is essentially neutral in reaction. Anything that changes the pH of the cell environment may inactivate or change the level of activity of the cellular enzymes. Inactivation of the enzymes results in cellular starvation and death of the cell. Among the many factors influencing the reaction of the cell is the nature of the minerals available to it from the extracellular fluids.

Some minerals are acid forming because they form an acid medium in solution. These elements are chlorine, sulfur, and phosphorus. The acid-forming properties of a food are determined by the components of its noncombustible mineral ash and not by the presence of organic acids such as citric acid found in fruits. These may give food an acid taste but are generally oxidized to form carbon dioxide, water, and energy. Thus they do not influence acid-base balance. The acid-forming elements predominate in foods containing protein, such as meat, fish, poultry, eggs, and cereal products. These are designated as acid-forming foods.

Mineral elements that are basic, or alkaline, in solution are calcium, sodium, potassium, and magnesium. These elements tend to predominate in fruits and vegetables. Thus even citrus fruits, such as grapefruit, lemons, and oranges, which have an acid taste because of the presence of organic acids, are base forming, since their organic acids are metabolized and the mineral ash predominates in potentially basic or alkaline elements. A few foods, such as cranberries, rhubarb, cocoa, and tea, are acid forming because they contain acids the body cannot metabolize—benzoic, oxalic, and tannic acid. The acid potential of these foods overbalances the alkalinity of their base-forming mineral elements.

Neither milk, which contains an internal balance of base-forming calcium and acid-forming phosphorus, nor pure carbohydrates and fats, which contain virtually no minerals, influence the acid-base balance of the body.

Most mixed diets contain a slight surplus of acid-forming mineral elements, but the body has mechanisms by which it can counteract this potential acidity. The excretion of carbon dioxide through the lungs and of a slightly acid urine through the kidneys rids the body of excess acid and helps to maintain the neutrality of its internal environment. However, strict vegetarians who consume a diet with a predominantly basic residue, persons on an extreme high-protein diet with a predominantly acid residue in the mineral ash, and those who make frequent use of sodium-containing antacids, which create an alkaline balance, may tax the body's ability to maintain neutrality.

The maintenance of body neutrality is so important to the survival of body cells that there are several ways in which an excess acid or base can be neutralized. The blood contains buffers, such as carbonates, phosphates, and proteins, which can react with either excess acid or excess base to prevent them from influencing the reaction of the blood and hence that of the fluids bathing the tissues. Bone can also release phosphates to act as buffers to remove hydrogen ions from surrounding fluids. If the buffers cannot neutralize the excess base, a reserve acid (carbonic acid) can be formed from the carbon dioxide and water of metabolism, which are normally excreted. This acid then neutralizes excess alkali-forming elements and prevents alkalosis. Similarly, excess acid may be neutralized by a reserve base formed from the NH_2 from deamination of protein plus water. This prevents acidosis. With all these mechanisms for coping with a diet producing an excess of either base-forming or acid-forming elements, an upset in acid-base balance can seldom be caused by dietary factors alone. However, diets that have either a predominately acid or predominately alkaline ash may be prescribed in the treatment of certain conditions. Carbohydrate-free diets, frequently promoted for weight reduction, are potentially acid forming.

Catalysts for biological reactions. Mineral elements are catalysts for many biological reactions. As such they are not part of the initial compounds or the end products but must be present for the reaction to take place. Minerals that catalyze the action of many of the body's enzymes can serve as the vital link between an enzyme and its substrate. Sometimes they are part of an enzyme known as a "metalloenzyme"; often they act to maintain the structure of the enzyme; or they can combine with the end product to modify the rate of the reaction. They catalyze many of the separate steps involved in the catabolism of carbohydrate, fat, and protein to carbon dioxide, water, and energy and in the anabolism, or synthesis, of fat and protein. The synthesis of essential body compounds such as hemoglobin depends on the presence of several mineral elements other than those that may become a part of the substance. In another example, the clotting of blood depends on the catalytic effect of calcium, but the clot does not contain calcium.

Fig. 6-1, which is by no means a complete tabulation, indicates the role of minerals in the metabolism of carbohydrate, fat, and protein in the body. It is obvious that many reactions are mineral dependent and that some of the elements listed are involved at several different stages.

The transport of substances across biological membranes, as in absorption of nutrients

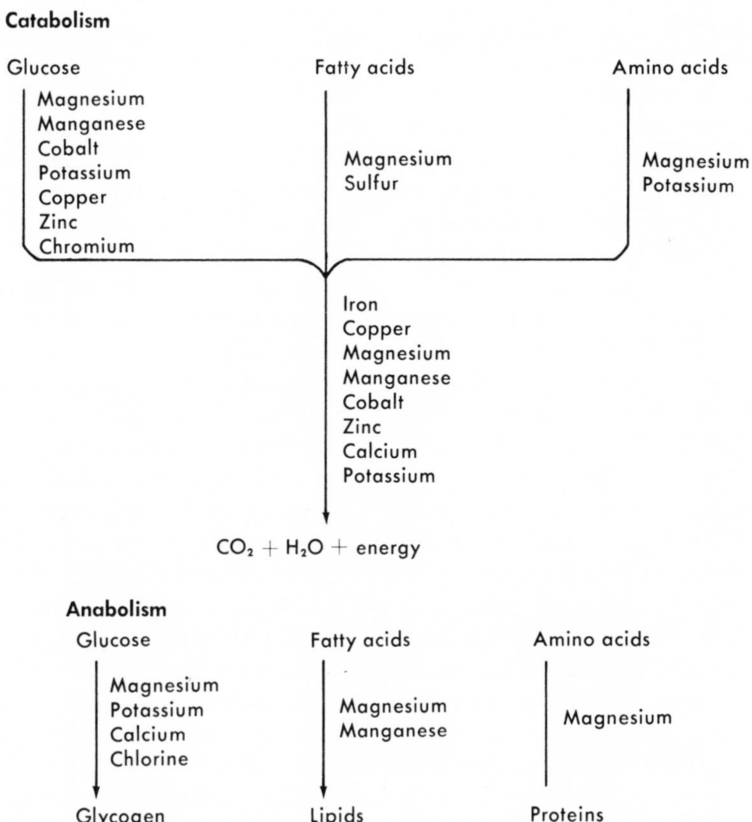

Fig. 6-1. Role of minerals in metabolism. Minerals act primarily as catalysts to enzyme action. Some function as essential parts of enzymes.

from the gastrointestinal tract or uptake of nutrients by the cell, is often a mineral-dependent reaction. For instance, calcium facilitates the absorption of cobalamin, or vitamin B_{12}, and magnesium and sodium facilitate the absorption of carbohydrate. Several digestive enzymes are activated by minerals, as in the case of activation of pancreatic lipase by calcium and magnesium. Chromium catalyzes the attachment of the hormone insulin to the cell wall. In many cases in which minerals act as catalysts it is possible to substitute one mineral for another, but the substitute is generally less effective.

Components of essential body compounds. Many of the hormones, enzymes, and other vital body compounds that are synthesized in the body and regulate its functioning contain minerals as integral parts of their structure. In the absence of the required mineral, the body will be unable to produce adequate amounts of the essential substance.

The production of thyroxin, which controls energy metabolism, depends on an adequate supply of iodine to the thyroid gland. The production and storage of insulin, which regulates carbohydrate metabolism, usually involves zinc. Hemoglobin, essential for the transport of oxygen to and carbon dioxide from the cells, is an iron-containing compound. Chlorine must be available for the production of the hydrochloric acid that is secreted into the stomach and creates the acid environment necessary for the action of digestive enzymes.

Minerals are an integral part of many enzymes in the body. These mineral-containing enzymes are sometimes designated as metalloenzymes, since if the metal is removed, the enzyme loses its effectiveness. To cite but a few examples: both copper and iron are part of the enzyme cytochrome oxidase involved in the release of energy; molybdenum is part of xanthine oxidase needed to release liver stores of iron for use by other tissues; and zinc is part of a protein-splitting enzyme, carboxypeptidase, secreted in the pancreatic juice to help digest protein.

In addition to the carbon, hydrogen, oxygen, and nitrogen that are part of the vitamins most essential for body functioning, some, such as thiamin with sulfur and cobalamin with cobalt, have minerals as integral parts of their structure.

Maintenance of water balance. Water, which comprises approximately 70% of the fat-free weight of the body and 60% of the total body weight, may be considered to be present in three "compartments" in the body, each separated from the other by a semipermeable membrane across which there is a free exchange of fluid. The compartmentalization is shown diagrammatically in Fig. 6-2. The intravascular compartment includes the fluid in all parts of the vascular system—arteries, veins, and capillaries. The walls of the vascular system separate the intravascular fluid from the intercellular, or extravascular, fluid that bathes the individual cells and tissues and provides the external environment from which the cells are nourished. The fluid or nutrients in the intercellular compartment must cross the membrane to enter the cell and become a source of nourishment. The intercellular compartment acts as a buffer area; its volume will adjust to prevent changes in the volume of either the intravascular or intracellular fluid. The term transcellular fluid has been applied to a fourth compartment—fluids such as the synovial fluid lubricating joints and the vitreous humor of the eyeball—but this represents a very samll portion of total body water and is not usually involved in fluid shifts.

The movement of fluid from one compartment to another is governed to a large extent by the concentration of minerals on either side of the membrane separating the compartments. Mineral elements in body fluids occur primarily as salts. However, these salts in solution dissociate into their component ions, one of which will have a positive charge and the other a negative charge. These charged ions are known as electrolytes and account for much of the osmotic pressure of the body fluids. As the concentration of electrolytes increases, the osmotic pressure

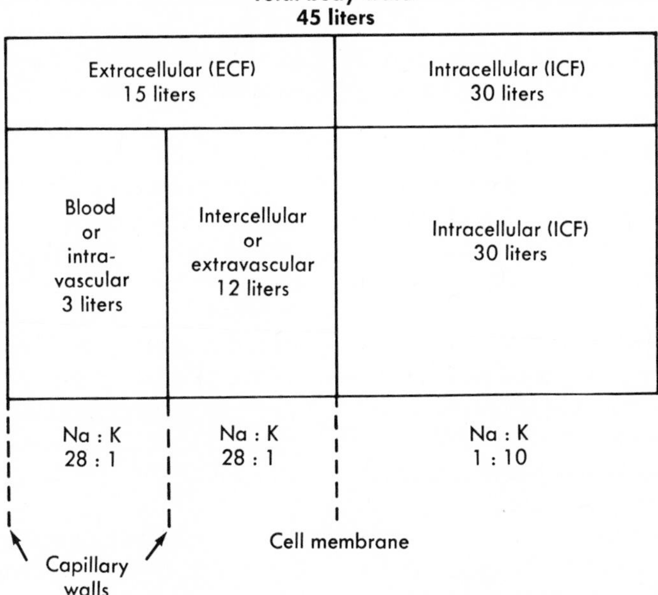

Fig. 6-2. Diagrammatic representation of three major fluid compartments of the body. A fourth division, the transcellular fluid compartment, is a subdivision of extracellular fluid and includes water in collagen, connective tissue, bone, synovial fluid, vitreous humor, and digestive secretions.

increases. Whenever the osmotic pressure of the fluid on one side of a semipermeable membrane becomes higher than that on the other, fluid is drawn from the side of the membrane with the lower concentration of electrolytes to that with the higher concentration until the osmotic pressure on each side is equalized. When the same number of molecules and ions per exact volume of fluid is present on either side of the membrane, the osmotic pressures are the same and the amount of fluid on either side remains relatively constant.

Under most circumstances the body is able to prevent a shift in electrolyte concentrations so that there is no marked change in water balance among compartments. However, in some cases the homeostatic mechanisms of the body are taxed, resulting in a noticeable change in salt and hence electrolyte concentration in one of the fluid compartments. For instance, when the sodium intake exceeds the ability of the kidneys to excrete it, the level of sodium in the blood and in the intercellular fluid increases. Since the cells cannot function in such a hypertonic environment, a series of changes occurs to restore normal electrolyte levels. The thirst center is stimulated to increase the water intake, and at the same time fluid is withdrawn from the cells to dilute the intercellular fluid. This causes an increase in the volume of blood and intercellular fluid. The former results in an elevated blood pressure and the latter in the accumulation of fluid in the intercellular spaces to produce a soft, spongy, edematous tissue. Conversely, if sodium levels fall, there is a contraction of blood volume, a drop in blood pressure, a decrease in intercellular fluid, and fluid is restored to the cells.

When sodium is lost from the extracellular compartment, as it may be following excessive perspiration, potassium is pumped out of the cells to replace the lost sodium and to establish electrolyte balance. At the same time some water leaves the cells. Loss of water and potassium from the cell produces the symptoms of weakness so common in heat prostration.

The mineral elements within each compartment vary, sodium being present in higher concentrations outside the cell and potassium within the cell. Chlorine, which crosses the cell membrane easily, quickly establishes an equilibrium between the cell contents and the extracellular fluid, thus helping to minimize fluid shifts.

Transmission of nerve impulses. Minerals play a vital role in the mechanism by which nerve impulses are conducted along nerve fibers. A nerve impulse is essentially an electrical stimulus that passes through a nerve fiber. During excitation, or stimulation, of nerve fibers the permeability of the membrane of nerve cells changes, allowing sodium to enter the cell more freely and potassium to leave. This creates a temporary change in the electrical charge on the membrane. This charge, in turn, changes the permeability of the next segment of the membrane, which changes the electrical charge again, and the message is passed down the fiber. It is, then, the exchange of sodium and potassium ions across the cell membrane that is responsible for the transmission of a nerve impulse. Anything that changes the mineral concentration of the fluids bathing nerve cells may interfere with their ability to transmit nerve impulses.

The transmission of a nerve impulse from one nerve cell to another is dependent on the presence of acetylcholine at the junction of the two fibers. The release of this compound is regulated by calcium.

Regulation of contractility of muscles. The muscles of the body are constantly bathed in a fluid—the interstitial fluid. For normal function of these muscles in contraction and relaxation, the composition of the interstitial fluid must represent a certain balance between elements that tend to stimulate muscular contraction, such as calcium, and those that exert a relaxing effect, such as sodium, potassium, and magnesium. This balance is steadfastly maintained under normal conditions. An upset in this balance is usually caused by the effect of the parathyroid hormone on the calcium levels. A drop in calcium levels without a concurrent decrease in the levels of the relaxing elements leads to a state of spasmodic contractions known as tetany. Conversely, an increase in calcium levels relative to the relaxing elements produces a state of tonic contractions known as calcium rigor.

During muscular contraction there is a release of potassium from the muscle cell, which is subsequently restored during the resting period. This seems to indicate an essential role for potassium in muscular contraction.

Growth of body tissue. Some mineral elements such as calcium and phosphorus occur in large concentration in bones and teeth and can rightly be considered as building constituents of body tissue. An absence of these raw materials will be reflected as stunted growth or in the development of tissue of inferior quality. Indirectly, other minerals are involved in the growth process through their catalytic action on many reactions involved in the synthesis of body compounds or in the release of energy.

In the following chapters the macronutrients will be discussed first, after which a detailed presentation of the information available on the most extensively studied microelements will be given.

BIBLIOGRAPHY

Camien, M. N., Simmons, D. H., and Gonick, H. C.: Critical reappraisal of "acid-base" balance, Am. J. Clin. Nutr. **22:**786, 1969.

Chesters, J. K.: Trace elements: Adventitious yet essential dietary ingredients, Proc. Nutr. Soc. **35:**15, 1976.

Food and Nutrition Board: Soil fertility and the nutritive value of crops, Nutr. Rev. **34:**316, 1977.

Hoekstra, W. G.: Recent observations on mineral interrelationships, Part I, Fed. Proc. **23:**1068, 1964.

Maugh, T. H.: Trace elements: a growing appreciation of their effects in man, Science **181:**253, 1973.

McCall, J. T., et al.: Implications of trace metals in human diseases, Fed. Proc. **30:**1011, 1971.

Miller, W. J., and Neathery, M. W.: Newly recognized

trace mineral elements and their role in animal nutrition, Bioscience **27:**674, 1977.

Reinhold, J. G.: Trace elements—a selected survey, Clin. Chem. **21:**476, 1975.

Schwarz, K.: Recent dietary trace element research as exemplified by tin, fluorine, and silicon, Fed. Proc. **33:**1748, 1974.

Ulmer, D. D.: Metals—from privation to pollution, Fed. Proc. **32:**1758, 1973.

Underwood, E. J.: Trace elements in human and animal nutrition, ed. 3, New York, 1971, Academic Press, Inc.

Wacker, W. E. C.: Metalloenzymes, Fed. Proc. **29:**1462, 1970.

7

Macronutrient elements

Study of the seven macronutrient elements is directed toward evaluation of the need to balance the intake of various pairs. Proper calcium/phosphorus ratios are critical for bone growth and stability, calcium/magnesium in control of neuromuscular functioning, and sodium/potassium relationships for maintenance of fluid balance. These elements occur in a limited number of foods; thus the need for a wide variety of foods in a nutritionally balanced diet is reemphasized.

CALCIUM

Calcium is a relatively inert inorganic mineral element usually associated with bone and tooth formation. The use of the term calcification to describe the process by which these structures assume strength and rigidity has tended to reinforce the importance of calcium in bone formation. Calcium does play an important role in this process, but it is only one of many nutrients necessary for effective bone and tooth formation. In addition, the role of calcium in bone and tooth formation is only one of its vital biological functions. Although many writers have chosen to discuss calcium and phosphorus together because of their intimate relationship in bone and tooth development, their unique and independent roles will be emphasized here by discussing them separately.

Distribution

In the adult body between 1.5% and 2% of the weight is calcium. Of this 850 to 1400 g, 99% is in the hard tissues—bones and teeth. The remaining 10 g are widely distributed. In the blood, calcium levels are maintained within a very narrow range of 9 to 11 mg/dl. About a third of the 5 to 6 g of calcium in blood is loosely bound to protein, and 5% is found as calcium citrate, bicarbonate, and phosphate, all of which are physiologically inert complexes. The remaining two thirds of blood plasma calcium is present in a physiologically active ionized form. Approximately 1 g of calcium is found in the extracellulur fluids and 4 to 5 g in soft tissues, where it is vital to normal cell functioning. Much of the calcium in soft tissue is concentrated in muscle, although the membrane and cytoplasm of every cell contain some. The roles of calcium in extracellular fluids and soft tissue are so important that it will be mobilized from reserves in the bones to maintain a functional level. In addition, when intakes are low, the body can adapt by absorbing a higher proportion of dietary calcium and excreting less. These adaptations reduce the effect of intakes below recommended levels.

Functions

Although specific deficiency symptoms can rarely be attributed to a lack of dietary calcium, scientists do have substantial evidence of several specific roles on the mineral in body metabolism.

Bone formation. Early in fetal development a strong but flexible protein matrix, or pattern, for bone begins to be formed. It bears the same general shape as the mature bone but lacks strength and rigidity. The **matrix** remains rather flexible until after birth, possibly to facilitate the birth process.

This matrix, which accounts for 30% of the bone, is composed of fibers of the protein **collagen** embedded in a gelatinous *ground substance* composed of a carbohydrate, mucopolysaccharide, and a glycoprotein. Shortly after birth this matrix gains strength and rigidity, primarily as a result of the deposition and growth of mineral crystals within the matrix in a process known as **ossification** or **calcification.** These crystals are either calcium phosphate or a combination of calcium phosphate and calcium hydroxide, which makes up a physiologically stable compound called hydroxyapatite ($Ca_{10}[PO_4]_6OH_2$). Since calcium and phosphorus are the predominant mineral elements in these compounds, an adequate supply of both must be present before they can precipitate from the fluids surrounding the bone matrix to grow in the bone tissue. This deposition of calcium compounds in the mature collagen matrix appears to begin eight to ten days after the collagen has been laid down by the osteocytes, or living bone cells. The transfer of calcium and phosphates into the matrix is facilitated by the mitochondria of these cells. Fig. 7-1 is a diagrammatic representation of a bone.

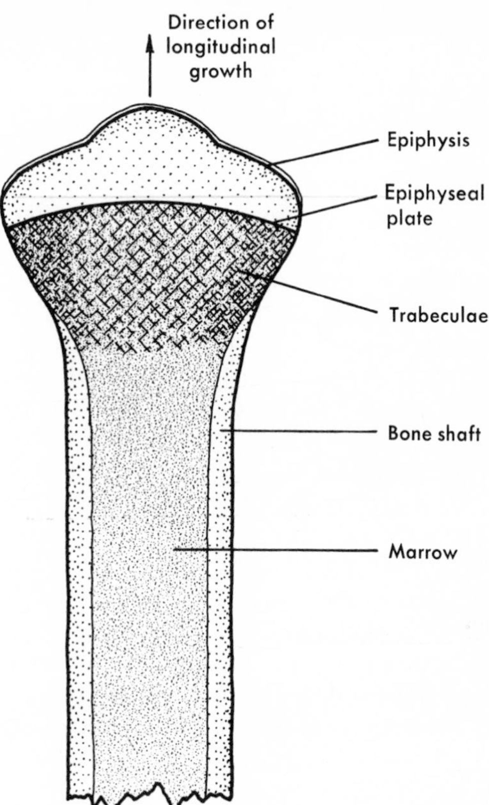

Fig. 7-1. Diagrammatic representation of bone structure.

The flexibility of the bone matrix can be readily demonstrated by soaking a bone in strong acid to leach these calcium compounds out of the bone (reverse calcification). The remaining collagen structure is the original "mold" of the bone.

Calcification apparently occurs when the product of the level of calcium and inorganic phosphorus in the blood and extracellular fluids exceeds 30 (that is, milligrams of phosphorus × milligrams of calcium per deciliter of blood > 30).

However, since normal blood serum is usually supersaturated with both calcium and phosphorus, it appears that some other factor is necessary to facilitate the calcification process.

The shaft of the long bones calcifies to become rigid and strong, capable of supporting the weight of the body before the infant begins to walk, sometimes as early as 8 months of age. Throughout the entire growth process there is a constant lengthening of this bone shaft as the formation of new collagen matrix is followed by its calcification. The ends and inside the shaft of the long bones contain a porous crystalline structure, known as the *trabeculae.* The trabeculae, which come in direct contact with the blood vessels in the bone marrow, provide a liberal supply of calcium that can be readily mobilized to maintain the critical blood calcium levels when dietary levels drop. Only when calcium reserves in the trabeculae have been depleted will decalcification of other parts of the bones occur. Under these conditions the pelvis and the spine are the first to release calcium.

During growth and throughout adult life there is a constant remodeling and reshaping of the bone in response to changing stresses from the weight of the developing body. This constant deposition and resorption of bone is the result of the activity of cells on the bone surface that act alternately as osteoblasts (bone-forming cells) and osteoclasts (bone-destroying cells). Once the osteoclasts have caused the destruction of the matrix and the resorption of the calcium phosphate crystals, these same cells act as osteoblasts to produce a new collagen mold that will be slightly different from the original. New crystals then grow in this mold to restore strength to the bone. The old collagen mold is degraded.

In an adult 20% of bone calcium is resorbed and replaced each year; thus every five years the calcium in the bone has been completely replaced. Approximately 600 to 700 mg of calcium are deposited each day in newly formed adult bone, replacing what has been resorbed. Knowledge of this dynamic, or changing, state of bone metabolism came only with the availability of radioactive isotopes of calcium that could be traced in their path through the body. About a third of the calcium in adult bone appears to be in equilibrium with that in the extracellular fluids; the rest is in a more stable complex.

The amount of calcium needed to meet demands for bone growth varies with the rate of skeletal development. The increase in calcium content of the body from 0.8% of body weight at birth (about 28 g) to 2% at maturity (about 1400 g) represents an average daily increment of 165 mg with a reported range of 70 to 400 mg, depending on the stage of bone growth. Maximum needs occur between 13 and 14 years of age, when the body acquires about 90 g of calcium a year, representing an increase of about 300 to 400 mg/day in body calcium. The rate at which body calcium accumulates with age is shown in Fig. 7-2. The need for calcium reflects growth in body height rather than weight.

In addition to calcium and phosphorus, vitamin A, magnesium, manganese, silicon,

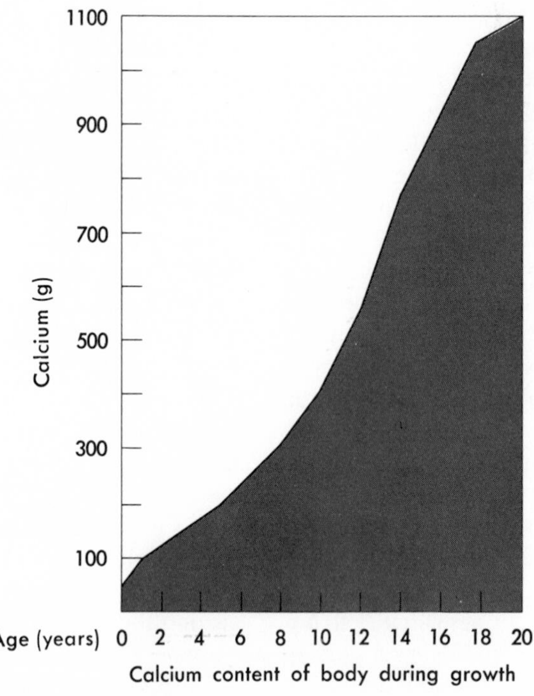

Fig. 7-2. Rate of accumulation of calcium in the body during growth.

copper, vitamin C, vitamin D, and protein all play a role in bone growth.

Tooth formation. The mineral that forms **dentin** and **enamel** is the same hydroxyapatite found in bones, but the crystals are more dense and the water content (<10%) lower. The protein in enamel is keratin, whereas that in dentin is collagen. In contrast to bones, which are relatively active metabolically, teeth undergo an almost imperceptible change once they have erupted into the oral cavity. The slow rate of exchange between the tooth calcium and that of the body is confined almost entirely to the dentin layer, although evidence is accumulating to suggest that there may be some microchemical reaction involving calcium exchange between the tooth enamel and saliva that is accentuated once tooth decay has been initiated.

Calcification of deciduous teeth begins by the twentieth week of fetal life, although it is completed only shortly before eruption into the oral cavity. Permanent teeth begin to calcify when the child is between 3 months and 3 years of age, whereas wisdom teeth, the last to erupt, may not begin to calcify until the eighth to tenth year of life. A full complement of adult teeth contains only 11 g of calcium, or about 1% of total body calcium.

Since teeth do not have the ability to repair themselves once they have erupted, there is no further need for a dietary source of calcium to maintain or repair teeth. A deficiency of calcium during the formative period for teeth may be reflected as a weakness in structure with increased susceptibility to tooth decay even though the teeth appear normal histologically. As in the case of bone, the integrity of tooth structure involves many nutrients in addition to calcium.

Growth. Although failure in growth is not a specific response to a dietary calcium deficiency, the observation that some persons raised on a diet traditionally low in calcium are frequently shorter than persons of the same race raised in a part of the world where the diet is adequate in calcium has led to the suggestion that calcium is necessary for normal growth. Since diets low in calcium also are frequently low in protein and since protein is a specific growth factor, it is difficult to argue that a lack of calcium is a primary cause of growth failure, although it may be a contributing factor.

Blood-clotting. The role of calcium in the blood-clotting mechanism is one of the more clearly understood of its functions. Once cells have been injured, ionized calcium, representing over half the total blood calcium, stimulates the release of a phospholipid, thromboplastin, from the blood platelets. Thromboplastin in turn catalyzes the conver-

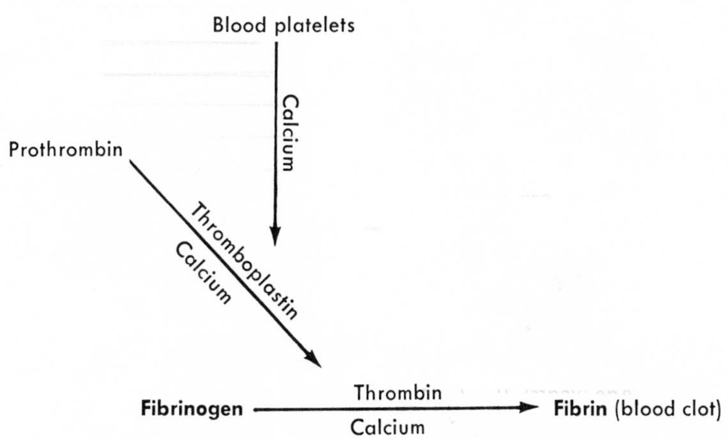

Fig. 7-3. Schematic representation of blood-clotting mechanism.

sion of prothrombin, a normal blood constituent, to thrombin. Thrombin then aids in the polymerization of fibrinogen to fibrin, the clot. A schematic representation of the blood-clotting mechanism (Fig. 7-3) shows that calcium must be present at each step in the series of changes needed for the formation of the clot. Under normal conditions blood calcium levels are maintained at a level sufficiently high to facilitate the blood-clotting process; therefore an increase in dietary calcium will have little direct effect on blood-clotting time.

Catalyst for biological reactions. Calcium is vital to normal body functioning through its role as a catalyst in many biological reactions. The absorption of cobalamin (vitamin B_{12}) through the intestinal wall depends on calcium. The fat-splitting enzyme of pancreatic lipase is activated by calcium, as are many of the enzymes involved in the release of energy from carbohydrates, fat, and protein. The cells of the pancreas that secrete insulin must have calcium in the intercellular fluid before they can respond to the stimulation from glucose. In addition, the formation and breakdown of acetylcholine, the substance necessary for the transmission of an impulse from one nerve fiber to the next, is dependent on calcium. The level of calcium needed to facilitate these reactions will be maintained at the expense of skeletal calcium; therefore, as in blood-clotting, the level of dietary intake will not have a direct effect on these reactions.

Maintenance and function of cell membrane. Calcium occurs in the cell membrane closely bound to the phospholipid lecithin. Here it governs the permeability of the cell membrane to various nutrients and thus controls the uptake of nutrients by the cell.

Regulation of muscular contraction and transmission of nerve impulses. As discussed on p. 128, calcium acts to stimulate muscle contractions and to facilitate the transmission of nerve impulses.

Regulation of strontium uptake. With the increased amounts of strontium 90 in the environment as a result of radioactive fallout, the possible protective value of a high-calcium diet in preventing the uptake of strontium has received much attention. Although similar chemically, calcium and strontium behave differently physiologically. Uptake of strontium by the body is often undesirable, since it can replace calcium in bone formation, where, because of its long half-life, it may continue to cause radiation damage. Present evidence indicates that if sufficient calcium is available, the body will preferentially absorb calcium by a factor of 9:1, but if less calcium is available, strontium will be taken up and will become an undesirable substitute for calcium in many compounds. Additionally, absorbed strontium interferes with the conversion of vitamin D into the form in which it enhances calcium absorption. The body excretes strontium in preference to calcium in the urine, by a factor of 4:1 and preferentially transfers calcium to milk and across the placental barrier to the fetus. Thus, when dietary calcium is high, the body absorbs less strontium and excretes more, reducing the amount retained by the body compared to conditions of limited calcium intake. Recent evidence shows that calcium has a similar role in protecting against lead toxicity.

Absorption

In comparison with the rat, which absorbs dietary calcium efficiently, the human adult is normally very inefficient, absorbing a maximum of 30% to 50% under optimal conditions and greatest need. The amount of calcium absorbed varies inversely with the amount in the diet. At intakes of 400 mg or more about 25% of dietary calcium is absorbed. The percentage increases to 35% at intakes of 300 to 400 mg and is as high as 60% if less than 150 mg is ingested. For adults an intake in excess of 1000 mg/day may be needed to maintain calcium balance. Normally, an absorption of 20% to 30% of ingested calcium is considered good, and frequently it is as low as 10%. In growing children, however, up to 75% of dietary calcium can be absorbed.

Before absorption takes place, vitamin D must be available to stimulate the synthesis of the one or two calcium-binding proteins (CaBP) that facilitate the uptake of the nutrient.

Most of the absorption occurs in the upper three fourths of the small intestine, where the digestive mass is likely to be more acid. Before being absorbed, calcium must be separated from any complex in which it may occur in food and must be ionized. Calcium is absorbed primarily by active transport, an energy-requiring process in which calcium attaches to the calcium-binding protein, enters the cells of the intestinal wall, and is transported across the cell and released through the membrane on the other side of the cell into the blood. Occasionally it is absorbed by passive diffusion, in which absorption occurs when calcium goes from an area of high concentration (intestine) to one of lower concentration (the blood). Any dietary calcium that is unabsorbed passes on through the digestive tract and is excreted as exogenous fecal calcium, along with some endogenous calcium that is secreted into the gastrointestinal tract in digestive juices.

The efficiency with which calcium is absorbed is a function of many factors. Under any set of conditions there are wide individual differences in the efficiency of calcium absorption. In general, absorption declines with age.

Factors favoring calcium absorption

Vitamin D. The effectiveness of vitamin D in facilitating the uptake of calcium from the intestine has been recognized since the early 1920s, but only recently has there been any evidence about its mode of operation. It is now established that a derivative of vitamin D formed in the kidneys catalyzes the synthesis of a protein carrier in the mucosal cells of the intestinal wall. Calcium then attaches to this carrier, specific for calcium, and is transported across the cells of the intestinal membrane to the blood. Glucocorticoids secreted by the adrenal gland and strontium interfere with conversion of vitamin D to a biologically active form, which results in depressed calcium absorption. When vitamin D is present, calcium is absorbed throughout a greater length of the intestine than when it is absent; thus more calcium will be absorbed before the food moves on to the colon, where no absorption occurs.

Acidity of digestive mass. Calcium is more soluble in acid and hence is more readily absorbed from an acid than from an alkaline medium. Since calcium is absorbed primarily from the small intestine, in which the contents must be rendered slightly alkaline before the intestinal enzymes can function, anything that increases the acidity of the digestive mass entering from the stomach and prolongs the time before the acid is neutralized should increase the possibility of calcium absorption. Hydrochloric acid normally secreted in the stomach is responsible for the acidity of the contents of the digestive tract as it enters the small intestine. When hydrochloric acid secretion is reduced, as it often is in old age, calcium absorption may be depressed. This may be partially compensated for by an increased intake of foods rich in ascorbic acid, which helps keep calcium ionized. The increase in calcium absorption noted on diets high in protein has been attributed by some to the action of the amino acids in forming a soluble complex with calcium to facilitate its absorption or prevent its precipitation as an insoluble complex. Although we have no explanation of why it is effective, there is experimental evidence to show that a high intake of the amino acid lysine will increase calcium absorption as much as 50%.

Lactose. There is ample evidence that the absorption of calcium is improved in the presence of the disaccharide lactose, with reports of increases ranging from 15% to 50%. Attempts to explain this effect on the basis of changes in the growth of microorganisms in the lower gastrointestinal tract, its slower rate of absorption, or changes in the acidity of intestinal contents as a result of the fermentation of lactose to lactic acid have failed. It has been suggested that the beneficial effects are caused by the formation of a soluble sugar-calcium complex in the intestine that keeps the calcium in a form in which it can be transported to and possibly across the intestinal wall. This complex also prevents the precipitation of calcium as an insoluble and hence unabsorbable complex as the contents of the gastrointestinal tract change from acid to alkali in the intestine. A relatively high ratio of lactose to calcium is necessary to form the soluble complex. Other sugars, such as the 5-carbon monosaccharide ribose and the 6-carbon monosaccharide fructose, also enhance calcium absorption, but lactose is the most effective. The benefits of obtaining calcium from milk, a food also high in lactose, are obvious.

Calcium/phosphorus ratio. The relationship between calcium and phosphorus levels in the diet plays an important role in the absorption of both. A dietary ratio of 1 part calcium to 1 part phosphorus promotes the highest level of absorption. A decreased Ca/P ratio is unlikely to occur on a normal diet unless large amounts of carbonated beverages with added phosphate are consumed. Because of the low intake of milk and the high intake of protein-rich foods and carbonated beverages, the current American diet has a calcium to phosphorus ratio of 1:4. For infants a Ca/P ratio of 1.3:1 is advised. Ca/P ratios below 1:2 and above 2:1 are not recommended.

Need for calcium. The extent to which calcium is absorbed may be influenced by the body's need for calcium. During pregnancy, lactation, and adolescence, when needs are greatest, absorption rates as high as 50% of ingested calcium have been observed. Similarly, on a consistently low calcium intake the body is able to compensate by absorbing a high percentage. When the demands for calcium are lower, a smaller portion of the ingested calcium will be absorbed. Frequently, smaller amounts are absorbed to a greater extent than are large doses.

Factors depressing calcium absorption

Oxalic acid. Oxalic acid is an organic acid found in several fruits and vegetables, such as rhubarb, spinach, chard, and beet greens. It combines in the digestive tract with calcium to form an insoluble complex, calcium oxalate, from which the calcium cannot be released for absorption. In most foods containing oxalic acid, there is also sufficient calcium present to tie up all the oxalic acid, leaving no surplus to bind calcium from other foods eaten at the same time. There is no evidence, for instance, to suggest that the oxalic acid of spinach will interfere with the absorption of the calcium in milk taken at the same time. The presence of 5% to 6% unbound oxalic acid in lower grades of cocoa led to reservations about the use of chocolate milk for children. Early misgivings were based on results of studies on rats, in which the addition of a low-grade cocoa to the diet caused as much as a 27% depression of calcium utilization. More recent work on college women at the University of Illinois showed that the women could tolerate a maximum of 28 g (1 oz) of cocoa without becoming nauseated. This did not cause any significant depression in calcium utilization on either a low or high calcium intake. Comparable studies have not been done on children, but one would expect results similar to those on women, indicating no reason for condemning chocolate milk on the basis of decreased calcium utilization.

Phytic acid. Another organic acid, phytic acid, found predominantly in the outer husks of cereals, lowers the utilization of calcium by binding it in an insoluble complex. Studies comparing the use of calcium in diets containing comparable amounts of farina, low in phytic acid, and oatmeal, high in phytic acid, showed up to 33% poorer utilization on the oatmeal diet. Humans lack the enzyme phytase to hydrolyze the phytate group and to release the calcium. Only in cases in which the consumption of calcium-poor foods is in conjunction with foods high in phytic acid would this inhibitory effect become a practical problem. There is evidence, too, of a rapid adaptation to diets high in phytic acid. This minimizes the depressing effect of phytic acid on calcium absorption.

Dietary protein. Contrary to earlier theories that a high-protein diet promoted a positive calcium balance and protected against osteoporosis, considerable evidence now exists that elevated protein intakes may increase the need for calcium.

Studies of adult males showed that an increase in the protein content of the diet had a limited effect in enhancing calcium absorption but had an unlimited effect on increasing calcium excretion in the urine. Thus a low-calcium, high-protein diet can result in a negative calcium balance. For instance, with a calcium intake of 500 mg and a protein intake of 95 g, levels that occur quite commonly in the United States, men showed a consistent loss of 59 mg/day, sufficient to reduce calcium reserves by 10% in ten years. There is now evidence of adaptation over time to high-protein intakes.

Fat. The evidence of the effect of fat on calcium absorption is somewhat contradictory. Some research indicates improved absorption resulting from the slower passage of food through the digestive tract.

The Food and Nutrition Board of the National Research Council concludes, however that in high-fat diets the formation of insoluble soaps of fatty acids and calcium results in steatorrhea (fatty stools) and a concurrent reduction in calcium absorption. Studies with infants showed that the use of whole cow's milk results in a lowering of calcium absorption. It appears that long-chain fatty acids depress calcium absorption while medium- and short-chain ones enhance it.

Emotional stability. The efficiency with which dietary calcium is absorbed can be influenced by the emotional stability of the individual. In one study a group of emotionally distressed young women were found to require a higher intake of calcium to maintain calcium balance than a comparable group of happy relaxed women. Another study of calcium metabolism of college men indicated a lowered absorption and increased excretion under conditions of stress such as examinations.

Increased gastrointestinal motility. Anything that increases the rate of passage of food through the intestinal tract decreases the absorption of calcium by reducing the time in which the contents of the intestinal tract are in contact with the intestinal wall. Laxatives and foods high in bulk may have this effect.

Lack of exercise. Persons who receive little exercise and bed-ridden persons who are essentially immobilized experience a loss of bone calcium of 0.5% of total stores a month and a reduced ability to replace it. This may be a cause, or at least a complicating factor, in the decalcification of bone so often experienced by older individuals. Evidence now indicates that it is the lack of weight on the legs rather than immobility per se that causes negative calcium balance during bed rest. Although the explanation of this is disputed, it is postulated that either the lack of weight on the legs or the decrease in vascularity accompanying the reduced muscle contraction leads to a decrease in stimulus for bone formation. Similarly, astronauts experienced negative calcium balance due to either weightlessness or immobility.

• • •

The factors affecting calcium absorption are summarized as follows:

- Factors favoring absorption
  - Adequate vitamin D
  - Acidity of digestive mass
  - Calcium/phosphorus ratios of 1:1
  - Parathyroid hormone
  - Lactose
  - Lysine
  - Growth hormone
  - Need for calcium
- Factors depressing absorption
  - Oxalic acid
  - Phytic acid
  - Intestinal alkalinity
  - Increased gastrointestinal motility
  - Emotional instability
  - Presence of dietary fat, especially long-chain fatty acids

Metabolism

Once calcium has been absorbed through the wall of the intestine, it is transported in the blood plasma and released to the fluids bathing the tissues of the body. From there the cells absorb whatever calcium is needed for their normal functioning and growth. Some calcium becomes a part of the digestive secretions in the stomach and intestine. Much of this calcium is reabsorbed, but endogenous fecal calcium amounts to about 130 mg, regardless of dietary intake. As the blood plasma is filtered through the kidneys, about 99% of the calcium (10 g/day) is resorbed. The remaining 1% excreted in the urine usually amounts to 100 to 175 mg/day.

As indicated earlier, most of the absorbed calcium is used in the calcification of bones to give strength and rigidity. The deposition of calcium in the bones is facilitated by a vitamin D metabolite and the enzyme phosphatase.

The calcium in the blood is in equilibrium with bone calcium, about a third of which is available to maintain adequate blood calcium levels (from 9 to 11 mg/dl). The parathyroid gland has a major role in maintaining these levels. If blood calcium levels fall below 7 mg/dl, the parathyroid secretes a parathyroid hormone, which has several regulatory functions. Within minutes the kidneys are stimulated to resorb more of the calcium that might normally be excreted in the urine; and within hours some of the exchangeable bone calcium has been released. Bone calcium is released as some of the carbohydrate of bone is metabolized to citrate and lactate, in which the calcium is soluble. This in turn increases the amount of calcium in the blood and the intercellular fluids to more normal levels. The parathyroid also stimulates a greater absorption of calcium from the gastrointestinal tract. This occurs after several days and results from stimula-

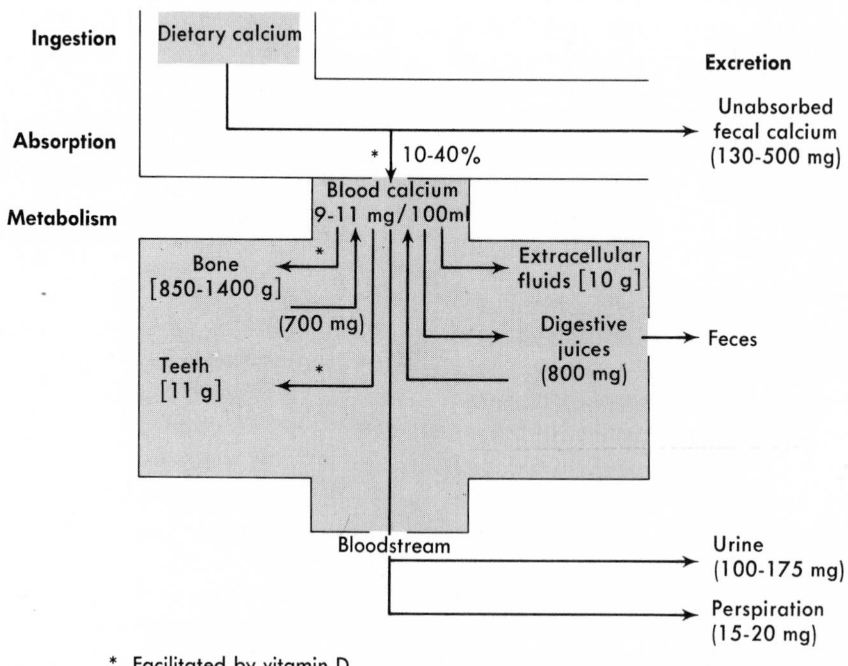

Fig. 7-4. Absorption and metabolism of calcium.

tion of the formation of vitamin D–active derivatives. When blood calcium levels return to normal, the secretion of the parathyroid gland also returns to normal.

Opposing the action of parathormone is a second hormone, **calcitonin** (formerly known as thyrocalcitonin), a polypeptide with thirty-two amino acids. It is formed in cells derived from a part of the thyroid gland. It is secreted when blood calcium levels become elevated and acts to lower both calcium and phosphate levels by inhibiting bone resorption. Thus the parathyroid gland, through its effect directly or indirectly on the secretion of these two hormones, is responsible for maintaining the level of calcium in the blood within the very narrow limits demanded by the body. Calcitonin is now available in synthetic form.

The regulatory effect of the parathyroid hormone is integrated with the action of the vitamin D derivative, which also stimulates the absorption of calcium from the intestinal tract, increases the retention of calcium by the kidneys, and allows the parathormone to act to release bone calcium to maintain blood levels. An excess of vitamin D may lead to decalcification of bone and an increased absorption of calcium from the gastrointestinal tract, with the resultant hypercalcemia.

The paths of the absorption and metabolism of calcium are shown schematically in Fig. 7-4.

Requirements

Controversy

In attempting to establish a recommended level for calcium intake, nutritionists have become involved in an intense controversy. Proponents of a lower allowance maintain that (1) there is no evidence of adverse effects from low intakes, (2) there is evidence that the body can adapt to low intakes, and (3) no clinical condition can be classified as a calcium deficiency. They maintain that conditions classified as calcium deficiency diseases are in reality the result of a vitamin D deficiency. On the other hand, those who believe that the present standard should be maintained are convinced that persons who have been on a restricted intake in their early years are more susceptible to osteoporosis, a debilitating bone disease, as they grow older, that there is no evidence of harm from intakes up to 2 g, that not all individuals are able to adapt to low intakes, and that the larger amounts are readily available in the food supply to provide these levels for the American population. Recent evidence of the effect of the high-protein content of the American diet in depressing calcium balance lends further support to maintaining a relatively high calcium intake.

Where less calcium is available in the food supply and the population has adapted to lower intakes, a lower dietary standard is justified. Low intakes are common in the tropics where available vitamin D helps to maximize absorption.

Calcium balance studies

Estimates of calcium needs have been based on the results of calcium balance studies in which the calcium content of the diet is compared to the amount of calcium excreted in the urine and feces. Urinary calcium represents that not resorbed by the kidneys; fecal calcium represents the endogenous calcium of the digestive secretions plus any unabsorbed dietary calcium. It has been assumed that when calcium intake exceeds calcium excretion, the body is in positive calcium balance and is storing calcium. When intake equals excretion, the body is in calcium equilibrium and is neither accumulating calcium or losing it. When excretion exceeds intake, the body is in negative calcium balance and is releasing more body calcium than it is replacing, resulting in a net loss from the body that reflects decalcification of bone tissue in most cases.

Limitations. There are several limitations to the use of calcium balance data. Measurement of intake seldom involves a determination of the calcium in water, which in tropical areas with a hard water supply is an appreciable amount. A considerable amount of calcium may be lost in perspiration and tears, which are not usually analyzed because techniques to do so have not been developed. Although under normal circumstances the loss of calcium in the sweat amounts to only 20 mg, for those living in the tropics this may amount to as much as 140 mg, and for those working hard at extremely high temperatures, as much as 1000 mg. This is sufficient to make a difference between positive and negative balance in many studies.

Since some persons adapt to a low calcium intake by conserving calcium either through a higher rate of absorption, a lower rate of excretion, or lessened secretions in the digestive juices, calcium balance data are meaningful only if there is information about dietary history. A person accustomed to an intake of 500 mg could maintain calcium balance of 400 mg more easily than could a person whose customary diet provided 1000 mg. The length of time required for adaptation varies. Some persons adapt within two months to a lower intake, others much more slowly, and some, never. In addition, it has been observed that in women a positive or negative balance that had prevailed for weeks could be reversed without any dietary change. Calcium balances have been reported to reflect the emotional state of the individual, becoming negative under stressful circumstances and positive again as stress passes.

Some evidence suggests that calcium balance data are useful only if considered in the light of phosphorus balance data. There is now good reason to believe that if calcium balance data were evaluated in relation to protein intake, the results of balance studies might not be so controversial or confusing.

In spite of the reservations that many

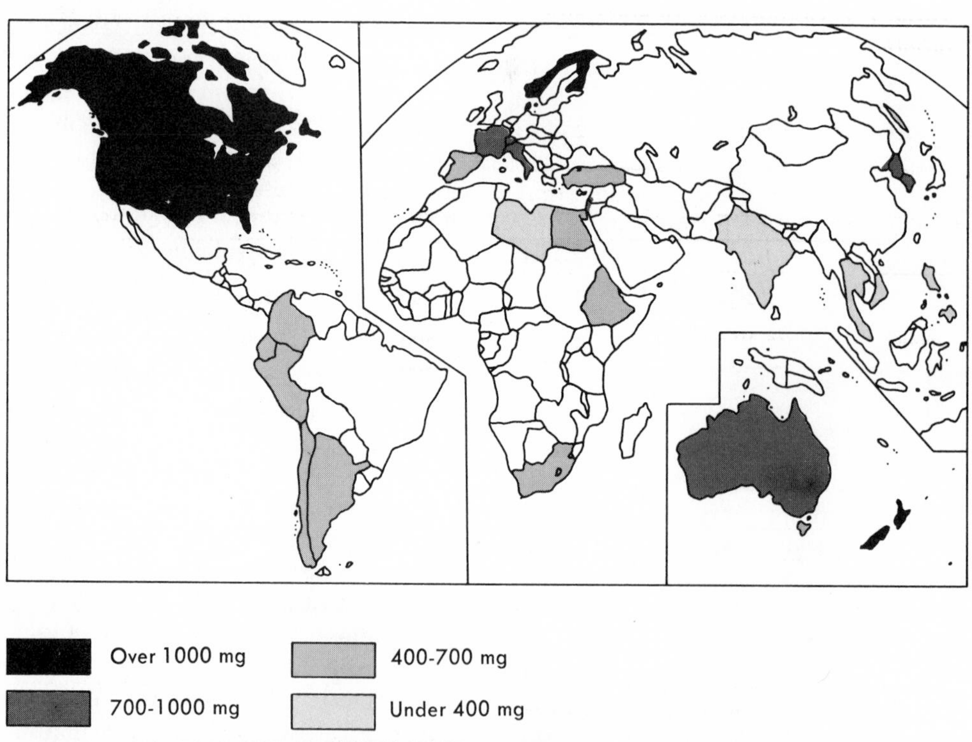

Fig. 7-5. Amounts of calcium per capita available in food supply in different parts of the world. (Based on data from Calcium requirements, Report of Joint FAO/WHO Expert Committee, WHO Techn. Rep. Ser. No. 230, Geneva, 1962.)

scientists have expressed about the validity of calcium balance studies, they remain a widely used criterion for establishing a standard for calcium intake. These data take into account previous calcium intake, adaptation, and physiological stress.

The use of ^{47}Ca, which has a relatively short half-life, has proved useful in studying calcium metabolism as a basis for estimating requirements.

Dietary allowances

The recommended allowances proposed by the Food and Nutrition Board of the National Research Council in 1974 have been set at a level the Council believes will meet the needs of essentially all healthy individuals and that can be readily achieved from the national food supply.

The Food and Agricultural Organization has released suggested practical calcium allowances. They believe these lower values represent a level that can more readily be achieved by a larger segment of the world's population, many of whom consume low amounts of calcium because of its limited availability in national food supplies. The FAO group, after evaluating all available data, suggested that there is no evidence that when vitamin D is adequate, there are any harmful effects from diets containing below 300 mg or more than 1000 mg of calcium/day. The wide variation in the calcium available in the diets of various countries is evident from Fig. 7-5.

A comparison of American, Canadian, British, and FAO recommendations listed in Table 7-1 shows that there is no general

Table 7-1. Comparison of standards for calcium intake for selected age and sex groups

	Age	Canadian dietary standard (1975)* (mg/day)	British† (mg/day)	NRC recommended dietary allowances (1979)‡ (mg/day)	FAO/WHO suggested practical allowances§ (mg/day)
Children	7-12 mo	500	600	540	500-600
	7-10 yr	500	700	800	600-700
Males	16-19 yr	1200	500	1200	500-600
	Adult	800	500	800	400-500
Females	16-19 yr	1000	600	1200	500-600
	Adult	700	500	800	400-500
	Pregnancy	1200	1200	1200	1000-1200
	Lactation	1200	1200	1200	1000-1200

*Dietary standards for Canada, Canadian Bulletin on Nutrition, vol. 6, No. 1, March, 1964; revised, 1975.

†Department of Health and Social Security: Recommended intakes of nutrients for the United Kingdom, Reports on Public Health and Medical Subjects, No. 120, London, 1969, Her Majesty's Stationery Office.

‡Food and Nutrition Board: Recommended dietary allowances, ed. 9, Washington, D.C., 1979, National Academy of Sciences–National Research Council.

§Calcium requirements, Report of Joint FAO/WHO Expert Committee, WHO Techn. Rep. Ser. No. 230, 1962.

agreement regarding the optimal level of calcium intake.

Infants. Relatively little data are available on calcium needs of infants. It is assumed that the breast-fed infant who receives about 60 mg/kg of body weight and retains two thirds of it receives adequate calcium. For the artifically fed infant who retains from 25% to 30% of the 170 mg/kg from cow's milk formula, an intake of 400 to 600 mg is recommended. If undiluted whole milk is fed, the amount of calcium absorbed is greatly reduced because of the relatively high fat content.

Children. The daily retention of 75 to 150 mg of calcium/day requires a daily intake of 800 mg of calcium for children 1 to 10 years of age. The rapidly growing skeleton of adolescents requires as much as 400 mg of calcium/day, calling for an intake of 1200 mg.

Adults. The recommended dietary allowances for the adult are based on the assumption that the mandatory endogenous calcium losses plus exogenous calcium losses and losses in sweat and in the urine total 320 mg/day. Assuming that 40% of dietary calcium is absorbed, it is suggested that an intake of 800 mg/day will meet the needs of essentially all healthy adults. Balance studies show that the average person achieves calcium equilibrium on an intake of 10 mg/kg of body weight; however, because of wide individual variations, 18 mg/kg would be needed to meet the needs of 95% of the population, and 22 mg would be needed to meet the needs of 99%.

Pregnancy and lactation. Although a child is born with poorly calcified bones, the full-term fetus contains approximately 28 g of calcium, which must be provided from the mother's reserves. There is need for an increased maternal intake, not only for the calcification of the fetal teeth and bones that occurs during pregnancy but also to build the storage reserves of the mother to meet the high demands during lactation. During the last seven months of pregnancy calcium is deposited in the fetal tissue at the rate of 25, 50, 85, 125, 175, 235, and 300 mg/day, respectively. Two thirds of fetal calcium is transferred from the mother to the fetus between the thirtieth and fortieth week of pregnancy, when fetal calcium increases from 10 to 28 g. Studies using radioactive isotopes of calcium in mothers' diets showed that 85% to 90% of the calcium in the fetal skeleton and in human milk comes from the mother's diet, and 10% to 15% of this is withdrawn from maternal reserves. Indications are that the ability to absorb calcium increases with need and that pregnant women may double their usual level and absorb up to 40% of dietary calcium. Even so, the National Research Council has recommended an additional 400 mg/day over normal requirements to meet both fetal and maternal demands. A retention by the mother of two to five times fetal needs has been reported in the sixth and seventh months, indicating that maternal reserves are being built up at this time. Research also suggests a sharp reduction in muscular cramps frequently encountered in pregnancy on administration of both vitamin D and calcium.

The transfer of calcium from mother to infant is greater during lactation than during pregnancy. About 50 g is secreted in milk during a six-month lactation period. Human milk contains about 30 mg of calcium/dl. To meet this demand for 200 to 300 mg/day for the production of 850 ml of milk without causing a severe depletion of the mother's reserves or a decrease in milk production, a maternal intake of 1200 mg has been advised. At a 40% utilization rate, 750 mg would be needed for milk production alone. This requires the use of large amounts of dairy products (a minimum of 1.5 liters of milk or its equivalent), plus generous use of other calcium-rich foods. Few women maintain calcium equilibrium during lactation but draw on the calcium reserves built up during pregnancy to help provide the calcium transferred to milk. The ability of some women to maintain a successful level of lactation on very low calcium intakes is unexplained.

Old age. There is no basis on which to

suggest an increase in calcium need with age, but all evidence points to the need for maintaining the adult intake of 800 mg/day throughout the later years to reduce the likelihood of demineralization of the skeleton, especially in women over 65 years of age.

Adequacy of calcium in the American diet. If the NRC recommended allowances are used as a criterion for adequacy, it is apparent from various studies of dietary intake that many persons in the United States fail to meet this standard. The extent to which the diets of Americans meet the National Research Council standards is shown in Fig. 7-6. This shows that men and boys are much more likely to consume adequate amounts than are women and girls. Milk was a major source of calcium in all diets, providing about three fourths of the calcium in most of the diets evaluated. Persons who do not drink milk, especially those who also restrict their use of other dairy products, find it virtually impossible to consume a diet reaching NRC standards. The inadequate intake in calcium in the diets of older women is of special concern because of the increased likelihood of osteoporosis in this group.

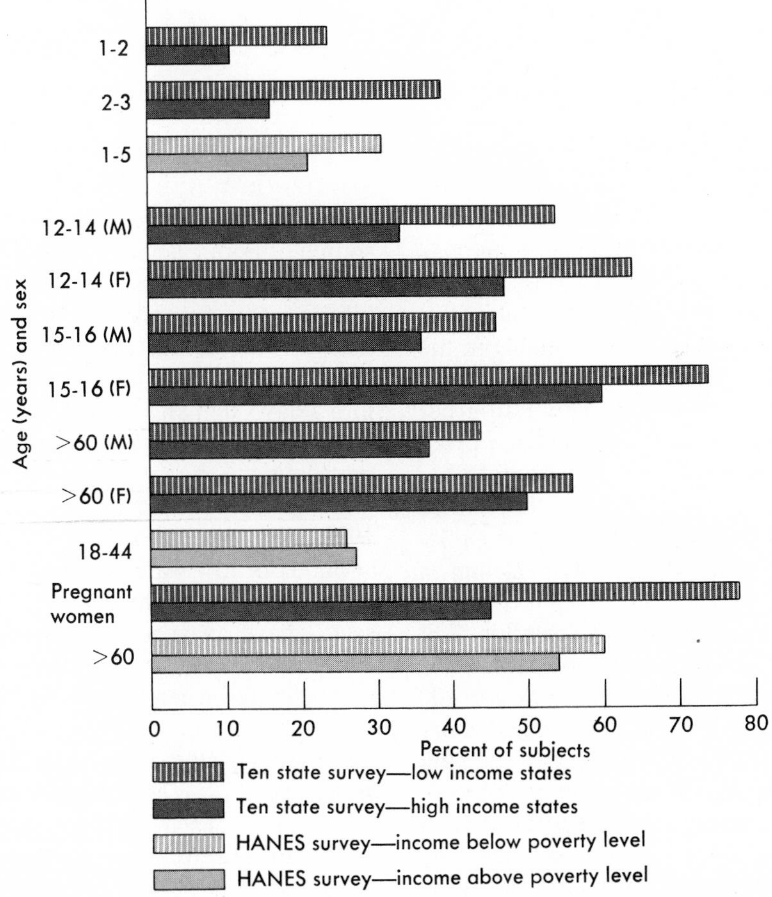

Fig. 7-6. Percentage of persons with dietary calcium intake below two-thirds RDA by age, sex, and income level. Data based on results of Ten-State Nutrition Survey (1968-1970) and preliminary findings of First Health and Nutrition Examination Survey (HANES) (1971-1972).

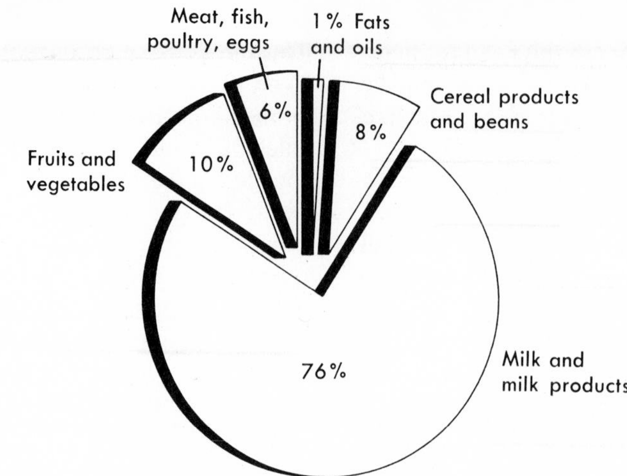

Fig. 7-7. Contribution of various food groups to the calcium content of the American food supply. (Based on Contribution of major food groups to nutrient supplies available for civilian consumption, National Food Review NFR-1, Washington, D.C., 1978, Economic Research Service.)

Food sources

Calcium is present in significant amounts in a very limited number of foods. Fig. 7-7 shows the contribution of various food groups to the total calcium available in the American diet. This amount has increased steadily from 0.86 g in 1906 to 1.16 g per capita per day in 1962. Milk and dairy products are the most dependable sources because of the many ways in which they can be consumed, their availability, and their relatively low cost. In addition, the calcium in milk is in complexes from which it is readily released. It becomes obvious from Fig. 7-8, showing the relative amounts of calcium from various food sources on the basis of 100 g and 100 kcal of food, that should dairy products be excluded from the diet, the bulk of other foods needed to supply comparable amounts of calcium would make their use as a major source of calcium difficult. As sources of calcium these other foods are also expensive.

Fish flour made from whole fish, including bones, has an extremely high calcium value both per 100 g portion and per 100 kcal. Although it may assume major importance as a source of both calcium and protein in countries where milk is not available, the possibility of its widespread use in the American diet is remote. Because only a limited amount could reasonably be incorporated into a day's diet and because there were still many problems relative to flavor and keeping qualities to be solved, the only processing plant in the United States was closed in 1974.

Foods of low water content, such as sardines, almonds, and seeds such as sesame seeds, have an appreciable amount of calcium in 100 g portions, but their value to the diet is limited when one considers their contribution relative to calories—an especially important consideration for persons on diets restricted in calories. Table 7-2 presents INQ for calcium for various food sources.

The most useful sources of calcium remain milk and milk products, which contribute 85% of the calcium in United States diets. The ultra-high temperature sterilization of milk does not affect the availability of milk calcium, nor do the more common practices

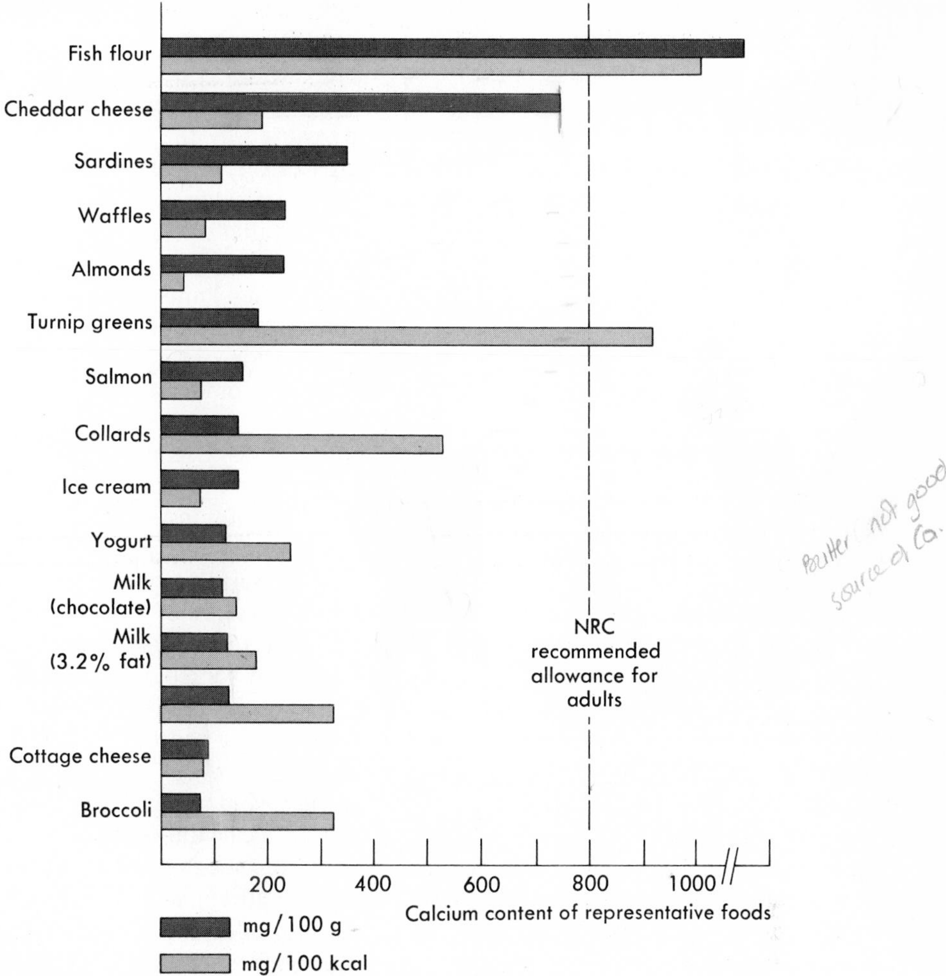

Fig. 7-8. Calcium content of some representative foods. (Based on Watt, B. K., and Merrill, A. L.: Composition of foods—raw, processed and prepared, Handbook No. 8, Washington, D.C., 1963, U.S. Department of Agriculture.)

of pasteurization or homogenization. The adding of chocolate to milk does not reduce significantly the availability of calcium.

Evidence that many adults of black and Oriental extraction lack the enzyme lactase necessary for the digestion of lactose explains the aversion to milk often reported by these groups. Promotion of the use of milk as a source of calcium cannot be justified under these conditions.

Nonfat milk and buttermilk are slightly better than whole milk as sources of calcium. This may be explained by the fact that when the fat portion, which is almost devoid of calcium, is removed, it is replaced by the calcium-containing portion of milk. When cost is a prime consideration, nonfat products will provide calcium at 50% to 80% of the price of whole milk.

One ounce of cheddar cheese provides as much calcium as a cup of milk and often is more acceptable than milk as a source of

Table 7-2. INQ for selected sources of calcium providing at least 15% of the U.S. RDA of calcium per serving

Cabbage	23.1
Turnip greens	19.3
Nonfat milk	7.6
Processed Swiss cheese	5.8
Yogurt (from partially skimmed milk)	5.4
Natural cheddar cheese	4.3
Whole milk	4.1
Natural cottage cheese	2.0
Waffle	2.0
Ice cream (with 10% fat)	1.7
White sauce	1.6

calcium for adults. Cottage cheese is a variable source of calcium, depending on the method of processing used. Rennin coagulation retains more calcium in the curd than either a combination of acid and rennin coagulation or acid coagulation alone. All methods are used commercially. Cream cheese is a poor source being made from the fat portion of milk that is low in calcium. One cup of ice cream can be substituted for one-half cup of milk as a source of available calcium.

The amount of calcium in milk from a particular species varies with the rate of growth of the offspring. It ranges from 0.02% in the milk of humans, whose babies double their birth weight in 180 days, to 0.12% in the milk of cows, whose calves double their weight in forty-seven days, to 0.32% in the milk of dogs, whose puppies achieve the same proportionate increase in weight in seven days.

Goat's milk contains slightly more calcium than cow's milk and is often substituted when an infant is allergic to cow's milk. Calcium-enriched soybean milk preparations in either powdered or liquid form are also a satisfactory source of calcium.

Broccoli and green leafy vegetables such as turnip greens and kale, which do not contain oxalic acid, have appreciable amounts of available calcium. The utilization of vegetable calcium is not as high as milk calcium because the increased gastrointestinal motility caused by the bulk of the vegetable increases the rate of passage of food through the intestinal tract. In green leafy vegetables the fact that calcium is contained within the cell whose cellulose wall is digested with difficulty often limits the availability of this calcium. Considerable calcium may be lost in preparation of vegetables if thick skins are removed or the dark green leaves discarded.

Soybeans become a significant calcium source when consumed in large amounts. In Indonesia, for instance, a fermented soybean product, tempeh, and a dried soybean milk powder, saridele, are being advocated as potential sources of calcium and protein. In Oriental countries soy sauce may represent a significant source of calcium.

Although bread has not been traditionally considered a source of calcium, the current trend toward use of dried milk solids and calcium-containing mold inhibitors raises its available calcium to the point at which many adults receive as much as one seventh of their daily requirement from bread. Similarly, the calcium value of baked products such as muffins, waffles, and cakes should not be overlooked. There is also the potential for increasing their calcium content by adding additional milk solids up to the level at which it interferes with palatability and quality. The optional enrichment of flour with 500 to 1500 mg of calcium per pound makes it a significant source, providing 20 to 60 mg per slice of bread from enriched flour. Data from food consumption studies in 1965 show that cereal products and beans contributed 21% of the calcium in the American diet.

In tropical areas where milk products are produced and consumed by only a small segment of the population, other less traditional sources of calcium may assume much greater importance, although there is virtually no information regarding the extent to which they are utilized by the body. Where water consumption is high, as is common in the tropics, and its mineral content is high (50 mg or more per liter), water may provide up to 200 mg of more of calcium per day. A California study showed hard water contributing 6% to 9% of daily calcium intake. Small whole fish or fermented fish pastes are high in calcium. The mill powder used in grinding rice may adhere to the kernel in sufficient quantities to contribute to the overall calcium intake. Lime used in making tortillas adds a significant amount of calcium to the diets in Mexico. Similarly, lime used by betel chewers adds to the calcium intake of these individuals, as does the ground rock, cal, used in porridges by the Peruvians. Even sweet potatoes, when they are a staple item in the diet as in the Papuan highlands of New Guinea, pro-

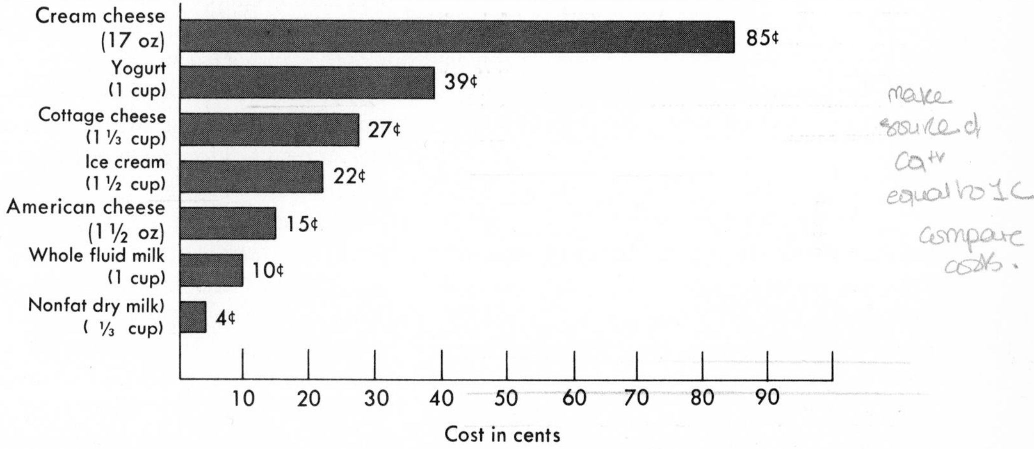

Fig. 7-9. Relative cost of calcium from various milk products (equivalent to 1 cup fresh whole milk, which provides 290 mg calcium).

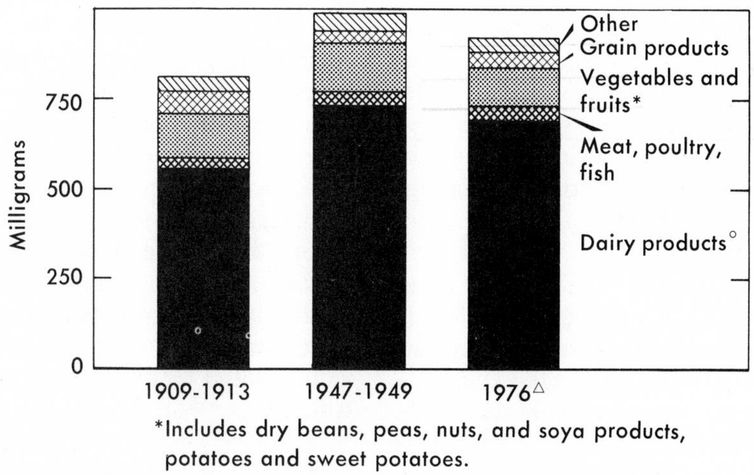

Fig. 7-10. Sources of calcium per capita per day in the American diet (1909-1976). (U.S. Department of Agriculture, 1977.)

vide sufficient calcium to meet minimum dietary needs. In China, eggs may contribute to a substantial proportion of the limited total calcium consumed, and in Malaya pregnant women eat a small shellfish that is ground up whole. These represent but a few of the ways in which various populations may acquire sufficient calcium, although they consume practically no dairy products.

Many diet supplements contain calcium salts, such as calcium carbonate, calcium gluconate, calcium lactate, and calcium citrate. These seem to be well utilized and may be of value during times of very high need such as pregnancy and lactation. However, the user is cautioned to read the label carefully, since multivitamin-mineral pills seldom contain significant amounts of calcium. It is usually necessary to take a separate calcium supplement to obtain any appreciable amount, and even then several large doses will be needed each day.

Purveyors of special food-blending devices are constantly promoting the consumption of pulverized eggshell as a feasible method of obtaining an adequate calcium intake. An eggshell does contain 2 g of calcium, but since there are no data on the utilization of calcium from this source, the reliance on eggshells may be risky.

For persons who have a restricted food budget, knowledge of the price of a nutrient from various sources may be helpful in planning an adequate intake at minimum cost. Fig. 7-9 gives such information for some representative sources of calcium. Trends in sources of dietary calcium are shown in Fig. 7-10.

High calcium intake

Although we have no evidence of deleterious effects from excessive intakes of calcium per se, popular literature suggests with increasing frequency that a high intake of calcium is undesirable. In the several studies to assess the effect of high oral calcium intakes (more than 2 g), it was found that they had no effect on the level of calcium in the urine of normal subjects, although high intakes would result in high urinary calcium levels (hypercalcuria) in numerous disease states. In addition, there is no evidence that high dietary calcium levels have any effect on kidney stone formation or lead to deposition of calcium in other soft tissues in the absence of metabolic abnormalities.

Calcification of soft tissues does not occur in normal, healthy individuals solely as a result of high intakes of calcium. If, however, blood calcium levels become high because of increased bone resorption, it may be helpful to reduce dietary calcium in an effort to reduce the amount available for calcification of soft tissues such as the kidney. The abnormal deposition of calcium in soft tissues is more likely a result of low magnesium than of high calcium.

Work on animals has suggested that excessively high intakes of calcium have a depressing effect on the utilization of other nutrients, such as phosphorus, fat, iodine, zinc, magnesium, and iron, when the latter are present at minimum levels. However, the ratios at which this can occur are far beyond those calcium intakes encountered in a normal diet. In adults high intakes of calcium lead to increased total absorption of calcium, although the efficiency of absorption is decreased. In children, however, an intake of 2300 mg of calcium and 2400 mg of phosphorus resulted in a depressed retention of calcium. This was accompanied by a marked increase in fat excretion in feces and may be caused by inhibition of the fat-splitting enzyme pancreatic lipase in the presence of high calcium concentration in the intestine.

Thus, although there is no evidence of additional benefits to be derived from calcium intakes in excess of recommended levels, neither is there any evidence of detrimental effects except for the small number of individuals with a tendency to deposit calcium in soft tissues.

Assessment of body calcium reserves

The major problem in assessing nutritional status in respect to calcium is the lack of a feasible method that is sensitive to changes in body calcium. Blood calcium levels are readily determined, but the action of the parathyroid gland in mobilizing bone calcium to maintain blood calcium at a level at least 7 mg/dl means that a drop in blood calcium is a more sensitive measure of the efficiency of the parathyroid than of calcium status. The hazards and cost involved in the use of radioactive isotopes of calcium restrict its usefulness to controlled studies on small numbers of subjects. Considerable work has been done to develop an x-ray measurement of bone density that will reflect the degree of mineralization of bones. Bones of the heel and finger, which have been investigated, do not show sufficient variation in mineralization within the normal range of human calcium intake to be of any use in assessing calcium nutriture. From 10% to 40% demineralization of bone may have occurred before the change will be reflected in x-ray measurements. The problem is further complicated by the fact that so far no deficiency symptoms can be attributed to a lack of dietary calcium.

Abnormalities of calcium metabolism

Osteoporosities. Osteoporosis is a condition found primarily among middle-aged and elderly women in which the mass, or amount, of bone in the skeleton has been diminished but the remaining bone mass is of normal composition. This is reflected in a shortening of stature, susceptibility to bone fracture, and low backache. Estimates of its incidence in persons over 50 years of age range from 10% to as high as 50%. Although there is no simple diagnostic test for osteoporosis, it is estimated that in 1965 there were 14 million cases of osteoporosis in the United States, 25% of which were severe and 80% of which were in women. Women lose as much as 8% of their bone mass per decade after age 40 compared to a 3% loss in men.

The high incidence of bone fracture among osteoporotic patients may be due to spontaneous fractures in which the break preceded the fall rather than being caused by it. Osteoporotic bone breaks at loads 40% less than normal, and the healing period for fractures is considerably longer than average. Over 80% of the 6 million spontaneous fractures annually occur in women.

Osteoporosis is now regarded as a condition of multiple origins. This has led to the proposal that it be referred to as the *osteoporosities.* The concept of multiple causation may help to explain why high dietary calcium levels are not necessarily protective and low levels not necessarily associated with bone loss. The osteoporosities have been attributed to a decrease in bone mass as the result of long-standing dietary inadequacy and poor absorption or utilization of calcium. Other possible causes considered are the action of the parathyroid in stimulating bone resorption, possibly in response to high-phosphate intake, the failure to synthesize the collagen matrix of bone, the effect of immobility, or a loss of the stimulus for bone formation provided by the estrogens. It is now believed that in osteoporosis the rate of bone formation is normal but bone resorption occurs at an accelerated pace, leading to a decrease in bone mass. The increased rate of bone resorption may occur to maintain normal blood levels of calcium when dietary intake is low or when dietary needs are abnormally high because of poor absorption.

People with osteoporosis usually have had a lower than normal intake of calcium over a long period of time. Older persons have been shown to absorb less calcium than do younger individuals, and those with osteoporosis less than do those free of the disease. In some cases persons with osteoporosis also excrete more, but in all cases the gain in body calcium has failed to compensate for the losses, which has led to a resorption of bone tissue to maintain normal blood levels. Those with osteoporosis do not have the ability to reduce urinary calcium excretion when dietary intake is low. Thus it appears that the people who develop osteoporosis are those who cannot adapt to a low level of dietary intake, have impaired absorptive mechanisms, or persistently lose body calcium.

A diet high in calcium (15.5 mg/kg of body

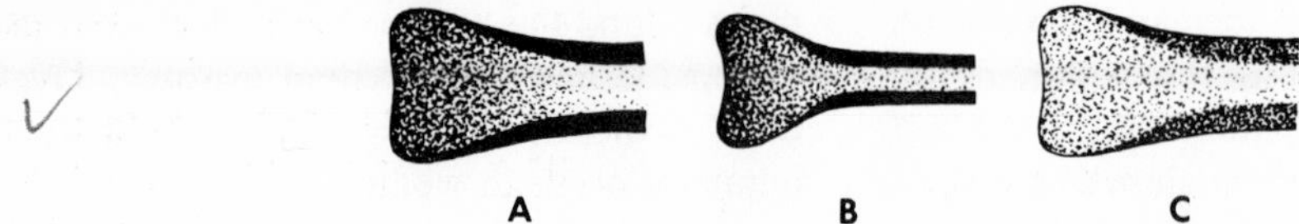

Fig. 7-11. A, Normal bone. **B,** Osteoporosis, in which there is a reduced amount of bone of normal composition. **C,** Osteomalacia, in which the amount of bone is normal but composition is abnormal.

weight), with 50 mg/day of sodium fluoride, and with adequate vitamin D has been shown to arrest the resorption of the bone and has led to the observation that the prevention of osteoporosis with lifelong adequate calcium intake is the best treatment. An accumulating body of evidence demonstrates that fluoride may protect against bone loss by stimulating bone formation and by substituting for the hydroxyl portion of the bone mineral, rendering it less susceptible to degradation.

Osteomalacia. Osteomalacia is a condition in which there is a reduction in the mineral content of the bone but not in the total amount of bone. It is most likely to occur among women living in areas of low sunshine, those whose clothing prevents exposure to sunlight, those whose diets are low in calcium, those taking anticonvulsive drugs, and those for whom the demands of successive pregnancies and prolonged lactation have depleted their mineral resources. Most cases respond to vitamin D therapy. The differences in bone changes in osteoporosis and osteomalacia are shown in Fig. 7-11.

Hypercalcemia. Hypercalcemia has been reported in infants as the result of high intakes of vitamin D or a diet in which the ratio of phosphorus to calcium is very high. These cases have been observed in connection with widespread supplementation of infant foods with vitamin D and the use of whole milk formulas in which the fat interferes with calcium absorption. It is best corrected by reducing the vitamin D intake rather than lowering the amount of calcium in the diet.

Tetany and calcium rigor. When the level of calcium in the blood (and hence in the extracellular fluids) drops below a critical level, there is a change in the stimulation of nerve cells, resulting in increased excitability of the nerve and spasmodic and uncontrolled contraction of muscle tissue. This condition is described as *tetany*. When calcium levels rise above normal, the muscle fibers enter a state of tonic contraction known as *calcium rigor.* Neither of these conditions is the result of abnormal dietary levels of calcium but rather both reflect an abnormality in parathyroid functioning.

PHOSPHORUS

Distribution

Since phosphorus constitutes 22% of the mineral ash in an adult body or 1% of the body weight, it is classified as a **macronutrient** element. Its role as a major constituent of bones and teeth is recognized by even the casual student of nutrition. The fact that it is often discussed in connection with calcium has further emphasized its role in the formation of hard tissues, with the result that its other equally vital roles are often overlooked or underestimated.

It is estimated that the adult body contains 12 g of phosphorus per kilogram of fat-free tissue. This amounts to about 670 g of phosphorus in the male and 630 g in the female. Of this phosphorus 85% to 90% is in the form of the insoluble calcium phosphate (apatite) crystals that give rigidity and strength to bones and teeth. The remaining 10% to 15% is distributed throughout all living cells of the body, with about half present in striated muscle. Specifically it is a part of the nucleus and the cytoplasm of every living cell, where as phospholipid it is a structural component of the cell and as organic phosphate it participates in cellular functions. In fact, practically all biological reactions involve phosphorus to some extent, since it is vital to any reaction that involves the uptake or release of energy.

Functions

Regulates the release of energy. Phosphate, a phosphorus-containing substance, is necessary for the controlled release of energy resulting from the combustion or oxidation of carbohydrate, fat, and protein. Energy is stored when a third phosphate molecule is attached to the compound ADP (adenosine diphosphate) to form ATP (adenosine triphosphate). This linkage is referred to as a high-energy phosphate bond. As energy is needed, the ATP is changed to ADP, and a phosphate molecule and the energy that held it to ADP is released to supply energy for many body reactions. If the cells were unable to convert energy into these high-energy bonds for storage, they would be incapable of regulating the rate at which it is available.

Facilitates absorption and transportation of nutrients. Phosphate is attached to many substances within the cell, such as monosaccharides in a process known as phosphorylation. Phosphorylation occurs in absorption from the intestine, release from the blood stream to the intercellular fluids, uptake into the cell, and uptake by the organelles of the cell. Fats, which are insoluble in water, are transported in the bloodstream as phospholipids, a combination of phosphate with the fat molecule that renders the fat more soluble. When glycogen is released from the liver or muscle storage sites to be used as a source of energy, it appears as a phosphorylated glucose compound, another manifestation of the essential nature of phosphorus.

Part of essential body compounds. The active forms of some vitamins contain phosphorus—thiamin pyrophosphate (B_1) is an example. Since all enzymes are proteins and many proteins contain phosphorus, the essentiality of this mineral is obvious. Even more crucial is the role of phosphate as an integral part of the nucleic acids DNA and RNA both of which are essential for cell reproduction through their vital roles in the replication of genes and in protein synthesis.

Calcification of bones and teeth. The initiation of the calcification process involves the fixation of phosphate to the matrix, indicating a primary role for phosphorus in bone formation. Although use of the term *calcification* has led to the belief that a lack of calcium is the major cause of failure in this process, failure of bone calcification is as often the result of unavailability of phosphorus as of calcium. In cases of poor calcification of bone there is an increase in the enzyme phosphatase, which facilitates the release of phosphorus from organic tissue compounds into the blood to create the proper calcium to phosphorus ratio for bone growth.

The low phosphorus levels in the body are more likely a reflection of excessive excretion of phosphorus in the urine than of inadequate dietary phosphorus.

Regulation of acid-base balance. Because of its ability to combine with additional hydrogen ions, phosphorus is important as a buffer to prevent a change in the acidity of body fluids as the result of anions is released in metabolism.

It is well beyond the scope of this presentation to attempt to enumerate all the biological reactions in which phosphorus plays a key role. Those mentioned merely illustrate the diversity of reactions in which phosphorus participates.

Absorption and metabolism

Since practically all phosphorus must be absorbed as free phosphate, that present in food as inorganic esters must be hydrolyzed, or split, from the complex in which it occurs in food. In the intestinal tract this is accomplished by enzymes known as phosphatases. The amount of phosphorus absorbed varies inversely with the amount of magnesium, iron, and other elements with which it forms insoluble complexes that are excreted in the feces. Fecal phosphorus also includes that which is part of substances secreted into the gastrointestinal tract. Unabsorbed phosphorus amounts to about 30% of dietary phosphorus. Phytic acid, a phosphorus-containing compound found in the outer husks of cereals, is poorly absorbed and also interferes with calcium absorption. However, when whole wheat is used in leavened bread, the calcium phytate, a combination of phytic acid and calcium, is changed to an absorbable form.

The control of the amount of phosphorus in the body is maintained through excretion of excess in the urine rather than by decreased absorption. Urinary phosphorus increases due to the release of phosphorus from the tissues during catabolism.

In addition to being associated in bone and tooth structure, calcium and phosphorus are influenced by the same factors during metabolism. The parathyroid, which regulates the level of calcium in the blood, affects the level of phosphorus in the blood and its rate of resorption from the kidneys. Vitamin D, which facilitates the absorption of calcium and phosphorus from the gastrointestinal tract, also increases the rate of resorption of phosphorus from the kidneys. In this way the levels of calcium and phosphorus, both needed for calcification of bone, are raised simultaneously. Blood levels of phosphorus range from 35 to 45 mg/dl, of which 3 to 5 mg is in the form of inorganic phosphorus. Like calcium, phosphorus is constantly being released and rebuilt into bone tissue in the remodeling processes typical of bone. Evidence now indicates that the phosphorus of tooth enamel is exchanged with that in the saliva and the phosphorus in the dentin with that of the blood supply.

Food sources

Foods rich in protein are also rich in phosphorus. Thus meat, fish, poultry, eggs, and cereal products are the primary sources of phosphorus in the average diet. The amount of phosphorus in some representative food is given in Table 7-3.

Table 7-3. Phosphorus content of representative foods*

Food	Phosphorus (mg/100 g)
Cheddar cheese	478
Peanuts	401
Cod, broiled	274
Beef, lean round	250
Pork, lean	249
Halibut, broiled	248
Bread, whole-wheat	228
Eggs	205
Cottage cheese	152
Peas, fresh	116
Milk, whole	93
Bread, white enriched	90
Lima beans	67
Oatmeal	57
Rice, cooked	28

*Based on Watt, B. K., and Merrill, A. L.: Composition of foods—raw, processed and prepared, Handbook No. 8, Washington, D.C., 1963, U.S. Department of Agriculture.

The high phosphorus content of carbonated soft drinks (up to 500 mg per 12 oz bottle) not only contributes to the phosphorus intake but also causes problems among those who consume large amounts by creating a calcium to phosphorus imbalance. Other uses of phosphorus-containing substances in processed foods are contributing to high phosphorus intakes, which in turn contribute to a low calcium/phosphorus ratio in the diet. The contribution of various food groups to the phosphorus content of the diet is shown in Fig. 7-12.

Deficiency

Because of the widespread occurrence of phosphorus in food there is no evidence of a deficiency in humans except among persons who consume large amounts of antacids, which interfere with phosphorus absorption or those who suffer excessive urinary losses. Symptoms such as fatigue, loss of appetite, and demineralization of bone result.

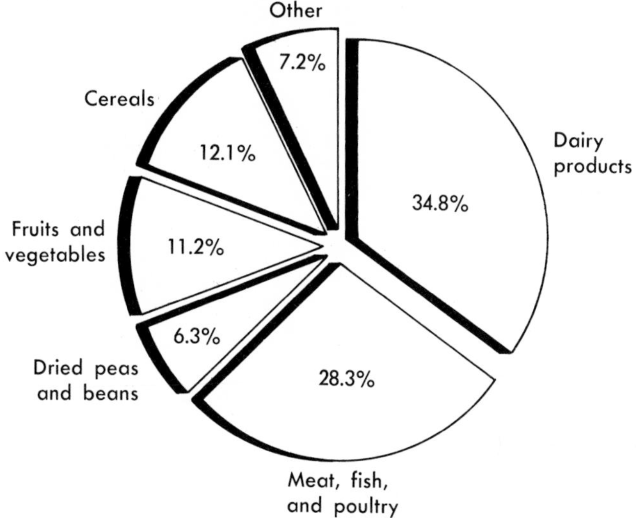

Fig. 7-12. Contribution of various food groups to phosphorus content of the American diet. (Based on data from National Food Review NFR-1, Washington, D.C., 1978, Economic Research Service.)

Requirements

The NRC recommended allowances suggest a phosphorus intake of at least 800 mg a day, equal to the calcium allowance indicated for the growth period, although bone growth requires a 1:2 ratio of phosphorus to calcium and tissue growth a 1:17 ratio of phosphorus to nitrogen. Such a ratio in the diet would be undesirable since there are obligatory urinary and fecal losses of phosphorus and the absorption varies with the source of phosphorus and the ratio of calcium to phosphorus in the diet. Diets adequate in protein invariably provide an adequate amount of phosphorus.

For infants under 6 months the recommended intake of phosphorus is two thirds that of calcium.

MAGNESIUM

The presence of magnesium in living organisms has been known since 1859. Although it had long been used as a healing substance, an anesthetic, and anticonvulsant, practically all the information on its biological functions has been gathered since 1950. By 1926 it had been identified as a dietary essential for mice and by 1932 as an essential for rats, but its role in human nutrition was much more difficult to establish. The effects of a magnesium deficiency in humans are difficult to study because of the sizable reserve of magnesium in bone, some of which can be liberated to help meet the needs of the soft tissues, and because the kidneys have the ability to resorb magnesium when needed. It is now, however, recognized as an essential element that occurs predominantly within the cell. In plant life magnesium is essential in the structure of chlorophyll, which enables the plant to trap the energy from the sun in photosynthesis. Chlorophyll chemically resembles hemoglobin, which is responsible for the ability of the blood to carry oxygen. They differ only in that chlorophyll contains magnesium, whereas hemoglobin contains iron.

Distribution and metabolism

The magnesium content of the infant's body at birth is approximately 0.5 g, most of which was transferred to the fetus in the latter part of pregnancy. However, since magnesium crosses the placental barrier freely, the amount will vary with the amount available from maternal tissue. In the adult the magnesium content of the body varies from 21 to 28 g, of which 60% is concentrated in bone, where it represents 0.5% to 0.7% of the bone ash. About a third of this magnesium is closely bound with phosphate, and the remainder is adsorbed on the bone surface, from which it can be mobilized to maintain normal blood and tissue levels. The remaining 40% of body magnesium is evenly distributed between muscle and soft tissues.

In the soft tissues, magnesium, like potassium, is concentrated within the cell; in the blood it occurs primarily in the red blood cells rather than in the serum. In serum, with half the magnesium free, a third bound to protein, and a sixth in other complexes, magnesium levels are maintained at 1 to 3 mg/dl. In a deficiency the level in the red blood cells drops; in an excess the serum level rises.

Magnesium is absorbed primarily in the small intestine. About 40% of an average intake is absorbed with a range from 25% on high intakes to 75% on low intakes. Absorption is further reduced by the presence of calcium, phytates, and fat but increased by dietary vitamin D and lactose. The absorption of magnesium is increased by the parathyroid hormone, which is secreted when serum magnesium drops.

Magnesium excretion is regulated through the kidneys by the hormone aldosterone secreted by the adrenal gland in response to changes in blood levels of magnesium. Urinary losses increase with the use of diuretics and with the consumption of alcohol. Little endogenous magnesium appears in the feces; most represents unabsorbed dietary magnesium. The amount lost in perspiration is only 15 mg/day but in high environmental temperatures may amount to 15% of magnesium losses. Since the gastric juice is relatively high in magnesium, vomiting may lead to large losses. That secreted in the pancreatic juice is almost all reabsorbed.

Functions

Within the cell, magnesium plays an important role as catalyst to several hundred biological reactions, a major portion of which take place in the mitochondrion. It activates the production of ATP and any changes of ATP to ADP. This change is necessary in all reactions involving the expenditure or release of energy, such as synthesis of body compounds, absorption and transportation of nutrients, and any physical activity. The importance of magnesium in cellular metabolism is evidenced by the fact that the level of intracellular magnesium in metabolically active muscle tissue and liver is seven times that in the blood.

Magnesium is crucial in cellular respiration, although in some reactions it may be replaced by other divalent elements such as manganese. Magnesium also influences protein synthesis by affecting the arrangement of the protein-synthesizing organelles of the cell, the ribosomes, and by facilitating the attachment of RNA to the ribosome. It is also necessary for the activation of amino acids so that they can be incorporated into protein molecules and for the synthesis, degradation, and stability of the genetic material DNA.

Although only 1% of magnesium occurs in extracellular fluids, it is one of the minerals involved in providing the proper environment in the extracellular fluid of nerve cells to promote the conduction of nerve impulses and to allow normal muscular contraction. In this situation, magnesium and calcium play antagonistic roles, calcium acting as a stimulator and magnesium as a relaxor substance. The relaxing effect of magnesium is evident from the fact that with increasing levels of the element in the blood, there is an increasing anesthetic effect. At extremely high serum levels, coma and eventually heart failure will result. These levels may be reached in kidney failure in which the excretion of magnesium is depressed. On the other hand, low serum magnesium levels are associated with irritability, nervousness, and convulsions as the result of stimulation of nerve impulses and increased muscular contraction. The competitive nature of the calcium-magnesium interrelationship is further evident during absorption and excretion. When a large amount of one is being absorbed or excreted, there is usually a reduction in the amount of the other.

Adequate magnesium may increase the stability of calcium in tooth enamel. It also influences the secretion of thyroxin and the maintenance of normal basal metabolic rate and facilitates adaptation to cold.

Deficiency

Symptoms of a magnesium deficiency are associated with starvation, which may cause renal excretion of up to 20% of body magnesium, persistent vomiting with resultant loss of magnesium-rich intestinal secretions, trauma of surgery, and with rapid transit of food through the gastrointestinal tract, which reduces absorption time.

A recognized form of magnesium deficiency is low-magnesium tetany similar to that produced when the blood calcium level drops. After twenty-five to a hundred days of a severely deficient diet the body's control over the contractions and relaxations of muscles is lost. The individual suffers from uncontrolled neuromuscular activity diagnosed early as tremors but progressing until convulsive seizures occur in the more severe cases of deprivation. These symptoms most often arise when a low dietary intake is superimposed on conditions that reduce the absorption and increase the excretion of magnesium. Alcohol increases the rate of magnesium excretion and may partially explain the loss of neuromuscular control diagnosed as magnesium tetany in alcoholics. Others who experience magnesium deficiency symptoms are infants suffering from kwashiorkor, persons maintained for long periods on magnesium-free fluids, as may occur postoperatively, or persons suffering prolonged losses because of nausea or diarrhea.

The increase in the undesirable calcification of soft tissues in magnesium deficiency may reflect the increase in calcium absorption that occurs when there is less magnesium to compete with calcium for the common carrier that transports them across the intestinal wall. This is often accompanied by an increase in the amount of calcium mobilized from the bone, which also increases the calcium available for deposition in soft tissues. High-calcium and low-magnesium diets also lead to an increase in magnesium excretion, further evidence of the antagonistic relationship between these two elements.

Animal studies have shown that in magnesium deficiency normal levels of fluoride will prevent the calcification of kidney tissue observed on low intakes. In humans, however, it has been shown that high fluoride intakes cause a depletion of calcium and magnesium by increasing excretion.

In the absence of adequate magnesium the cardiovascular system and the renal system are also affected, with symptoms such as vasodilation and skin changes being frequent. Intramuscular injections of magnesium sulfate relieve these symptoms.

New methods of measuring magnesium in body fluids have demonstrated that magnesium depletion occurs more commonly than previously assumed.

Assessment of reserves

Serum levels of magnesium do not provide a sensitive indication of the level in cells, since about 35% of the blood magnesium is bound to a protein and is not measurable with current analytical techniques. In addition, tissues may be depleted of magnesium while serum levels remain normal.

Bone formed when there is adequate magnesium available contains about 16% of its magnesium as a reserve that can be released to maintain blood levels when dietary magnesium drops. However, bone formed when little magnesium is available will have little or no magnesium and will tend to take up magnesium when the mineral becomes available from the diet, thus keeping blood levels low for a longer time.

The levels of magnesium found in the red blood cells reflect the amount of magnesium available as the cells were formed. Administration of a load of magnesium parenterally followed by the measurement of the amount excreted in the urine is considered the most sensitive test for children. Retention of more than 40% is believed to indicate a magnesium deficiency.

Requirements

The Food and Nutrition Board of the National Research Council recommends an intake of 300 mg/day for women and 350 mg for men, or approximately 5 mg/kg of body weight. These amounts were recommended after considering data from balance studies. It is estimated that a typical American diet provides 120 mg/1000 kcal—a level that will barely provide the recommended intake. In one study, when intakes were increased to 10 mg/kg in an experimental situation, there was a period of high magnesium retention, which later dropped, apparently after body stores were replenished.

The absence of magnesium deficiency symptoms in the American population may be explained by the fact that the deficit is very slight and that it becomes significant only when a condition of stress or a disease state is superimposed. Such situations may be the increased excretion that occurs with alcohol consumption, the impaired absorption accompanying the increased use of diuretics, or the decreased intake of magnesium by patients on fluid feedings.

Recommended allowances are presented in Table 7-4. Canadian standards are about 15% lower.

Table 7-4. Recommended dietary allowances for magnesium in the United States

Age	Magnesium (mg)
1 to 10 yr	60-250
11 to 14 yr	300-350
15 to 18 yr	300-400
Adult men	350
Adult women	300
Pregnancy	450
Lactation	450

Food sources

Table 7-5 classifies some common foods on the basis of their magnesium content. Precise figures are not given, since in several instances only single determinations have been

Table 7-5. Classification of some representative foods as sources of magnesium

Rich sources (>100 mg/dl)	Good sources (50-100 mg/dl)	Fair sources (25-50 mg/dl)	Poor sources (<25 mg/dl)
Cocoa	Clams	Oysters	Lobster
Nuts	Cornmeal	Crab	Pork
Soybeans	Spinach	Fresh peas	Lamb
Whole grains		Liver	Milk
Molasses		Beef	Eggs
Spices			Veal
			Most fruits and vegetables
			Fowl

made. When the magnesium content of food is expressed in relation to its caloric content, vegetables are the best source followed by legumes, seafood, nuts, cereals, and dairy products. The high chlorophyll content of green leafy vegetables accounts for their value in providing 30% of dietary magnesium. Absorption is reduced in diets high in calcium, fat, or phytic acid, normally found in the outer husks of cereal grains such as rice or oats. The magnesium in foods high in oxalic acid may be found in an insoluble complex.

Although milk is a relatively poor source of magnesium, it appears adequate to meet the needs of either breast- or bottle-fed infants, who absorb from 33% to 85% of the magnesium present.

Oriental diets with appreciable amounts of magnesium from rice, soybeans, and fish provide sufficient amounts to maintain magnesium balance. This observation is interesting in the light of findings that those persons with high magnesium intakes are less susceptible to cardiovascular disease than those on low intakes and that Orientals are less susceptible than Westerners.

Seawater contains 1300 ppm of magnesium compared to 1 to 16 ppm in fresh water, and soft water contains considerably more than hard water.

The contribution of various food groups to the magnesium content of the diet is shown in Fig. 7-13.

SODIUM

The necessity of salt, a major source of sodium, has been recognized for centuries, and many of the major conquests of the world revolved around a search for a salt supply. Trading in salt has had many social, political, and economic consequences. However, it was not until 1937 that the role of sodium as a dietary essential was established. In many countries the only source of salt is the evaporation of seawater, which is frequently carried out on a small scale in the home.

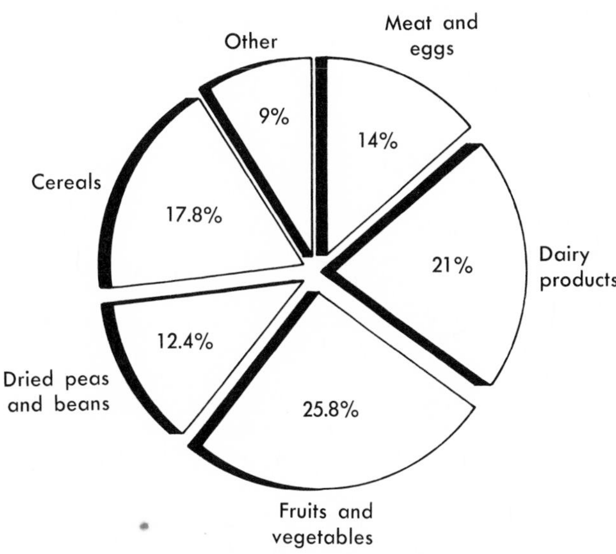

Fig. 7-13. Contribution of various food groups to the magnesium content of the American diet. (Based on data from National Food Review NFR-1, Washington, D.C., 1978, Economic Research Service.)

Distribution in body

Sodium is a monovalent cation present in the body primarily in the extracellular fluids—the fluids within the blood vessels and the intercellular fluids surrounding the cells. About 57 g, or 50% of the total body sodium, is found in these fluids, where it represents an important part of the cell's environment. Under normal conditions as little as 10% of body sodium is present within the cell, although the body must work constantly to pump sodium out of the cell. The remaining 40% of body sodium is found in the skeleton bound in the surface of bone crystals. Here about half of it acts as a reserve of exchangeable sodium available to the extracellular fluids when less dietary sodium is available or when losses from the body are high. Except when low intakes occur in conjunction with increased demand due to losses, it takes a long period of sodium restriction to use up all the body reserves.

Absorption and metabolism

Normally from 3 to 7 g of sodium or 7.5 to 18 g of salt are ingested daily, although the amount varies greatly with the extent to which table salt (sodium chloride) is added during cooking and at the table. Two teaspoons of table salt will provide 4 g of sodium. The body has an ability to handle considerably larger amounts. Although sodium can be toxic if consumed in excessive amounts (35 to 40 g of sodium chloride), levels sufficiently high to become toxic are extremely unpalatable and unlikely to be consumed voluntarily.

A small portion of sodium is absorbed in the stomach, but most of it is absorbed rapidly from the small intestine. The absorption of sodium is an active (energy-requiring) process. Absorbed sodium is carried through the bloodstream to the kidneys, where sodium is filtered out and returned to the bloodstream in amounts to maintain the blood levels within the narrow range required by the body. Any excess, which amounts to 90% to 95% of ingested sodium, is excreted in the urine. This regulation of sodium metabolism by the kidneys is controlled by aldosterone, a hormone secreted by the adrenal gland in response to blood sodium levels.

When the need for sodium increases, the secretion of aldosterone increases. This stimulates the resorption of sodium by the kidneys. Conversely, when blood sodium levels are high, the secretion of aldosterone diminishes and less sodium is retained. The level of sodium in the urine reflects dietary intake—being high when intake is high, and low when intake is low. Some sodium is also deposited in bone to become a reservoir available in time of need.

Since there is a limit to the amount of sodium that can be excreted in a certain volume of urine, blood levels and extracellular fluid levels will rise if dietary intake exceeds the kidneys' ability to excrete it. When blood sodium levels rise, the thirst receptors in the hypothalamus of the brain react by stimulating the thirst sensation. This leads to greater fluid consumption, which in turn allows the kidney to excrete more urine and more sodium. Blood sodium levels drop, followed by a diminution of thirst.

Sodium is also lost from the body through perspiration. Normally, these losses are minimal (< 1 g), but under environmental conditions or fever leading to excessive perspiration the loss of sodium and water by this route may be appreciable. One investigator reported losses of 5 to 6 g of sodium chloride per day in the summer in the tropics. If losses through the skin become great, aldosterone secretion again stimulates the kidneys to retain more sodium to help minimize the effects of this loss.

An additional intake of 2 g of salt for every liter of fluid lost in excess of 4 liters is recommended to help replace the lost sodium, although the acclimated person may need less and the unacclimated two to three times as much.

The loss of body sodium leads to low levels in the extracellular fluids. In an attempt to equalize the osmotic pressure from electrolytes on either side of the cell membrane, potassium and water leave the cell. It is this cellular dehydration and loss of potassium that causes the feeling of fatigue that accompanies sodium depletion.

In contrast to potassium, sodium is an integral part of digestive secretions, such as bile and pancreatic and intestinal juices, which contain approximately 3 g/L. A large amount (20 g/day) is secreted into the gastrointestinal tract by this route, but most of this is reabsorbed. Only under abnormal conditions, such as diarrhea, in which the digestive mass passes through the digestive tract rapidly, or with vomiting, in which sodium-rich digestive fluids are lost, is there a major sodium loss from the intestinal tract.

Functions

Sodium plays a vital role in performing the general functions of minerals discussed in Chapter 6.

As a cation in the extracellular fluids it helps maintain osmotic pressure on the outside of the cell membrane to counteract the similar effect of potassium within the cell, which is essential to maintain normal water balance. If the sodium concentration within the cell rises when the cell cannot pump it out quickly enough, water will be taken in to dilute the sodium to normal concentrations; the resulting waterlogged cells are described as edematous. This same uptake of water by the cell occurs if the water in the extracellular fluid increases without a concurrent increase in sodium. Water, which can cross the cell membrane freely, then enters the cell to dilute cellular potassium, reestablishing an equilibrium on either side of the cell wall. If very marked uptake of water occurs, the condition is described as water intoxication. When sodium loss is accompanied by water loss, the amount of fluid in the extracellular tissues diminishes, resulting in low blood volume and hence low blood pressure, muscle cramps, and a high concentration of red cells (hematocrit) within the blood.

Sodium accounts for 90% of the basic ions in the extracellular fluids and helps to maintain body neutrality by counteracting the effect of the acid-forming elements. When an excess of acid-forming elements appears in the body fluids, sodium can be released from the sodium reserves in the bone to offset the acid. One of the major causes of alkalosis, or an excess of base-forming elements, is the ingestion of sodium-containing antacid preparations.

In the transmission of nerve impulses a change in the permeability of the nerve cell membrane allows sodium to enter, and for a temporary period this changes the electrical charge on the membrane. This charge travels down the nerve fiber as a nerve impulse, or message. If the balance between sodium outside and inside the cell were upset, this transmission of nerve impulses could not occur. Similarly, the contraction of muscles involves a temporary exchange of sodium and potassium in the contracting muscle cell. Sodium is also essential for the absorption of glucose and in the transport of other nutrients across membranes.

Requirement

The dietary requirement for sodium has not yet been determined, but it is generally observed that the usual intake far exceeds needs. The requirement for sodium is determined by the needs for growth, estimated at 1.8 g/kg of new tissue, the losses in sweat and other secretions, and the amount of potassium in the diet.

The obligatory losses of sodium, which represent the minimum amount that would have to be replaced, have been estimated at 40 to 185 mg/day. This includes 5 to 35 mg lost in the urine, 10 to 125 mg lost in the stools, 25 mg through nonsweat losses from the skin, and 25 mg in sweat. The usual intake of 3 to 7 g, therefore, represents many times the minimum requirement. Since a diet that provides only 100 to 150 mg would be extremely unpalatable to most persons, the likelihood of an insufficient intake is remote.

The suggested requirement of 5 g represents as much as ten times the amount on which adequate sodium balance can be maintained.

Food sources

Dietary sources of sodium fall into two main categories: that present in food naturally and that added primarily as salt during processing and preparation.

Sodium is present in food in widely varying amounts, more generally being found in foods of animal origin than in those of plant origin. The sodium content of some representative foods is shown in Table 7-6. The amount found in a diet is as much a function of the amount of salt and other sodium-containing compounds added in processing as of the amount present in the food. For instance, raw potatoes have only 1 mg/100 g, but the same weight of potato chips has 340 to 1000 mg. Cured ham has twenty times as much sodium as raw pork. Similarly whereas fresh peas have less than 1 mg of sodium/100 g, frozen peas have 100 mg and canned peas 230 mg. This is exclusive of any sodium added as table salt or salted butter. In countries where monosodium glutamate (MSG) is used extensively as a flavor enhancer it contributes appreciable amounts of sodium to the diet. Since a large and growing proportion of food is commercially prepared and processed, there is an increase in the use of salt by industry and a decrease in home use. Considerable evidence exists that a taste for salt can be modified over a period of time.

In some areas the sodium content of the water supply may be sufficiently high to make it a major source of sodium, perhaps exceeding that provided by food. Many of the ion exchange units used as water softeners also produce water with a high sodium content. There is some evidence associating high sodium levels in the water with the incidence of atherosclerosis.

Sodium restriction

Under certain conditions, such as hypertension and kidney disorders, it has been considered important to restrict dietary sodium intake. The degree of restriction varies with the severity of the condition. Mild restriction, with intake limited to 500 to 700 mg, can often be accomplished by limiting the use of salt at the table.

For a strict limitation to 200 mg, it is neces-

Table 7-6. Sodium content of representative foods (23 mg = 1 mEq)*

Low sodium	mg/100 g	Moderate sodium	mg/100 g	High sodium	mg/100 g
Apples	1	Milk	50	Canned salmon	540
Asparagus, cooked	1	Chicken		Graham crackers	670
Grapefruit	1	Light meat	64	Cornflakes	1000
Pineapple	1	Dark meat	86	Processed cheese	1100
Egg noodles	5	Celery	100	Cured ham	1100
Sweet potato	10	Egg	122	Sauerkraut	1750
Broccoli, frozen	15	Tomato juice, canned	200	Bacon	1770
Raisins	25			Olives, green	2400
Carrots	50	Cottage cheese	290		
Shredded wheat	10	Sardines, canned	510		

*Based on Watt, B. K., and Merrill, A. L.: Composition of foods—raw, processed and prepared, Handbook No. 8, Washington, D.C., 1963, U.S. Department of Agriculture.

sary to choose foods naturally low in sodium, eliminate all foods in which sodium is used in processing, and use sodium-free salt substitutes and low-salt milk from which much of the sodium has been removed by a process using an exchange of ions. Spices, except celery salt, parsley flakes, and vegetable salts, may be used, since they contain virtually no sodium.

The long-standing use of low-sodium diets to treat toxemia of pregnancy is now being challenged. Clinical studies on humans indicate that moderate-sodium rather than low-sodium diets are effective in preventing or relieving the symptoms of toxemia—high blood pressure, edema, proteinuria, and blurred vision. Extensive studies in rats have indicated an increased need for sodium during pregnancy, as evidenced by a decreased excretion of the element. The animals were better able to maintain normal bone and muscle sodium levels and gave birth to more and healthier young on elevated rather than reduced sodium intakes. Those on restricted intakes showed signs of sodium deficiency—general lethargy, debility, and a reduced amount of sodium in the blood and tissues.

There has been concern that infants who received diets high in sodium because of the early introduction of solid foods are unable to excrete the excess sodium and thus develop a predisposition to hypertension. As a result processors of baby foods have either eliminated all added salt from their products or have voluntarily restricted it to 0.25%. In addition, they advise parents to refrain from adding salt to make the food more acceptable to their adult tastes. Studies have shown that infants do not discriminate between salted and unsalted food.

Excess sodium

Although it is obvious that sodium is an essential element, there is also evidence that excessive amounts may be detrimental. In some, but not all, persons large intakes are associated with increased blood sodium levels. Similarly, restriction in sodium intake results in lowering blood pressure to normal in only some individuals. It is generally conceded that the usual sodium intake of the American public is generous and for some it would be desirable to restrict sodium to somewhat lower levels. However, there is no need to suggest therapeutic levels of 300 mg for the general population.

POTASSIUM

Distribution

Potassium is a positively charged ion with chemical properties similar to those of sodium, but physiologically unlike sodium in that potassium is concentrated inside the cell rather than in the extracellular fluid. A sodium to potassium ratio of 1:10 is maintained within the cell, compared to 28:1 in the extracellular fluids. Most of the 250 g of potassium normally present in the body is within the cells; therefore blood potassium is a poor indicator of potassium status.

The amount of potassium in the blood plasma reflects the nature of cellular metabolism rather than body reserves. Plasma potassium rises when there is a breakdown of body tissue (catabolism) and also in acidosis, which occurs with diarrhea, as an indication that potassium is leaving the cell to help establish a normal acid-base balance. It decreases when the rate of protein synthesis or glycogen deposition within the cell increases or in alkalosis, indicating that potassium is entering the cell. If the level of potassium in the blood, and hence in the extracellular fluids, increases above 7 mEq or 0.5 g/L, muscular coordination is disturbed, and in severe cases cardiac arrest occurs. This is usually the result of failure of the kidneys to excrete potassium.

The body is less efficient in conserving or resorbing potassium than many other constituents; therefore there is normally a loss of about 7% of blood potassium in the urine. The presence of chlorine aids in the conservation of potassium.

Potassium levels in the body have been found to be constant in lean body tissue and thus to reflect body composition. This relationship has become the basis of a fairly simple and promising method of determining lean body mass, the *whole body counter.* In this method an estimate of the amount of radioactive potassium 40 in the body is made by a special human whole body counter. Since potassium 40 represents a constant percentage of the total dietary potassium, it is assumed that the same ratio holds in the body. By determining the amount of radioactive potassium in the body and from this the total amount of potassium, it is possible to estimate the amount of lean body mass. The difference between this value and total body weight provides information on total body fat. A drop in body weight without a concurrent drop in total body potassium indicates a loss of adipose tissue rather than lean body mass.

Functions

Within the cell potassium acts as a catalyst in many biological reactions, especially those involved in the release of energy and in glycogen and protein synthesis. If the sodium level increases in the intracellular material, it may counteract the catalytic effect of potassium and may interfere with cellular metabolism, especially protein synthesis. Potassium is a major factor in maintaining the osmotic pressure of the cell essential to the regulation of fluid balance. Its presence within the cell is important in the maintenance of acid-base balance, although it is not as readily mobilized as sodium to be a reserve base in offsetting an excess of acid-forming elements. It also plays a role in the transmission of nerve impulses and in the release of insulin from the pancreas. Potassium acts along with magnesium as a muscular relaxant in opposition to calcium, which stimulates muscular contraction.

Deficiency

Potassium-deficiency symptoms are fairly well documented but seldom occur as a result of suboptimal dietary intakes. A deficiency state may occur in infants suffering from diarrhea when the passage of the intestinal contents is so rapid that there is a decreased absorption of dietary potassium and an increased loss of potassium not resorbed from digestive secretions. Vomiting, the use of diuretics, severe protein-calorie malnutrition, and surgery may also lead to potassium depletion. Overall muscle weakness, poor intestinal tonus with resultant abdominal bloating, heart abnormalities, and weakness of respiratory muscles are characteristic. Infants suffering from kwashiorkor respond to treatment only when potassium therapy is given along with an increased protein intake.

Because of the antagonistic relationship between sodium and potassium, an excessive intake of sodium may have the same effect as a suboptimal level of potassium.

A magnesium deficiency also leads to decreased retention of potassium.

Requirements

The amount of potassium in the American diet has been estimated at 2 to 6 g/day, or 0.8 to 1.5 g/1000 kcal. Since potassium is distributed in a great many foods, its presence in the diet tends to parallel the caloric value of the diet. Although it has been established that potassium is a dietary essential, there is little information on minimal needs, which are estimated to be about 2.5 g/day. There is no evidence that the amount generally found in the diet is suboptimal. The potassium content of some representative foods is shown in Table 7-7. Potassium in food occurs in very soluble form, increasing the possibility that a considerable amount may leach into the cooking water. Similarly, potassium is lost in whey in making cheese.

Because plants are rich in potassium, it is sometimes necessary to provide salt licks for herbivorous animals, such as cattle and sheep, to prevent a sodium-potassium imbalance.

CHLORINE

Chlorine, present as 0.15% of body weight, is widely distributed throughout the body, but is found in highest concentration as

Table 7-7. Potassium content of average servings of some representative foods

>500 mg	300-500 mg	100-300 mg	<100 mg
Avocado	Banana	Grapefruit	Lemonade
Dried apricots	Liver	Orange	Egg
Cantaloupe	Pork	Apple	Cottage cheese
Lima beans	Chicken	Citrus juice	Bread
Potato	Salmon	Tuna	Cereals
	Molasses, dark	Ham, cured	Sugar
	Potato	Frankfurters	Cheddar cheese
	Peanut butter	Ice cream	
	Milk	Cabbage	
	Broccoli	Carrots	
		Tomato	
		Beef	
		Pork	

chloride in the cerebrospinal fluid and in the secretions into the gastrointestinal tract. Muscle and nerve tissue are relatively low in chlorine.

As a part of hydrochloric acid, chlorine is necessary to maintain the normal acidity of the stomach contents needed for the action of gastric enzymes. It is an acid-forming element, and along with the other acid-forming elements phosphorus and sulfur, helps to maintain acid-base balance in the body fluids. Chloride ions are able to pass out of the red blood cell into the blood plasma easily. They contribute to the ability of the blood to carry large amounts of carbon dioxide to the lungs. As carbon dioxide is taken up and released from the blood, chloride shifts in and out of the plasma to counteract any change in the acid-base balance that might otherwise occur. This ready transfer of chloride in and out of the red blood cell is called a chloride shift.

Chlorine in the diet is provided almost exclusively by sodium chloride; therefore when salt intake is restricted, the chlorine, level, first in urine and then in the tissue, drops. Whenever there are excesssive losses of sodium, as in diarrhea, sweating, or vomiting, concurrent losses of chloride ions occur.

SULFUR

Sulfur, which represents 0.25% of body weight, is present in every cell of the body. It is concentrated in the cytoplasm. The highest concentration of sulfur is found in the hair, skin, and nails, as evidenced by the characteristic odor of sulfur dioxide given off when these keratin-containing tissues are burned. The sulfur-containing amino acids, cystine and methionine, are characteristic of keratin and are found in high concentration in these tissues.

Sulfur in combination with hydrogen (SH) plays an important role in metabolism, since it is readily oxidized—a reaction essential for the formation of a blood clot. It is also able to form high-energy compounds that make it important in the transfer of energy. It is part of at least four vitamins—thiamin, pantothenic acid, biotin, and lipoic acid—which act as coenzymes necessary to activate several enzymes. Compounds containing sulfur act as detoxifying substances by combining with poisonous substances to convert them into harmless compounds that are excreted. Sulfur appears necessary for collagen synthesis and the formation of many mucopolysaccharides.

Sulfur is available to the body primarily as

the organic sulfur in the amino acids, methionine and cystine. Inorganic sulfur, or sulfur as sulfate, can contribute to the pool of sulfur in the body, but its availability depends on the ratio of organic to inorganic sulfur. Any excess of the element is excreted in the urine.

BIBLIOGRAPHY

Calcium

Alveoli, L. V.: Intestinal absorption of calcium, Arch. Intern. Med. **129:**345, 1972.

Calcium requirements, Report of Joint FAO/WHO Expert Committee, WHO Techn. Rep. Ser. No. 230, 1962.

Copp, D. H.: Endocrine control of calcium metabolism, Annu. Rev. Physiol. **32:**61, 1970.

Council on Foods and Nutrition: Symposium on human calcium requirements, J.A.M.A. **185:**588, 1963.

Engelmann, D. T., Sie, T. L., and Draper, H. H., et al.: Effect of a high protein intake on calcium metabolism in the rat, J. Nutr. **105:**475, 1975.

Heaney, R. P., Recker, R. R., and Saville, P. D.: Calcium balance and calcium requirements in middle-aged women, Am. J. Clin. Nutr. **30:**1603, 1977.

Hegsted, D. M.: Nutrition, bone, and calcified tissue, J. Am. Diet. Assoc. **50:**105, 1967.

Irwin, M. I., and Kienholz, E. W.: A conspectus of research on calcium requirements of man, J. Nutr. **103:**1019, 1973.

Jowsey, J., Riggs, B. L., and Kelly, P. S.: New concepts in the treatment of osteoporosis, Postgrad. Med. **52:**62, 1972.

Leitch, I., and Aitken, F. C.: An estimation of calcium requirement; a re-examination, Nutr. Abstr. Rev. **29:**394, 1959.

Lutwak, L.: Tracer studies in intestinal calcium absorption in man, Am. J. Clin. Nutr. **22:**771, 1969.

Lutwak, L., and Whedon, G. D.: Osteoporosis—a mineral deficiency disease? J. Am. Diet. Assoc. **44:**173, 1964.

Malm, O. J.: Calcium and magnesium, Prog. Food Nutr. Sci. **1:**173, 1975.

Margen, S., Chu, J.-Y., Kaufmann, N. A., and Calloway, D. H.: Studies in calcium metabolism. I. The calciuric effect of dietary protein, Am. J. Clin. Nutr. **27:**584, 1974.

Rassmussen, H., and Pecht, M. M.: Calcitonin, Sci. Am. **223:**4, 1970.

Shenolikar, I. S.: Absorption of dietary calcium in pregnancy, Am. J. Clin. Nutr. **23:**63, 1970.

Spencer, H., Kramer, L., Osis, D., and Norris, D.: Effect of phosphorus on the absorption of calcium and on the calcium balance in man, J. Nutr. **108:**447, 1978.

Walker, A. R. P.: The human requirement of calcium: Should low intakes be supplemented? Am. J. Clin. Nutr. **25:**518, 1972.

Walker, R. M., and Linkswiler, H. M.: Calcium retention in the adult human male as affected by protein intake, J. Nutr. **102:**1297, 1972.

Magnesium

Caddell, J. L.: Magnesium in the nutrition of the child, Clin. Pediatr. **13:**263, 1977.

Caddell, J. L: Magnesium deficiency in extremis, Nutr. Today **2**(3):14, 1967.

Krehl, W. A.: Magnesium, Nutr. Today **2**(3):16, 1967.

Malm, O. J.: Calcium and magnesium, Prog. Food Nutr. Sci. **1:**173, 1975.

Schroeder, H. A., and Nason, A. P.: Essential minerals in man—magnesium, J. Chronic Dis. **21:**815, 1969.

Seelig, M. S.: Magnesium interrelationships in ischemic heart disease: a review, Am. J. Clin. Nutr. **27:**59, 1974.

Seelig, M. S.: The requirement of magnesium by the normal adult, Am. J. Clin. Nutr. **14:**342, 1964.

Shils, M.: Experimental human magnesium depletion. I. Clinical observations and blood chemistry alterations, Am. J. Clin. Nutr. **15:**133, 1964.

Wacker, E. C., and Parisi, A. F.: Magnesium metabolism, N. Engl. J. Med. **278:**658, 712, 722, 1968.

Potassium

Darrow, D. C.: Physiological basis of potassium therapy, J.A.M.A. **162:**1310, 1956.

Sodium

Bloch, M. R.: Social influence of salt, Sci. Am. **209:**88, July, 1963.

Earley, L. E., and Daugharty, T. M.: Sodium metabolism, N. Engl. J. Med. **281:**72, 1969.

Pike, R. L.: Sodium intake during pregnancy, J. Am. Diet. Assoc. **44:**176, 1964.

8

Micronutrient elements

Some trace elements such as iron and iodine have been recognized as essential for many years. As sensitive techniques have been developed for study of these elements, which generally amount to less than 5 ppm in both food and the body, it has become evident that many other elements are needed. Almost yearly scientists either identify a new essential element or learn more about the ways known trace elements function. Knowledge of the amounts in food and some provisional estimates of human requirements have raised questions about the adequacy of these elements in the American diet. These questions are of special concern as a larger portion of our diet consists of processed foods.

IRON

The element iron was first recognized as a constituent of body tissue in 1713. Since that time it has been determined that iron represents about 0.004% of the body weight—an amount that varies from 3 to 5 g, depending on age, sex, size, nutritional status, general health, and size of iron stores. Virtually all iron exists in combination with protein in transport, storage, enzymes, or respiratory compounds. These respiratory compounds capitalize on the ability of iron to accept and release oxygen and carbon dioxide readily. Such reactions are essential to life and represent the primary biochemical role of iron.

Distribution

Iron is concentrated in the blood, but some is present in every living cell. The distribution of iron throughout various body tissues is shown in Table 8-1. About 70% of the iron in the body is considered functional iron. The majority of this is present in the hemoglobin molecule of the red blood cell. A small portion exists as part of **myoglobin,** the iron-containing protein in muscle, which differs from **hemoglobin** only in the nature of the protein. The rest of the functional iron exists in the tissue enzymes, notably cytochrome oxidase and catalase, which are present in every living cell and are essential for cellular respiration, involving the exchange of oxygen and carbon dioxide.

Functional iron amounts to about 35 mg/kg of body weight. The remaining 30% of body iron stored in the liver, spleen, and bone marrow is designated as storage or nonessential iron. Storage iron is quite variable but generally amounts to 15 mg/kg of body weight or from 0.1 to 1.5 g in men. Stores in women are usually much lower (0.3 g) and may represent from 0% to 20% of total body iron. Storage iron is present in the liver and spleen as a soluble iron complex, ferritin, with a 20% iron content or as hemosiderin, an insoluble iron-protein complex, containing 35% iron. Both are capable of releasing stored iron.

In addition to the hemoglobin iron, the blood contains about 4 mg of iron that is being transported from the site of absorption or the liver to the cells, tightly bound to the protein transferrin. This transport iron is turned over so rapidly that as much as 35 to 40 mg is exchanged each day. Another iron-containing substance, ferritin, is present in

Table 8-1. Distribution of iron throughout the body

	Total (%)	Approximate amount (mg)	
		Male	Female
Hemoglobin	60-75	2100	1750
Myoglobin	3	100	100
Storage iron (liver, spleen, and bone marrow)	0-30	1000	400
Tissue iron	5-15	350	300
Transport iron	1	4	4
Serum ferritin	1	0.3	0.1
TOTAL		3554.3	2554.1

the blood serum in equilibrium with storage iron. A very small amount of iron is present loosely bound to other substances.

Since the body has no mechanism for excreting iron, the level of both functional and storage iron is regulated through absorption. The body is extremely efficient in conserving iron and will avidly retain or salvage any iron that results from the catabolism, or breakdown, of iron-containing substances. Iron is absorbed in response to a need.

Functions

Carrier of oxygen and carbon dioxide. The basic biochemical role of iron is to permit the transfer of oxygen and carbon dioxide from one tissue to another. It accomplishes this primarily as a part of both hemoglobin and myoglobin, which are iron-containing proteins in the blood and muscle, respectively. It is also part of several other compounds and enzymes that are also essential for the uptake and release of oxygen and carbon dioxide. Since these reactions are involved primarily in release of energy within the cell, iron is essential for energy metabolism.

Blood formation. Hemoglobin is an essential component of the red blood cells, or erythrocytes. These cells are formed in the bone marrow in response to the presence of the hormone erythropoietin, produced in the kidneys. The level of erythropoietin increases to stimulate the production of more cells when the oxygen-carrying capacity of the blood decreases with a reduction in the number of red blood cells.

Erythrocytes begin as nucleated immature cells, known as erythroblasts. As these cells mature in the bone marrow, heme, an iron-containing protein, is synthesized in the presence of vitamin B_6 (pyridoxine) from the amino acid glycine and iron. The heme unites with another protein, globin, synthesized simultaneously from other amino acids. These hemoglobin-containing immature red blood cells, known as reticulocytes, are released into the bloodstream, where they lose their nuclei to become mature non-nucleated red blood cells capable of functioning as carriers of carbon dioxide and oxygen.

Because red blood cells have no nucleus they cannot synthesize the enzymes essential for their life. As a result, they live only as long as the enzymes present at maturity remain functional—usually about four months. As the red blood cells die, they are removed from the bloodstream by the cells of the reticuloendothelial system—the liver, bone marrow, and spleen. In the spleen the iron and the amino acids of the hemoglobin molecule are removed. The iron is stored as hemosiderin and ferritin in the liver and spleen or is returned to the bone marrow, where it is incorporated into new hemoglobin molecules. This turnover of iron amounts to about 20 mg/day. The amino acids are returned to the amino acid pool in the blood, making them available for the synthesis of new protein or for deamination before being used as a source of energy. The remaining portion of the erythrocytes is excreted in the bile. By this mechanism, iron is carefully conserved and reused. The rate at which red blood cells break up is accelerated in dietary deficiencies of ascorbic acid, vitamin E, and vitamin B_{12} (cobalamin), all of which favor hematopoiesis (formation of red blood cells) and hemoglobin synthesis.

The adult male has 15 g of hemoglobin per deciliter of blood and the adult female 13.6 g/dl. Therefore the total hemoglobin content of the 5 liters of blood in the adult male is 750 g. This amount of hemoglobin contains 2500 mg of iron (0.34%). Since erythrocytes live only 120 days on the average, 1/120 of these cells are replaced every day. This means that 1/120 of the total iron, or approximately 20 mg, is released each day from old cells and is incorporated into the 5 to 6 g of hemoglobin in the cells that replace them. As will be discussed later, it would be impossible to provide this amount of iron from dietary sources; therefore the process of conserving iron is essential to the survival of the organism.

A small amount of the total body iron is incorporated into tissue enzymes. The mechanism for this is not as well understood as is that for hemoglobin synthesis. There is ample evidence that in a dietary deficiency the level of iron-containing tissue enzymes drops before the hemoglobin level of the blood drops.

Other functions. There is considerable evidence that iron is important in many functions other than those associated with blood formation and the transport of oxygen. These nonheme functions include catalyzing the conversion of beta-carotene, the precursor of vitamin A, to vitamin A; the synthesis of purines, an integral part of nucleic acid; clearance of blood lipids; collagen synthesis; antibody production; and detoxification of drugs in the liver. Studies of the role of iron as an anti-infective agent suggest two conflicting roles. Although iron is necessary for the growth of microorganisms, it is an essential part of enzymes and immune substances needed to destroy invading infectious organisms. Since it is essential for the growth of microorganisms, if iron is available potentially harmful bacteria will be able to grow. On the other hand, if iron is not available there will be a decreased production of iron-containing enzymes and other immune substances, which are needed to destroy infectious organisms. For instance, lactoferrin in breast milk is an iron-containing substance especially effective against *E. coli* organisms in the gastrointestinal tract of infants apparently because it binds iron so that it is not available for growth of this bacteria.

Need for dietary iron

Replacement of losses of body iron. Although iron is avidly conserved once it has been absorbed and there is no mechanism for excreting iron, there is some loss each day that must be replaced. Since iron is present in every cell of the body, any loss of cells will represent a loss of iron. Thus the desquamation, or sloughing, of surface cells, the loss of cells lining the gastrointestinal tract, and the shedding of hair or nails all contribute to the loss of body iron. A small number of red blood cells, containing less than 0.1 mg of iron, appear in the urine. Perspiration is also believed to contain some iron. Losses in the urine, perspiration, and desquamated cells vary from 0.2 to 0.5 mg. Daily fecal losses from the sloughing of iron-containing mucosal cells lining the intestine are estimated at up to 0.5 mg/day.

These small losses of 0.7 to 1 mg/day are the only ones that the adult male must replace. Women, however, must replace the iron lost in menstruation. Although this amount varies greatly among women, it is fairly consistent from month to month in the same woman, amounting to 16 to 32 mg/mo, or 0.5 to 1 mg/day calculated over the month. About 95% of women have a menstrual loss

Table 8-2. Summary of iron requirements (mg/day)

Age group	Losses in feces	Losses in urine, perspiration, and desquamation	Needs for menstruation	Needs for growth	Needs for pregnancy	Total needs
Adult men	0.7	0.2-0.5				0.9-1.2
Adult women	0.7	0.2-0.5	0.5-1.0			1.4-2.2
Pregnant women	0.7	0.2-0.5			1.0-2.0	1.9-3.2
Children	0.7	0.2-0.5		0.2		1.1-1.4
Adolescent girls	0.7	0.2-0.5	0.5-1.0	0.5-1.0		1.9-3.2

of less than 1.4 mg/day. When these needs are added to other adult needs, it becomes apparent that before menopause women must absorb from 1.2 to 2 mg daily to replace their losses, which are almost twice those of men.

Growth. Need for iron during growth is the result of an increase in blood volume with a concurrent increase in hemoglobin and in tissue mass, calling for more myoglobin and iron-containing enzymes. The increase in body iron from 0.5 g at birth to 5 g in the adult represents an increase of 4.5 g during the twenty-year growth period. Assuming a uniform rate of growth, this would amount to 225 mg/yr, or 0.6 mg/day. This is in line with observations that infants over 3 months of age retain 0.5 mg, older children 0.2, and adolescents 0.5 to 1 mg/day. Others have estimated growth needs at 35 mg/kg increase in body weight.

It is recognized that the physiological iron needs for growth, menstrual losses, and other losses are great. Table 8-2 summarizes our knowledge about iron needs.

Blood donation. The gift of 0.5 liter (1 pint) of blood represents a loss of 250 mg of iron that must be replaced. The blood volume and the cell number will return to normal quickly, but the return of hemoglobin to previous levels can occur only at the expense of storage iron. To replace the amount of iron lost would require the absorption of an additional 0.7 mg of iron a day for a year.

Absorption

Mechanism

Iron from food is absorbed primarily in the oxidized form, **ferric iron** (Fe^{+++}), although some **ferrous iron** (Fe^{++}) is used. Both occur in food attached to organic compounds, from which they must be released before being absorbed. The body can utilize either form, but evidence indicates that naturally occurring ferrous iron is used more efficiently than ferric iron and that most iron is reduced to ferrous iron before being absorbed. This is facilitated by the acidity of the stomach contents. Iron present in food in the porphyrin portion of the hemoglobin is referred to as **heme iron.** All other dietary iron is called **nonheme iron.**

The absorption of iron occurs in regulated amounts in the upper part of the small intestine, usually in the duodenum. The rapid rate of absorption has been indicated by studies with radioactive iron, which showed that significant amounts were absorbed within four hours after ingestion and appeared in the erythroblasts within twenty-four hours. From 2% to 10% of the iron content of food is absorbed. The many factors that influence this will be discussed later.

Since the body has no mechanism for excreting iron, the iron content of the body is regulated through controlled absorption. The exact nature of the mechanism is still being debated, but it now appears that dietary iron linked to a carrier substance becomes attached to the surface of the cells lining the upper intestinal tract. From there it enters the cell and is handled in one of two ways. It may be carried quickly across the cell and released on the other side to the blood. There, if the carrier protein in the blood, **transferrin**, is not already saturated with iron, the dietary iron is released from the cell, attaches to the carrier, and is absorbed into the general circulation. Otherwise the iron may remain within the mucosal cells that line the intestinal wall, attached to the intracellular carrier form for iron. Alternatively, it may be changed to ferric iron and transferred to a larger molecule, apoferritin, as long as free apoferritin is formed within the cells. The combination of iron and apoferritin is known as ferritin, the form in which much iron is temporarily stored in the epithelial cells.

The rate at which iron is released from the mucosal cell to the general circulation depends on the amount and saturation of transferrin (a beta-globulin) in the blood. This protein, capable of binding 2 atoms of iron per molecule, is able to carry iron to the tissues, bone marrow, and storage sites. When transferrin is saturated up to about a third of its total iron-binding capacity (TIBC) of 0.3 mg/dl of plasma, no more iron is absorbed from the mucosal cells except under conditions of excessive intakes in which iron absorption is no longer under control. However, whenever there is more unbound transferrin, the iron in the epithelial cell recombines with a carbohydrate or amino acid carrier to again form an iron chelate. This iron-containing complex passes from the epithelial cell into the blood plasma, where it releases its iron to transferrin which has attached to the cell wall.

Once the transferrin has picked up the iron, it controls its distribution to other tissues. It delivers large amounts to tissues, such as bone marrow and the placenta that have high requirements and protects those with low requirements from taking up too much. If the iron is needed, it passes quickly into the bloodstream. If not needed, it remains in the epithelial cells and will be lost from the body through fecal excretion when these cells die and slough from the wall of the intestinal tract. From 50 to 80 g of these cells are lost each day, with complete renewal of the lining of the gastrointestinal tract occurring in less than four days.

In contrast to inorganic iron, iron contained in heme is absorbed as a heme molecule. The iron is then released into the bloodstream from heme by action of the enzyme xanthine oxidase within the mucosal cell.

Factors affecting absorption

Body's need for iron. The need for iron is indicated by the unbound transferrin level of the blood and possibly the amount of messenger iron in the mucosal cells of the intestinal wall. This messenger iron reflects the amount of iron available at the time the cell was formed. When unbound levels rise, indicating that iron has been removed from the blood to tissues or storage sites, more iron is absorbed to maintain a constant level in the blood. When the transferrin is saturated with iron, representing a decreased demand for iron on the part of the body cells, less is absorbed. Thus the iron absorption mechanism responds to the body's need for iron.

A person with normal hemoglobin levels absorbs from 2% to 10% of dietary iron. A person with low hemoglobin levels and probably high demands for iron may absorb as much as 35% of dietary iron from heme found only in animal foods. One study using the whole body counter for radioactive iron showed that iron-deficient subjects absorbed 29% of ingested iron, whereas normal subjects absorbed 10%. Progressive increase in iron absorption is noted in the latter half of pregnancy, when the demands of the fetus on maternal iron are great. Children may also absorb iron at a rate up to twice that of adults.

The need for iron is increased under any condition such as exercise where the production of red blood cells is speeded up. Similarly, when a person suffers from hypoxia, or loss of oxygen, in the brain, the need for oxygen is reflected in an increased synthesis of red blood cells, presumably to increase the amount of oxygen available to the brain cells.

Form of iron. Although the body can absorb both the reduced ferrous (Fe^{++}) and the oxidized ferric (Fe^{+++}) iron, absorption is greater when iron is available in the ferrous form. The ferric iron that predominates in food is usually reduced to the ferrous form prior to absorption, although during absorption it may be oxidized and reduced several times. The presence of any reducing substance, such as acid, is believed to enhance iron absorption. The hydrochloric acid secreted in the stomach keeps iron in the more readily available reduced form. Utilization of ferric iron is reduced up to 50% in persons with a decreased secretion of hydrochloric acid in the stomach, known as achlorhydria. This is often associated with increasing age or with the consumption of alkaline powders in large amounts, as by ulcer patients. The addition of hydrochloric acid to the diets of those suffering from achlorhydria had no beneficial effect on iron absorption, suggesting that the decreased hydrochloric acid secretion may well be a result and not a cause of poor iron absorption. The low pH maintained under normal gastric secretions may facilitate the formation of an iron complex that remains soluble at the higher pH of the intestinal contents.

Organic acids in food, such as ascorbic acid (vitamin C) found in citrus fruits, enhance iron absorption by helping reduce ferric to ferrous iron. These acids may play an important role in diets of older individuals, in whom they may compensate for the reduced hydrochloric acid level. Since studies have shown that an increase in dietary vitamin C without an increase in iron is beneficial in iron-deficiency conditions, vitamin C is often included with iron supplements. Amino acids, especially cysteine, increase the proportion of dietary iron absorbed.

Composition of the meal. The absorption of iron depends on whether a food is eaten alone or in combination with other foods. Only 5% of the iron in most vegetable foods such as rice, corn, spinach, and wheat is absorbed, whereas 20% of that in meat such as veal and 10% in fish are absorbed.

The consumption of meat in conjunction with vegetables increases the absorption of iron from the vegetables twofold or threefold—apparently because of the enhancement of inorganic iron absorption by the sulfur-containing amino acid cysteine. This amino acid, released during digestion of meat, probably acts through the formation of soluble iron chelates. The synergistic effect of meat on iron absorption is reflected in the WHO recommendation that adult women whose diets contain less than 10% of the calories from animal foods receive 28 mg of iron whereas those with 25% of the calories from animal foods require an intake of 14 mg.

The beneficial effects of ascorbic acid on iron absorption suggest that a source of vitamin C be consumed at each meal that provides a dietary source of iron. It acts not only by maintaining iron in a reduced form but also by forming a complex that remains soluble at the pH of the small intestine where iron is absorbed. The effect of interaction of various foods on iron absorption raises a question about the value of data on the absorption of individual foods rather than mixed meals.

Bulk in diet. High bulk in the diet depresses the utilization of iron, which may account for the reports of poor absorption of 1% to 2% often noted from green leafy vegetables such as spinach. On the basis of this it has been suggested that iron supplements should be taken before meals to minimize the interference that the bulk of the diet may exert on iron absorption.

Size of dose. The percentage of iron absorbed varies inversely with the size of the dose. An intake of iron at a level of 0.25 mg/kg of body weight resulted in 32% utilization, whereas at 4 mg/kg only 4.1% was utilized. The administration of supplemental iron in smaller divided doses three or four times a day at a level commensurate with the body's ability to absorb it results in much better utilization than does a single large dose.

Other factors. Phytic acid is an organic acid found in some whole-grain cereal products, such as oatmeal. It combines with iron to form an insoluble iron complex that the body cannot utilize. The presence of phytic acid is not a cause for concern in a normal mixed diet, but should oatmeal or other foods high in phytic acid become staple items in the diet, the adverse effects on iron absorption may become significant. Excess phosphorus may also have an inhibitory effect on iron absorption.

Steatorrhea, an abnormal condition in which higher than normal amounts of fat appear in the feces, is associated with a decreased rate of iron absorption.

The altitude at which a person lives also influences the extent of iron absorption. An increase occurs at high altitudes, whereas less is absorbed at lower altitudes.

Transportation and metabolism

Once iron has been absorbed from the epithelial cells into the blood, it is carried throughout the body bound to the protein carrier transferrin. From the blood it may be removed by several pathways. In response to the demands of all body cells it will be released for use in the synthesis of respiratory enzymes and other vital cellular constituents that require iron. Much of the iron in transit in the blood plasma, which may come either from dietary sources, from the breakdown of body cells, and/or from the storage depots, will be removed by the bone marrow to be used in the manufacture of hemoglobin for red blood cells. About 20 mg of iron is used in the 5 to 6 g of hemoglobin liberated daily

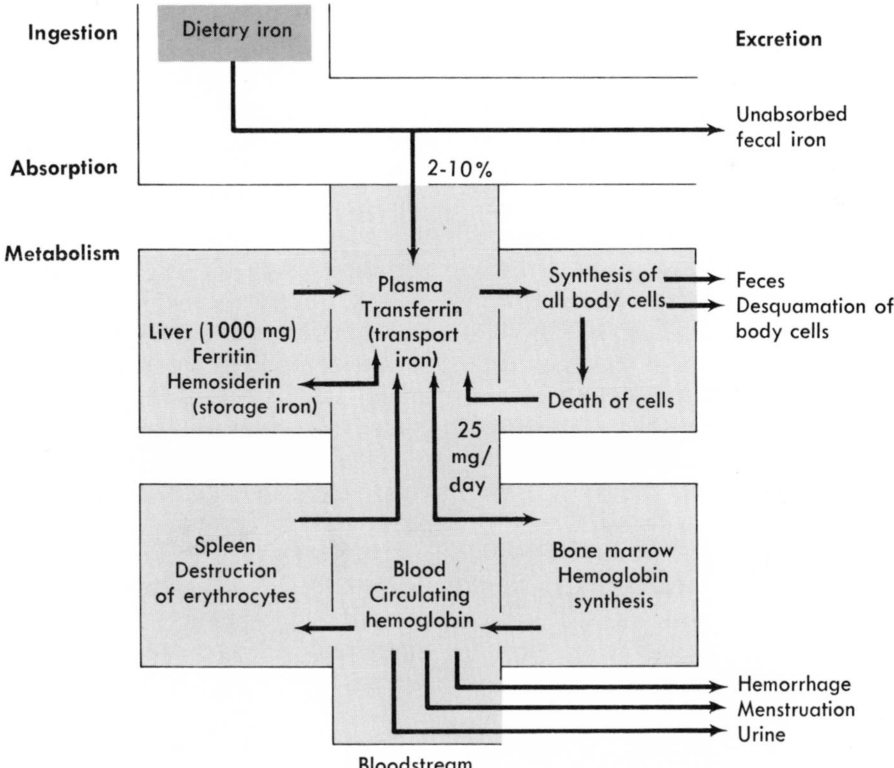

Fig. 8-1. Schematic representation of absorption and metabolism of iron.

from the bone marrow in the newly formed red blood cells. Iron in excess of immediate needs of cells and bone marrow will be deposited in the iron storage sites of the body. Of approximately 1000 mg (1 g) of iron stored in the body at any one time, 30% is in the liver, 30% in the bone marrow, and the rest in the spleen and muscles.

If the dietary iron absorbed from the intestinal tract coupled with that obtained from the breakdown of red blood cells is not adequate, iron will be mobilized from the reserves in the liver, will be bound to transferrin in the blood, and will be recirculated throughout the body. If necessary, up to 50 mg/day can be mobilized from storage iron. Only when the body's reserves of iron have been depleted will there be any evidence of iron deficiency symptoms. In infants the liver stores are adequate to last three to six months. A reserve of 1000 mg in the adult lasts a male 1000 days and a woman over 500 days. The absorption and metabolism of iron are summarized diagrammatically in Fig. 8-1.

Table 8-3. Recommended dietary allowances for iron for "reference" men and women

Country	Allowance (mg/day)	
	Male	Female
Australia	10	10
Canada	10	14
Central America and Panama	10	10
Columbia	10	15
East Germany	10	15
West Germany	10	12
Japan	10	10
Netherlands	10	12
Norway	12	12
South Africa	9	12
United Kingdom	12	12
United States	10	18

Recommended dietary allowances

Adults. The National Research Council recommended allowances for iron for adults are based on the assumption that an adult male must obtain approximately 0.7 to 1 mg of iron a day to replace body losses and the adult female, from 1.2 to 2 mg/day. Since the average rate of iron absorption is 2% to 10% of ingested iron, it has been recommended that men obtain 10 mg and women 18 mg from dietary sources. For women this represents a narrow margin of safety and may actually fail to meet the needs of some women.

The extent to which various advisory groups differ in their recommendations for desirable iron intake is evident from Table 8-3. In some cases differences can be attributed to differences in philosophy, in others to differences in interpretation of available data.

Pregnancy. An evaluation of iron requirements during pregnancy shows that 300 mg are needed for the growth of the fetus, 70 mg for the placenta, and 500 mg for the synthesis of hemoglobin associated with the increase in blood volume that occurs at this time. Iron accumulates in the fetus at a rate of 0.5 mg/day in the first trimester but increases to 3 to 4 mg/day in the last two trimesters. Even with the increase in the extent to which iron is absorbed, it is almost impossible for a woman to obtain the required amount of iron from food alone, especially since the increase in calorie requirement is relatively small. As a result the Food and Nutrition Board of the National Research Council recommends that pregnant women in addition to obtaining 18 mg from dietary sources, take a supplement providing from 30 to 60 mg of iron.

Iron is stored rapidly in fetal tissue during the latter half of pregnancy when the fetus is parasitic on the mother for iron. Iron will be transferred to fetal blood in an irreversible fashion even if the mother's hemoglobin level drops. The apparent drop in hemoglobin levels of the mother during pregnancy often reflects an increase in blood volume rather than an absolute drop in the amount of hemoglobin. The normal level for newborns is 18 to 22 g of hemoglobin per deciliter of blood. Twins, who must share a maternal iron supply, and premature infants are usually born with hemoglobin levels below the normally high infant levels. Since the reserve of iron is usually lower also, it may be necessary to supplement their diet with iron at an earlier age than for a full-term infant.

Lactation. Human milk, which contains about 0.2 μg/ml (about twice the amount in cow's milk), is still a relatively poor source of iron. The amount in hind milk produced at the end of a feeding is significantly higher than that at the beginning of the nursing period. In all cases this iron is well absorbed. The amount present is not influenced by the amount in the maternal diet. As a result, the recommended intake during lactation is the same as for the adult woman.

Infants and children. The reserve of iron in the liver of a full-term infant is sufficient to last from three to six months, during which time the infant doubles its birth weight. Thus the National Research Council sees no need to recommend a dietary source of iron other than milk until at least three months of age. The very high hemoglobin values in newborn infants drop rapidly to 12 g at 4 to 6 months of age and are maintained close to this level throughout childhood before rising in late adolescence to adult levels.

No advantage apparently results from maintaining the high birth levels. In fact, attempts to supplement the infant diet to prevent a drop have been unsuccessful, since little iron is absorbed in early infancy unless there is a physiological need for it. Although the current trend of adding iron to infant formula from birth does not prevent the drop in hemoglobin levels, it may provide some protection against anemia after 3 months of age.

For infants over 4 months of age, dietary iron should be provided in adequate amounts for the synthesis of hemoglobin required by the increasing blood volume and the demands of newly formed cells for iron. (The Academy of Pediatrics recommends that infants be given iron-fortified milk throughout the first year of life.) Needs of infants for dietary iron are greater per unit of body weight than adult needs and remain relatively high during childhood. Recommended iron intakes then increase in proportion to the increase in body size up to physical maturity, after which iron is needed only for replacement of iron lost from the body.

The recommended dietary allowances for iron proposed by FAO/WHO vary, depending on the proportion of the recommended calorie intake that is provided by animal foods. This reflects the fact that absorption of dietary iron is increased as the proportion of heme iron increases.

Table 8-4. Iron content of different types of cooked liver*

Liver	mg/100 g
Chicken	8.5
Beef	8.8
Calf	14.2
Lamb	17.9
Pork	29.1

*From Watt, B. K., and Merrill, A. L.: Composition of foods—raw, processed and prepared, Handbook No. 8, Washington D.C., 1963, U.S. Department of Agriculture.

Food sources

A diet adequate in most other nutrients will provide only 6 mg of iron/1000 kcal. Because of this it is difficult to obtain the recommended 18 mg of iron for the adult woman, especially if caloric intake is below 3000 kcal. The extent to which the American diet meets these standards is illustrated in Fig. 8-2.

The iron content of some representative foods in the American diet is given in Fig. 8-3. Liver is the only very rich source of iron, and as noted from Table 8-4 a sizable difference exists, depending on the type of liver

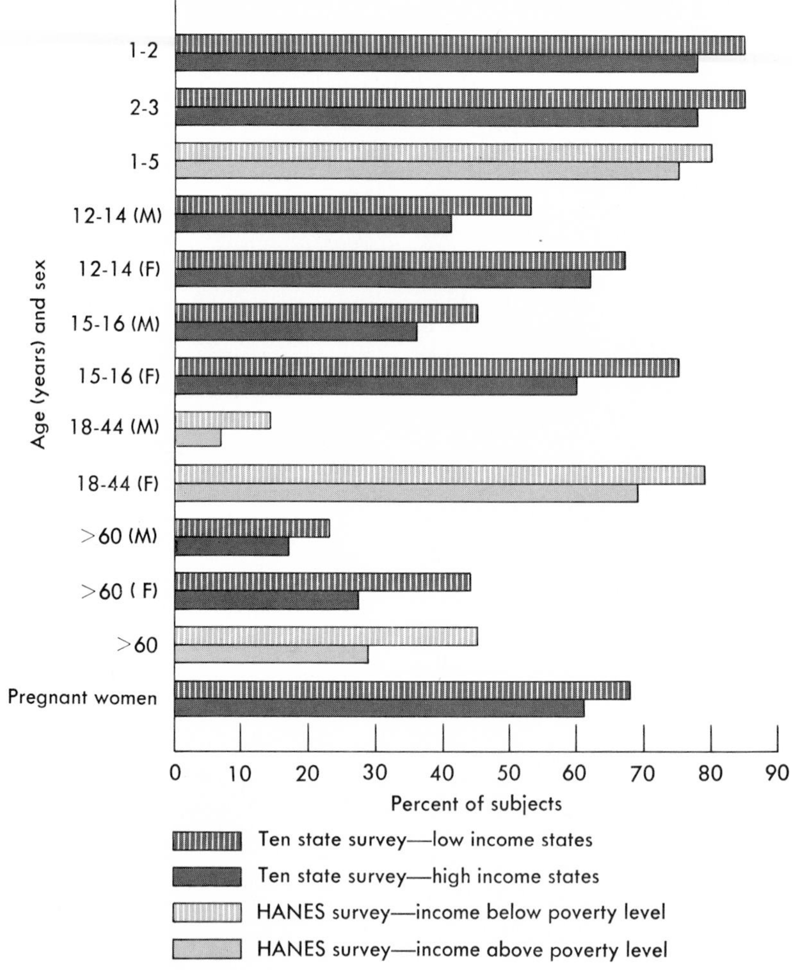

Fig. 8-2. Percentage of persons with dietary iron intake below two-thirds RDA by age, sex, and income level. Data based on results of Ten-State Nutrition Survey (1968-1970) and preliminary findings of First Health and Nutrition Examination Survey (HANES) (1971-1972).

used. In any species the amount found in the liver will reflect the storage of iron by the animal.

Since nutritionists have been singularly unsuccessful in increasing the popularity of liver in the American diet, most persons depend on other sources. As there are virtually no other very rich sources, a variety of moderately good sources must be combined to meet needs.

From Fig. 8-4, showing the contribution of various food groups to the iron in the nation's food supply, it is clear that no one group is responsible for a large share of the iron in the diet, but that the meat, cereal, and fruit and vegetable groups make comparable contributions. INQ for representative iron sources are given in Table 8-5.

Because of wide differences in the degree to which iron from various sources is absorbed, knowledge of the iron content of foods does not always give a true picture of its availability. Absorption depends on many factors, including the composition of the diet

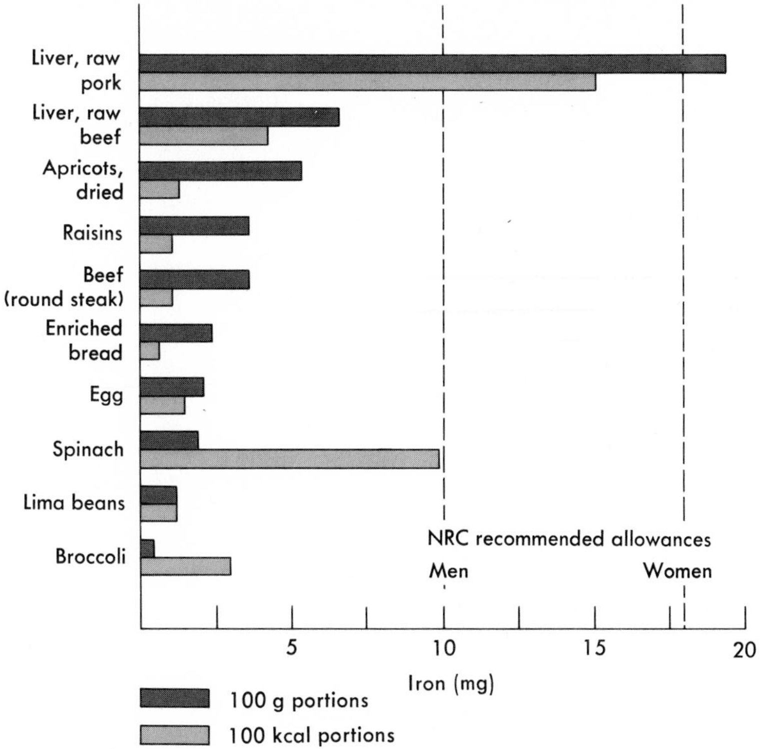

Fig. 8-3. Iron content of 100 g and 100 kcal portions of representative foods. (Based on Watt, B. K., and Merrill, A. L.: Composition of foods—raw, processed and prepared, Handbook No. 8, Washington, D.C., 1963, U.S. Department of Agriculture.)

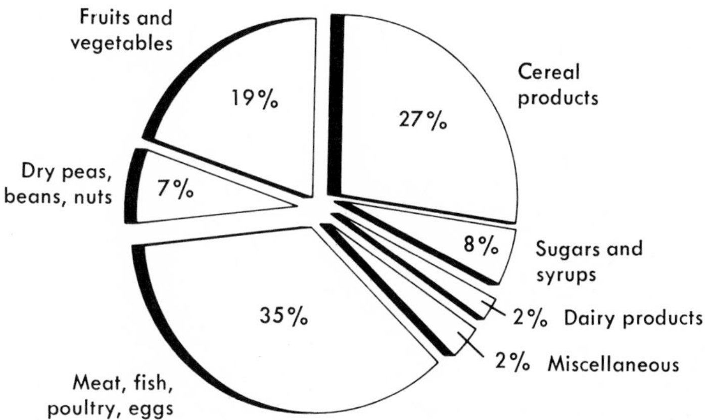

Fig. 8-4. Relative contribution of various food groups to total iron in American food supply. (Based on Contribution of major food groups to nutrition supplies available for civilian consumption, National Food Review NFR-1, Washington, D.C., 1978, Economic Research Service.)

Table 8-5. INQ for selected sources of iron providing at least 15% of the U.S. RDA

Bran flakes (40% bran)	15.0
Spinach	12.8
Asparagus	11.6
Clams	10.2
Molasses	9.1
Beans, snap	8.2
Dandelion greens	6.8
Prune juice	6.7
Beef heart	4.0
Apricots	2.7
Roast beef	2.5
Ground beef	2.1
Chili con carne	1.6
Whole wheat bread	1.6
Seedless raisins	1.5

and the needs of the individual. Difficulties inherent in determining the utilization of iron are responsible for the lack of agreement concerning the rate of iron absorption. Variations in results occur even with the use of radioactive iron biologically incorporated into food and when balance studies are done with meticulous care. In all cases, absorption by iron-deficient subjects averaged 20%, whereas that by subjects with normal hemoglobin levels averaged 2% to 10%, but a wide range of values is reported for each food tested. Interpretation of data on iron absorption is further complicated by the fact that they are different when a food is eaten alone than when it is eaten as part of a meal. Meat and citrus fruit in a meal enhance absorption, whereas eggs tend to depress it. Certain characteristics of the individual also influence absorption. The extent to which iron from various sources is absorbed is illustrated in Fig. 8-5.

The iron found in meat, described as heme iron, reflects the iron in both blood and muscle hemoglobin and as much as 35% may be absorbed. In eggs the iron is concentrated almost entirely in the yolk, but only from 4% to 10% is absorbed. The iron in chicken is well absorbed, with values up to 30% reported.

Fruits and vegetables are fairly good sources of iron, but often the bulk of the cellulose they contain results in relatively poor utilization. The iron content of vegetables is influenced by soil and climatic conditions so that there is a wide range of values reported for the same product. Vegetables provide about three times as much iron in the American diet as fruits. Fruits and juices are rated as poor iron sources, potatoes and green stalks and leaves as good sources, and leguminous plants as excellent sources.

Studies to determine the use of iron have not given consistent results. The pulp of fruits such as tomatoes and oranges contains twice as much iron as the juice. Occasionally canned fruits and vegetables or acid foods cooked in an iron container will pick up additional iron, which is as available as naturally occuring iron. Legumes such as peas and beans are relatively good sources, especially when the dry mature seed, which has had a prolonged growing period during which to accumulate iron, is used. Most plants have an upper limit of 10% of iron available. For soybeans 20% is available.

Although raisins and other dried fruits are often recommended for their iron content, they will have no more iron than the original fruit from which they were derived. It should be remembered that the amount of dried fruit needed to make a significant contribution of iron also makes a significant contribution of calories. For instance, one fourth cup of raisins, which provides 1.4 mg of iron, also provides 115 calories, giving an INQ for women of 1.5.

About 28% of the dietary iron is available as the result of the fortification of foods with iron. Although only thirty states have laws requiring the enrichment of flour, about 90% of the flour and bread sold in the United States has been enriched with iron salts at a level that makes it comparable in iron content to the unrefined cereal from which 20% of the iron is removed in milling. Evidence on the effectiveness of absorption of these

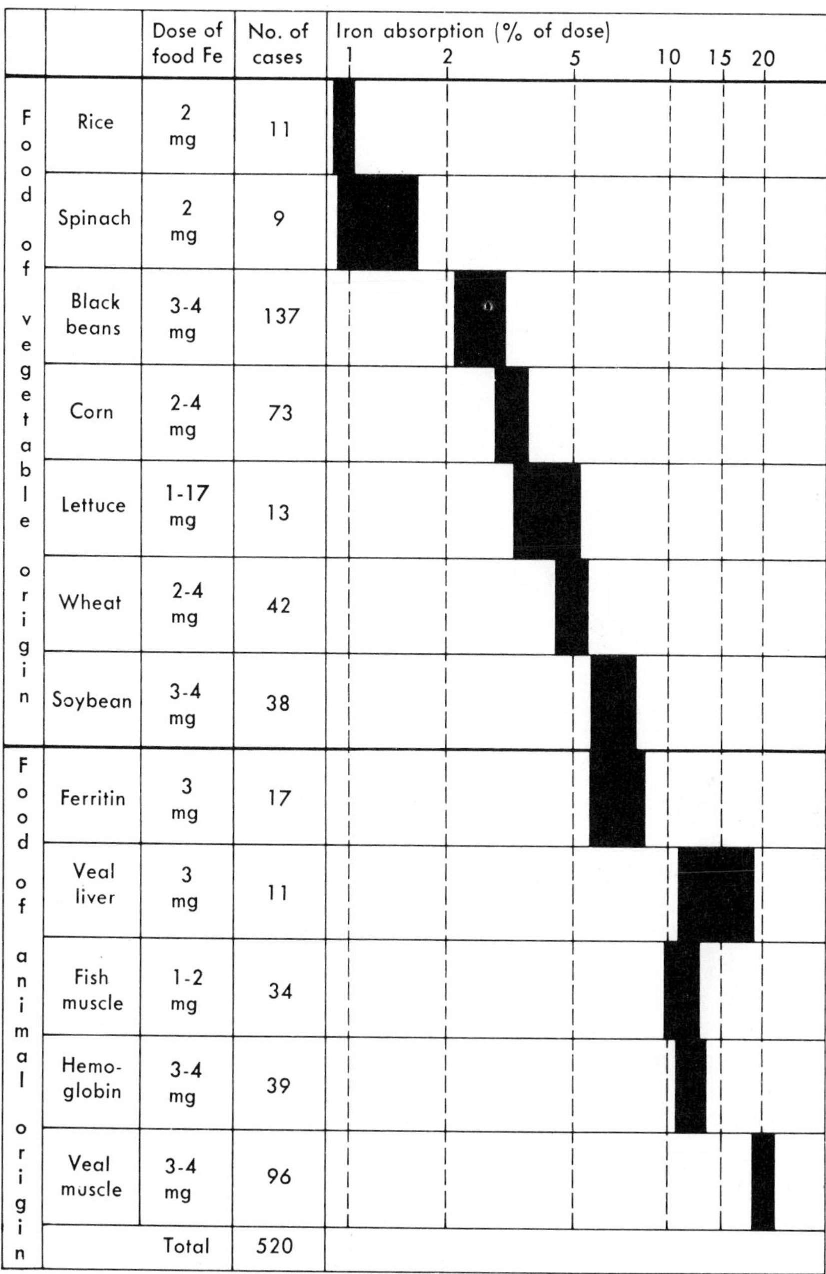

Fig. 8-5. Iron absorption from various plant and animal foods. (Data from Layrisse, M., and Martinez-Torres, C.: Prog. Hematol. **7:**137, 1971.)

added salts is fragmentary. As a result of findings indicating widespread anemia, the FDA proposed a revision of its standards for enrichment of bread and cereals to require the addition of almost three times as much iron as previously (40 mg/0.45 kg of flour and 25 mg/0.45 kg of bread). This regulation, which was to have been effective April, 1974, led to much controversy. Supporters maintained that this is the most effective way to reduce the incidence of anemia, which they assume is due to iron deficiency. The opponents feel that there is little basis to support the claim that such supplementation is or will be effective and that there has been insufficient study concerning possible harmful effects. Implementation of the regulation has been delayed and there appears to be little evidence that it will be enacted.

Cereals, either enriched or whole grain, provide small amounts of iron per unit of weight, but because of the extent to which they may be consumed by certain groups, such as adolescent boys and families on restricted food budgets, they often make a significant contribution to the day's iron intake even although only 0.5% to 6.5% is absorbed. Enriched bread, macaroni, and corn grits contain slightly less iron than the whole-grain cereal from which they were derived. It is estimated that the use of enriched bread and cereals in place of refined cereals has increased the iron content of the diet by 14%. For other cereal products, however, iron can be added at any level within safe limits as long as the amount is declared on the label. Processors of such products as infant cereals and some prepared dried cereals have chosen to enrich their products at an extremely high level. This likely represents excessive enrichment to promote the sale of the product, and the consumer may be able to utilize only a small fraction of the added amount.

The only food group characterized as a poor source of iron is milk and milk products. The small amount of iron in milk is well utilized but still makes an insignificant contribution to the total dietary intake.

Some food sources that are relatively rich in iron but do not make a major contribution to the diet because of the infrequency with which they are consumed are oysters (6.3 mg per 3 oz serving), clams (6.1 mg per 3 oz serving), and cocoa (1 mg per tablespoon).

Iron in the drinking water (present as ferric hydroxide) is a significant source only when iron values of water exceed 5 mg/L.

Blackstrap molasses, a by-product of the sugar-refining process, contains about 2.5 mg per tablespoon. But because of the bitter flavor of the product it is questionable whether it can be considered a significant dietary item.

In 1965 the average per capita consumption of iron was placed at 16.3 mg/day. Of all families 90% reported an intake of over 12 mg per person per day, and 42% reported over 20 mg/day, indicating intakes capable of meeting the needs for most adults. However, results of the Ten-State Survey in 1970 showed median intakes ranging from 9 to 13 mg per person per day for different age and sex groups.

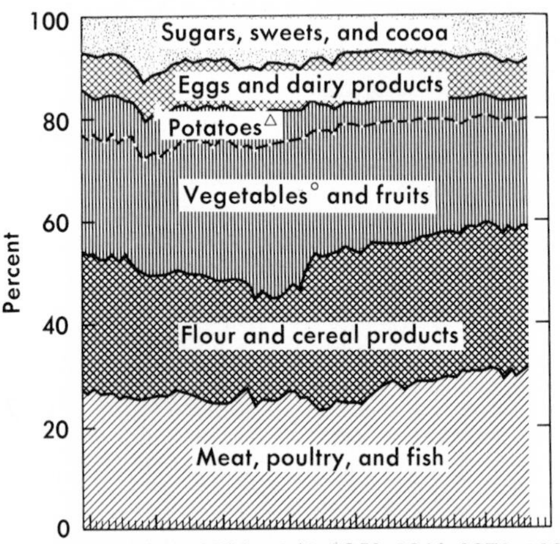

Per capita civilian food supply. 1977 preliminary data. △Includes sweet potatoes. °Includes dry beans, peas, nuts, soya products.

Fig. 8-6. Trends in dietary sources of iron from 1910 to present. (From Agricultural charts, Washington, D.C., 1978, U.S. Department of Agriculture.)

Effect of cooking. Loss of iron in cooking arises from loss by solution into cooking water, which is discarded, and the removal of peelings, with the loss of the iron concentrated near the skin. Any cooking method that minimizes the possibility of iron dissolving in the cooking water, such as the use of relatively large pieces of food, cooking with skins on, and the use of simmering rather than boiling water, will increase the amount of iron available in the diet. Steamed vegetables have more iron than boiled vegetables; those cooked for a short time in a small amount of water have more than those cooked for a longer period and in a large amount of water; and those cooked in their skins have more iron than peeled ones. The use of vegetable stock in soups or gravies also helps minimize iron losses. Trends in dietary sources of iron in the American diet are shown in Fig. 8-6.

Iron fortification

In the United States iron enrichment of cereal has been considered an effective means of improving iron nutriture. The fortification of both salt and sugar with iron have proved effective vehicles in developing countries but have limited potential in the United States. A Swedish study has demonstrated that heme iron salvaged from the blood waste materials of slaughterhouses is a potential for readily available iron for food fortification.

Based on biological assays with rats, it is evident that various iron salts differ in their effectiveness as enrichment compounds. Ferric orthophosphate is only a tenth as available as ferrous sulfate or reduced iron with a particle size less than 10 μm. The availability of ferrous sulfate is considerably less in baked products than in solution, and when eaten as a baked roll in a meal containing meat, approximately 10% is absorbed. In all tests with humans wide ranges of absorption have been observed as have variations from day to day in the same subject. Coated ferrous sulfate is more stable and less likely to be destroyed by oxidation than uncoated compounds.

Evaluation of iron deficiency

Measurement of hemoglobin content of the blood has been the traditional method of assessing the adequacy of dietary iron. It use has several limitations. First, little agreement exists among hematologists regarding what level of hemoglobin is characteristic of iron deficiency; standards range from 10 to 12 g/dl. Second, hemoglobin levels fluctuate over a twenty-four hour period, and a single determination may give erroneous information. Third, hemoglobin levels drop only after stores have been depleted; therefore low hemoglobin values represent an advanced stage of iron deficiency. Last, anemia may be due to a deficiency of other nutrients.

Since there seems to be considerable overlap in hemoglobin values between individuals with normal iron status and those that can be considered iron depleted, many attempts have been made to identify a more sensitive test for iron status. One such test involves administering an iron supplement, for example, 60 mg of iron a day for three months, on the theory that those who are truly anemic will respond. "Nonresponders," who are not anemic, will show no increase in hemoglobin levels. On the basis of these data on populations it would be possible to calculate a cut-off point so that only a small percentage of nonresponders would be treated and a small percentage of responders would be missed.

The assessment of iron stores, a more sensitive indicator of iron status, includes several measurements. An increase in the amount of the transport protein transferrin or the total iron-binding capacity (TIBC) is indicative of a depletion of iron stores. If this is not accompanied by an increase in serum iron, the saturation of the iron-carrying capacity of the blood decreases. An iron-binding capacity of less than 15% compared to normal values of 30% to 40% indicates that iron reserves are inadequate to meet the needs for iron and the individual is said to suffer from "latent iron deficiency." This may be due to iron depletion or the result of fever or chronic infection.

The most sensitive indicator of iron stores

is serum ferritin, an iron-protein complex that is present in normal serum in very small amounts (nanograms) yet reflects the amount of storage iron. Unfortunately the method for taking this measure is complex and costly to set up, which has so far limited its usefulness as either a diagnostic or survey tool. Normal levels are 94 ng/ml for men and 32 ng/ml for women.

Iron stores can be determined by an analysis of a bone marrow aspirate, usually obtained from the sternum. This is a rather delicate procedure that does not lend itself to screening population groups.

In another test an increase in protoporphyrin, a precursor of heme (the iron-containing porphyrin of hemoglobin in red blood cells) indicates that heme synthesis has been depressed due to lack of iron.

The combination of measuring plasma iron, total iron-binding capacity, red blood cell protoporphyrin, and serum ferritin can define iron status with considerable precision. Hemoglobin determinations are insensitive to the early stages of iron deficiency but are useful in assessing the severity of anemia.

Deficiencies

Since the body is extremely efficient in conserving iron supplies, simple iron deficiencies occur only during the growth period or when intake fails to meet needs after loss of blood or in women who have experienced frequent pregnancies in rapid succession. In iron deficiency, however, there is a gradual and well-defined sequence of changes that ultimately results in anemia. In the first phase there is a depletion of iron stores (a decrease in serum ferritin) and a compensatory increase in iron absorption, transferrin, or iron-binding capacity. This is followed by a stage in which iron stores are exhausted, transferrin saturation is reduced, the amount of the heme precursor protoporphyrin that can be converted to heme decreases, and serum ferritin drops. In the third stage anemia characterized by low hemoglobin levels develops.

In addition to changes in components of the blood, iron deficiency is associated with a drop in heme iron-containing enzymes and metalloflavoproteins, which play critical roles in cellular metabolism and in the functioning of compounds that require iron as a cofactor.

Evidence of these deficiencies may show up in decreased work capacity, altered behavior as apathy and irritability, decreased secretion of hydrochloric acid, and altered susceptibility to infection.

Anemia, a condition in which a deficiency occurs in the quantity and/or quality of red blood cells, is the most easily recognized manifestation of iron deficiency.

Diagnosis. Anemia can be diagnosed by comparing blood hemoglobin levels measured as grams of hemoglobin per dl of blood and red blood cell counts measured as the number of red blood cells per cubic millimeter of blood to established standards. Standards for hemoglobin are 15 g of hemoglobin per deciliter of blood for men and 13.6 g for women. Clinical laboratories frequently report hemoglobin levels as a percentage of the standard. Thus a hemoglobin level of 90 means that the blood contained 90% of the standard. Red blood cell standards are 5 million/ml^3 of blood for men and 4.5 million for women. The total number of red blood cells in the body is so large that it defies comprehension—over 25 trillion. The number replaced every second is a mere 2.5 million.

Anemia can be classified into two categories based on the underlying cause—nutritional and hemorrhagic.

Nutritional anemia. Nutritional anemia is caused by the absence of any dietary essential involved in hemoglobin formation or by poor absorption of these dietary components. The most likely causes are lack of either dietary iron or high-quality protein. However, anemias have been reported associated with a lack of pyridoxine (vitamin B_6), which catalyzes the synthesis of the heme portion of the hemoglobin molecule; lack of ascorbic acid, which influences the rate of iron absorption and the release of iron from transferrin to the tissues; and lack of vitamin E, which affects the stability of the red blood cell membrane. Experimentally the omission of copper from the diet causes low hemoglobin values. Copper is not part of the hemoglobin molecule but apparently facilitates its formation by influencing either the absorption of iron, its release from the liver, or its incorporation into a hemoglobin molecule.

Nutritional anemia is usually characterized as hypochromic and microcytic. This broad classification suggests a lack of the pigment hemoglobin and the presence of small cells. Failure of the cell to grow in the absence of hemoglobin synthesis produces the small cells. As a result, nutritional anemia occurs primarily during the growth period when demands of growing cells and increased blood volume are not met by dietary intake of nutrients needed for hemoglobin synthesis. It is most pronounced in adolescent girls when the growth demands superimposed on the menstrual losses are difficult to meet by dietary means. This condition is sometimes described as *chlorosis* because of the greenish cast it gives the skin. A cursory diagnosis of hemoglobin status can often be made by a visual examination of the mucous membranes, especially on the underside of the eyelid or in the mouth, where the blood vessels are close to the epithelial surface. Pale membranes usually signify low hemoglobin values.

In adult males nutritional anemia is not likely to develop once normal levels have been reached because of the minimal need for iron and the relatively large liver reserves.

Nutritional anemia occurs frequently in young infants who are maintained on a diet consisting solely of milk after the three- to six-month period during which fetal liver reserves are adequate. Infants utilize little dietary iron during the first three months of life, but after that the addition of enriched cereal, egg yolk, and meat to the infant's diet or the use of iron-fortified formula for bottle-fed babies provides good sources of iron. One study of nutritional intake of infants showed that unless the diet contained enriched cereals, it would fail to meet the recommended allowances for iron. Meat, fruits, and vegetables in the amounts consumed by these infants were not capable of meeting the iron need without the use of cereal products.

Pernicious anemia. Pernicious anemia is a form of nutritional anemia in which the number of red blood cells, not the hemoglobin level, is low. It is caused primarily by failure in the absorption of vitamin B_{12}, or cobalamin, rather than lack of a nutrient. It will be discussed in Chapter 12.

Hemorrhagic anemia. Hemorrhagic anemia is caused by an excessive loss of blood. This may occur after surgery, bleeding of wounds, internal hemorrhaging, excessive menstrual losses, blood donations, or as a result of intestinal parasites. After a blood loss the blood volume is restored almost immediately, followed by an increase in the number of red blood cells and finally by the restoration of hemoglobin levels.

The loss of blood represents a loss of 0.5 mg of iron/ml of blood or 250 mg/0.5 L. Even with the increased rate of iron absorption that occurs after blood loss, it takes at least fifty days to restore normal hemoglobin levels following the donation of 0.5 liter of blood. This period may be reduced to thirty-five days if iron supplements and ascorbic acid are given. The wisdom of limiting blood donations to 2 to 3 liters a year, especially for women, is obvious.

Treatment. When iron-deficiency anemia with its symptoms of pallor, easy fatigue, decreased resistance to infection, soreness in the mouth, and palpitation after exercise is diagnosed, the use of a diet high in iron-rich foods with a concurrent intake of appreciable amounts of ascorbic acid is indicated. The use of iron salts in therapeutic doses is likely justified to speed the restoration of hemoglobin levels to normal, and in many cases it is the only way in which hemoglobin synthesis is adequately stimulated. Over thirty iron salts, both organic and inorganic, such as ferrous gluconate, ferrous sulfate, ferrous citrate, ferric ammonium citrate, and ferrous fumarate, have been promoted by pharmaceutical firms. So far no preparation has been shown to be superior to ferrous sulfate, which contains 36% iron and is the least expensive of all these forms, costing from 1 to 15 cents per daily dosage. Therapeutic doses may contain as much as 250 mg of iron, which may be absorbed at the rate of 150 mg/day to bring about a maximum rate of increase in hemoglobin levels of 0.3 g/day. To provide this level of iron requires 0.8 g of ferrous sulfate or 1.2 g of ferrous gluconate. It is wise to build up therapeutic dosages slowly to develop a gradual tolerance to the iron and to prevent gastrointestinal upsets. Once normal hemoglobin levels are reached, the continued use of iron salts is not justified from either a nutritional or an economic point of view, if the quality of diet has improved.

Excess

The theory that the absorption of iron was regulated in the intestinal mucosa suggested that the uptake of excess iron was impossible. This theory was questioned when it was reported that an African tribe, the Bantu, suffered from siderosis or hemochromatosis, a disease in which the iron reserves were found to be up to thirty times the normal 1 g reserve. The source of iron, which amounted to 200 mg/day, is thought to be the kettles in which the large amount of beer they consume is fermented. An excess absorption as small as 3 mg/day will result in 1 mg of storage iron daily, which can accumulate to a sizable amount over a period of years. A similar iron toxicity has been reported among persons who are overzealous in their use of therapeutic iron readily available in drugstores. There are many reports of ferrous sulfate toxicity in infants who have been given 3 to 10 g daily. Under these conditions the excess iron accumulates in the normal storage sites—liver and spleen; this condition is known as hemosiderosis or siderosis.

In siderosis, iron increases in the mitochondria of cells, reflecting increased tissue iron; serum iron increases, and the bone marrow becomes hyperplastic. The failure of the absorption mechanism to regulate iron absorption occurs at very high levels of iron intake. Under these circumstances the transferrin of blood is saturated at three times its normal level and is incapable of binding all the absorbed iron in a harmless complex. It is then that the excess iron may stimulate the growth of pathogenic organisms in the blood, resulting in an increased susceptibility to infection.

Hemochromatosis is another form of iron-storage disease that occurs in less than 0.1% of the population (about 22,000 individuals in the United States). These persons have an inherited defect in the regulation of iron absorption, which allows them to absorb unusually high amounts and to store it in tissues that normally do not store iron. Opponents of the increased level of iron proposed for bread enrichment feel that this may intensify the problem of regulating iron uptake in persons with hemochromatosis even though it cannot increase the number with the disease, since it is an inherited problem.

Some evidence of iron overload has been noted in persons who have had successive blood transfusions. Even though the transfused blood is providing iron, iron is absorbed in a manner characteristic of an iron-deficient individual.

IODINE

Distribution

The essential trace mineral element iodine is present in the body in minute amounts, about 0.00004% of body weight (15 to 23 mg) or a hundredth of the amount of iron in a healthy human adult. Like iron, iodine is present in every living cell of the body. Similarly, from 70% to 80% (about 10 mg) is concentrated in a single tissue, the thyroid gland. Here the level of iodine used in the synthesis of the hormone thyroxin is twenty times that of the blood supplying it.

The thyroid gland consists of two lobes, or parts, located in the neck area on either side of the trachea just below the larynx, as shown in Fig. 8-7. It weighs about 25 g or 0.2% of body weight. The two sides of the thyroid

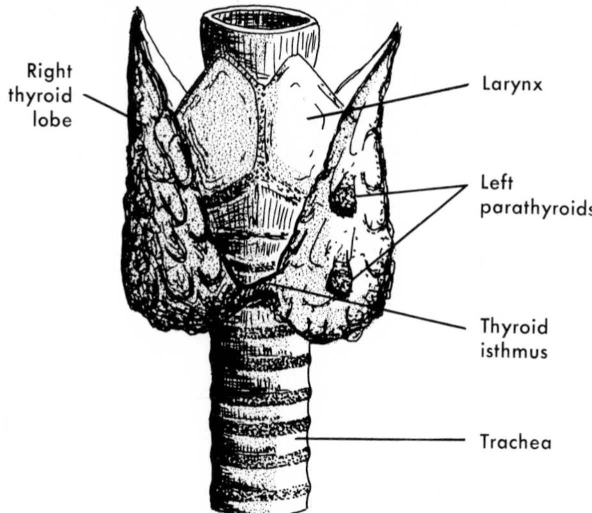

Fig. 8-7. Diagrammatic representation of location of thyroid and parathyroid glands.

gland are joined by a thin strip of tissue, sometimes called the thyroid isthmus.

Knowledge of iodine metabolism has been advanced with the use of radioactive isotopes of iodine, especially ^{131}I, and the development of analytical methods sufficiently sensitive to determine the minute amounts of this element found in biological material.

Absorption

Iodine occurs in food primarily as the reduced iodide but also in lower amounts as inorganic iodine or as an organically bound complex. The latter is freed from its organic component, and the free iodine is reduced to iodide before its rapid absorption. Inorganic iodide is absorbed in all parts of the gastrointestinal tract but primarily in the small intestine. Some organically bound iodine is not absorbed and may be excreted in the feces, but it represents a maximum of 2% of ingested iodine. Even smaller amounts are excreted by the sweat glands. Iodine may also be absorbed through epithelial cells of the skin and inhaled as a contaminant from the combustion of fossil fuels.

Once absorbed, the iodine appears immediately in the bloodstream, where it constitutes the major part of the "iodide pool"—all extracellular iodide. About 30% of the iodide in the blood plasma is absorbed by the thyroid gland, and the rest is taken up by the kidneys to be excreted in the urine. The excretion of iodine not used by the thyroid gland provides a protection against the accumulation of toxic levels in other tissues.

Metabolism

The iodide picked up, or "trapped," by the thyroid gland is immediately oxidized to iodine within the gland. In this form 1 or 2 molecules unite with the amino acid tyrosine, which is part of the protein thyroglobulin. Two iodated tyrosine molecules unite to form either thyroxin (T_4), with 4 atoms of iodine, or thyronine (T_3), with 3 atoms of iodine. These active hormones are released from storage in thyroglobulin by a protein-splitting enzyme, itself released under the stimulus of the thyroid-stimulating hormone (TSH) of the pituitary gland, and enter the circulation. Thyronine is a much more active form of the hormone than thyroxin but is present in relatively small amounts (1:4) in the blood. There is some evidence that once thyroxin enters the individual cell, it becomes deiodated by the removal of 1 atom of iodine to form the more active thyronine with 3 atoms of iodine.

Function

Part of thyroxin. As part of the thyroid hormone thyroxin secreted into the circulating plasma, iodine plays a major role in regulating the growth and development of the organism and its rate of metabolism. The stimulating effect of thyroxin on metabolism can be appreciable, up to 30% above normal, with the effects of a single dose persisting for six days or more. When the rate of metabolism increases, more oxygen is used up by the cells, indicating that more energy is being released from glucose and fatty acids to provide for the needs of the more active cells. Much of this energy appears as heat rather than ATP.

Although most attention has been focused on the role of thyroxin in energy metabolism, an increasing number of direct and indirect effects of thyroxin on metabolic functions are becoming apparent. The conversion of carotene, the precursor of vitamin A, to the active form of the vitamin, the synthesis of protein by ribosomes, and the absorption of carbohydrate from the intestine are more efficient when thyroxin production is normal. The synthesis of cholesterol is influenced by thyroxin levels, with above-normal cholesterol levels occurring in **hypothyroidism** and below-normal levels in **hyperthyroidism.** Additionally, it is essential for reproduction.

Before the Food and Drug Administration ruled that thyroxin preparations would be available through prescriptions only, unscrupulous peddlers of weight-reducing aids were using thyroid extract on the theory that it facilitated weight loss. It does, indeed, but the undesirable side effects that accompany its uncontrolled use make such a practice potentially hazardous.

Requirements

The Food and Nutrition Board of the National Research Council has suggested that an intake of 1 μg of iodine/kg of body weight is adequate for most adults. To assure a margin of safety to provide for individual variations, the NRC recommends a daily intake of 100 μg for women and 130 μg for men. For pregnant and lactating women the need is 25 and 50 μg higher. If the salt intake is unadvisedly restricted during pregnancy, eliminating a major source of iodine in the diet, precautions should be taken to see that sufficient iodine is available from other sources. A wide range of intakes between 50 and 100 μg is considered safe.

The need of growing children, especially girls, may exceed the suggested level of 1 μg/kg of body weight.

Food sources

Both food and water provide iodine in the human diet. The amount present in the water varies from one area to another and tends to parallel the iodine content of the soil. An iodine content of less than 2 μg/L is associated with iodine-deficiency conditions and that of 2 to 15 μg with the absence of iodine deficiency. In the United States the iodine content of fresh water varies from 0.5 to 2.0 ppb, being the lowest in glacial rivers and lakes, and that of seawater varies from 17 to 50 ppb or μg/L.

Seafoods, such as lobster, shrimp, and oysters, are among the richest dietary sources, but because of the relatively minor role they play in the diet (except among persons living in coastal regions), they do not make a major contribution to the iodine content of many diets. Saltwater fish contain from 300 to 3000 μg of iodine/kg of flesh compared to 20 to 40 μg in freshwater fish. Saltwater fish have an amazing capacity to concentrate this relatively small amount of iodine within their tissue.

The amount of iodine in dairy products and eggs is extremely variable and reflects the season of the year and the iodine content of the soil on which the rations of the animals were grown. The iodine content of milk rapidly reflects the addition of iodine to the cow's diet as a result of use of iodized salt in feeds.

Most cereal grains, legumes, fruits, and vegetables are low in iodine content. Although iodine is not essential for plant growth the amount present depends on the iodine content of the soil in which they were grown. The amount of iodine in the soil in the United States varies from 0.6 to 6.0 mg/kg with the lowest amounts being found in soils of glacial orgin. In general, the leaves of plants have higher iodine concentrations than the roots. Spinach leaves have the highest iodine content of all plants (1 to 2 mg/kg). Because corn is extremely low in iodine, populations who rely on corn as a major part of their diet may be susceptible to iodine deficiency conditions.

The variation in iodine content of vegetables from various sources can be illustrated by values of 240, 407, and 1283 μg/kg of dry weight of carrots grown in Florida, Oklahoma, and Louisiana, respectively. Modern marketing practices in which the food supply of any one community comes from widely separated geographical areas have done much to assure a more uniform and more nearly adequate level of iodine for the average American.

The use of iodized salt in cooking has proved the most effective method of increasing the amount of iodine in the diet. It is added to salt as potassium iodate at a level of 100 mg/kg, or 1 part per 10,000 parts salt, a level established to be completely safe and yet valuable in combatting goiter. However, it is ten times higher than the 1 part of 100,000 recommended by the World Health Organization. This provides the person who consumes 6 g of table salt with 500 μg/day. Between 1949 and 1968 Canada, Guatemala, and fourteen of the seventeen Latin American countries passed legislation to require the iodization of salt at levels ranging from 1 part iodine to 10,000 parts salt to 1 part in 66,000. All have not been successful in implementing their programs. In Europe 1 part iodine to 100,000 parts salt is used. Mandatory iodization has been recommended by the Food and Nutrition Board in the United States, but currently it is a voluntary measure on the part of the salt producers, who must comply only with the labeling requirements of the Food and Drug Administration.

The FDA requires that iodized salt bear the legend "This salt contains added iodine, an essential nutrient"; noniodized salt must be labeled to indicate "This product does not contain iodine, an essential nutrient."

The cost of iodized salt in the United States is estimated at a half to three cents per person a year.

Currently 55% of the salt sold in the United States is iodized, although 75% of all families report using it and only 4% say they never use it. One study showed that some persons thought they were buying iodized salt when they actually had the uniodized form. The 25% drop, from 4.2 to 3.2 g of iodized salt per person daily, has been attributed to the fact that Americans are preparing less food at home and relying more on processed foods, which in general do not use iodized salt because of technical and quality control problems. The trend toward eating more meals away from home has also contributed to the decline.

Contrary to popular opinion, sea salt is not a good source of iodine. However, kelp, a form of seaweed, does contain appreciable amounts (0.8 to 4.5 g/kg). The evidence of iodine deficiency uncovered in the National Nutrition Survey indicates that we have failed in our efforts to control the iodine deficiency disease goiter through the use of iodized salt.

Other methods of increasing the iodine intake of population groups in low-iodine areas have met with varying degrees of success. Russian scientists have reported success with the use of iodized starch. The addition of iodine to water supplies has been abandoned because of its failure to benefit people in rural areas and others with private water supplies. Although they provide measured amounts of iodine, iodized tablets or candies are rarely satisfactory because their success depends on complete cooperation of a number of individuals. Where bread is a staple in the diet, the use of iodized salt and an iron-containing dough conditioner in commercial bread has been fairly effective. Failure of food processors to use iodized salt in packaged food products may be partially responsible for the suboptimal intake of many.

In Tasmania enrichment of flour with potassium iodide resulted in an increased potassium intake but led to concern about the possibility of thyrotoxicosis among older persons with goiter who ate large amounts of bread.

In areas of endemic goiter intramuscular injection of poppy-seed oil fortified with 37% iodine every three to four years has proved to be an effective measure at a cost of approximately 15 cents per person yearly. Oral doses of lipiodol, which are easier to administer, also provide adequate protection against goiter. The use of both should, however, be replaced by an effective salt iodization program as soon as possible.

Recent data from Argentina showed that a twenty-year program of adding iodine to salt at a level of 1 part in 30,000 resulted in a decreased incidence of goiter in school children from 46% to 3%. At the same time urinary excretion of iodine rose and the uptake of ^{131}I decreased as further evidence of improved iodine nutriture.

In countries such as Japan where seaweed is consumed as a regular dietary item, it is a major source of iodine, containing from 0.4% to 0.6% of iodine on a dry weight basis. The value of recommending seaweed, or kelp, for consumption in a culture unaccustomed to its use is doubtful. Excessive intakes may contribute to a form of goiter.

One study based on the chemical analysis of the iodine content of American diets showed intakes varying from 65 to 529 μg/day, the principal contribution being from vegetables and dairy products. The use of calcium and potassium iodates in continuous dough process in breadmaking contributes up to 4 mg/0.45 kg or 23 to 40 μg/slice. A study of the uptake of iodine suggests intakes ranging from 260 to 740 μg. Data showed that the intake of men is about one third higher than that of women. Similar data on school children showed that they were receiving approximately 100 μg from bread, 32 to 90 μg / cup of milk, and 76 μg from 10 g of salt.

Evaluation of nutritional status

Since the dietary intake of iodine includes that in water as well as in food, the difficulties of conducting iodine balance studies to assess iodine nutriture are greater than those for nutrients provided only by food. To obtain some assessment of the adequacy of iodine nutriture, use has been made of the determination of the iodine excretion in a single sample of urine in relation to the amount of creatinine excreted. In areas of low available iodine an excretion of about 25 μg of iodine per gram of creatinine occurs, whereas in areas of high available iodine the excretion is at least 50 μg. Some excretion rates are as high as 1000 μg per gram of creatinine. The uptake of iodine by persons with a normally functioning thyroid is also useful in assessing iodine status.

Thyroxin

Since most of the iodine in the body is used in thyroxin synthesis, a convenient way to study iodine metabolism is to study thyroxin metabolism.

Measurement. The rate of thyroxin production can be measured in several ways. The basal metabolic rate as determined by indirect calorimetry (described in Chapter 5) is closely related to the level of thyroxin production. A basal metabolic rate elevated at least 15% above the level predicted on the basis of body surface area or metabolic body size is indicative of a state of hyperthyroidism in which there is an excess production of thyroxin. On the other hand, a depressed basal metabolic rate reflects a state of hypothyroidism and a decreased rate of thyroxin production.

A simpler, less costly method of assessing thyroxin level is the protein-bound iodine (PBI) test. This method has an advantage over basal metabolism in that it is not influenced by previous meals or activity and is less costly. A positive relationship exists between the amount of iodine bound to protein circulating in the blood and the level of thyroxin produced. About 90% of the protein-bound iodine is in thyroxin, which is 65% iodine by weight. Normally PBI levels fall between 4 and 8 μg/dl of blood. PBI blood levels above 11 μg/dl are indicative of hyperthyroidism and levels below 3 μg indicate hypothyroidism. It is not possible to calculate the exact change in energy expenditure using this method, but the relative level of basal metabolism can be determined.

Radioactive isotopes have proved useful in assessing the state of thyroxin production. The amount of orally administered radioactive iodine taken up by the thyroid gland is determined by measuring radioactivity in the neck region. That taken up by other tissues is determined by a radioactivity reading in the thigh area. In hyperthyroidism a very rapid uptake of iodine by the thyroid is followed by a gradual drop after 24 hours. Under conditions of normal thyroid function the uptake of radioactive iodine is gradual. In hypothyroidism the rate of uptake is rapid, and the iodine remains in the thyroid gland for much longer periods.

Regulation. The functioning of the thyroid gland is controlled by a thyroid-stimulating hormone (TSH) secreted by the pituitary gland in response to the level of thyroxin in the blood. This, in turn, may reflect the availability of iodine for thyroxin synthesis. Many factors may influence the amount of TSH produced and hence the activity of the thyroid gland. When dietary iodine falls to a level inadequate for sufficient thyroxin synthesis, more TSH is produced. Over a period of time this results in an increase in size of the thyroid gland, a condition known as simple goiter, in which both the size and number of thyroid cells increase.

Several antithyroid drugs, such as thiourea and thiouracil, inhibit thyroxin formation. They may either interfere with the ability of the thyroid gland to trap iodine, block the oxidation of iodide to iodine, or block the organic binding of iodine. Thiocyanates used in the treatment of hypertension inhibit the ability of the thyroid gland to concentrate iodine and to produce thyroxin.

The salivary gland may play a role in regulating the level of thyroxin in the blood. It has the capacity to remove iodine (deiodate) from thyroxin, thus inactivating it. The iodine is secreted in the saliva and can be reabsorbed in the gastrointestinal tract. Work with guinea pigs suggests that thyroid function is disrupted in an ascorbic acid deficiency.

Goiter

Iodine is recognized as an effective agent in the treatment of simple goiter, a condition characterized by a swelling in the neck, reflecting the enlargement of the thyroid gland. The gland enlarges as it attempts to compensate for the lack of iodine essential to its major role in the synthesis of thyroxine. Enlargement begins when the concentration of iodine in the thyroid drops to half the normal 0.2% of dry weight. Both cell number and cell size increase.

Simple goiter is a painless condition but has some undesirable effects on physical appearance.

Contrary to earlier belief, it has now been established that appropriate iodine therapy will lead to a slow reduction in the size of the enlarged thyroid gland, characteristic of goiter. If the thyroid gland continues to grow, pressure from the growth of thyroid tissue on either side of the trachea could lead to difficulty in breathing. Under these circumstances, treatment involves thyroidectomy, the surgical removal of part of the thyroid gland. This operation, which accounts for 0.4% of the operations in the United States, is complicated by the fact that the parathyroid gland, vital in the control of calcium metabolism, is embedded in the surface of the thyroid gland. Ligating (tying off) an artery leading to the thyroid has occasionally been effective in controlling the growth of the gland.

A deficiency of iodine is the primary but not the only cause of simple goiter. Goiter may also be caused by factors that interfere with the availability of dietary iodine, impose abnormal demands on the thyroid gland, or interfere with the utilization of iodine by the thyroid. These factors include chemicals present in some foods (present either naturally or purposely introduced for therapeutic reasons) or defects in an enzyme system necessary for the synthesis and release of thyroxin. In all these cases the thyroid gland enlarges to compensate for the lack of iodine needed for its normal functioning. Of the estimated 200 million cases of simple goiter in the world today, the majority are caused by a dietary lack of iodine and tend to occur in definite geographical regions.

Incidence. There is increasing evidence that an interaction between low-iodine intake with other factors such as polluted water or other elements in the soil may be involved in the development of simple goiter. The incidence of goiter is regional, occurring primarily in areas where the soil is of glacial origin or where flooding or tropical rains have leached the iodine from the soil. It is almost nonexistent in areas where iodine-laden vapors from the sea condense and deposit iodine on the soil. As shown in Fig. 8-8 in the United States the areas of highest incidence are those bordering the Great Lakes—Michigan, Wisconsin, and Ohio—and the Rocky Mountain states. Coastal areas are relatively free of the condition, as are the southern states. Studies of the iodine content of the soils and water supplies of goitrous areas showed a very low concentration.

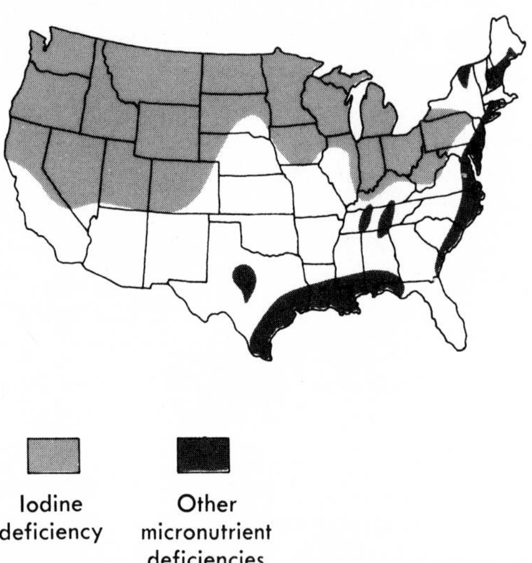

Fig. 8-8. Distribution of micronutrient element deficiencies in soil in the United States. Some other micronutrient deficiencies also occur in scattered parts of goitrous areas. (Modified from Beesom, K. C.: In Lamb, C. A., Bentley, O. G., and Blathic, J. M.: Trace elements, New York, 1958, Academic Press, Inc.)

Treatment. Most goiters respond to iodine therapy. The use of iodine in the treatment of goiter was recognized as early as 1820, and thirty years later the lack of iodine was associated with low iodine levels in the soil and water. However, the suggestion of the French botanist Chatin that iodine be added to water in areas where goiter occurred was not then accepted. Toward the turn of the century, when it was shown that iodine was a normal constituent of the thyroid gland, there was a renewed interest in the use of iodine therapy in the treatment of goiter. Several investigations confirmed that endemic goiter could be controlled by raising dietary iodine intakes.

The increase in incidence of goiter reported by 1915 led to the first large-scale study on the control of goiter in humans. In Ohio from 1916 to 1920 the addition of iodine tablets to the water supply twice a year effectively reduced the incidence of goiter in adolescent girls, the group most susceptible to the disease. Other methods, such as feeding iodized salt to cows in an effort to increase the amount appearing in the milk, the iodization of the water supply, and the iodization of salt, have been used. Of these, only the iodization of salt has proved an effective method for reaching the majority of the population. The cost of adding iodine to the salt supply is so small that in most cases the manufacturers absorb the cost.

In Michigan, where goiter among 47% of school children in 1921 constituted a major public health problem, an intensive educational campaign to promote the use of iodized salt was launched. The results were encouraging. By 1925 the incidence had dropped to 32%, and by 1951 only 1% of the population had simple goiter. Michigan's experience, however, has shown that it is necessary to maintain the educational program to keep the condition under control, since a letup in educational efforts resulted in a 6% incidence by 1970. In 1970 a nutritional status survey in ten states revealed that in some areas as many as 7.2% of the population were afflicted—an incidence considered endemic. Among 7500 10- to 15-year-olds the incidence ranged from 4.5% to 9.9% in four different areas. A follow-up study, however, showed that many of the persons with enlarged thyroids had intakes that met established standards and iodine excretions indicating that intake exceeded need. This indicates a prevalence of goiter unrelated to iodine deficiency.

Certain foods contain substances called goitrogens which predispose a person to goiter. They act in much the same way as the antithyroid drugs by blocking the absorption or utilization of iodine. Foods of the cabbage family, such as rutabagas, turnips, and cabbage, contain a heat-stable substance, *progoitrin*, and a heat-labile activator that converts progoitrin to *goitrin*. In raw foods the goitrin that interferes with iodine utilization is formed; in cooked foods, however, the conversion cannot take place unless an activator is formed by bacterial synthesis in the intestine. Evidence of the presence of such an enzyme in the gastrointestinal tract is increasing, which means that the progoitrin in cooked foods may also be converted to a goitrin.

Ground nuts, or peanuts, contain a substance called *arachidoside* that also interferes with iodine utilization. The presence of this substance is one of the drawbacks to the use of nuts to improve protein quality of the diet. Similarly, a goitrogen in soybeans and cassava may be a deterrent to their use.

Sulfonamides, widely used antibiotics, reduce the conversion of iodide to iodine and are potentially goitrogenic but at the levels used in treating infection they have little effect on thyroid activity. The vitamin-like substance para-aminobenzoic acid (PABA) has a similar effect. Some evidence also exists to

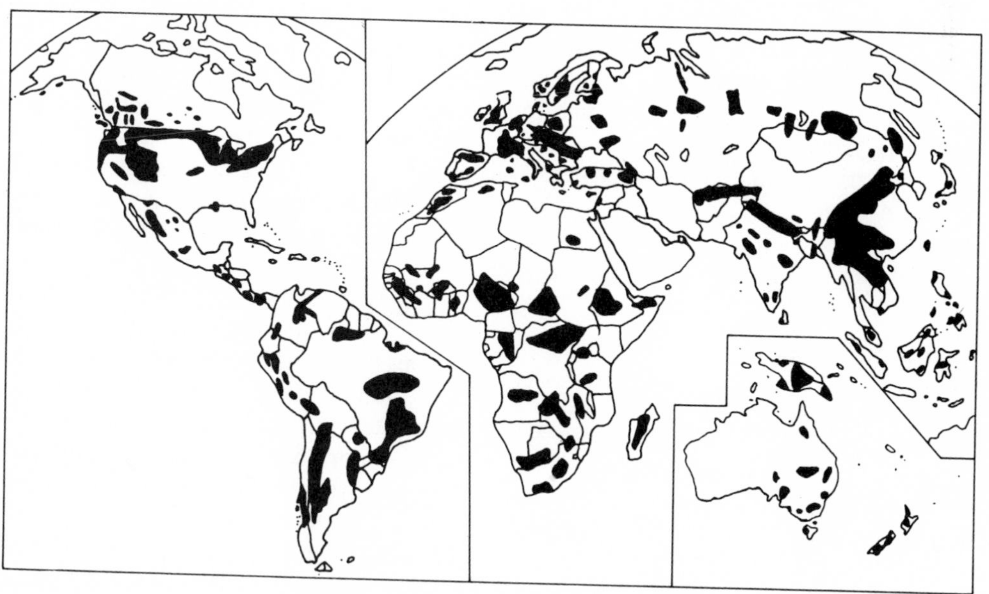

Fig. 8-9. Goitrous areas of the world.

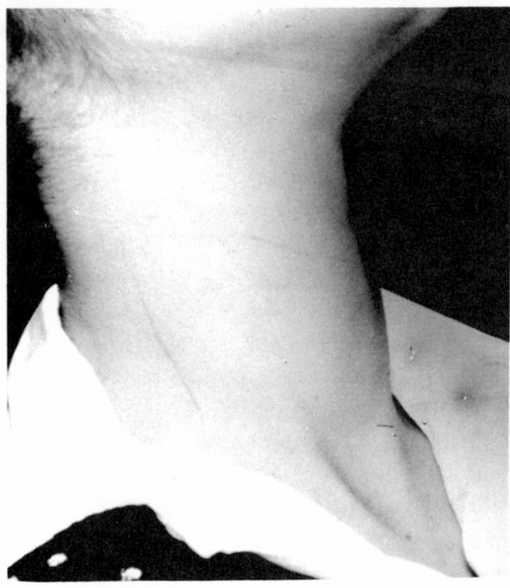

Fig. 8-10. A typical case of adult goiter with swelling in throat region, identified in the 1970 National Nutrition Survey. (Courtesy Dr. W.J. McGanity. University of Texas, Galveston, Texas.)

support the theory that both high-calcium and high-fat diets may be goitrogenic.

The incidence of goiter is about six times as high in females as in males, and the most susceptible groups are adolescent girls and pregnant women. Practices of limiting the use of iodized salt in an effort to control adolescent acne and the restriction of salt intake in pregnancy may be questioned because of the risk of stimulating the growth of the thyroid gland.

The distribution of goiter areas in the world is shown in Fig. 8-9 and a typical case of goiter in Fig. 8-10.

Other abnormalities

Cretinism is frequently encountered among children born to mothers who have had a limited iodine intake during adolescence and pregnancy and who live in areas where goiter is endemic. Since the mother's need for iodine takes precedence over those of the developing fetus, cretins have suffered from an intrauterine iodine deficiency as well as one in postnatal development. These children who suffer from hypothyroidism are physically dwarfed and mentally retarded and have thick dry pasty skin and enlarged protruding abdomens. If treatment is started soon after birth, many of the symptoms of cretinism are reversible, but if the condition persists beyond early childhood, permanent mental and physical retardation cannot be prevented.

Adults who have had symptoms of hypothyroidism throughout their developmental period suffer from **myxedema.** These persons have coarse sparse hair, dry yellowish skin, poor tolerance for cold, and a low husky voice. This can be due to a defect in the thyroid gland or in the pituitary, which produces the thyroid-stimulating hormone.

Both cretinism and myxedema are still found, but the use of iodized salt has greatly reduced the incidence in countries such as Switzerland where the soil and water are extremely low in iodine. A similar program in the Andes would undoubtedly lower the incidence in this mountainous low-iodine area.

Hyperthyroidism, in which the basal metabolic rate may be elevated as much as 100% above normal, is also known as Graves' disease and exophthalmic goiter. Persons suffering from overactivity of the thyroid gland experience nervousness, weight loss, increased appetite, intolerance to heat, tremors when the hand is outstretched, and protruding eyeballs. The increased rate of metabolism that accompanies increased thyroxin production puts an increased load on the cardiovascular system.

OTHER MICRONUTRIENT ELEMENTS

Essentiality

The use of the term *trace elements* to describe this group of micronutrients is unfortunate, since it may imply a lack of nutritional importance. Its use stems from the era when analytical techniques were sufficiently sensitive to detect their presence but not to measure the minute amounts needed. The use of atomic absorption spectrophotometry and neutron activation as analytical techniques has made it possible to detect amounts as low as 1 ppb in natural material. Additionally, the use of radioactive isotopes has made it possible to study the metabolism of trace elements in the body. The extremely small concentrations at which these elements are functional is illustrated by the fact that 1 part in 10 million is active. The occurrence of micronutrient element deficiences in the soil in the United States is shown in Fig. 8-8.

In addition to the seven macronutrient elements discussed in the previous chapter and the micronutrient elements iron and iodine discussed in this chapter, twelve other mineral elements present in the body in small and variable amounts have been shown to play an essential role in human metabolism. In the human body they almost always occur bound to organic compounds rather than as free inorganic elements. These include copper, manganese, zinc, fluorine, cobalt, molybdenum, selenium, chromium, nickel, tin, vanadium, and silicon.

Seven others whose essential nature has not yet been established on the basis of these criteria may perform some functions similar to those deemed essential and may eventually be classified as essential.

A trace element is considered essential when the following are repeatedly demonstrated: (1) a significant growth response to dietary supplements of this element alone, (2) the development of a deficiency state on diets otherwise adequate, (3) a correlation of the deficiency state with the occurrence of suboptimal levels of the element in the blood or tissues of animals, (4) consistent occurrence in healthy tissue (especially fetal tissue), and (5) homeostatic control of rate of uptake and excretion.

Because some aspects of metabolism are common to many of these microelements, they will be discussed as a group, followed by a brief discussion of unique aspects of several of them.

Role in the body

The small amounts of micronutrients needed bear no relationship to their importance; a lack of one of these micronutrients can be equally as serious as a lack of an element needed at a level many hundred times higher. Some may be catalysts to biological reactions, acting as a link between the enzyme and its substrate; others are part of essential body compounds, such as hormones and enzymes; and others are involved in the growth of tissue.

In some cases the action of an essential element such as chromium is facilitated by a nonessential element. In others nonessential elements can satisfactorily replace essential elements in some enzymes.

Because of the varied geographical sources of food in the average diet and the fact that the amount of these micronutrient elements present in food is a function of the soil on which they are grown, there is little evidence of naturally occurring dietary deficiences of these nutrients. (Exceptions occur where the diet consists of a limited number of foods from a restricted geographic area where the soil is deficient or when the diet consists largely of highly processed foods.)

It has been difficult but not impossible to formulate experimental diets to the point at which an inadequate level of one nutrient and an adequate amount of all others are present. As a result, most of the evidence of the biological role of trace elements has been established by animal studies in which the diet has been developed by using purified nutrients known to be essential for the species. Once the role of the nutrient has been elucidated in animals, it has often been possible to demonstrate a similar function in human nutrition. Frequently it is necessary to interfere with the absorption or to stimulate the excretion of an element as well as to eliminate it from the diet for long periods to demonstrate a deficiency.

Interrelationships

One of the major difficulties in acquiring precise information on the function of many mineral elements has been the extent to which the presence or absence of one element may influence the role of a second and modify the requirement of another.

The interactions among minerals may occur in the diet, during absorption in the intestine, at the sites of excretion in the kidneys, intestine, or lungs, and at specific sites within the body cells. The interactions may be either synergistic or competitive.

As an example of this interrelationship, an increase in the molybdenum content of the diet without a simultaneous increase in the copper or sulfur content results in depressed growth and restricted hemoglobin production. The copper-molybdenum antagonism is apparently reciprocal. As further examples, increased copper interferes with iron and zinc metabolism, high levels of manganese affect iron metabolism, and excess cobalt interferes with the synthesis of the iodine-containing hormone thyroxin. Zinc-deficiency symptoms can be precipitated by diets high in calcium relative to zinc and can be relieved by correcting the imbalance without changing the amount of zinc.

Abnormally high levels of some elements can displace other elements that are essential parts of enzymes and can lead to failure to produce a biologically active enzyme. In addition, they may also interfere with the use of the effective enzyme. The utilization of one mineral element can be evaluated only in the light of the availability and utilization of other nutrients with which it may have a close dietary and metabolic interrelationship.

The ability of one element to replace another in key compounds and render it inactive is one of the hazards of using some of the multimineral supplements on the commercial market. Too often the basis of the formula is to give the producer a competitive advantage rather than any consideration of the nutritional needs of the individual. Unbalanced mineral supplements are potentially harmful. The Food and Drug Administration has suggested that calcium, iron, and iodine are the only mineral elements that can be justified in dietary supplements and in 1973 successfully supported its legislation to restrict the amounts that can be included only to have its authority to do this withdrawn.

Because of the complexities of the interrelationships among trace mineral elements, it is necessary to assess the whole pattern of nutrient intake in studies of deficiency, toxicity, or requirements. Simple and uncomplicated deficiencies of single micronutrient elements seldom occur under normal conditions.

Toxicity

Some trace mineral elements essential in small amounts may be toxic when present at higher levels. Most of the cases of toxicity from trace minerals have been the result of exposure to an environment saturated with the element, since minerals can enter the body through the respiratory tract and the skin as well as through the gastrointestinal tract. The manganese and selenium toxicity found among miners is believed to be caused by aspiration of air containing above-normal concentrations of the elements. Fluorine toxicity, which takes the form of a dental fluorosis, or mottled enamel, is the result of ingesting large quantities of water containing over 2.5 ppm of naturally occurring fluorine.

Selenium poisoning in animals is common in areas where the selenium content of the soil is high. High urinary levels are found in humans in the same area, although no definite evidence of selenium poisoning exists.

There are some trace elements such as lead and cadmium for which no biological function has been established and which are known to exert toxic effects. For instance, high levels of cadmium are associated with hypertension. In addition, some essential trace elements play a role in combating toxic or deleterious effects of high amounts of nonessential trace elements.

Deficiencies

Deficiencies of most trace mineral elements become evident only after prolonged dietary inadequacies and usually then only when associated with some defect in absorption and a change in other dietary components that leads to increased need. Generally the first evidence of an inadequacy appears in a reduction of enzymes of which the mineral is an essential part or a reduction in the activity of enzymes catalyzed by the element. Changes in blood levels of trace elements usually reflect the level of body stores rather than dietary intake, since body stores will be mobilized to maintain blood and tissue levels in the event of a dietary deficiency. Only when these are depleted and intake is inadequate will blood levels drop.

Requirements

Until 1979 there had been no attempt to estimate the human requirement for trace elements. However, it is anticipated that in the ninth revision of the Recommended Dietary Allowances, the Food and Nutrition Board will use the available evidence to establish provisional dietary standards.

The widespread presence of trace elements in foods, the minute amounts involved, the limited occurrence of any deficiency states that can be attributed directly to lack of the nutrient, and the interrelationships among trace elements have made the assessment of dietary needs difficult. In addition, modification of the level of other nutrients of the diet, such as protein, may influence the amount of the element needed.

Food sources

The amount of trace elements present in vegetable foods is primarily a function of the amount present in the soils in which the crops were grown and whether or not the element is essential for plant growth. Since these elements must be in the inorganic form before they can be used by the plant, those in "organic fertilizers" must be freed from the organic matter. In the case of animal foods the amount of some elements reflects the diet of the animal, whereas for others—especially those essential for the particular species—the animal may be able to regulate the amount present in its tissue by regulation of excretion. In any case, the ultimate source of the trace elements in food is the soil.

The possibility of a trace mineral element deficiency is greatly reduced with modern marketing techniques that lead to the consumption of a diet from widely scattered areas rather than from a restricted geographic region. However, the increased use of highly refined, fabricated, or processed foods may result in a marginal intake of some trace elements. On the other hand, some elements may be introduced into foods through contamination during processing or from containers.

Milk is a relatively poor source of most micronutrient elements. In addition, since it has been shown that the trace element content of human milk decreases as lactation progresses, it may be desirable to add foods to an infant's diet after 3 or 4 months of age.

ZINC

Although zinc, an element present at 50 ppm in the earth's crust and at 23 ppm in plants, was recognized as a dietary essential for rats in 1934, it was not until 1961 that there was evidence of zinc deficiency in humans. At that time retarded growth, delayed sexual maturity, and slow healing of wounds were identified as symptoms clearly associated with a lack of dietary zinc. These symptoms could be reversed by the addition of zinc to the diet. Since then, many of the roles of zinc in human nutrition have been identified but in only a few instances has the mechanism of action been clarified.

In Egypt and Iran, where zinc deficiency has been studied most effectively, it has been associated with a diet of unleavened whole wheat flour with little animal protein, complicated by respiratory losses of zinc due to high environmental temperatures. Additionally, in Egypt the deficiency has been further aggravated by hookworm infection and in Iran by geophagia, the practice of eating a clay that apparently binds zinc. In the United States some cases of retarded growth have been attributed to a lack of dietary zinc, failure to absorb zinc, or use of the drug penicillamine in the treatment of diseases such as Wilson's disease.

In 1974 knowledge of the metabolic role of zinc, its importance in human nutrition, and food sources of the nutrient had advanced to the point at which the Food and Nutrition Board of the National Research Council was confident enough to include it among those nutrients for which it made recommendations on dietary intake. The extent to which scientists have become involved in further study of its role in nutrition is evident from the fact that at a single scientific meeting in 1978 there were sixty-seven papers pertaining to zinc.

When zinc deficiency is produced experimentally in animals, there is a very rapid loss of appetite. This is followed by a decreased rate of growth that is attributed partly to the lack of food and partly to the lack of zinc needed for many biological functions.

Distribution

The human body contains from 1.4 to 2.3 g of zinc with about 70% or 1 g, concentrated in the skeleton at a level of 0.2 mg/g. There is also a high concentration in the skin, hair, and testes, tissues which seem particularly affected by a lack of zinc. In the blood 75% to 85% of the zinc occurs in the red blood cells, 3% in the white blood cells and platelets, and the remainder in the serum. About a third of the serum zinc is tightly bound to the protein macroglobulin and the remainder is loosely bound to the protein albumin, except for a very small amount bound to the amino acids histidine and cysteine. Blood serum levels are usually maintained within a range of 70 to 125 μg/dl of blood but fall below these levels during infections, pernicious anemia, hyperthyroidism, and pregnancy and in women using oral contraceptives.

Absorption

It is known that zinc is absorbed in the upper part of the small intestine but little is understood about the mechanism. Absorption does appear to be regulated by the cells in the intestinal wall, which respond to zinc levels in the plasma. In the average adult from a third to a half of the 10 to 15 mg provided in the diet is absorbed. Unabsorbed zinc along with that secreted in the intestinal enzymes appear in the feces.

Absorption of zinc is increased when blood levels fall or in the presence of vitamin D. The increased needs during pregnancy and lactation are reflected in up to a twofold increase in absorption. On the other hand, absorption is decreased as the stores of zinc increase or when the diet contains the outer husk of whole grains in which either phytic acid or fiber bind zinc in an insoluble complex. High levels of dietary calcium or copper also result in a lowered absorption of zinc but this does not appear to be a problem with normal dietary intakes.

It is not clear how zinc is distributed from the blood to the cells, but there is evidence that in humans it can appear in the tissues within 15 minutes of intake. Tissues such as liver, kidneys, lungs, pancreas, and testes release absorbed zinc rapidly, whereas the brain muscle and red blood cells turn it over slowly and hair and bone even more slowly.

Zinc is excreted primarily through the gastrointestinal tract in the feces, but again the mechanism is still unknown. Fecal zinc varies in proportion to dietary zinc but always includes about 1.5 mg from pancreatic secretions. A small amount (0.3 to 0.7 mg) is lost in the urine and about 1 mg in sweat.

Biological role

Zinc is essential in the composition or function of at least fifty-nine enzymes involved in digestion and metabolism, although the presence of all have not been demonstrated in humans. In some of these, zinc is an integral part of the enzyme (metalloenzyme) and in others it serves to catalyze the action of the zinc-dependent enzyme. As a result zinc is essential to many vital body functions. For example, as part of carbonic anhydrase in red blood cells it functions in the maintenance of acid-base balance by facilitating the catabolism, or breakdown, of carbonic acid. This is necessary for the transport and elimination of carbon dioxide, essential aspects of respiration. As part of the protein-splitting enzyme of the pancreatic juice cocarboxypeptidase plays a role in digestion. As part of alkaline phosphatase it is involved in bone metabolism, and as part of alcohol dehydrogenase in the liver it functions in the oxidation and detoxification of ethanol. Perhaps the most critical role of zinc is as an integral part of the enzymes DNA and RNA polymerase. These are necessary for the synthesis of DNA and RNA; they are also important for RNAase, which is involved in the breakdown of RNA. Zinc's essential roles in cell duplication and protein synthesis have been clearly established in animals but have yet to be established in humans, although it is reasonable to expect zinc to have a role in human metabolism also.

Since zinc is involved in a large number of enzymatic reactions, many tissues of the body can be affected by a zinc deficiency, especially at times when growth of the tissue is greatest. Some of the best documented roles of zinc will be discussed here.

Reproduction

Since zinc has its most profound influence on rapidly growing tissues, its effect on reproduction is significant. The importance of zinc in reproduction is emphasized by studies of zinc-deficient rats in which 99% of the fetuses were either resorbed or born with congenital malformations such as clubbed feet, hydrocephalus, cleft palate, or heart problems or with serious defects in the central nervous system and brain. The effect of prenatal zinc deficiency on brain development is similar to that of a deficiency in early infancy and has adverse effects on behavior and learning that persist into adulthood. In humans maternal zinc deficiency is clearly associated with low–birth weight infant and is suggested as a cause of malformation of the central nervous system. The increased absorption of zinc by pregnant and lactating rats likely represents a response to an increased need at a critical time in development. Observations of zinc-deficient humans have shown retarded gonadal development in males and impaired sexual maturity in both sexes. Severely deficient animals are not able to reproduce.

The drop in serum zinc as a result of the use of oral contraceptives may be a cause for concern in subsequent pregnancies, if a woman enters pregnancy with depleted reserves.

Skin health

Zinc has been associated with wound healing for some time. It is now believed that zinc, which concentrates in wound tissue, plays a role in the incorporation of methionine into the protein of the skin, although there is some evidence that it may function by stabliizing the cell membranes through decreasing lipid peroxidation. Studies on humans showed that zinc is most critical in the latter part of the healing process when the epidermal layers are healing. Supplementary zinc is effective in promoting more rapid healing only when zinc levels have been depressed. There is no added advantage from high levels, which may account for contradictory reports on the effectiveness of zinc.

A study of the role of oral zinc in the treatment of acne showed that a supplement of 135 mg of zinc as zinc sulfate resulted in a decrease in acne scars from 100% to 15% in four weeks. Similarly there are reports of the successful treatment with oral zinc sulfate of an often fatal genetic defect known as acrodermatitis enteropathica. The symptoms of this condition—diarrhea, dermatitis, and loss of hair—are believed to be due to malabsorption of zinc. This usually appears within the first few months of life and is associated with the change from breast milk to formula. Skin rashes are common in infants with low plasma zinc levels.

Gustatory system

Low blood levels of zinc have been associated with hypogeusia (loss of the sense of taste) usually accompanied by loss of appetite and hyposmia (loss of the sense of smell). These conditions often occur under the stress of burns, long bone fractures, and infections and may partially account for the poor appetite of hospitalized patients. Under circumstances in which depressed appetite is caused by low dietary zinc, the administration of 2 mg of zinc sulfate per kilogram of body weight daily has been helpful in restoring taste and appetite. This may be critical in the recovery of the patient.

Growth

Growth in humans suffering from zinc deficiency is severely stunted, often to the point of dwarfing. A diet high in animal protein supplemented with zinc results is a very rapid growth response.

Other roles

Many other seemingly unrelated roles have been identified for zinc. It is essential in normal glucose tolerance, apparently through its role in facilitating the action of insulin. Although evidence is contradictory, there is reason to believe that zinc may play a role in the mobilization of vitamin A from its storage site in the liver. The rapidity with which symptoms develop during zinc deficiency and are alleviated on its administration suggests that zinc may be involved in the transport of metabolites across cell membranes. The fact that the release of LEM (leukocyte endogenous mediator) in response to infections, toxins, and tissue damage is followed by a decline in zinc taken up by the liver may explain the effect of an inflammatory response on zinc levels. Observations that the biochemical and clinical symptoms of zinc deficiency found in persons with sickle cell anemia respond to supplementation with zinc sulfate (660 mg) suggests that zinc may be beneficial in the treatment of this disease, although the long-term effects of such large intake must still be evaluated.

Requirement

Only recently has it been recognized that the American diet may not provide optimal amounts of zinc. It has been reported that most diets provide from 10 to 15 mg/day, of which 20% to 30% is absorbed. However, the incidence of hypogeusia, delayed wound healing, and growth failure, all manifestations of zinc deficiency, adds support to the notion that inadequate intakes may be more common than suspected and that a significant portion of the population may have marginal intakes.

Table 8-6. Recommended dietary allowances for zinc*

	Age	Amount
Infants	0-6 mo	3 mg
	7-12 mo	5 mg
Children	1-10 yr	10 mg
Males	11+ yr	15 mg
Females	11+ yr	15 mg
Pregnant		20 mg
Lactating		25 mg

*From Food and Nutrition Board, National Research Council: Recommended dietary allowances, ed. 8, Washington, D.C., 1974.

Infant growth is stimulated by a level of zinc similar to that in human milk. Supplementation of formula with 4 mg of zinc/L results in increased growth in both height and weight and fewer gastrointestinal problems for males but not for females. This suggests that supplementation corrects an underlying deficiency. Greatest growth was associated with highest plasma zinc levels. Males may have higher zinc requirements than do females.

The currently recommended intakes are presented in Table 8-6; the values are based on the assumptions that 20% of dietary zinc is available, zinc is needed for growth, some is lost in the urine, and about 0.5 mg/L is lost in sweat. Need for bone growth is not included.

Food sources

The zinc content of some representative foods is shown in Table 8-7. From this it is

Table 8-7. Dietary sources of zinc (mg/100 g)*

Nuts	3.4†	Seafood	1.75†
Cashews	4.4	Oysters	148.7
Peanuts	3.2	Lobster	7.9
Almonds	2.6	Tuna	1.7
Coconut	0.03	Shrimp	1.5
Meat	3.1†	Vegetables	1.1†
Round steak	5.7	Green beans	4.2
Lamb chops	5.3	Lima beans	3.5
Chicken leg	2.9	Asparagus	1.0
Pork liver	1.9	Potatoes	0.9
Eggs	2.1†	Peas	0.7
Cereals	1.8†	Spinach	0.2
Wheat germ	16.7	Cabbage	0.2
Whole wheat	3.6	Dairy products	0.86†
Quick oats	3.2	Nonfat dried milk	3.51
Rye bread	1.3	Homogenized milk	0.01-0.05
Cornmeal	0.9	Fats and oils	0.84†
Refined	0.8		
White bread	0.5		

*Data from Sandstead, H. H.: Zinc nutrition in the United States, Am. J. Clin. Nutr. **26:**1251, 1973; and Freeland, J.E., and Cousins, R.J.: Zinc content of selected foods, J. Am. Diet. Assoc. **68:**526, 1976.
†Average amount for food group.

evident that the best sources of zinc, seafood and meat, are expensive foods. Less expensive foods such as cereals and legumes contain significant amounts of zinc, but they also contain phytic acid and other substances that can appreciably interfere with intestinal absorption of zinc. In addition, up to 80% of the zinc in whole-grain cereal may be lost in milling. The availability of zinc from leavened whole wheat bread is enhanced 30% to 50% compared to that from unleavened bread.

The observation that the low-income segment of the population may have suboptimal intakes was confirmed in an analysis of the diets of preadolescent low-income girls who were ingesting diets providing only 4.7 mg, an amount considerably below the recommended 15 mg. Fruits and vegetables have a relatively low zinc content. The amount of zinc in foods is affected by the zinc content of the water used in preparation and by the type of utensils used to prepare and store food. Cooking acid foods in galvanized utensils increases the zinc content.

The zinc content of plant protein, such as soybean or sesame oil meal is less available than that in animal protein. Phytic acid as found in cereals depresses the absorption of zinc, as shown by an increased excretion in the feces. The action of leavening in bread destroys phytic acid and increases the absorption of zinc.

The zinc concentration of early human milk is 16 mg/L but drops to 0.65 mg/L by 6 months. This is less than the level in cow's milk.

Diagnosis of a deficiency

Several tissues have been used in attempts to identify a sensitive test for zinc status. Since plasma levels may not drop even in severe zinc depletion, they are of limited usefulness. Zinc levels in the red blood cell, urine, and hair are more sensitive to decreased intakes. Urinary values reflect current intake whereas the others,which deplete more slowly, are indicative of long-term status. Balance studies, involving measurement of intake and excretion and the monitoring of ^{65}Zn in the blood following a test dose, are sensitive but expensive indices of zinc status. Measuring the level of some certain zinc-dependent enzymes such as alkaline phosphatase appears to be a promising diagnostic tool for zinc deficiency, as does the monitoring of the zinc content of the saliva.

Toxicity

Although so far there have been no reports of toxicity from the oral ingestion of zinc sulfate, even with therapeutic doses up to 200 mg (three times the amount needed to reverse deficiency symptoms), there is concern that there has not been adequate opportunity to assess effect over months or years. For this reason, unsupervised supplementation with zinc should be discouraged. The ingestion of excess zinc resulting from the storage of food and beverage in galvanized containers has resulted in fever, nausea, vomiting, and diarrhea, and toxicity has been associated with the inhalation of zinc chloride from industrial pollution. Among the metabolic changes are a loss of iron from the liver, which may amount to 50% in three days, followed by a loss of copper much later. Both of these changes may result in anemia.

MANGANESE

Although no deficiency of manganese has been demonstrated in humans, it is considered an essential nutrient on the basis of our knowledge of its biochemical reactions within the body. It is necessary for normal skeletal and connective tissue development. Manganese acts as a catalyst or as part of the essential enzymes involved in the synthesis of fatty acids and cholesterol; in the formation of urea, by which nitrogen is excreted; in the release of lipid from the liver; and in the structure and function of the mitochondrion of the cell, essential for the release of energy.

Absorption and metabolism

Manganese is believed to be absorbed by a mechanism similar to that involved in iron absorption. A specific protein carrier, transmanganin, is available to transport manganese in the blood. Of the 10 mg stored in the body, most is concentrated in the pancreas, bone, liver, and kidneys. Little of the element is excreted in the urine. The major path of excretion is the bile, from which a significant amount is reabsorbed. Absorption increases in iron deficiency and is inhibited by iron. Large intakes of calcium depress manganese absorption. Animal studies showed

Table 8-8. Dietary sources of manganese

Rich sources (>20 ppm)	Moderate sources (1-5 ppm)	Poor sources (>1 ppm)
Nuts	Green leafy vegetables	Animal tissues
Whole-grain cereals	Dried fruits	Poultry
Dried legumes	Fresh fruits	Dairy products
Tea	Nonleafy vegetables	Seafood

that manganese crosses the placental barrier freely.

Requirement and food sources

Although the requirement for manganese has not been established, the 2 to 4 mg/day found in a typical Western diet is considered adequate. About 10% is retained.

Whole-grain cereals and green vegetables are among the better sources of manganese, but the amount present depends on the part of the plant and the geographical source. Tea (150 to 990 ppm) is an extremely rich source and in English diets is estimated to provide 3.3 mg of manganese. Relative values of common foodstuffs are given in Table 8-8.

Toxicity

Although the accumulation of excessive amounts of manganese is toxic, it is usually the result of inhalation of industrial contamination rather than a high dietary intake. Weakness and psychological and motor difficulties are manifestations of high tissue levels. Iron metabolism is also adversely affected. High levels of dietary protein protect against manganese toxicity.

COPPER

Copper was first recognized as a dietary essential in 1928 when it was observed that anemia could be prevented only if both copper and iron were available. Since that time, many metabolic functions of copper have been identified but often have been difficult to assess because of the interaction of copper with other trace elements, such as zinc, molybdenum, and sulfur.

Absorption and metabolism

Typical diets provide from 2 to 5 mg of copper, about 30% of which is absorbed, with reported values ranging from 15% to 97%. Copper is taken up rapidly from the stomach and upper intestine, where the contents are still acid. Its absorption from the intestine is dependent on a copper-binding protein, metallotheonein, which also functions in the absorption of cadmium and zinc. This decreases when intakes of ascorbic acid are high, implicating high vitamin C intakes with copper deficiency.

Absorbed copper appears in the bloodstream in as little as 15 minutes after ingestion. Initially it appears loosely bound to albumin or to some amino acids. Both these chelates, a combination of a trace element with another substance, represent the transport form of copper, and the amino acid chelate appears to have the special function of facilitating the transport of copper across membranes into the cells. This transport copper represents only 7% of serum copper.

Copper is removed from the serum by the liver. There copper is either excreted into the bile, stored in a protein complex containing 2% copper, or used in the synthesis of ceruloplasmin, another protein-copper complex that is released again into the blood, where it accounts for 93% of serum copper. Serum copper values are normally from 90 to 150 μg/dl with higher values found in women than in men. Serum copper levels increase twofold in pregnancy or with the use of oral contraceptives, in persons with pellagra (a deficiency of the vitamin niacin), and in both chronic and acute liver disease.

The release of copper from the liver is controlled by the adrenal gland through its influence on the synthesis of the protein needed for its removal. Some serum copper enters the bone marrow, where it is used in the synthesis of erythrocuprein, which accounts for 60% of the copper within the red blood cells. Erythrocuprein has been identified as the same compound as hepatocuprein in the liver and cerebrocuprein in the nerve tissue. To reduce the confusion about nomenclature it has been suggested that these compounds be called either *cytocuprein,* reflecting its structure, or *superoxide dismutase,* reflecting its function as an enzyme in red blood cells.

Another nonerythrocuprein copper compound that accounts for the rest of the copper in the red blood cells may also be produced in the bone marrow or may arise from the serum copper directly.

Copper is excreted by two pathways. Fecal copper represents unabsorbed, dietary copper and copper released in the bile and that lost through the intestinal wall in the albumin-copper complex of the serum. Urinary copper of 5 to 24 mg daily accounts for a mere 4% of copper loss.

The total copper content of the body is estimated at 75 to 150 mg. About 50% of this is concentrated in the bones and muscles, but on a weight basis the liver, which stores 10% of body copper, is the most concentrated site of copper, followed by the brain, heart, and kidneys. The newborn infant has liver stores five to ten times those of the adult, but they drop to adult levels as early as three months of age. A high level of copper in fingernails of infants is associated with cystic fibrosis and shows promise as a routine screening technique.

Functions

Copper has already been identified as an essential component of many enzymes and the list is growing constantly. Only a few of its many roles will be discussed here.

The role of copper in preventing anemia has been attributed variously to its effectiveness in facilitating iron absorption, in stimulating the synthesis of heme or globin fractions of the hemoglobin molecule, or in releasing stored iron from the ferritin in the liver. It now appears that as part of a multifunctional enzyme known as ceruloplasmin or ferroxidase I or II copper plays an important role in the oxidation of ferrous to ferric iron. This reaction takes place at many points from the time iron is absorbed until it is incorporated into the hemoglobin molecule and then again as it is returned to the iron pool.

In addition to its role in preventing anemia, copper is required for the synthesis of the phospholipids essential in the formation of the myelin sheath surrounding nerve fibers. It is part of the respiratory enzyme cytochrome oxidase, necessary for the release of energy in the cell. Copper is part of the enzyme tyrosinase, needed for the conversion of the amino acid tyrosine to melanin, the dark pigment of hair and skin. The absence of this enzyme is associated with albinism. In conjunction with ascorbic acid (vitamin C), copper maintains the activity of the enzymes involved in the synthesis of both elastin, a protein in the wall of the aorta, and the connective protein collagen. It is necessary in the last stage of synthesis when the cross-linkages between the polypeptide chains are established. Lack of copper to catalyze this reaction results in defective bone matrix, which in turn shows up as fragile bones susceptible to fractures.

Requirement

A dietary intake of 2 mg of copper daily appears to maintain copper balance in the adult. It is recommended that copper intake be 0.03 mg/kg of body weight. Infants have an exceptional need for copper of 0.08 mg/kg.

Food sources

Copper is widely distributed in foods in varying concentrations. To a certain extent the amount is a reflection of the copper content of the soil on which the plant or animal was raised; higher levels reflect copper available beyond that needed for growth. Amounts in the soil reportedly vary from 2 to 60 ppm. Copper content of representative foods is given in Table 8-9. The use of copper pipes in water systems may be a source of some ingested copper.

Deficiency

Copper deficiency has been described in 7- to 9-month-old infants on a milk diet who were hospitalized with malnutrition associated with severe diarrhea. It was recognized by a drop in ceruloplasmin levels and low blood copper levels. Symptoms included depressed iron absorption, decreased number of white blood cells, demineralization of bone, and defective red blood cell formation. Since infants are born with stores of copper that last until foods other than milk are introduced at 3 to 6 months, it appears that the

Table 8-9. Dietary sources of copper*

Rich sources (>8 ppm)	Intermediate sources (2-8 ppm)	Poor sources (<2 ppm)
Liver	Leafy vegetables	Milk
Shellfish (especially oysters)	Eggs	Butter
Nuts	Muscle meat	Cheese
Cocoa	Fish	Sugar
Cherries	Poultry	Fresh fruits and vegetables
Mushrooms	Peas	
Whole-grain cereals	Beans	
Gelatin	Fresh fruit	
	Refined cereals	

*From Pennington, J. T., and Calloway, D. H.: Copper content of foods, J. Am. Diet. Assoc. **63:**143, 1973.

copper deficiency reported here may have been due to the failure to reasorb the copper secreted in the bile.

The importance of copper in normal elastin and collagen formation to maintain the health of the cardiovascular system is evident by the massive internal hemorrhages that result from rupture of a major blood vessel such as the aorta. These hemorrhages occur in a copper deficiency as a result of defects in these intercellular proteins.

The copper content of the hair decreases with age and appears to reflect nutritional status in some age groups.

An inherited condition known as Menke's kinky hair syndrome, characterized by slow growth, degeneration of brain tissue, and peculiar stubby white hair, is associated with low serum copper and ceruloplasmin levels. The condition results from defective copper absorption when copper taken up by intestinal cells is not released into the bloodstream. It thus appears that copper may be important in treatment of the disease.

Toxicity

Copper is toxic to humans when it exists as the unbound copper ion. In this way it acts as an inhibitor to many enzyme systems. There is no evidence of toxicity as the result of environmental contamination. The ingestion of copper salts at levels ten times that found in a normal diet leads to nausea and vomiting, possibly as a result of a disturbance of the balance between absorption and excretion. Chronic copper toxicity occurs in the hereditary condition Wilson's disease, in which the level of ceruloplasmin is greatly reduced in the presence of a positive copper balance. The increased synthesis of a metal-binding protein with an affinity for copper results in an accumulation of copper in the liver, brain, kidneys, and cornea of the eyes, where it is identified visually by brown or green rings. Successful control involves the reduction of dietary copper to the point its accumulation in these tissues is inhibited. Penicillamine, a penicillin derivative that promotes the excretion of copper, has been used to help reduce these stores to normal levels.

High copper intakes are associated with decreased levels of plasma retinol.

MOLYBDENUM

Molybdenum, which has long been recognized as essential for plant growth, is now considered an essential element in human nutrition.

Biological role

Molybdenum is an essential part of two enzymes—xanthine oxidase and aldehyde oxidase. Xanthine oxidase is involved in the formation of uric acid from the purines hypoxanthine and xanthine and also aids in mobilizing iron from the liver reserves. Aldehyde oxidase is necessary for the oxidation of aldehydes. Evidence has been accumulating that molybdenum may act in conjunction with fluoride in the prevention of dental caries, possibly by promoting the retention of fluoride. It is unconfirmed, however, that the human cannot accomplish all these biochemical roles in other ways that do not require molybdenum. On this basis there was a reluctance to classify molybdenum unequivocally as an essential nutrient. Evidence of molybdenum toxicity at high levels includes diarrhea, a depressed growth rate, and anemia associated with failure of the red blood cell to mature or a decrease in its life span.

Interrelationships

Most of the interest in molybdenum nutriture has centered around its metabolic interrelationships with copper and sulfate. The toxicity manifest in animals as depressed growth and hemoglobin production from high levels of molybdenum can be overcome by the addition of copper to the rations. Similarly, a high molybdenum intake simulates a copper deficiency either by interfering with the removal of copper from the blood or the synthesis of ceruloplasmin needed to transport copper. High intakes of molybdenum also alter the activity of alkaline phosphatase and produce certain bone abnormalities.

Absorption

Molybdenum is readily absorbed from the gastrointestinal tract and is excreted mainly in the urine, but the amount absorbed and excreted is influenced to a large extent by the amount of sulfate in the diet. High-sulfate diets increase urinary but not fecal excretion levels.

The 9 mg of molybdenum in the body is found in highest concentration in liver, kidneys, adrenals, and blood cells.

Legumes such as peas and beans (3 to 5 ppm) and meat (2 to 5 ppm) are relatively rich sources; whole-grain cereal (0.6 to 5 ppm) and fruits and vegetables are poor sources.

Requirement

The provisional recommended allowance has been estimated to be between 0.15 and 0.5 mg/day for adults. Since the usual intake is estimated at 335 μg, there seems little likelihood of a deficiency except among vegetarians and persons eating a diet composed largely of highly refined foods.

SELENIUM

Selenium is unique among mineral elements in that it may be present in a diet of natural foods in such small amounts that deficiency symptoms develop or in such large amounts that it is toxic or possibly carcinogenic. It is both the least abundant of all elements in food essential to mammals and the most toxic.

The amount of selenium in food is a function of the selenium content of the soil in which it is grown. In the United States soils in the eastern part have low selenium content while those of the Great Plains and Rocky Mountain areas, described as seleniferous, are characterized by high selenium content. The high selenium levels in these areas were first associated with toxic symptoms in cattle in 1934. It was not until 1957, however, that a biological role and hence a nutritional need for selenium was identified in relation to deficiency symptoms associated with the use of animal feeds low in selenium.

Biological role

Initial studies suggested that selenium functioned as an antioxidant capable of sparing vitamin E in many metabolic reactions. It is now well established that selenium is an essential part of the enzyme glutathione peroxidase, which protects against damage from the peroxides produced when lipids or fats are oxidized. This enzyme acts much like vitamin E in protecting against the destruction of red blood cells when the fat in the membrane is oxidized to form peroxides. It is now evident that selenium also plays a unique role in preventing degenerative changes in the pancreas and exudative diathesis in chicks, a condition associated with low levels of the enzyme glutathione peroxidase due to a selenium deficiency. At low levels it also exerts a protective effect in retarding growth of cancer tissue.

Selenium resembles sulfur biochemically and hence frequently replaces it in sulfur-containing amino acids such as methionine, cystine, and cysteine. This may account for the beneficial effect of selenium salts used in conjunction with dietary protein in enhancing the growth response in the treatment of children with kwashiorkor.

The role of selenium in protecting the red cell membrane and hemoglobin against oxidative changes is distinct from the role of vitamin E. Selenium also provides protection against mercury and cadmium toxicity. It may function as part of the enzyme that is responsible for destroying the undesirable peroxides derived from unsaturated fatty acids.

Absorption and metabolism

All tissues contain some selenium but the kidneys, hair, and liver have the highest levels. Well over 90% of dietary selenium is absorbed, suggesting that any control over the amount in the body is through the excretion rather than the uptake of the nutrient. Blood levels of selenium remain amazingly constant, but when intake is low the red blood cells contain about three times the amount in the serum. Excess selenium is excreted in the urine, feces, and sweat. Some is also excreted by the respiratory system.

Food sources

While the amount of selenium in food varies greatly from one area to another, analysis shows that seafood (including tuna), meat, and cereals, especially wheat, contain the largest amount. In areas where the selenium content of the soil is high, cow's milk may contain up to 1.27 ppm, a level that may be injurious to health. Selenium usually occurs in conjunction with protein in plants. In contrast, the amount in human milk is maintained within a very narrow range of 0.2 ppm, a level believed to be safe for the human infant. In cereals the element is distributed evenly throughout the endosperm, which accounts for the fact that many analyses show no difference between whole-grain and refined products. Vegetables contain practically no selenium.

Selenium is a volatile substance and may be lost in cooking.

Requirement

The requirement for selenium is estimated to be 0.05 to 0.2 mg or 0.1 to 0.3 ppm and may increase as the unsaturated fatty acid content of the diet increases. There have been no reports of dietary deficiencies in humans. One beneficial effect of low intake has been observed when the consumption of alcohol is high. Under these circumstances the normally observed increase in fatty livers is inhibited.

Clinical uses

Although there have been periodic claims that selenium is effective in preventing cancer, increasing human fertility, improving memory, or increasing resistance to infection, currently there are no scientific data to support any of these claims.

Toxicity

At high levels of intake (5 to 10 ppm) selenium is toxic, apparently because of its capacity to replace sulfur in biological compounds and to inhibit the action of some enzymes. Likelihood of selenium poisoning in humans is confined to persons exposed to industrial dusts containing the element. Toxicity is reduced by diets high in protein.

While studies on chicks and rats have raised questions about a possible carcinogenic effect of high selenium intakes, epidemiological evidence on the incidence of cancer in human populations shows no relationship with the selenium content of the blood. In areas where selenium levels are high, discolored teeth, skin eruptions, brittle nails edema, gastrointestinal disorders, and partial or total loss of hair have been observed in humans. The higher incidence of dental caries observed in children in these high selenium areas has been attributed to the fact that selenium becomes incorporated in the protein matrix of the enamel and prevents normal mineral deposition. After the tooth has erupted, the selenium in the saliva may increase the susceptibility of the tooth to decay.

Although there seemed to be much evidence to suggest that chicken feed should be supplemented with selenium, the possibility of toxicity from high levels kept the Food and Drug Administration from approving such a measure until 1974, when they agreed to allow its use at levels of 0.1 to 0.2 ppm. This judicious use should allow growth in animals without the risk of developing cancer.

CHROMIUM

Chromium, first identified as an essential element for mammals in 1959 and first associated with human dietary deficiency in 1966, is now considered an essential element in human nutrition.

Biological role

Although its biochemical role has not been clearly defined, it has been identified as part of the glucose tolerance factor required for optimal utilization of glucose. There is some evidence that it acts to facilitate the binding of insulin to the cell, which in turn facilitates the uptake of glucose from the cell.

The amount of chromium in the body (1.7 mg) in the United States is much lower than in people in the Far East (9 mg). From 1% to 20% of dietary chromium is absorbed, and it is excreted primarily in the urine. It tends to accumulate in the skin, muscle, and fat. The amount of chromium in the hair is a sensitive indicator of chromium nutriture.

Deficiency

Low intakes of chromium have been associated with a reduced tolerance to glucose and an increasing incidence of diabetes, both of which occur with increasing age. Many cases of mild glucose intolerance can be treated successfully with chromium. Studies of chromium in the body show that the fetus obtains a generous supply from the maternal organism but that in the United States there is a steady decline throughout life. A similar decline has not been observed in other countries.

Other symptoms observed in chromium deficiency include decreased glycogen reserves, retarded growth, disturbed amino acid metabolism, and increased aortic lesions associated with elevated blood cholesterol levels. In the United States it has been observed that chromium is absent from the aorta but not other tissues of persons with coronary heart disease. A role in lipid metabolism is postulated.

Food sources

Chromium is found almost exclusively in foods of plant origin. The amount varies with species, soil, and season. Vegetables provide from 30 to 55 ppm, whole grains and cereals from 30 to 70 ppm, and fruits 20 ppm. White sugar and raw sugar contain indetectable amounts, while brown sugar and commercial syrups have appreciable amounts. Typical American diets contain from 50 to 400 μg daily, an amount sufficient to meet the provisional Recommended Allowance for Adults of 50 to 200 μg and the minimum requirement of 10 to 20 μg. Lower intakes have been associated with the use of refined sugars and cereals, which contain much smaller amounts of the element than do less refined products.

Toxicity

Inhalation of chromium, a contaminant from industrial waste, can be toxic, and the ingestion of excess chromium in drinking water has resulted in subacute toxicity. There is no evidence of toxicity from excessive dietary intakes. However, since the effects are known to vary with the form of chromium available, and since there are many uncertainties about the effect of excessive amounts and imbalances with other nutrients, the use of supplements should be discouraged.

COBALT

Biological role

In human nutrition the major role of cobalt is as an essential part of vitamin B_{12}, or cobalamin, which is necessary to prevent pernicious anemia. Humans do not have the ability to synthesize the vitamin and must depend on animal sources of the nutrient. These animal sources have been synthesized by microorganisms in the intestine of animals that can incorporate the cobalt obtained from the plants they eat. The cobalt content of plants reflects the cobalt of the soil in which they are grown.

There is increasing evidence that cobalt may be essential in the functioning of several other essential enzymes. It is absorbed primarily from the jejunum in the upper intestine by the same pathway as iron. About 85% is excreted in the urine and a small amount in the feces and sweat.

Food sources

The average American diet contains about 300 mg of cobalt. Cobalt is so widely distributed in foods that there is little likelihood of a deficiency in humans. The cobalt of some representative foods is given in Table 8-10. In spite of the large amount taken in, only the 0.04 mg required in vitamin B_{12} is needed.

Toxicity

There is some evidence that high intakes of cobalt may have toxic effects. One that has been observed is the goitrogenic effect after the prolonged ingestion of cobaltous chloride. The enlarged thyroid gland returns to normal after the cessation of cobalt administration. High intakes in animals have been observed to cause polycythemia (increase in the number of red blood cells) and hyperplasia (increase in quantity) of bone marrow, which are believed to be the result of the production of erythropoietin, the hormone that stimulates red blood cell formation in the bone marrow.

Polycythemia is also seen in cobalt toxicity with beer drinking. A synergistic effect between cobalt and ethanol has been identified as the causative factor in the cardiac problems observed in persons who drink large quantities of beer to which cobalt has been added to control foaming. The vasodilation observed in high dosages of cobalt has led to the use of cobalt to treat hypertension in humans.

VANADIUM

The possibility that vanadium is an essential element for humans was considered only recently. There is now sufficient evidence to

Table 8-10. Dietary sources of cobalt listed according to micrograms per grams dry weight

Excellent (>5)	Good (1.5-5)	Poor (<0.05)
Liver	Lean beef	Cereal grains
Kidney	Lamb	Leguminous seeds
Oysters	Veal	Green leafy vegetables
Clams	Poultry	Yeast
	Saltwater fish	
	Milk	

class it as a dietary essential. It is a constituent of human tissues. About 60% of the absorbed vanadium is excreted in the urine, and the remainder is retained in the liver and bones.

Estimates of the vanadium content of the average American diet indicates that it is about ten times the estimated requirement of 0.1 to 0.3 mg. An intake of 100 to 125 mg/day in humans may inhibit the synthesis of cholesterol by counteracting the stimulating effect of manganese. However, failure to demonstrate this cholesterol-lowering effect in middle-aged men has discouraged its use as an anticholesterolgenic agent.

Studies on animals indicate that vanadium plays an essential role in growth, iron and lipid metabolism, reproduction, and bone development.

There is some evidence to indicate that vanadium may be exchanged for phosphorus in the apatite crystals of tooth enamel, thus contributing to resistance to tooth decay.

TIN

Since tin is neither found in the tissues of the newborn nor widespread in the animal kingdom, there is still some controversy as to whether or not it is an essential micronutrient. However, in 1970 it was fairly well established that rats exhibit a definite growth response when 1 ppm of tin is present compared to when the diet contains little or none. Symptoms of deficiency range from poor growth and loss of hair to dermatitis. This evidence is suggestive of a definite metabolic role and it has been postulated that tin may function in maintaining the structure of protein or in oxidation reduction reactions.

Since there is very little information on the tin content of food, it is not surprising to find estimates of intakes ranging from 3 to 17 mg/day. Needs are estimated at 3 to 6 mg/day. Stannous sulfate, the most commonly available form, is absorbed poorly and is excreted in the feces. Although up to 114 ppm may be dissolved from unlacquered cans into some acid-containing juices, there seems to be no basis for concern about possible toxicity.

NICKEL

The understanding of the role of nickel in metabolism has led to its inclusion in the list of mineral elements considered essential. It is present in all human tissues, in which it is firmly associated from DNA and RNA. It is also found in human blood serum as a metalloprotein.

Studies on chicks have demonstrated the role of nickel in maintaining cellular structure and functioning and on pigs for normal growth and reproduction.

There is little likelihood of a deficiency in the human diet, although a diet devoid of fruits and vegetables would only provide marginal amounts. Malabsorption might further reduce the nickel available.

SILICON

Until recently interest in silicon centered on silicosis or silicon toxicity as the result of the absorption of excessive amounts of the element. It is now evident that silicon plays a role in stimulating growth, initiating calcification of bone, and promoting the synthesis of connective tissue, collagen. Although most of the evidence on a metabolic role has come from research on rats and rabbits, there is general agreement that it is essential in human nutrition. The human requirement is unknown and information on food sources is scanty. Unrefined cereals are good sources and animal foods poor sources. Beer has a high concentration of silicon.

FLUORINE

Although the role of fluorine in controlling tooth decay has been recognized for some time, it has only been in the last few years that fluorine has been considered an essential nutrient. The exact nature of its metabolic role has not been established, but there is evidence that growth and possibly reproduction in animals is retarded when the diet is deficient in fluorine.

Historical background

Fluorine is one of the most abundant elements in the earth's crust and as such it is widely distributed throughout nature.

Interest in the possible nutritional role of fluorine dates back to 1931 when it was established that in communities where residents had a remarkable freedom from tooth decay but suffered from an undesirable brownish appearance on the tooth surface, the water contained considerably more fluorine than did most communal water supplies. The efforts to identify the factor had started in 1902 when a dentist in Colorado Springs became curious about the brown stain known as "Colorado brown stain" on the teeth of many of his patients.

Once fluorine had been identified as the substance in the water supply responsible for the brown staining and the absence of dental caries, other studies soon showed that somewhat lower levels of fluorine in the water were responsible for a markedly decreased incidence of tooth decay without the undesirable mottling of tooth enamel (dental fluorosis) illustrated in Fig. 8-11. The relationship between the fluorine content of the water and the rate of tooth decay was established in 1942. A water supply containing 1 ppm of fluorine was associated with a 50% to 60% lower incidence of tooth decay without any opacity or chalkiness in the tooth enamel. Only when the fluorine content of the water rose above 2.5 ppm did evidence of dental fluorosis occur.

Recognizing dental caries as a major public health problem and seeking some effective means of controlling it, the United States Public Health Service in 1945 initiated a study to determine if the addition of sufficient fluorine to the water supply to raise the natural fluorine content to 1 ppm would afford the same degree of protection against tooth decay as would a natural fluoride level of 1 ppm. Newburgh, on the Hudson River in New York, was chosen as the experimental city, and Kingston, across the river with a population of similar economic, racial, and cultural background and a low-fluorine wa-

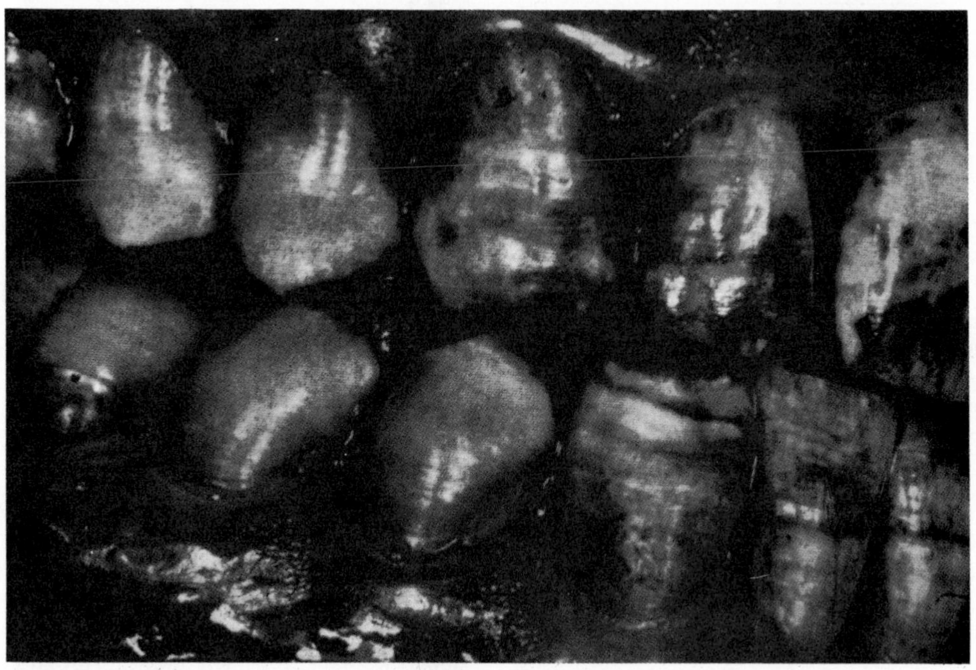

Fig. 8-11. Appearance of teeth in dental fluorosis. (From Duckworth, R.: Proc. Nutr. Soc. **22:**79, 1963.)

Table 8-11. Reductions in decayed, missing, and filled permanent teeth (DMF index) reported among children in communities after ten years of fluoridation*

Community	Age studied	Percentage reduction
Grand Junction, Colo.	6	94.0
New Britain, Conn.	6-16	44.6
District of Columbia	6	59.1
Evanston, Ill.	6-7-8	91.3-64.6-62.6
Fort Wayne, Ind.	6-10	>50.0
Hopkinsville, Ky.	? (Children)	56.0
Louisville, Ky.	First 3 grades	62.1
Hagerstown, Md.	7, 9, 11, and 13	57.0
Grand Rapids, Mich.	6-7-8	75.0-63.0-57.0
Grand Rapids, Mich.	9-10	50.0-52.0
Newburgh, N.Y.	6-9	58.0
Newburgh, N.Y.	10-12	57.0
Newburgh, N.Y.	13-14	48.0
Newburgh, N.Y.	16	41.0
Charlotte, N.C.	6-11	60.0
Chattanooga, Tenn.	6-14	70.8
Marshall, Texas	7-15	54.0
Brantford, Ont.	6-7-8	60.0-67.0-54.0
Brantford, Ont.	9-10	46.0-41.0
Brantford, Ont.	11-13	44.0
Brantford, Ont.	14-16	35.0

*From Dunning J. M.: Current status of fluoridation, N. Engl. J. Med. **272:**30, 1965.

ter supply, was the control city. Careful records were kept of the incidence of tooth decay in both cities. At the end of a ten-year period a report showed that children under 10 years of age had received the greatest protection, having a DMF index* (Table 8-11) 60% to 65% below those of their counterparts in Kingston. Children 12 to 14 years old who consumed fluoridated water from early childhood but not since birth had a 48% reduction in tooth decay, and 16-year-olds who had consumed fluoridated water for an even shorter time had only a 40% reduction. A fifteen-year report on the same communities showed a similar degree of protection with no detectable adverse effects.

*DMF index is the number of decayed, missing, and filled teeth. It considers only the number of teeth involved, but not the extent of the decay.

A comparison of 6-year-olds in the two communities in 1962 showed that 33.9% of those in Newburgh were caries free compared to 16.4% in Kingston. In addition, comparable DMF rates were 0.09 and 0.65 per child, respectively. These findings, showing that the earlier a child has an available source of fluoride the greater the protection it will provide, have since been confirmed and reconfirmed in fluoridation studies in many other communities.

The effect of the fluoridation of the water supply on the dental health of children in various communities is shown in Table 8-11. The observed reduction of 50% to 60% approaches that observed in communities whose natural fluorine content is similar. Reports of studies from Holland show that the addition of fluorine to the water affords greater protection for the exposed surface of the tooth than it does for the pits and fissures.

Several reports have shown an increase in tooth decay when a community drops a fluoridation program that has been in effect for several years. Such reports indicating beneficial effects from the addition of fluorine and a reversal of these in its withdrawal help establish the fact that the benefits are caused by fluorine rather than other unidentified factors.

In addition to the benefits a pregnant woman passes on to her child by drinking fluoridated water, there may be other benefits that accrue to the adult from the ingestion of fluorine-containing water. For instance, fluorine, by increasing the stability of the skeleton, may protect it against losses of calcium that often occur at menopause, under conditions of immobility, and, as recently observed, in space flight.

Metabolism

Soluble fluoride is absorbed readily from the stomach, although some continues to be taken up by the intestine. About 75% of that ingested appears in the bloodstream within 1 hour and 90% within 8 hours. Of this, about 50% is excreted in the urine within 24 hours, and the other half is taken up readily by teeth and bones, where it apparently becomes an integral and important part of the tooth and bone structure. Regardless of the amount ingested, blood levels remain amazingly constant, reflecting the ability of the kidneys to control the levels in body tissues by excreting amounts in excess of the body's needs. The amount of fluorine appearing in other tissues, including soft tissue, saliva, milk, and fetal blood, parallels that in the blood at a slightly lower level. The amount in soft tissue remains a relatively constant 0.5 ppm, which does not fluctuate with age or fluorine intake.

Sources

Almost all the fluorine in water and from 50% to 80% of that in food is absorbed. In addition to water, from which an adult usually ingests 1 mg daily in nonfluoridated areas and 2 to 3 mg in fluoridated areas, another 1.3 to 1.8 mg comes from tea and solid foods. Fish products are reasonably good sources. There is increasing evidence that the amount of fluorine in processed or cooked foods may be two to three times higher than that in fresh foods if fluoridated water has been used in preparation. The determination of the fluorine content of food is tedious. Results of some efforts are shown in Table 8-12.

Table 8-12. Fluorine content of some representative foods*

Food	mg/100 gm
Tea	0.475
Coffee	0.250
Rice	0.07
Buckwheat	0.17
Soybeans	0.40-0.67
Spinach	0.02
Onions	0.05
Lettuce	0.01

*From Gordenoff, T., and Member, W.: Fluorine, World Rev. Nutr. Diet. **2**:213, 1962.

Fluoridation of public water supplies

As soon as communities began to consider the fluoridation of their water supplies, groups began to oppose it for a wide variety of reasons, most of which revolved around its hazards, its ineffectiveness, and ethical considerations of so-called compulsory medication. Social issues assumed more importance than health issues. The opponents claimed that fluorine was toxic and that fluoridation of water supplies was a violation of the right of the individual; through a variety of highly emotional attacks on the program they created doubt regarding the motives of the proponents of the measure.

Any possibility of fluorine toxicity has been thoroughly investigated by the United

States Public Health Service, which has been unable to find any evidence of detrimental effects from the addition of 1 ppm of fluorine to the drinking water no matter how large the water consumption. Based on the health records of 2 million people in artificially fluoridated areas, no evidence exists of increased deposition of fluorine in soft tissues, such as the kidneys or heart, no increase in mortality and morbidity rates, no growth depression or abnormalities, no increase in cancer or nephritis, and no increase in birth rate of mongoloids, all of which have been claimed by the antifluoridation forces. Claims that fluorine interfered with cell growth and protein synthesis have been discredited by studies showing that cellular reproduction continues in the presence of an amount of fluorine far in excess of the amount that can be brought into the circulating fluids by oral intakes of fluorine. On the contrary, in addition to a reduction in tooth decay, a reduction in the amount of periodontal disease, a 30% reduction in the incidence of malocclusion was found.

Fluorine is toxic but only at levels well above that at which it is added to communal water supplies. Mottled enamel, or dental fluorosis, which presents only aesthetic problems, may occur at concentrations of 2 to 8 ppm, osteosclerosis at 8 to 20 ppm, growth depression at 50 ppm or more, and fatal poisoning at 2500 times recommended levels. Extreme precautions and constant surveillance of the level of fluorine in the water assure the public that the level in their water could not approach toxic levels. As an added precaution, it is suggested that in tropical areas where water consumption may be higher, the level of fluoridation should be reduced to 0.7 ppm.

In spite of the evidence that the addition of fluorine to the water supply to provide a total fluorine content of 1 ppm has no adverse effects at this level, and in spite of the endorsement of fluoridation by every medical and dental group in the United States, the United States Public Health Service, and many Asian and European countries, fluoridation remains a controversial issue. The antifluoridation groups have become so vocal that in many cases in which fluoridation has come up for a public referendum, it has been defeated. In 1974 slightly less than half the persons on public water systems were receiving fluoridated water. Another 6% were consuming naturally fluoridated water. Of 1899 communities that had considered fluoridation up to 1966, 1126 rejected it. In most cases in which it has been rejected, the decision was made at public referendum, and those in which it has been accepted, the decision was generally an administrative or legislative one.

In 1965 Connecticut became the first state to require fluoridation of the water supply in all cities over 50,000 population. By 1967 this had been extended to cities of 20,000 or more. Seven other states have passed similar legislation. By 1969 over 75% of the populations of fifteen states were drinking fluoridated water. In a few cases fluoridation has been terminated after a period of successful use. In spite of the efforts of the antifluoridation forces, by 1974 over 80 million people in over 4000 communities including Chicago and New York City were consuming water to which fluorine had been added, and another 10 million were drinking water in which the natural fluorine content was at a protective level. In all cases where it has been introduced, a significant reduction occurred in tooth decay among children, a protection that carries over into adulthood. Currently in thirty-two of the fifty states, mostly in the central and eastern part of the country, over 50% of the population is on public water supplies with natural or controlled fluoridation. Illinois with 99% of its population ranks highest whereas Colorado with 2.7% ranks lowest.

Different forms of fluoride—sodium fluoride, sodium silicofluoride, and fluorosilicic acid—have all been used effectively to provide the fluoride ions as active agents in the water supply. None of these appears to influence the odor, taste, color, or hardness of the water, and all can be readily introduced into the community water system without causing a depreciation in plumbing equipment. The cost of fluoridation varies, depending on the chemical chosen and the engineering complexity of the water system, but most cities report a cost of from 10 cents to $1.15 per person per year. In the light of the fact that over 95% of the population without fluorine experience tooth decay and will stand to benefit financially as well as through a reduction in physical discomfort accompanying tooth decay, the cost seems small. In Philadelphia it was estimated that fluoridation had saved 360,000 teeth valued at over $2 million in dental bills during a thirteen-year period. In Newburgh the cost of the initial dental care of 5- to 8-year-old children who had been on fluoridated water all their lives was less than half and annual dental costs slightly more than half that of their counterparts in Kingston. Defluoridation, or the removal of natural fluorine from the water, has been undertaken in some communities where fluorine is naturally present at a level that causes mottling of tooth enamel. It has cost $1.00 per person per year.

Other methods of acquiring fluorine

Fluoridation of the water supply has proved the most feasible means of providing protection against tooth decay, but for persons who either do not have access to a community water supply or who live in communities that have not introduced it, other methods of obtaining the benefits of fluorine have been tried. The most frequent method is the use of sodium fluoride tablets. A year's supply of 2 mg tablets to be taken daily that will release 1 mg of fluorine costs only 15 cents per person, but distribution costs add another $3.50 per year. A major deterrent to the success of tablets is the failure of parents to continue to provide them throughout the whole growth period or at least for the first ten years. In Hawaii, where tablets were distributed free, 90% of the parents provided them for their children at the beginning of the program, but four years later only 12% were still using them. In Switzerland the use of tablets proved more successful, with only a 20% to 35% reduction in use reported. For infants the tablets must be dissolved in the formula or fruit juice, and care must be taken to see that they do not inadvertently get an overdose. Many of the commonly used infant vitamin supplements have fluorine added, but in areas where the water supply is fluoridated, their sale is restricted to prescription distribution.

Two studies on the feasibility of adding fluorine to the water supply in the schools in communities that did not have a community fluoridation program showed that a reduction in dental caries incidence of 33% could be achieved in an eight-year period by the addition of either 3 or 5 ppm of fluorine. This higher level was used to compensate for the fact that the children had access to the water supply for only part of the day, five days a week. There was no incidence of dental fluorosis.

A proposal that fluorine can be injected into the gum area just prior to the time that the teeth erupt, when they are most receptive to the uptake of fluorine ions, has received some scientific backing.

Topical applications of 8% stannous fluoride solution to the dry surface of teeth shortly after they erupt has been relatively successful, providing about 40% protection against caries, but the professional time involved makes the yearly treatment relatively expensive and hence unavailable to many who would benefit most. Success has been enhanced by applying a plastic coating over the fluoride application to reduce the dilution with saliva and keep the fluoride in contact with the tooth surface longer. The application of a phosphate fluoride every two years has resulted in a 70% reduction in caries. Although successful, these methods have limited value because of a shortage of dentists needed to carry out the process.

In Switzerland an attempt to add fluorine to salt was unsuccessful, especially since infants who need fluorine are seldom given salt. Attempts to add fluorine to the milk supply were also of limited usefulness.

The value of fluoridated dentifrices that contain about 0.1% fluorine is still being evaluated, and at the present time the evidence seems controversial. One problem revolves around the observation that fluorine content decreases with storage. It is possible that fluorine inhibits the action of enzymes or bacteria involved in the formation of acid in the mouth. It has been shown that the plaques that form on teeth, on which it is believed that bacteria act to produce the acid which initiates the solution of enamel and tooth decay, contain almost twice as much fluorine where there is a 2 ppm in the water supply compared to a fluorine-free area. Apparently the enamel surface is capable of taking in some fluorine ions from the fluids to which it is exposed in the mouth.

With concern over the waste that occurs when only 1% of the fluoridated water is used for human consumption, the possibility of adding fluorine to a staple food item such as salt, flour, bread, milk, or sugar has been investigated. Of these, flour and salt seem to be utilized most effectively, although some limitations in their usefulness have been indicated.

Since the addition of fluoride to the diet of pregnant women does little to protect the primary teeth of the infant against caries, the use of supplements during pregnancy is not recommended. However, since it is critical that fluoride be available for the formation of caries-resistant primary teeth, and since milk is low in fluoride, it is recommended that infants receive a supplement of 0.25 to 0.50 mg/day during the first year of life. If the formula is made with fluoridated water, no supplement is necessary.

The affinity of bone for fluorine has given rise to concern over possible skeletal toxicity from the deposition of excess fluorine in the skeleton after ingestion of water with a high-fluorine content. The homeostatic mechanism that maintains blood levels at a constant value undoubtedly prevents this situation. Efforts to identify such an effect have shown that a lifelong ingestion of water containing 4 ppm of fluorine has no detrimental effects on bone formation. With continued exposure to high fluorine intakes, the bone ceases to take up more fluorine. Some evidence exists that fluorine delays the excretion of calcium, a factor that is advantageous in maintaining calcium balances. In fact, a dose of 50 mg of fluorine daily has proved effective in improving calcium balance, increasing bone formation, and preventing osteoporosis without any toxic effects.

Mode of action

The mechanisms by which fluorine imparts greater resistance to tooth decay have been studied extensively. It appears that where fluorine is available, some crystals of fluoroapatite replace the crystals of hydroxyapatite normally deposited during tooth formation. The presence of fluorine increases not only the size but the perfection of the tooth crystals. Fluoroapatite in tooth enamel is apparently less soluble in acid and more resistant to the cariogenic action of acids in the oral environment. Fluorine content of the outer layer of the enamel, up to 10,000 ppm, is much higher than the 50 to 200 ppm found in the inner layers where caries activity is less likely to be initiated. The levels in both parts are considerably lower when fluoridated water is not available.

Fluorine is known to stimulate the action of some enzymes and to inhibit that of others. There is considerable evidence that fluorine may exert a protective effect on teeth by inhibiting the formation of acid by bacterial enzymes in the plaque on the teeth of persons receiving fluoridated water. This plaque contains up to 250 times the concentration of fluoride in the saliva. Even small differences in the pH of plaque will influence the extent to which the enamel may be dissolved.

The enamel surface is still capable of taking up fluorine shortly after eruption, during the final stages of tooth calcification. Fluorine available in the saliva is presumably preferentially absorbed on the tooth surface, adding strength and rigidity. In addition, some evidence exists that fluorine promotes the precipitation of calcium phosphate from saliva, which may facilitate the remineralization of teeth after decalcification in the oral environment during the initial stages of tooth decay.

Larger, more nearly perfect crystals in bone have been observed as fluorine concentration of human bone increases. As much as 5000 to 6000 ppm in bone does not constitute a physiological hazard.

In addition to its effect on tooth structure, fluorine has been shown to protect against the effects of a magnesium deficiency.

Osteoporosis and bone disorders

Considerable evidence exists that ingestion of fluorine at the relatively high level of 4 ppm during adult life gives protection against osteoporosis in later life.

Fluorine also protects against the breakdown of the bone in the jaw area often associated with loss of teeth and other forms of peridontal disease. This effect is undoubtedly due to the inhibition of bone resorption by reducing the solubility of the mineral in the bone.

The possible beneficial roles of fluorine in increasing the rate of wound healing and enhancing iron absorption when iron intake is marginal need further investigation.

Toxicity

Although there has been some concern over the possibility of fluorine toxicity associated with fluoridation of the water supply, there is little evidence that this is a practical problem since the kidneys appear capable of excreting any excess. Under experimental conditions it has been observed that high levels of fluorine are associated with a mottling of bone, higher calcium retention, and interference of collagen formation. These effects are more common in conjunction with low calcium, low protein, and low ascorbic acid intakes. There is no evidence that a high fluorine intake is involved in hypercalcification, although it has been suggested that the kidneys, which are involved in the excretion of excess fluorine, may be in special jeopardy. Acute toxicity, which requires an intake of 2 to 10 g, is rare. Chronic toxicity, although more common, occurs infrequently, usually as the result of prolonged ingestion of water with high natural fluorine content that provides 20 to 80 mg/day or from industrial contamination. Any danger from the consumption of artificially fluoridated water can be discounted, and the continued use of this water and processed foods with higher fluorine contents should have beneficial rather than detrimental effects.

BIBLIOGRAPHY

Iron

Beaton, G. H., Thein, M., Milne, H., and Veen, M. J.: Iron requirements of menstruating women, Am. J. Clin. Nutr. **23:**275, 1970.

Charley, P. J., Still, C., Shore, E., and Soltman, P.: Studies in the regulation of intestinal iron absorption, J. Lab. Clin. Med. **61:**397, 1963.

Cook, J. D., Minnich, V., Moore, C. V., Rasmussen, A., Bradley, W. B., and Finch, C. A.: Absorption of fortification iron in bread, Am. J. Clin. Nutr. **26:**861, 1973.

Cook, J. D., and Monsen, E. R.: Food iron absorption in man. II. The effect of EDTA on absorption of dietary nonheme iron, Am. J. Clin. Nutr. **29:**614, 1976.

Cook, J. D., and Monsen, E. R.: Food iron absorption in human subjects. III. Comparison of the effect of animal proteins on nonheme iron absorption, Am. J. Clin. Nutr. **29:**859, 1976.

Council on Foods and Nutrition: Iron deficiency in the United States, J.A.M.A. **203:**407, 1968.

Council on Foods and Nutrition: Iron in enriched wheat flour, farina, bread, buns, and rolls, J.A.M.A. **220:**855, 1972.

Crosby, W. H.: Fortification of food with carbonyl iron, editorial, Am. J. Clin. Nutr. **31:**572, 1978.

Crosby, W. H.: Current concepts in nutrition: Who needs iron? N. Engl. J. Med. **297:**543, 1977.

Czaika-Nardins, O. M., Haddy, T. B., and Kallen, D. J.: Nutrition and social correlates in iron-deficiency anemia, Am. J. Clin. Nutr. **31:**955, 1978.

Elwood, P. C.: Evaluation of the clinical importance of anemia, Am. J. Clin. Nutr. **26:**958, 1973.

Finch, C. A.: The role of iron in hemoglobin synthesis, Conference on Hemoglobin, Publication No. 557, Washington, D.C., 1957, National Academy of Sciences.

Finch, C. A.: Iron-deficiency anemia, Am. J. Clin. Nutr. **22:**512, 1969.

Forth, W., and Rummel, W.: Iron absorption, Physiol. Rev. **53:**724, 1973.

Frieden, E.: The ferrous to ferric cycles in iron metabolism, Nutr. Rev. **31:**41, 1973.

Gardner, G. R., Edgerton, V. R., Senewiratne, B., Barnard, R. J., and Ohira, Y.: Physical work capacity and metabolic stress in subjects with iron-deficiency anemia, Am. J. Clin. Nutr. **30:**910, 1977.

Haddy, T. B., Jurkowski, C., Brody, H., Kallen, D. J., and Czajka-Narins, D. M.: Iron deficiency with and without anemia in infants and children, Am. J. Dis. Child. **128:**787, 1974.

Hegenauer, J., Saltman, P., and Winberg, E. D.: Iron and susceptibility to infectious disease, Science **188:**1038, 1975.

International Nutritional Anemia Consultative Group: Guidelines for the eradication of iron-deficiency anemia, Washington, D.C., 1977, The Nutrition Foundation.

Jacobs, A., and Greenman, D. A.: Availability of food iron, Br. Med. J. **1:**673, 1969.

Kasper, C. K., Whissel, V. E., and Wallerstein, R. O.: Clinical aspects of iron deficiency, J.A.M.A. **191:**359, 1965.

Leibel, R. L.: Behavioral and biochemical correlates of iron deficiency. A review, J. Am. Diet. Assoc. **71:**398, 1977.

Linman, J. W.: Physiologic and pathophysiologic effects of anemia, N. Engl. J. Med. **279:**812, 1968.

Man, Y. K., and Wadsworth, G. R.: Dietary intake and urinary loss of iron, Proc. Nutr. Soc. **27:**12A, 1968.

Mirahmodu, K. S.: Serum ferritin level, J.A.M.A. **238:**601, 1977.

Monsen, E. R., and Cook, J. D.: Food iron absorption in human subjects. IV. The effects of calcium and phosphate salts on the absorption of nonheme iron, Am. J. Clin. Nutr. **29:**1142, 1976.

Perutz, M. F.: Hemoglobin structure and respiratory transport, Sci. Am. **239**(6):92, 1978.

Pollitt, E., and Leibel, R. L.: Iron deficiency and behavior, J. Pediatr. **88:**372, 1976.

Strauss, R. G.: Iron-deficiency infections and immune functions; a reassessment, Am. J. Clin. Nutr. **31:**660, 1978.

Swiss, L. D., and Beaton, G. H.: A prediction of the effects of iron fortification, Am. J. Clin. Nutr. **27:**373, 1974.

Vaghefi, S. B., Ghassemi, H., and Kaighobadi, K.: Availability of iron in an enrichment mixture added to bread, J. Am. Diet. Assoc. **64:**275, 1974.

Waddell, J., Sassoon, H. F., Fisher, K. D., and Carr J. C.: A review of the significance of dietary iron on iron storage phenomena, Washington, D.C. 1972, Food and Drug Administration.

White, W. H.: Iron deficiency in young women, Am. J. Public Health **60:**659, 1970.

Iodine

Cullen, R. W., and Oace, S. M.: Iodine: current status, J. Nutr. Ed. **8:**101, 1976.

Dunn, J. T.: Thyroglobulin and other factors in the utilization of iodine by the thyroid. In Endemic goiter and cretinism: continuing threats to world health, Washington, D.C., 1974, Pan-American Health Organization, WHO.

Gillie, R. B.: Endemic goiter, Sci. Am. **224:**92, 1971.

Kelp diets can produce myxedema in iodide sensitive individuals, Med. News **233:**9, 1975.

Kevany, J. and Chopra, J. G.: The use of iodized oil in goiter prevention, Am. J. Public Health **60:**919, 1970.

Koutras, D. A.: Iodine metabolism in endemic goitre, Ann. Clin. Res. **4:**55, 1972.

Matovinovic, J., Child, M. A., Nichaman, M. Z., and Trowbridge, F. L.: Iodine and Endemic Goiter: In Endemic goiter and cretinism: continuing threats to world health, Washington, D.C., 1974, Pan-American Health Organization, WHO.

Oddie, T. H., Fisher, D. A., McConahey, W. M., and Thompson, C. S.: Iodine intake in the United States: a reassessment, J. Clin. Endocrinol. Metab. **30:**659, 1970.

Thilly, C. H., Delange, F., and Ermans, A. M.: Further investigations of iodine deficiency in the etiology of endemic goiter, Am. J. Clin. Nutr. **25:**30, 1972.

Trowbridge, F. L., Hand, K. A., and Nichaman, M. Z.: Findings related to goiter and iodine in the Ten-State Nutrition Survey, Am. J. Clin. Nutr. **28:**712, 1975.

Vought, R. L., and London, W. T.: Dietary sources of iodine, Am. J. Clin. Nutr. **14:**186, 1964.

Vought, R. L., and London, W. T.: Iodine intake and excretion in healthy nonhospitalized subjects, Am. J. Nutr. **15:**124, 1964.

Zinc

Burch, R. E., and Sullivan, J. F.: Clinical and nutritional aspects of zinc deficiency and excess, Med. Clin. North Am. **60:**675, 1976.

Catalanotto, F. A.: The trace metal zinc and taste, Am. J. Clin. Nutr. **31:**1098, 1978.

Evans, G. W., and Johnson, P. E.: Determination of zinc availability in foods by the extrinsic label technique, Am. J. Clin. Nutr. **30:**873, 1977.

Halsted, J., Smith, J. C., and Irvin, M. I.: A conspectus of research on zinc requirements of man, J. Nutr. **104:**345, 1974.

Keen, C. L., and Hurley, L. S.: Zinc absorption through skin: correction of zinc deficiency in the rat, Am. J. Clin. Nutr. **30:**528, 1977.

Michaelson, G., Juhlen, L., and Valquist, A.: Effects of oral zinc and vitamin A in acne, Arch Dermatol. **113:**31, 1977.

Osis, D., Kramer, L., Wiatrowski, E., and Spencer, H.: Dietary zinc intake in man, Am. J. Clin. Nutr. **25:**582, 1972.

Prasad, A. S.: A century of research on the metabolic role of zinc, Am. J. Clin. Nutr. **22:**1215, 1969.

Prasad, A. S.: Importance of zinc in human nutrition, Am. J. Clin. Nutr. **20:**648, 1967.

Prasad, A. S., and Oberleas, D.: Zinc: human nutrition and metabolic effects, Ann. Intern. Med. **73:**631, 1970.

Prasad, A. S.: Zinc deficiency in man, Am. J. Dis. Child **130**:359, 1976.

Sandstead, H. H.: Zinc as an unrecognized limiting nutrient, Am. J. Clin. Nutr. **26**:790, 1973.

Sandstead, H. H.: Zinc nutrition in the United States, Am. J. Clin. Nutr. **26**:1251, 1973.

Vallee, B. L.: The metabolic role of zinc, J.A.M.A. **162**:1053, 1956.

Westmoreland, N.: Connective tissue alterations in zinc deficiency, Fed. Proc. **30**:1001, 1971.

Copper

Al-Rashid, R. A., and Splangler, J.: Medical intelligence: neonatal copper deficiency, N. Engl. J. Med. **285**:841, 1971.

Burch, R. E., Hahn, H. K. J., and Sullivan, J.: Newer aspects of the roles of zinc, manganese and copper in human nutrition, Clin. Chem. **21**:501, 1975.

Carnes, W. H.: Role of copper in connective tissue metabolism, Fed. Proc. **30**:995, 1971.

Cartwright, G. E., and Wintrobe, M. M.: Copper metabolism in normal subjects, Am. J. Clin. Nutr. **14**:224, 1964.

Dowdy, R. P.: Copper metabolism, Am. J. Clin. Nutr. **21**:887, 1969.

Evans, G. W.: Copper homeostasis in the mammalian system, Physiol. Rev. **53**:535, 1973.

Klevay, L. M.: The ratio of zinc to copper in the United States, Nutr. Rep. Int. **11**:237, 1975.

Pennington, J. T., and D. H. Calloway: Copper content of foods, J. Am. Diet. Assoc. **63**:143, 1973.

Sandstead, H. H.: Some trace elements which are essential for human nutrition: zinc, copper, manganese, and chromium, Prog. Food Nutr. Sci. **1**:371, 1975.

Seelig, M. S.: Proposed role of copper-molybdenum interaction in iron-deficiency and iron-storage diseases, Am. J. Clin. Nutr. **26**:657, 1973.

Seelig, M. S.: Review: Relationships of copper and molybdenum to iron metabolism, Am. J. Clin. Nutr. **25**:1022, 1972.

Sturgeon, P., and Brubaker, C.: Copper deficiency in infants, Am. J. Dis. Child. **92**:254, 1956.

Molybdenum

Schroeder, H. A., Balassa, J. J. and Tipton, I. H.: Essential trace metals in man: molybdenum, J. Chronic Dis. **23**:481, 1970.

Selenium

Food and Nutrition Board; Selenium and human health, Nutr. Rev. **34**:347, 1976.

Hadjimarkos, D. M., and Bonhorst, C. W.: The selenium content of eggs, milk and water in relation to dental caries in children, J. Pediatr. **59**:256, 1961.

Hadjimarkos, D. M., and Shearer, T. R.: Selenium in mature human milk, Am. J. Clin. Nutr. **26**:538, 1973.

Levander, O. A.: Selenium and chromium in human nutrition. A review, J. Am. Diet. Assoc. **66**:338, 1975.

Schroeder, H. A., Frost, D. V., and Balassa, J. J.: Essential trace metals in man: selenium, J. Chronic Dis. **23**:227, 1970.

Scott, M. L.: The selenium dilemma, J. Nutr. **103**:803, 1973.

Stadtman, T. C.: Biological function of selenium, Nutr. Rev. **35**:161, 1977.

Thompson, J. N., Erdod, P. and Smith, D. C.: Selenium content of food consumed by Canadians, J. Nutr. **105**:274, 1975.

Chromium

Hambridge, K. M.: Chromium nutrition in man, Am. J. Clin. Nutr. **27**:505, 1974.

Masironi, R., Wolf, W., and Mertz, W.: Chromium in refined and unrefined sugars—possible nutritional implications in the etiology of cardiovascular diseases, Bull. WHO **49**:322, 1973.

Mertz, W., Toepfer, E. W., Roginski, E. E., and Polansky, M. M.: Present knowledge of the role of chromium, Fed. Proc. **33**:2275, 1974.

Mertz, R.: Chromium occurrence and function in biological systems, Physiol. Rev. **49**:163, 1969.

Schroeder, H. A.: The role of chromium in mammalian nutrition, Am. J. Clin. Nutr. **21**:230, 1968.

Schroeder, H. A., Nason, A. P., and Tipton, I. H.: Chromium deficiency as a factor in atherosclerosis, J. Chronic. Dis. **23**:123, 1970.

Cobalt

Schroeder, H. A., Nason, A. P., and Tipton, I. H.: Essential trace metals in man: cobalt, J. Chronic. Dis. **20**:869, 1967.

Underwood, E. J.: Cobalt, Nutr. Rev. **33**:65, 1977.

Vanadium

Hopkins, L. L., and Mohr, M. E.: Vanadium as an essential nutrient, Fed. Proc. **33**:1773, 1974.

Silicon

Carlisle, E. M.: Silicon as an essential element, Fed. Proc. **33**:1958, 1974.

Nielsen, F. H., and Sandstead, H. H.: Are nickel, vanadium, silicon, fluorine, and tin essential for man? A review, Am. J. Clin. Nutr. **27**:515, 1974.

Schwarz, K.: Silicon, fibre and atherosclerosis, Lancet **1**:454, 1977.

Fluorine

American Academy of Pediatrics: Fluoride as a nutrient, Pediatrics **49**:456, 1972.

Ast, D. B., Cons, N. C., Carlos, J. P., and Polans, A.: Time and cost factors to provide regular, periodic dental care for children in a fluoridated and nonfluoridated area, Am. J. Public Health **57**:1635, 1969.

Blomquist, C. H., Singer, L., Pollock, M. E., McLaren, L. C., and Armstrong, W. D.: Sodium fluoride and cell growth, Br. Med. J. **1**:486, 1965.

Bonner, F.: Fluoridation—issue or obsession? Am. J. Clin. Nutr. **22**:1346, 1969.

Conchie, J. M.: Fluorides in dental practice: a review, J. Can. Dent. Assoc. **35:**255, 1969.

Duckworth, R.: Fluoridation, Proc. Nutr. Soc. **22:**79, 1963.

Dunning, J. M.: Current status of fluoridation, N. Engl. J. Med. **272:**30, 84, 1965.

Evans, C. A., and Pickles, T.: Statewide antifluoridation initiatives: a new challenge to health workers, Am. J. Public Health **68:**59, 1978.

Korns, R. F.: Relationship of water fluoridation to bone density in two New York towns, Public Health Rep. **84:**815, 1969.

Latham, M., and Grech, P.: The effect of excessive fluoride intake, Am. J. Public Health **57:**651, 1967.

Murray, J.: Fluoridation studies and dental caries, Br. Dent. J. **129:**467, 1970.

Sapolsky, H. M.: Social science views of a controversy in science and politics, Am. J. Clin. Nutr. **22:**1397, 1969.

Schlesinger, E. R.: Dietary fluorides and caries prevention, Am. J. Public Health **55:**1123, 1965.

Smith, E. H.: Fluoridation of water supply, J.A.M.A. **230:**1569, 1974.

Sognnaes, R. F.: Fluoride protection of bones and teeth, Science **150:**989, 1965.

Wolinsky, I., and Guggenheim, K. Y.: The effect of fluoride on the mechanical strength of bone, Baroda J. Nutr. **3:**177, 1976.

9

Water

Water is the most important of all nutrients but the one most often taken for granted. The adverse effects from loss of body water that occur in some weight-reduction diets and when athletes rely on water loss to change their weight rapidly have focussed attention on the importance of water in body functioning.

If it is possible to say that one essential nutrient is more essential than another, it would have to be conceded that it is water. And yet it is the nutrient most often taken for granted to the point that it is sometimes even omitted from a list of essential nutrients. Humans can live for weeks and even years without an intake of some essential vitamins and minerals but will survive only a few days in the absence of water. Because of this need, the body possesses rather involved mechanisms for conserving water when the supply is short. The longest time a human has survived without water is seventeen days, but two or three days is the usual limit.

With 6% of the water in the adult body and 15% of that in the infant's body turned over each day, the exchange of water far exceeds that of any other nutrient. Although up to 3.6 kg (8 pounds), or 3.8 liters (4 quarts), of water may be taken in and another 3.8 liters may be lost each day from the body, homeostatic mechanisms are so sensitive that the variation in body weight seldom exceeds 150 g a day due to change in body fluids.

DISTRIBUTION

Water constitutes 60% of the total body weight in adults and 70% of the lean body mass, or fat-free tissue. The proportion in the body will, however, vary from 50% to 75%, decreasing with age and the amount of body fat. It is over 75% at birth and declines to 50% by age 60. Water is a constituent of every cell of the body. As shown in Fig. 9-1, it is present in widely varying concentrations in different tissues, constituting 72% of muscle, 20% to 35% of adipose tissue, and 10% of tooth and 25% of bone and cartilage.

The distribution of fluids in the body is described in terms of an *intracellular compartment* representing the water within the cells, which accounts for two thirds of the total body water, and an *extracellular compartment* (all fluid outside the cells), comprising the other third. The compartments were shown in Fig. 6-2. The intracellular fluid is enclosed inside the cell membrane of each individual cell. The extracellular component is usually further subdivided into two compartments: the intravascular and the intercellular. The intravascular fluid, amounting to about 3 liters, includes the water in the blood vessels, arteries, veins, and capillaries and accounts for 4.5% of body weight and 7.5% of total body water. The intercellular (extravascular, or interstitial) fluid (about 12 liters) includes that which has left the blood vessels and is present in the spaces between and surrounding each cell. Exchange of fluids between the cell and the fluid surrounding it and between the latter and the intravascular compartment (all of which are separated by a semipermeable membrane),

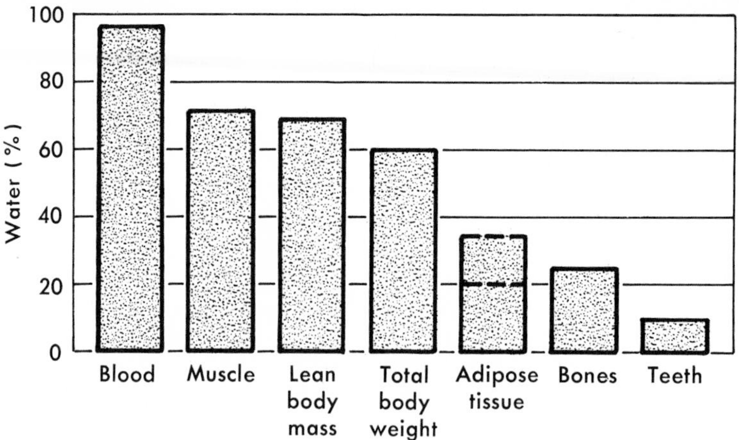

Fig. 9-1. Water content of representative body tissues.

occurs freely and is regulated by many factors, including the relative concentrations of protein and electrolytes such as sodium and potassium. The direction and the rate of exchange are determined by (1) osmotic pressure due to the presence of electrolytes (number of ionizable particles), (2) oncotic pressure due to the presence of other substances such as protein, and (3) hydrostatic pressure due to the force exerted by the pumping action of the heart on the fluid in the blood vessels. As much as 48 liters of fluid cross the membranes each day.

There are two other fluid compartments that do not participate as extensively in the dynamic exchange of fluid. *Transcellular water* is present in such fluids as the spinal fluid, the ocular fluid in the eyeballs, the synovial fluid that lubricates joints, and the fluids in the mucous secretions of the linings of the respiratory tract, the gastrointestinal tract, and the genitourinary tract. It comprises 2.5% of total body water. The water in dense connective tissue, cartilage, and bone is part of its structural material and accounts for 15% of total body water.

FUNCTIONS

Solvent. From 3 to 5 liters of fluid are present in the arteries, veins, and capillaries where the fluid acts as a solvent for the nutrients—monosaccharides, amino acids, fats (as phospholipids), vitamins, and minerals—and for the hormones secreted by the glands. All of these must be transported to all parts of the body if the individual cells are to be adequately nourished and function properly. This intravascular fluid also acts as a solvent and transporter of the waste products of metabolism, such as carbon dioxide, ammonia, and electrolytes, which must be carried from the cells to the lungs, skin, or kidneys to be excreted.

The 12 liters of fluid in the extravascular, or interstitial (between cells), compartment carry nutrients that have left the blood vessels into close proximity to the membrane of the cell. It also collects waste products and hormones or other substances that may be secreted by the cell. Much of this fluid reenters the circulatory system, being pulled back when the oncotic pressure built up by the blood proteins that do not leave the bloodstream exceeds the hydrostatic pressure that forced the fluid out of the intravascular compartment. Any remaining intercellular fluid in excess of normal amounts is accumulated by the lymphatic system and is eventually returned to the bloodstream. The amount of water in the extravascular, or intercellular, compartment fluctuates more than that in other compartments, since it can tolerate greater variations than other compartments. The blood volume is usually maintained at a fairly constant level at the expense of the intercellular fluid. Similarly, the intracellular fluid, which must also be maintained at a constant level to prevent the swelling or shrinking of cells, draws on the intercellular fluid. The intercellular fluid may thus be thought of as a buffer zone.

Within the cell water acts as a solvent for nutrients that must be transported from one organelle to another within the cell as well as for the waste products that must be eliminated.

Body builder. Within the cell intracellular water is used as a body builder, being incorporated in the synthesis of a new material. Glycogen, the form in which carbohydrate is stored, is about two-thirds water. The deposition of fat involves the accumulation of an additional 20% water and muscle 75%.

Catalyst. Water also acts as a catalyst in many biological reactions within the cell and in the stomach and small intestine, where digestion of food occurs. The water is necessary for the reactions required to break the complex nutrients into their simpler component parts, since most of these reactions are hydrolytic (water requiring).

Lubricant. In the synovial fluid of the joints the prime function of water is to act as a lubricant.

Temperature regulator. Another important role of water is in the regulation of body temperature. Although some heat is lost by radiation and conduction from the skin, especially at low environmental temperatures, the evaporation of water from the surface of the body is the most effective method of ridding the body of extra heat produced in the metabolism of carbohydrate, fat, and protein. Some of this heat is required to maintain body temperature at 37° C (98.6° F), the temperature at which all enzymes crucial to metabolic processes operate most effectively. Because of its ability to conduct heat, water assists in the even distribution of heat throughout the body. But the metabolism of nutrients to provide energy for chemical, muscular, and osmotic work in the body yields as a by-product more heat than is necessary to maintain normal body temperature. If this is not released promptly, the body temperature increases to a point at which all cellular enzymes will be inactivated. The evaporation of 1 kg of fluid from the skin requires 600 kcal of energy in the form of heat, and the body is constantly cooling itself by causing water to be lost through evaporation. The loss of heat through the skin represents about 25% of the total caloric expenditure. This water loss, which amounts to 350 to 700 ml/day under normal conditions of temperature and humidity, is referred to as "insensible perspiration loss." The greater the body surface area, the greater the amount of heat that can be lost through the skin. A layer of subcutaneous fat that acts as an insulating material, reducing the speed with which heat is lost from the body, is an advantage in the winter and a disadvantage in the summer. Heat loss may also be affected by the proximity of the circulating fluids to the surface of the skin.

Work performance. Studies to determine limiting factors in the work output of an individual suggested that a lack of water had a much more profound effect on work production than a lack of food. A reduction of 4% to 5% in body water will result in a decline of 20% to 30% in work performance. This is of special significance to wrestlers who too often lose weight by stimulating water loss to compete in a lower weight class. In addition, if water loss exceeds 10% of body weight, there is a possibility of circulatory failure.

In addition to these well-established roles of water in the body, it is becoming increasingly evident that the amount of water in the diet exerts a definite influence on the metabolism of other nutrients. When 20% water was added to diets containing 6%, 9%, or 12% protein, a significant gain occurred in the protein efficiency ratio (PER), the weight gain per gram of protein.

WATER BALANCE

Sources of body water. In contrast to all other nutrients, which can be provided by food alone, water is available to the body from several sources.

The major source is the fluids consumed as beverages. The amount of fluids will vary from one individual to another. Infants consume more per unit of body weight than do adults. Persons living in the tropics, where there is greater evaporation from the skin, consume more than those in temperate climates, and persons engaged in strenuous physical activity consume more than sedentary individuals. The amount consumed by adults as fluids varies from 900 to 1500 ml, with an average intake of 1100 ml under normal circumstances. However, intakes in excess of 800 ml/hr exceed the rate at which water can be absorbed from the stomach.

Depending on its origin, water may be a significant source of trace elements such as fluorine, zinc, and copper. Macroelements such as calcium and magnesium may be present in hard water but are removed in the ion exchange processes used to soften the water supply. Two liters of hard water may provide as much as 240 mg of magnesium. Since water is such a good solvent and as such may also be the source of toxic materials, constant monitoring of the water supply is essential to safeguard the health of the public.

So-called solid foods, the second most important source of water, vary from 0% to 96% water. The water content of some representative foods is given in Table 9-1, from which it is evident that many "solid" foods contain over 70% water. A 2000 kcal diet chosen according to a typical food plan provides from 500 to 800 ml of water.

Table 9-1. Water content of representative foods*

Food	Water (%)
Lettuce	96
Asparagus	92
Milk	87
Oranges	86
Potatoes	80
Cottage cheese	79
Veal	66
Chicken	63
Beef	47
Cheddar cheese	37
Bread	36
Butter	15
Gelatin	13
White sugar	0.5

*From Watt, B. K., and Merrill, A. L.: Composition of foods—raw, processed and prepared, Handbook No. 8, Washington, D.C., 1963, U.S. Department of Agriculture.

The end products of combustion of carbohydrate, fat, and protein include water, referred to as water of metabolism, in addition to carbon dioxide and energy. A constant amount of water is released during the oxidation or burning of each of these—1 g of carbohydrate yielding 0.6 g of water; 1 g of protein, 0.42 g; and 1 g of fat, 1.07 g. This amounts to 15, 10.5, and 11.1 g, respectively, from the metabolism of 100 kcal from carbohydrate, protein, and fat. Thus, for an individual utilizing 2000 kcal a day, 50% of which came from carbohydrate, 35% from fat, and 15% from protein, the water of metabolism would amount to 264 ml/day, as shown in the calculation in Table 9-2. This amounts to 13.2 g/100 kcal.

When either muscle or liver glycogen is mobilized to be used for energy, the additional water stored with it is also released. Thus an athlete who relies on this energy source during intense physical activity may produce as much as an additional liter of water as a result of metabolizing 500 g of glycogen.

Loss of body water. To counterbalance the intake of water and maintain fluid equilibrium, water is lost in several ways—urinary losses, respiratory losses through the lungs, and evaporation losses through the skin.

Losses in urine. Once is has been absorbed, water is taken up by the bloodstream, which is 80% water; it is carried to the kidneys, where it serves as a solvent for

Table 9-2. Calculation of water of metabolism produced on a 2000 kcal diet

Source of kcal	Percent of kcal provided	Distribution of kcal in 2000 kcal diet	Weight of nutrient (g)	Water of metabolism (ml/g)	Total water of metabolism (ml)
Carbohydrate	50	1000	250	0.6	150
Fat	35	700	77	1.07	82
Protein	15	300	75	0.42	32
					264

waste products from the body; and finally it is excreted as urine, which is 97% water. The fluid is filtered through the kidney tubule at the rate of 125 ml/min, which amounts to 120 to 190 L/day. Here sufficient water is resorbed to retain normal blood volumes, and the rest, 1 ml/min, is excreted. If the fluid intake is high, urine volume is increased above the normal level of 1 to 2 liters, and the concentration of excretory products in the urine will be low. Such urine has a low specific gravity. When fluid intake is low, more must be resorbed to maintain blood volume, and a much smaller amount will be used in the urine as a solvent for the excretory products. Since there is a limit to the extent that the kidneys can concentrate urine, there is a minimum urine volume necessary to rid the body of waste products. This minimum has been estimated at between 300 and 500 ml but depends on the solute load, primarily electrolytes and urea, to be excreted. If less than this amount of fluid is available for urine formation, waste products of metabolism will be retained in the tissue, where they may accumulate to toxic levels.

Under circumstances such as disasters and manned space flights when the fluid available is extremely limited and must be conserved, the mandatory excretion through the kidneys can be reduced by limiting the intake of foods that normally give rise to metabolites, which must be excreted in the urine. Restricting protein and salt intake are the easiest, most effective methods of reducing the necessary urine volume. The provision of sufficient carbohydrate (100 g) to prevent ketosis will help reduce the solute load of ketones and electrolytes. Young infants with poorly developed kidney function can excrete very small amounts of electrolytes. For this reason they should not be given excessive salt, a high-protein intake, or too concentrated a formula, all of which increase the work of the kidneys.

During starvation or when a carbohydrate-free diet is ingested an excessive loss of body water, potassium, and sodium occurs through the urine. This accounts for the rapid initial weight loss and weakness often reported by persons on such reducing diets. In extreme cases the loss of potassium may result in heart failure. A small amount of carbohydrate prevents this undesirable change in body fluid volume and electrolytes by preventing the accumulation of ketones.

Through skin. Loss of water through the skin amounts to 350 to 700 ml each day. It has been reported as high as 2500 ml/hr, and 500 ml/hr is not uncommon at high environmental temperature and low humidity. Infants experience a high rate of evaporation from the skin, which compensates for small urinary losses.

Through lungs. Water along with carbon dioxide is constantly being lost through the lungs. The amount released this way is 300 ml

Table 9-3. Water exchange in gastrointestinal tract

Source	ml	
Gastric secretions		8200
Saliva	1500	
Gastric juice	2500	
Bile	500	
Pancreatic juices	700	
Intestinal juices	3000	
Water intake		2000
Total intake		10,200
Reabsorbed	10,000	
Fecal loss		200

Table 9-4. Typical water balance in adult

Sources and loss	ml
Sources of water	
Liquid food	1100
Solid food	500-1000
Water of oxidation	300-400
TOTAL	1900-2500
Loss of water	
Urine	900-1400
Insensible perspiration	500
Perspiration and evaporation from lungs	300-500
Feces	200
TOTAL	1900-2500

but will increase at high altitudes because of increased respiration rates. Where the atmosphere is unusually dry, the total lost through the lungs and skin equals urinary losses.

Through digestive juices. During a 24-hour period as much as 8 to 10 liters of water (with 3700 ml considered a minimum) may be secreted into the digestive tract as digestive juices (Table 9-3). These secretions include saliva, gastric juices, intestinal and pancreatic juices, bile, and secretion of lymph glands. Practically all of this is reabsorbed as it passes down the gastrointestinal tract so that as little as 200 ml will be excreted in the feces.

Diarrhea will markedly increase the water content of the feces. Under these conditions dehydration is a severe problem if the fluid and sodium are not replaced quickly.

The volume of digestive juices secreted is determined to a certain extent by the moisture content of the food. When food is dry, the secretion of saliva is increased, exerting a maximum lubricating effect on the food to facilitate swallowing and the action of digestive enzymes. Secretion of bile is stimulated by ingestion of large amounts of fat, and the volume of the gastric, pancreatic, and intestinal juices may fluctuate in response to the variation in moisture content of the food.

In summary, it becomes obvious that to compensate for water losses in the urine and feces and through the skin and lungs, fluid intake must be at least 2 liters from food and beverages. Even under the most favorable conditions of low solute load, minimal physical activity, and absence of sweating, the total water from food, drink, and metabolic water should be at least 1.5 L/day. About 40% of the liquid comes from tap water; the rest comes from milk and other beverages. Table 9-4 summarizes water balance within the body.

REQUIREMENTS

The need for fluid in relation to body weight varies with age; the younger the person, the greater is the fluid requirement per unit of body weight. Fluid requirements under various conditions of age and environmental temperatures are shown in Table 9-5.

As a guide it is suggested that adults consume 1000 ml of water for every 1000 kcal in the diet and infants, 1500 ml. Usually about two thirds of this comes from beverages and the remainder from solid food. Since this is considerably less than the 4700 to 17,000 ml of water that may be turned over in the body each day, the body must have extensive mechanisms for conserving water.

Table 9-5. Fluid requirement per kilogram of body weight

Classifications	ml/kg
Infants	110
10-year-old children	40
Adults	
22.2° C (72°) F	22
37.8° C (100°) F	38

Regulation of fluid balance. Fluid balance within the body is achieved in two ways—regulation of fluid intake through changes in thirst sensations and regulation of fluid loss through the kidneys.

When excessive fluid is lost, the concentration of electrolytes, particularly sodium, in the extracellular fluid increases. This increase will cause water to be absorbed from the saliva, leaving a dry sensation in the mouth that stimulates fluid intake. In addition, the hypothalamus in the brain responds to the higher sodium content of the blood in two ways. It stimulates the thirst sensation and signals the release of the antidiuretic hormone (ADH) from the pituitary gland, which influences the kidneys to resorb more water, restoring blood volume to a normal level. As water is resorbed, the concentration of the urine will rise. Conversely, when the level of sodium in the fluid being filtered through the kidneys is too low, the kidneys release a substance that triggers another hormone, aldosterone. This hormone causes the kidneys to retain more sodium. Stimulation of thirst and secretion of ADH respond to changes in sodium concentration of as little as 1%.

Disturbances in water metabolism. Water is an essential part of cell cytoplasm, and the functioning of the cell depends on a certain concentration of nutrients in the internal environment of the cell. Any loss or accumulation of fluid in cells can lead to acute metabolic difficulties. This may result from abnormal loss, such as in diarrhea, nausea, or fever; abnormal retention; a defect in intestinal absorption; or an altered distribution of fluids within the body. When body fluids are reduced as much as 10%, symptoms of severe dehydration appear, a 20% reduction is fatal. An increase to levels 10% above normal result in edema.

Under conditions of high environmental temperature the body loses large amounts of water through perspiration. Along with the water loss an appreciable reduction in sodium occurs. The loss of water will stimulate the thirst center, leading to an increased consumption of water. If this water intake is not accompanied by a source of sodium to replace that lost in perspiration along with the water, the individual suffers from a condition known as *water intoxication,* in which the sodium concentration in the extracellular fluids becomes very diluted. Water then enters the cell (or potassium leaves the cell) to help equalize the concentration of electrolytes within and outside. Overhydration of the cell causes cramps, and a decrease in the extracellular fluid (as the fluid enters the cell) causes a drop in blood pressure and weakness. To protect against this, industries in which employees work at high temperatures frequently require that the workers take salt tablets (usually containing 1 g of sodium) when they drink water. Travellers in tropical areas who are unaccustomed to high temperatures may find it necessary to use salt tablets to avoid the weakness that accompanies a loss of sodium from the body. A similar precaution may be necessary for persons who engage in strenuous physical exercise even in a temperate climate. Severe muscle cramps may result from the loss of electrolytes during sweating.

Another form of water intoxication, in which the intake of water exceeds the maximum rate of urine flow of 16 ml/min, results in an uptake of the extra water by the cells, again causing a dilution of the cellular constituents in addition to the swelling of cells. When this occurs in brain cells, convulsions, coma, and death can result.

BIBLIOGRAPHY

Anderson, B.: Thirst and brain control of water balance, Am. Sci. **59:**408, 1971.

Brooke, C. E., and Anast, C. S.: Oral fluid and electrolytes, J.A.M.A. **179:**792, 1962.

Johnson, R. E.: Water and osmotic economy, J. Am. Diet. Assoc. **45:**124, 1964.

Robinson, J. R.: Water and life, World Rev. Nutr. Diet. **12:**172, 1970.

Robinson, J. R.: Water, the indispensible nutrient, Nutr. Today **5:**16, 1970.

Walker, J. S., Margolis, F. J., Teate, H. L., Weil, M. L., and Wilson, H. L.: Water intake of normal children, Science **140:**890, 1963.

10

Vitamins

A mere fifty years ago vitamins were of interest only to a small group of scientists who were recognizing them as substances present in food in extremely small amounts yet essential for health. They were curious about how many there were, where they were found, and how they functioned in the body. Today the vitamins are common words in most households. Scientists are concerned about the intricacies of the interrelationships among vitamins and possible adverse effects from their misuse, while food technologists are directing their efforts to assuring that vitamins in food are retained during processing.

DISCOVERY

Vitamins were the last group of dietary essentials to be recognized. This is easy to understand, since they are needed in such small amounts. Their presence in food is correspondingly low and hence was easily overlooked in the early analyses of foods. The minimum need for a vitamin varies from a low of a few micrograms to a high of 30 mg; those needed in the smallest amounts are equally as important as those needed at a hundred or a thousand times that level.

Vitamins are now defined as organic substances, needed in very small amounts, that perform a specific metabolic function and must be provided in the diet of the animal. Those substances considered vitamins for a species that cannot synthesize them may not be vitamins for another species that has the ability to synthesize its own. For instance, vitamin C must be provided in the diet of humans, monkeys, and guinea pigs but is synthesized by rats, rabbits, dogs, and other animals. Plants can manufacture vitamins from the elements available to them from the soil. In general, the more complex the animal, the more vitamins it must obtain from food.

The term *vitamine* was coined by Casimir Funk in 1912. Searching for the elusive substance in rice bran that had the power to cure the condition beriberi, he confirmed Eijkman's hypothesis that disease could be caused by lack of a dietary constituent. This substance he correctly believed to be necessary for life (vita) and, in the case of the antiberiberi factor, nitrogen containing (amine); hence the term *vitamine.* He suggested, again correctly, that it was likely vitamins existed to protect against pellagra, scurvy, and rickets. Subsequent work showed that many "vitamines" existed, but only a few were "amine" in nature, and so the final *e* was dropped, giving the familiar term *vitamin.*

Shortly after Funk postulated his vitamin hypothesis, Osborne and Mendel and McCollum and Davis, two teams working independently, reported that there was an elusive, unidentified substance in fat that was necessary for growth and reproduction in animals. This they designated fat-soluble A to differentiate it from the water-soluble B, believed to be responsible for preventing and curing beriberi.

From this simple classification of vitamins has grown a list of four completely different fat-soluble vitamins and eleven water-solu-

Table 10-1. Discovery, isolation, synthesis, and nomenclature of vitamins

	Discovery	Isolation	Synthesis	Other names*
Water-soluble vitamins				
Thiamin (B_1)	1921	1926	1936	Aneurine Antineuritic factor Antiberiberi factor
Inositol	1928	1928		Muscle sugar
Choline	1930	1962		
Ascorbic acid (C)	1932	1932	1933	Antiscorbutic factor Cevitamic acid
Riboflavin (B_2)	1932	1933	1935	Yellow enzyme Vitamin G Lactoflavin Hepatoflavin Ovoflavin
Pantothenic acid	1933	1938	1940	Pantotheine Pantothenol Antichromomotriclia factor
Biotin		1935	1942	Anti–egg-white injury factor Bios II Vitamin H
Pyridoxine (B_6)	1934	1938	1939	Pyridoxic acid Pyridoxal Pyridoxol Pyridoxamine
Niacin (B_3)	1936	1936		Nicotinic acid Nicotinamide or niacinamide Pellagra-preventive factor
Folacin	1945	1945	1945	Adermin Folic acid Citrovorum factor Pteroylglutamic acid *Lactobacillus casei* factor Vitamin M Vitamin B_c Factor U
Cobalamin (B_{12})	1948	1948	1973	Antipernicious anemia factor Cyanocobalamin Hydroxycobalamin Erythrocyte maturation factor Animal protein factor (APF)

*Terms appearing in the literature, many of which are no longer recognized as correct terminology.

Table 10-1. Discovery, isolation, synthesis, and nomenclature of vitamins—cont'd

	Discovery	Isolation	Synthesis	Other names*
Fat-soluble vitamins				
Vitamin A	1915	1937	1946	Axerophthol Retinoic acid Retinal Retinol Dehydroretinol
Vitamin D	1918	1930	1936	Antirachitic factor Cholecalciferol Ergocalciferol
Vitamin E	1922	1936	1937	Tocopherol Antisterility factor
Vitamin K	1934	1939	1939	Phytylquinone Multiprenylmenaquinone Farnoquinone Antihemorrhagic factor Menadione (synthetic) Synkayvite (synthetic) Hykinone (synthetic)

ble substances that have been grouped together as the vitamin B complex and vitamin C. As our knowledge of the chemical and physical properties and the physiological roles of vitamins has grown, and the unique features of each member of the B complex has been clarified, an effort has been made to drop such designations as vitamin B_1, B_2, B_6, which imply a common functional or biochemical relationship. Since virtually no direct relationship exists except that they are all water soluble and most operate as coenzymes in metabolic reactions, terms that more adequately designate their composition or structure, such as thiamin, riboflavin, pyridoxine, folacin, and cobalamin, are being used now. It will undoubtedly be some time before the old terminology disappears from the literature, but by pointing out the various systems of nomenclature, we hope to minimize the confusion.

Table 10-1 presents in historical sequence the discovery of vitamins. Gaps in the alphabetical and numerical designations can be explained by the fact that scientists, thinking they had discovered a new nutritional principle, would label it as a vitamin, only to discover later that either it did not have vitamin activity or was identical to another factor. Contrary to periodic reports in lay literature, no new vitamins have been elucidated in the last thirty years. Biochemists, physiologists, and nutritionists believe they can establish normal growth, reproductive capacity, and a high level of health by feeding a synthetic diet based on the now known nutritional principles in which the balance of nutrients approximates that in natural foods. However, one can never dismiss the possibility that other factors will be discovered. This is especially true as biochemical techniques and instruments become more refined and sensitive.

In spite of the fact that individual vitamins of the fat-soluble group (vitamins A, D, E, and K) and the water-soluble group (all oth-

Table 10-2. General properties of fat-soluble and water-soluble vitamins

Fat-soluble vitamins	Water-soluble vitamins
Soluble in fat and fat solvents (water-miscible derivatives available)	Soluble in water
Intake in excess of daily need stored in the body	Minimal storage of dietary excesses
Not excreted	Excreted in urine
Deficiency symptoms slow to develop	Deficiency symptoms often develop rapidly
Not absolutely necessary in diet every day	Must be supplied in diet every day
Have precursors or provitamins	Generally do not have precursors
Contain only elements carbon, hydrogen, and oxygen	Contain the elements carbon, hydrogen, oxygen, and nitrogen and in some cases others, such as cobalt or sulfur
Absorbed into lymphatic system	Absorbed into blood
Needed only by complex organisms	Needed by simple and complex organisms

ers) have unique functions, a few characteristics generally differentiate the two groups. These are summarized in Table 10-2.

RELATED SUBSTANCES

Two groups of compounds chemically related to vitamins are of nutritional importance—vitamin **precursors** (provitamins) and antagonists (antivitamins).

Provitamins, or precursors, are substances that are chemically related to the biologically active form of the vitamin but have no vitamin activity until the body converts them into the active form. The conversion of the precursor to the active form takes place in different parts of the body with varying degrees of efficiency, depending on the vitamin, the form of the precursor, and the complexity of the reactions required to convert it to the active form. For instance, carotenes are converted to vitamin A in the intestinal wall. Catalyzed by the ultraviolet rays from the sun, 7-dehydrocholesterol is converted to vitamin D in the skin and to the active form in the liver and the kidneys. Tryptophan is converted to niacin in the liver. Folic acid, or folacin, as it occurs in food, is actually the precursor of the biologically active form. In this case the conversion, which likely occurs in the cell, requires two other vitamins—ascorbic acid and niacin.

Antivitamins, vitamin antagonists, or pseudovitamins are usually but not always chemically related to the biologically active vitamin. In this case the body does not discriminate between the useful form of the vitamin and the antagonist and therefore incorporates either into essential body compounds. The active vitamin, as part of enzymes or coenzymes, allows biochemical reactions to occur normally. The antagonist not only does not function in the enzyme system but also stubbornly refuses to be replaced by the proper substance, which would allow the reaction to proceed. The situation is analogous to putting a key in a lock only to find that it does not work and cannot be removed so that the proper key can be used. Vitamin antagonists have been used to produce experimental vitamin deficiencies, especially of nutrients so widespread in nature that it is difficult to produce a diet sufficiently low in them to establish deficiency symptoms or to determine their metabolic role. Medically these are also proving useful in retarding the undesirable growth of tissues. A folacin antagonist, for instance, has shown some promise in retarding the growth of the rapidly growing leukocytes in leukemia but must be used with caution, since it also inhibits the growth of desirable cells.

FUNCTIONS

In spite of current knowledge of the chemical structure of the vitamins and observations on the effects of their absence on body biochemistry, scientists still have been unable to determine the exact biochemical role of many of the vitamins. Those whose functions have been determined serve primarily as coenzymes needed to facilitate the action of enzymes. Chemical changes that occur in the products of digestion of food after they have been absorbed, which lead either to their incorporation into body structure or release of energy, take place in individual cells. Each cell contains at least 500 enzymes that catalyze these changes. Some enzymes work alone to bring about the required changes; others require the help of **coenzymes,** most of which are vitamins attached to a protein, called an apoenzyme. The vitamin portion of the coenzyme is usually responsible for the attachment of the enzyme to the substrate. If the vitamins are not available to form the coenzymes, the sequence of chemical changes cannot proceed; the product whose change is blocked accumulates in the tissues or blood, or metabolism is diverted in another direction. In many cases the accumulated intermediary product of the biochemical changes that occur in a normal pattern is responsible for many of the symptoms associated with lack of a specific vitamin. Although the biochemical defect resulting from a vitamin deficiency is similar for all species, the clinical symptoms may vary considerably.

DEFICIENCIES

Vitamin deficiencies may arise from one or several causes. Most common is the lack of the nutrient in the diet. Individuals show wide variation in normal needs; an amount adequate for one person may be insufficient for another. For instance, some adults can function with 0.2 mg of thiamin, whereas others require as much as 0.8 mg. It is to provide for the needs of the latter that the National Research Council allows such a wide margin of safety over average needs in establishing its recommended dietary allowances.

Failure of the body to absorb the nutrient provided in food makes it unavailable to perform its function in the cells. For instance, persons whose secretion of bile is limited or absent usually absorb lower amounts of the fat-soluble vitamins than those who have an adequate amount of bile to facilitate fat absorption. A defect of gastric mucosa acid secretion precludes the absorption of cobalamin. Rapid passage of food through the gastrointestinal tract also inhibits absorption.

Increased need for a vitamin may precipitate symptoms on an intake that would normally be adequate. For instance, alcoholics experience an increased need for thiamin, persons with tuberculosis need more vitamin C, and now evidence is suggesting that an infant can be conditioned to need an abnormally high amount of pyridoxine or vitamin C if maternal tissues were saturated during fetal development.

Unusually high losses from poor methods of harvesting, storage, or preparation of the food reduce the actual content of the diet below expected levels. For this reason, care should be taken in the preparation and storage of foods to preserve the vitamin content.

SUPPLEMENTS

Knowledge of the beneficial effects of an adequate intake and the detrimental effects associated with an inadequate intake has resulted in an undue concern over the vitamin content of the diet. Many purveyors of vitamin supplements have capitalized on this concern and have created doubts on the part of the American public regarding the possi-

Table 10-3. United States recommended daily allowances (U.S. RDAs) and permissible compositional ranges for dietary supplements of vitamins and minerals*

	Unit of measurement	Children under 4 years of age†			Adults and children 4 or more years of age			Pregnant or lactating women		
		Lower limit	U.S. RDA	Upper limit	Lower limit	U.S. RDA	Upper limit	Lower limit	U.S. RDA	Upper limit
Vitamins										
Mandatory										
Vitamin A	IU	1250	2500	2500	2500	5000	5000	5000	8000	8000
Vitamin D‡	IU	200	400	400				400	400	400
Vitamin E	IU	5	10	15	15	30	45	30	30	60
Vitamin C	mg	20	40	60	30	60	90	60	60	120
Folic acid§	mg	0.1	0.2	0.3	0.2	0.4	0.4	0.4	0.8	0.8
Thiamin	mg	0.35	0.70	1.05	0.75	1.50	2.25	1.50	1.70	3.00
Riboflavin	mg	0.4	0.8	1.2	0.8	1.7	2.6	1.7	2.0	3.4
Niacin	mg	4.5	9.0	13.5	10.0	20.0	30.0	20.0	20.0	40.0
Vitamin B_6	mg	0.35	0.70	1.05	1.00	2.00	3.00	2.00	2.50	4.00
Vitamin B_{12}	mg	1.5	3.0	4.5	3.0	6.0	9.0	6.0	8.0	12.0
Optional										
Vitamin D	IU				200	400	400			
Biotin	mg	0.075	0.150	0.225	0.150	0.300	0.450	0.300	0.300	0.600
Pantothenic acid	mg	2.5	5.0	7.5	5.0	10.0	15.0	10.0	10.0	20.0
Minerals										
Mandatory										
Calcium	g	0.125	0.800	1.200	0.125	1.000	1.500	0.125	1.300	2.000
Phosphorus‖	g	0.125	0.800	1.200	0.125	1.000	1.500			
Iodine	mg	35	70	105	75	150	225	150	150	300
Iron	mg	5	10	15	9	18	27	18	18	60
Magnesium	mg	40	200	300	100	400	600	100	450	800
Optional										
Phosphorus‖	g		1.0	1.5	1.0		3.0	0.125	1.300	2.000
Copper	mg	0.5	8.0	12.0	7.5	2.0	22.5	1.0	2.0	4.0
Zinc	mg	4.0				15.0		7.5	15.0	30.0

*From Federal Register **41** (203): 46172, Oct. 19, 1976.

†When labeled for use by infants, a dietary supplement shall contain not less than the lower limit designated for a nutrient in this set of columns, nor more than 100% of the infant U.S. RDA for a nutrient in sec. 125.1 (b) except that the level of biotin, when used, shall be 0.05 mg daily recommended quantity.

‡Optional for adults and children 4 or more years of age.

§Optional for liquid products.

‖Optional for pregnant and lactating women. When present, the quantity of phosphorus may not be greater than the quantity of calcium.

bility of obtaining sufficient amounts of vitamins from food. In addition, they market supplements that contain vitamins at levels well beyond any conceivable need. As a result, many persons are buying and consuming vitamins in excess of their daily requirement. Aside from the economic waste involved, little harm results from excess amounts of the water-soluble vitamins. However, as will be discussed later, excessive intakes of fat-soluble vitamins may have definite harmful effects, and indiscriminate use of such supplements should be discouraged. It is interesting and perhaps appalling to find that the United States produced 675 kg of ascorbic acid in 1972, enough to provide 20 mg per person per day for a year for everyone in the world. Some was used in food to preserve and maintain food quality eventually to end up in the diet, but an undue amount went into vitamin pills to be consumed by an overzealous public.

Recent attempts by the Food and Drug Administration to limit the sale of vitamin supplements without prescription to those containing less than 150% of the United States Recommended Daily Allowance (U.S. RDA) was overruled by the government. Although the FDA believed there was no evidence of benefits under normal circumstances from intakes above this level and considerable cause for concern over indiscriminate use of large amounts, opponents maintained that any such restrictions were an infringement on individual rights. Thus as of January, 1978, it is permissable to sell nutrient supplements singly or in combination at any level for adults. However, products designed for children and pregnant and lactating women may not contain over 150% of the U.S. RDA for any nutrient (Table 10-3). Those that are promoted as multinutrient preparations must contain a specified number of nutrients at a specified level of supplementation. This regulation is designed to encourage more balanced composition of supplements and to preclude the omission of critical nutrients on the basis of price or complication of processing. Current standards are presented in Table 10-3.

BIBLIOGRAPHY

Nomenclature policy: Generic descriptors and trivial names for vitamins and related compounds, J. Nutr. **108:**7, 1978.

11

Fat-soluble vitamins

Although the last of the four fat-soluble vitamins, A, D, E, and K, was identified in 1939, there is still little information about the biochemical roles each plays. As a result, there are many unsubstantiated claims about the clinical effects of these vitamins. Because intakes in excess of need are stored in the body, there is as much concern about toxicity from the ingestion of large amounts as there is about a deficient intake or failure to absorb these nutrients. Vitamins A and K occur in a relatively large variety of foods, whereas vitamins D and E are present in a limited number.

VITAMIN A

Shortly after Funk designated the then-unknown accessory substances in food as "vitamines," two groups of scientists working independently recognized a fat-soluble substance in food necessary for growth in animals. This "vitamine," the first to be identified, was designated as fat-soluble A. It is still known as vitamin A, but it has since been established that there is a complex of chemically related substances, rather than one single active compound, with varying degrees of vitamin A activity. The term *axerophthol,* reflecting the role of one form of the vitamin in treating a condition known as xerophthalmia, has been applied occasionally to this same substance.

In 1912 Osborne and Mendel, working at Yale, reported that animals grew normally on diets containing milk fat but failed to grow when the milk fat was withdrawn. Growth failure was followed by an eye disease. Simultaneously, at the University of Wisconsin, McCollum and Davis were studying the growth of rats on a purified ration of carbohydrate, casein, minerals, and lard. They observed that after periods ranging from 70 to 120 days, growth ceased. They were able to restore growth and relieve the accompanying eye symptoms with an ether extract of butter, cod-liver oil, or egg yolk. Both groups concluded that a fat-soluble substance was necessary for normal growth in animals.

It was not until 1919 that Steenbock, also working in Wisconsin, recognized a similar growth-promoting property in diets containing a yellow vegetable pigment. He was stimulated in his work by Wisconsin dairy farmers' reports of better growth and improvement in fertility when cows were fed yellow corn rather than white corn. As a result of his observations, he was able to attach nutritional significance to the yellow coloring matter in plants such as corn, carrots, and sweet potatoes. By 1928 carotene, one of the yellow pigments of plants, had been identified as a potent precursor of vitamin A.

The term *vitamin A* is now used to refer to all forms of the vitamin—the alcohol, aldehyde and acid—all of which are biologically active.

Until 1967 the vitamin A activity of plant and animal tissue was expressed in terms of International Units (IU) or United States Pharmacopeia (USP) units. These were equivalent in potency and represented the amount of preformed vitamin A or its pre-

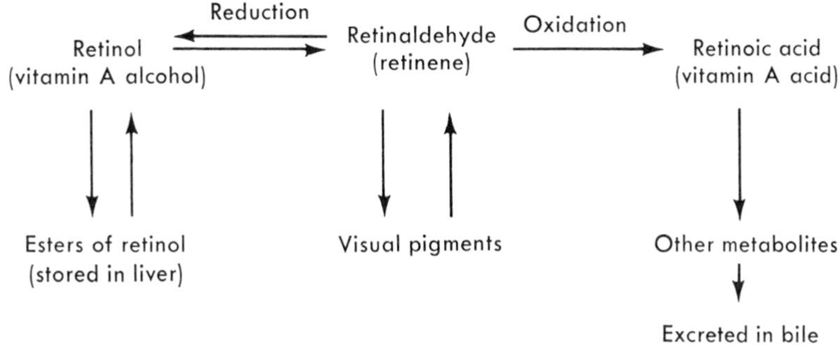

Fig. 11-1. Relationship of biological forms of vitamin A.

cursor, carotene, that caused a specific growth response in rats whose reserves of vitamin A had been depleted. In 1967 the FAO/WHO committee recommended that *retinol equivalents* (RE) be introduced as the unit of measurement of vitamin A. With the publication of the 1974 Recommended Dietary Allowances, the United States joined Great Britain and several other countries in adopting retinol equivalents as the unit of measurement of both vitamin A activity of foods and vitamin A requirements. The advantage of this system of nomenclature is that it takes into account the variation in absorption and conversion of different precursors into vitamin A. One retinol equivalent is equal to 1 μg of retinol, 6 μg of beta-carotene, and 12 μg of other carotenoid precursors. Similarly, when vitamin A is expressed in IU 1 retinol equivalent equals 3.33 IU retinol and 10 IU beta-carotene.

In spite of its early discovery, not until 1930 to 1932 did Swiss and British scientists identify the chemical structure of vitamin A. In 1937 it was crystallized from halibut-liver oil, which has a potency ranging from 2 million to 36 million IU per gram. By 1946 a method of synthesizing vitamin A had been developed. Synthetic vitamin A has a potency of about 4.5 million IU per gram at a cost of about 20 cents. This amounts to 6 cents for a year's supply for an adult. It is now used in enrichment of many food products and in vitamin supplements. A water-miscible form is available for enrichment of nonfat

Table 11-1. Effectiveness of various forms of vitamin A in various functions of the vitamin

	Retinol	Retinal	Retinoic acid
Growth	+	+	+
Epithelial tissue	+	+	+
Bone	+	+	+
Vision	+	+	−
Reproduction	+	+	−

products, such as dried milk solids. Over 747 metric tons of synthetic vitamin A were produced in the United States in 1976.

Vitamin A is an almost colorless substance soluble in fat or fat solvents. Vitamin A occurs in food and functions in the body in several chemical forms—retinol (the alcohol), retinal (the aldehyde), and retinoic acid (the acid). The relationship among these three forms is shown in Fig. 11-1. Whereas retinol and retinal can be reversibly oxidized and reduced, once retinoic acid has been produced by oxidation, it is impossible to reduce it back to either of the other two forms.

This explains why studies on the roles of vitamin A have shown that some forms are effective in certain functions and others in different functions. Retinoic acid, which plays a role in a limited number of functions and unlike the other forms cannot be stored, is sometimes referred to as a *partial vitamin.*

Table 11-1 presents a summary of the functions performed by each of the forms of the vitamin.

With the exception of a small amount found in spinach, the preformed biologically active form of vitamin A is found only in foods of animal origin. Many plants, however, are rich in a group of compounds, carotenoids, which are chemically related to vitamin A. They are known as precursors, or provitamins. Ten of these carotenoids have been identified in foods. Of these, alpha-, beta-, and gamma-**carotene** and cryptoxanthine are the most important in human and animal nutrition. It is from these carotenoid compounds that animals are able to form vitamin A. The presence of the biologically active provitamins parallels the presence of green, orange, and yellow pigments in fruits and vegetables—a direct relationship existing between degree of pigmentation and potential vitamin A value. The green pigment chlorophyll is not itself a precursor but occurs universally in food in association with the yellow pigment that is. Since chlorophyll is darker, it masks the yellow pigment. Yellow pigments such as lycopene in tomatoes and xanthophyll in corn do not themselves have vitamin A potency, although both these foods do contain other vitamin A precursors.

Beta-carotene, a vitamin A precursor with a pronounced yellow color in its purified form, was produced synthetically in 1954. It is currently one of the few yellow pigments approved by the Food and Drug Administration for the artificial coloring of food. It is used extensively in gelatin, margarine, soft drinks, cake mixes, and cereal products. The use of beta-carotene exceeded 100 metric tons in 1978.

Functions

In spite of the fact that it was the first vitamin to be discovered and has been chemically identified for about forty years, the metabolic roles of vitamin A are not well understood. Vitamin A is required only by complex organisms, which makes it more difficult to study; thus scientists are only now gaining some information on the nature of its biological role. It has been positively identified as essential for at least three distinct physiological functions—vision, growth, and reproduction. It is inferred that a common metabolic factor must exist in its effect on cartilage, bone, and epithelium, but so far no one has been able to identify the biochemical nature of this role. The clinical effects of vitamin A are many and seem to involve all human cells in one way or another, possibly through its effect on DNA synthesis.

Maintenance of visual purple for vision in dim light. The biochemistry of the action of vitamin A in dark adaptation is the only one of its functions that has been clearly defined. In the form of the aldehyde retinal oxidized from the retinol provided from the blood, vitamin A combines with the protein opsin to form visual purple, or **rhodopsin**. This pho-

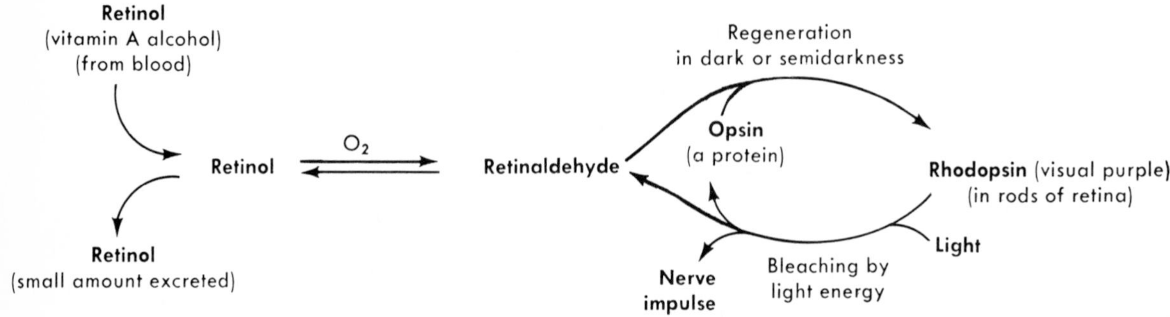

Fig. 11-2. Role of vitamin A in dark adaptation.

toreceptor pigment occurs in the special cells known as rods in the retina of the eyes, which are responsible for vision in dim light. As light strikes the retina, the visual purple is bleached to visual yellow, and retinaldehyde is separated from opsin. With this action a stimulus is transferred from the retina through the optic nerve fibers to the brain. During the process some vitamin A is split off from the protein and reduced to retinol, most of which is reconverted to retinaldehyde to recombine with opsin to regenerate visual purple, or rhodopsin. A small amount of retinol is lost, and vitamin A to replace it must come from the blood. The amount available in the blood determines the rate at which the rhodopsin is regenerated and is available to act again as a receptor substance in the retina. Until the cycle has been completed, vision in dim light is not possible. The mechanism involved is shown in Fig. 11-2.

Two good examples of this phenomenon are the visual reaction of persons on entering a dimly lit theater from a brightly lit street and the temporary blindness experienced by a driver at night after meeting a car with bright headlights. In both cases the bright light has caused excessive bleaching of rhodopsin, and vision in dim light will be possible only when a sufficient amount of visual purple has reformed . This process known as dark adaptation is illustrated in Fig. 11-3. The speed with which the eye adapts after exposure to bright light is believed to be directly related to the amount of vitamin A available to regenerate rhodopsin. The "dark adaptation" test, the speed of recovery of visual acuity in dim light as measured by an especially designed apparatus, was long considered the most sensitive measure of vitamin A status. It is now believed to be of limited usefulness.

Vitamin A is also part of other photoreceptor substances (opsins) in the cells of the retina known as cones, which are responsible for color vision in bright light. The cones, however, are not as sensitive to changes in the amount of vitamin A available as are the rods. In spite of the importance of vitamin A in visual processes, only 0.01% of the vitamin is found in eye tissue. Vitamin A supplementation, therefore, would not be expected to improve normal vision but only poor vision caused by a vitamin A deficiency.

Growth. The role of vitamin A in growth is the result of its effect on (1) the development and maintenance of epithelial tissue and (2) the development of bone. The role of the vitamin in promoting growth is best demonstrated by the observation that animals deprived of vitamin A will cease to grow when the reserves of the vitamin have been depleted (Fig. 11-4). This growth failure will occur before any other symptoms of the deficiency.

Development and maintenance of epithelial cells. Epithelial cells are found not only in the outer protective layer of the skin but also in the genitourinary tract.

Most epithelial cells secrete mucus, and there is considerable evidence that in a vitamin A deficiency this capacity is lost. This effect may be the result of the role of vitamin A in the formation (or differentiation) of the mucus-secreting cells. Since epithelial cells are constantly being lost and replaced, the need for vitamin A in maintaining healthy epithelial tissue is constant. In the absence of vitamin A dry hardened (keratinized) cells develop, which cannot preform the functions of healthy mucus-secreting cells.

In addition to losing the ability to form and secrete mucus, which keeps the linings of the body moist, keratinized cells lack the cilia, or hairlike projections, that prevent the accumulation of foreign material on the surface of the cells. Keratinized cells may also block the openings that allow material to enter or leave the body.

All these changes associated with the development and functioning of epithelial cells can account for many of the effects of vitamin A deficiency, which will be discussed later. The changes in epithelial cells are shown diagrammatically in Fig. 11-5.

Bone development. It is well established that vitamin A is essential for normal bone growth, since in a deficiency bones fail to

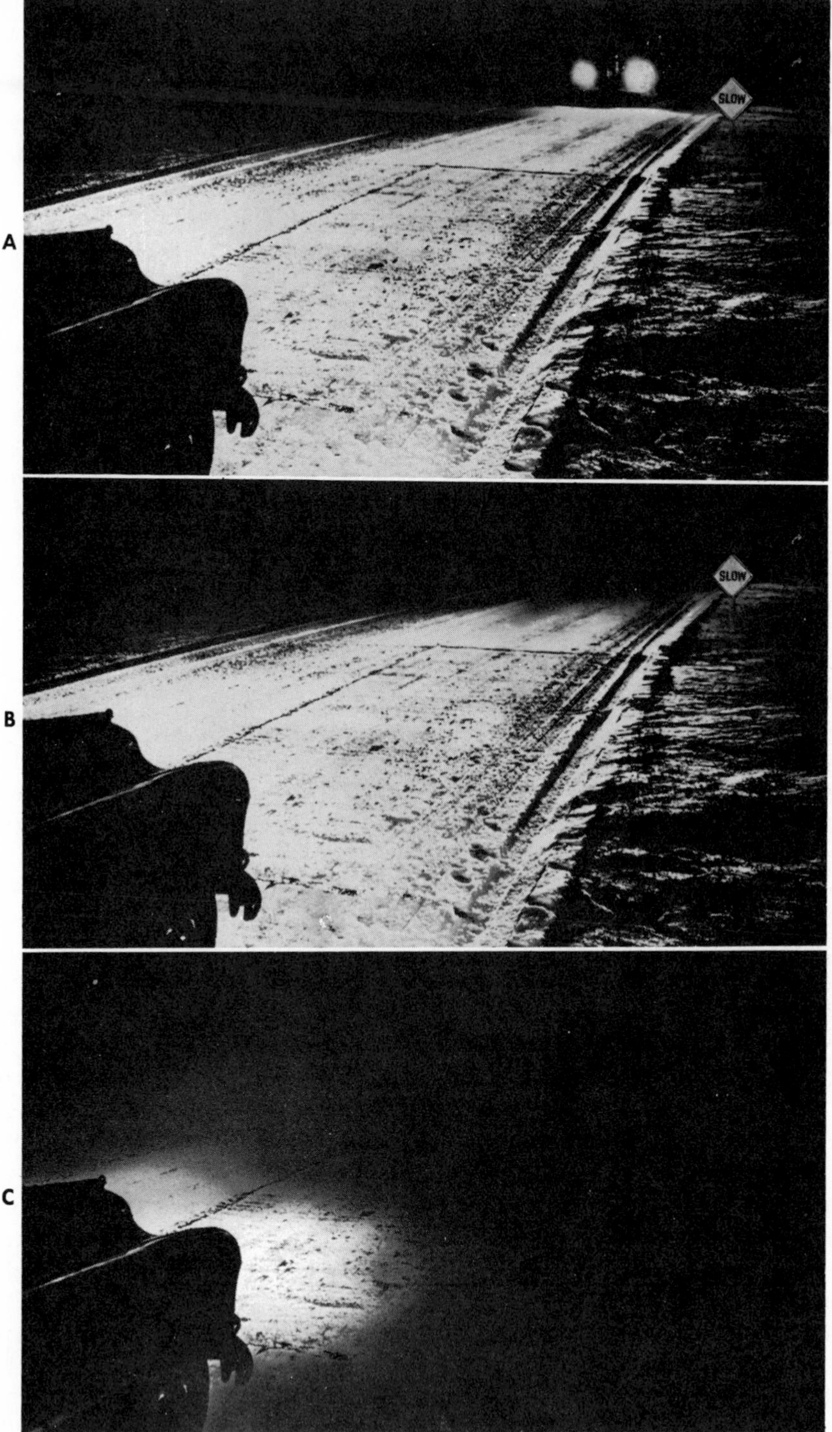

Fig. 11-3. Night blindness. This loss of visual acuity in dim light after exposure to bright light is illustrated here. **A,** Both normal individual and vitamin A-deficient subject see headlights of an approaching car. **B,** After car has passed, normal individual sees a wide stretch of road. **C,** Vitamin A-deficient subject can barely see a few meters ahead and cannot see road sign at all. (Courtesy The Upjohn Co., Kalamazoo, Mich.)

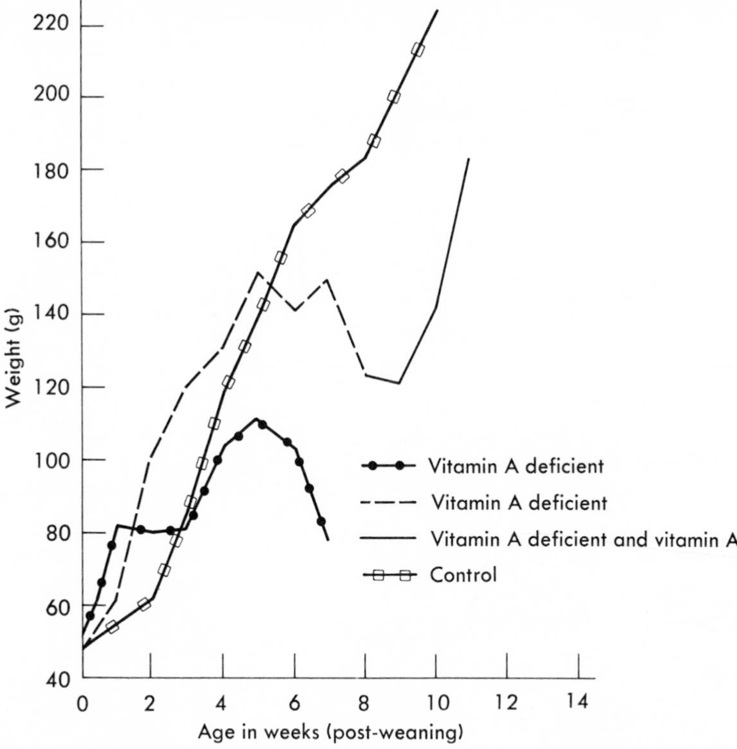

Fig. 11-4. Growth response of weanling albino rats to a diet deficient in vitamin A.

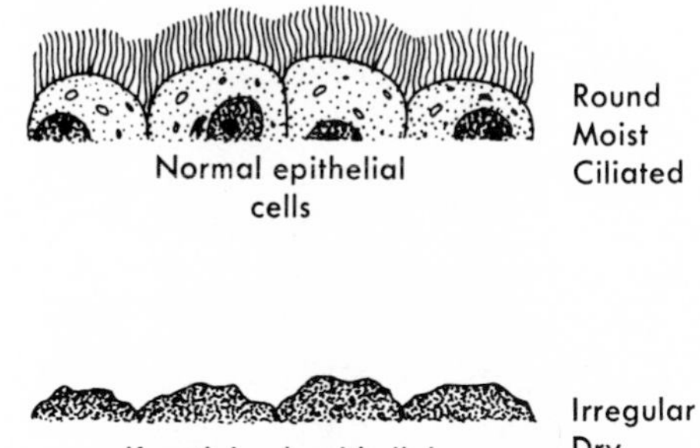

Fig. 11-5. Schematic representation of changes in epithelial cells in vitamin A deficiency.

grow in length, the remodeling process that is an essential phase of bone growth is poorly controlled, and the skull and spinal column do not continue to enlarge to accommodate the growing nervous system. The function of vitamin A in bone growth has been attributed to its role in the conversion of immature cells to osteoblasts, which are responsible for the increase in the number of bone cells, and to osteoclasts, which are necessary for the breakdown of bone cells as bone is remodelled during growth. There is considerable evidence that retinoic acid is the active form of vitamin A involved in the development of both bone and epithelial tissue.

Reproduction. The role of vitamin A in promoting fertility in animals was one of the first discovered. Either vitamin A alcohol (retinol) or its aldehyde derivative (retinaldehyde) is necessary for normal reproduction in rats. In the absence of vitamin A failure of spermatogenesis occurs in the male, and fetal resorption occurs in the female. The exact biochemical mechanism is unknown, but it has been shown that although the alcohol form of vitamin A is effective in stimulating normal reproduction, vitamin A acid will permit conception but will not prevent fetal resorption. A decrease in estrogen synthesis observed in vitamin A deficiency when there is a failure to convert cholesterol to the hormone may be related to the abnormalities in reproduction in the female. In the male vitamin A acts directly on testes rather than through hormones.

Other functions. Studies have indicated that vitamin A (either as acid or alcohol) is necessary for the release of proteolytic, or protein-splitting, enzymes from particles in the cell known as lysosomes. These enzymes must be released to act on the cartilage of bone tissue during bone remodeling, causing a breakdown of the protein structure and the dissolution of the matrix itself. An excess of vitamin A may cause complete disintegration of the matrix by releasing too many enzymes too fast. An imbalance between the rate of breakdown of bone and bone formation is reflected in abnormal bone structure.

In addition to participating in reactions involving the stability of the membranes of subcellular particles, such as the lysosomes and mitochondria, vitamin A is involved in the stability of cell membranes. Some retinol is necessary to maintain a stable membrane, but excessive amounts make the membranes abnormally susceptible to rupture. This phenomenon is believed to be one factor in vitamin A toxicity. Although there is no conclusive proof for a role of vitamin A as a coenzyme, there is considerable evidence to suggest such a role in stimulating the incorporation of sulfate and glucose into the mucopolysaccarides that are essential components of the mucus secreted by epithelial cells. Similarly, there is reason to believe that vitamin A fulfills the role of a coenzyme in the synthesis of hormones from cholesterol.

The loss of appetite in a vitamin A deficiency has been attributed to changes in the taste buds. This may be due to a decrease in mucopolysaccharide synthesis or to clogging of pores of taste buds with keratinized cells.

Many of the changes associated with a vitamin A deficiency can be explained on the basis of changes in cell proliferation. This has led to the theory that vitamin A plays a role in redirecting cell differentiation through its influence on RNA and DNA.

Absorption and metabolism

Absorption. From the time it is ingested until it is either used or excreted from the body, vitamin A changes its chemical form many times. Most of the preformed vitamin A in food appears in combination with the fatty acid palmitic acid as retinyl palmitate. Before it can be taken up from the intestine into the cells lining the intestine, it must be split by enzymes secreted in the pancreatic juice or produced in mucosal cells to form free retinol. Bile is necessary for the uptake of retinol by the mucosal cells. Once retinol is within the mucosal cell, it combines with fatty acid, usually palmitic, and is incorporated in the small transport particles of fat called chylomicrons.

Since vitamin A is fat soluble, factors that promote the absorption of fat enhance vitamin A absorption; conversely, factors that depress fat absorption depress vitamin A absorption. In addition, vitamin E enhances the absorption of vitamin A and increases the amount stored in the liver.

The absorption of vitamin A from foods is decreased in liver injury or in any condition in which the bile duct is obstructed. Mineral oil has an affinity for both vitamin A and carotene, and since it is unaffected by digestive enzymes and passes through the digestive tract, it will carry with it much of the potential vitamin A in the diet. For this reason the practice of using mineral oil as a low-calorie dressing on salad greens, one of the potentially good sources of vitamin A activity, is to be condemned. The intake of polyunsaturated fatty acids with carotene results in rapid destruction of carotene unless antioxidants are also present.

These are then released into the lymphatic circulation, which eventually enters the regular blood system to be carried to the liver. The presence of retinoic acid in food is minimal. In the intestine a small part (less than 10%) of the retinol from food is oxidized first to retinal and then to retinoic acid, which is readily absorbed. As opposed to retinol, which is transported into the body by the lymph system, retinoic acid attaches to the protein albumin to increase its solubility in blood and enters the general circulation through the portal vein.

Metabolism. As the remains of the chylomicrons containing vitamin A pass through the liver, the vitamin A is removed and combines with a protein to be stored in the liver as a lipoprotein. Before it can be released from storage, vitamin A must be released from this complex. It is then attached to a transport protein known as retinol-binding protein, which is synthesized in the liver. As this complex enters the blood plasma, it is attached to another protein, prealbumin, also produced in the liver and present in the blood. In this form it is transported to the tissues where it is needed. Together these two proteins make retinol more soluble to facilitate its transport and at the same time make it a larger molecule to protect it against being filtered out and lost through the kidneys. Most retinol is retained in storage in the liver until needed.

In addition to the intestine, which converts some dietary retinol to retinoic acid, both the kidneys and liver have similar enzymes capable of converting some absorbed retinol to retinoic acid. Retinoic acid from both sources is rapidly converted to a variety of metabolites (especially compounds called glucuronides) that are excreted either through the kidneys in the urine or through bile into the intestine. About 80% of the retinoic acid in the bile is reabsorbed, and the remainder is excreted in the feces.

The depressed utilization of vitamin A observed in protein deficiency can be explained by the number of proteins involved in its metabolism. Enzymes are needed at many stages. Vitamin A is stored in a protein complex and is transported in the blood attached to a protein. In a protein deficiency the synthesis of all these proteins is depressed. Thus protein appears necessary for the mobilization of vitamin A reserves from the liver. This may explain why low blood levels of vitamin A found in kwashiorkor increase when protein but no additional vitamin A is given.

Carotene. The four major vegetable precursors of vitamin A—alpha-, beta-, and gamma-carotene and cryptoxanthine—are absorbed intact in the presence of bile salts from the intestine after having been released from the plant cell during digestion. They are converted in the intestinal wall to retinol. The conversion of carotene to vitamin A, which involves splitting the carotene molecule into two parts, is not complete, with some unchanged carotene being absorbed and entering the circulation, where normal carotene levels approximate 150 IU/dl of blood. Blood carotene levels reflect dietary carotene and not the storage of vitamin A; therefore in decreased intakes a rather rapid drop in carotene values occurs. Carotene levels have little significance as indicators of vitamin A status, nor does unconverted carotene perform any biological function. Unconverted carotene is stored in the fat depots and adrenals rather than in the liver of humans.

The amount of vitamin A formed from the precursor depends on the nature of the precursor. Beta-carotene is a symmetrical molecule made up of 2 vitamin A molecules. It is changed into 2 molecules by breaking in the center. The other precursors can yield only 1 molecule of vitamin A. Conversion of carotene to retinol is enhanced by both thyroxin and vitamin E. Approximately a third of the carotene in food is converted to vitamin A; carotenes in carrots and root vegetables undergo less than one-fourth conversion and those in leafy vegetables about half. The conversion of carotene to vitamin A occurs primarily in the intestinal wall, although some may take place in liver and lungs. Once converted into vitamin A, it is handled in the same way as is the preformed vitamin.

The concentration of vitamin A in human liver (which has 90% of body stores) reflects long-term dietary intakes. The small number of studies reported have given values from 100 IU/g in Great Britain, 420 IU/g for Americans, and 980 for Canadians to a high of 1000 IU/g among New Zealanders who live on a diet high in butter. It is estimated that a healthy person stores 500,000 IU in his liver, an amount that may last several years. Autopsy data on livers of Canadians, however, showed that 10% had no measurable reserves and 20% had no more than normally found at birth. About 20% to 30% of the populations were judged to be at risk.

Food sources

The vitamin A value of some representative foods is shown in Fig. 11-6.

Preformed vitamin A is available only in

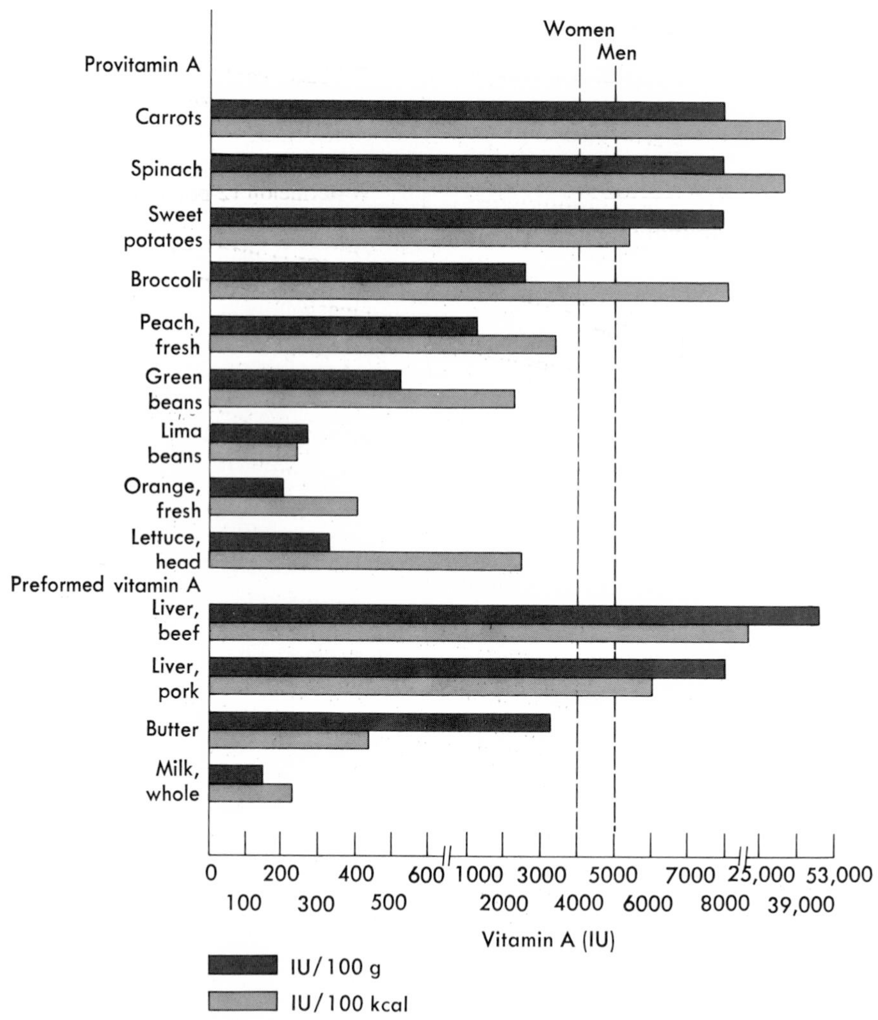

Fig. 11-6. Vitamin A value of 100 g and 100 kcal portions of some representative foods. The vertical broken lines at 4000 and 5000 IU indicate the NRC recommended allowances for women and men, respectively. (Based on Watt, B. K., and Merrill, A. L.: Composition of foods—raw, processed and prepared, Handbook No. 8, Washington, D.C., 1963, U.S. Department of Agriculture.)

animal products in which the animal has metabolized the carotene of its food into vitamin A and has concentrated it in certain tissues. Liver, representing the storage site for vitamin A, reflects the dietary intake of the animal. It ranges from 2,000,000 IU/100 g in polar bear liver to 45,000 IU/100 g in beef liver to 12,000 IU/100 g in pork liver. Fish-liver oils are extremely rich, and until recently concentrates of these were the most widely used therapeutic sources of vitamin A.

Egg yolk with 3300 IU or 1000 RE/100 g is a good source of vitamin A in the form of retinol and is the one usually introduced first into the diet to replenish the fetal reserves of an infant. Since preformed vitamin A is colorless, the color of the yolk is no indication of its potency in the yolk. A deep yellow color may reflect unconverted carotene, but more often it represents xanthophyll, which has no vitamin A activity. It is possible to increase the amount of vitamin A in an egg yolk by increasing the amount fed to the hen.

The vitamin A value of butter varies with the breed of animal and its diet and shows a definite seasonal variation. In winter, butter averages 1900 IU or 570 RE/kg; in the summer, values may exceed 33,000 IU, the amount with which margarine in the United States is usually fortified. In neither case is color an indication of vitamin A value.

In milk the vitamin A is present in the fat portion; this is absent in nonfat milk. Fresh fluid nonfat milk and dried nonfat milk solids are generally fortified with vitamin A. The average value for milk is 390 IU per cup, which is relatively low, and the loss of vitamin A when nonfortified nonfat milk replaces whole milk becomes important only when milk is the sole item in the diet, as it is for infants. Any yellow color in milk is due to presence of carotene, reflecting inefficient conversion to vitamin A by the cow. The amount of vitamin A in cheese is the same as that in the milk from which it was made. Aside from milk products, eggs, and liver, animal products contain virtually no vitamin A. Muscle meats are devoid of vitamin A value.

Table 11-2. Vitamin A values of representative foods

Food	IU of vitamin A activity
Fruits and vegetables[1]	
Spinach (½ cup)	10,600
Carrots, diced (½ cup)	9065
Kale (½ cup)	4610
Broccoli (½ cup)	2550
Asparagus (½ cup)	910
Peas (½ cup)	575
Brussels sprouts (½ cup)	260
Lima beans (½ cup)	230
Cabbage, cooked (½ cup)	75
Apricots, dried (½ cup)	8195
Apricots, canned (½ cup)	2260
Papaya (½ cup)	1595
Watermelon (2-pound wedge)	1265
Peaches, raw (½ cup)	1115
Orange (1 medium)	290
Banana (1 medium)	95
Pineapple, raw (½ cup)	90
Dairy products[2]	
Milk, fresh whole (1 cup)	390
Cheese, cheddar (1 ounce)	378
Butter (1 tablespoon)	230
Margarine (1 tablespoon)	230
Milk, fresh nonfat (1 cup)	10
Meat, fish, poultry, and eggs[2]	
Egg, whole	590
Egg yolk	580
Liver (3 ounces)	
Beef	45,450
Lamb	43,000
Chicken	27,000
Calf	19,000
Pork	12,000

[1]For retinol equivalents divide by 10.
[2]For retinol equivalents divide by 3.3.

Fruits and vegetables contain no preformed vitamin A, only precursors. Because of this, tables of food composition report vitamin A activity or vitamin A value of foods, reflecting the potential vitamin A available from the food based on ability of the body to make the conversion.

Generally, as seen from Table 11-2, the vitamin A value of fruits and vegetables is directly proportional to the amount of carotene or chlorophyll present in the food. Thus the deeper the orange, yellow, or green color of fruits and vegetables, the higher the vitamin A value. In addition, if one examines the vitamin A values of a food such as a head of lettuce, one finds a tenfold increase as one progresses from the inner bleached leaves to the outer leaves higher in chlorophyll and carotenoids. Unfortunately, a high concentration of chlorophyll is often accompanied by an astringent bitter taste, as in very dark green endive leaves, so that a potentially rich source of vitamin A is unpalatable. In some fruits, such as mangos, the carotene content increases with storage.

The yellow pigments lycopene, found in watermelon and tomatoes, and xanthophyll, found in corn and egg yolk, do not have vitamin A value. Another yellow pigment in corn, cryptoxanthine, does have vitamin A potential of about 3.5 IU/g. In countries where red palm oil is used in cooking, its carotene content represents a major cource of vitamin A activity, with 800 IU/g.

The ability of the body to utilize carotene varies with the food and the form in which the food is ingested. For instance, grated carrots have greater value than carrot slices. Utilization varies from 30% to 70% of available vitamin A.

Vitamin A is stable to heat and alkali, but unstable to light, acids, and oxidation. Little is lost under normal conditions of food preparation. Excessive temperatures in frying oils high in carotene, such as palm oil, that are used extensively in tropical countries, may cause its destruction, as will the oxidation that occurs in rancid fats. The small amount of green and yellow pigment that may appear in cooking water from fruits and vegetables represents an insignificant portion of that present in the food. Sun-drying of fruits and other forms of dehydration may lead to some loss of vitamin A.

The contributions of various food groups to the vitamin A content of the American diet are shown in Fig. 11-7, and Fig. 11-8 depicts the change in the contribution of the various food groups to vitamin A value between 1909 and 1968. Results of the National Nutrition Survey show that vitamin A is the nutrient for which intakes are most often below recommended levels and that blood

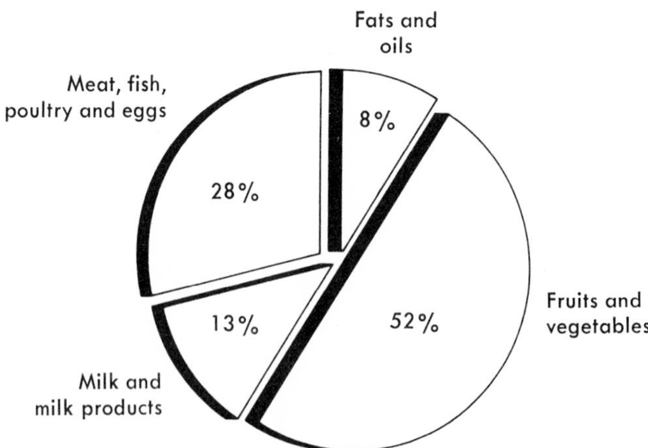

Fig. 11-7. Contribution of various food groups to vitamin A content of American food supply. (Based on Contribution of major food groups to nutrient supplies available for civilian consumption, National Food Review NFR-1, Washington, D.C., 1978, Economic Research Service.)

levels often fall below expected norms.

In the United Sates the average daily intake is 7500 IU, 50% of which comes from vegetable sources, compared to about 4300 IU in Britain, two thirds of which is from animal sources. In Central and South America 93% of the vitamin A comes from the precursor and a third of this from yellow maize. In India the intake is less than 1000 IU a day, and the simultaneous low-protein intake keeps the level of utilization low. In the tropics the 900,000 metric tons of palm oil used yearly provide substantial amounts. The INQ for vitamin A value of various food sources is given in Table 11-3.

Table 11-3. INQ for selected sources of vitamin A providing at least 15% of the U.S. RDA per serving

Cooked spinach	167.7
Carrots	123.7
Liver	107.1
Broccoli	46.0
Baked sweet potatoes	26.4
Papayas	21.0
Asparagus	20.1
Tomatoes	20.0
Tomato juice	19.9
Apricots	16.4
Peaches	15.8
Lettuce, iceberg	11.5
Spaghetti (meatballs and tomato sauce)	2.2
Butter	2.1
Orange juice	2.1

Recommended allowances

The National Research Council recommended allowances for vitamin A have been established assuming that a third of the vita-

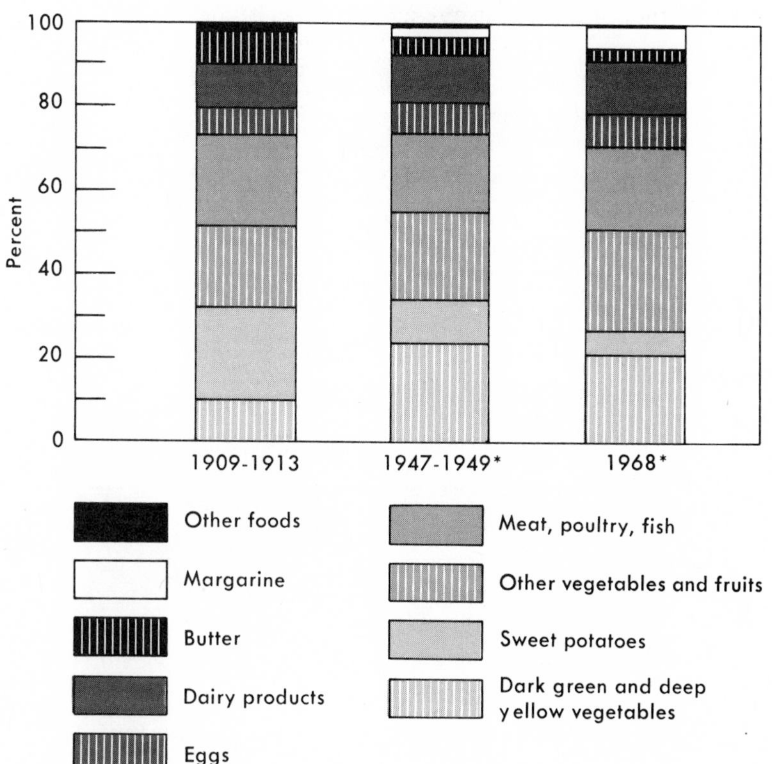

Fig. 11-8. Trends in consumption of dietary sources of vitamin A value from 1909 to 1968. *Includes fortification. (From Agricultural Research Service, U.S. Department of Agriculture, 1969.)

min A value of a mixed diet comes from animal sources and two thirds from vegetable sources. The recommended allowances have been set at 5000 IU (1000 RE) for an adult male each day. For women, 4000 IU (800 RE) are recommended. During pregnancy the recommendation is increased to 5000 IU (1000 RE), and in lactation 6000 IU (1200 RE) is deemed adequate. The recommended amounts for other age groups are shown in Appendix C. The extent to which diets in the United States fail to provide these levels is shown in Fig. 11-9.

The discrepancies in recommended levels of vitamin A intake expressed as IU in various standards result from assumptions of different proportions of vitamin A and carotene in diets and different interpretations of the efficiency with which carotene is converted into vitamin A. The use of retinol equivalents as the unit of measurement overcomes this problem.

The need for vitamin A varies under different conditions. Tiring work, especially in hot weather, tends to raise needs. This may be a manifestation of the decreased ability to

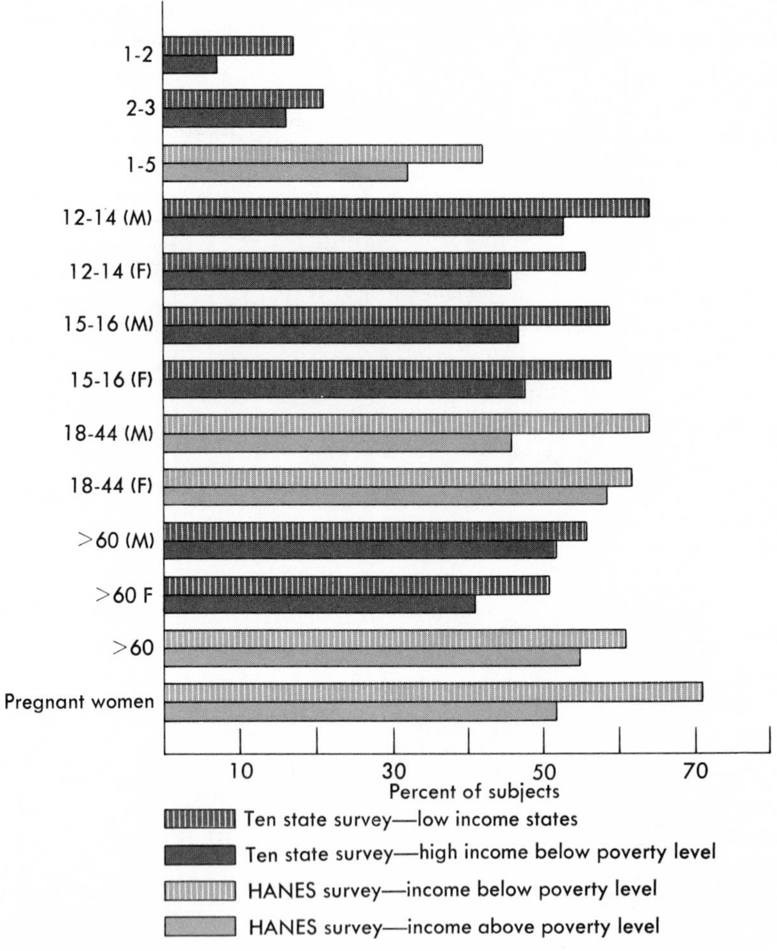

Fig. 11-9. The percentage of persons with dietary vitamin A intake below two-thirds RDA by age, sex, and income level. Data based on results of Ten-State Nutrition Survey (1968-1970) and preliminary findings of first Health and Nutrition Examination Survey (HANES) (1971-1972).

convert carotene into vitamin A at higher temperatures. Also, more vitamin A is needed after removal of the gallbladder, in hypothyroidism, and in conditions of impaired intestinal absorption.

Deficiency

Vitamin A deficiency symptoms show up only after liver reserves, which are determined by previous dietary intake, have been depleted. In animals, growth ceases when the reserves of vitamin A have been used up. Most symptoms of a vitamin A deficiency as seen in humans are a reflection of its role in maintaining the health of epithelial cells. They may result from low dietary intakes, interference with absorption and storage, interference with conversion of carotene to vitamin A, or rapid loss of vitamin A.

Night blindness. One of the earliest symptoms of vitamin A deficiency is night blindness. At low intakes the liver reserves drop, followed by a drop in blood levels and a subsequent drop in the level available in the retina of the eye for formation of the visual pigment rhodopsin. This eventually shows up in a slow dark adaptation time and finally night blindness.

Changes in the eye. The cornea of the eye is affected early. The lachrymal gland fails to secrete tears, possibly as a result of decreased ability to synthesize mucopolysaccharide or of a blocking of the lachrymal duct. In addition, there are distinct changes resulting from dryness of the film covering the cornea. This is followed by a keratinization, opacity, and sloughing of epithelial cells of the cornea, with eventual rupturing of the corneal tissue. Infection apparently sets in, pus is exudated, and the eye will hemorrhage. This condition is known as Bitot's spots in its mildest form, as xerosis conjunctivae in moderately severe form, and as xerophthalmia in advanced states. These conditions were prevalent in children in Denmark during World War I when occupation troops deprived them of dairy products, their most dependable source of vitamin A. It is now reported frequently in Indonesia and other tropical countries where a low protein intake may also be a contributing factor. Typical eye symptoms of severe vitamin A deficiency are shown in Fig. 11-10. Total blindness is a common result and most frequently affects children. Many children probably succumb to other forms of vitamin A deficiency or resultant infection before xerophthalmia develops.

Respiratory infections. Vitamin A has often been designated as the anti-infective vitamin because of the high incidence of respiratory ailments associated with a deficiency. Since vitamin A does not directly attack the infective organism, the use of this term has been questioned. However, evidence exists that when the epithelia of the trachea and bronchi become keratinized, deciliated, and deprived of their mucous secretions and a break occurs in the integrity of the mucous membranes, they become a good harbor for microorganisms that would not normally penetrate a healthy epithelial layer. In animals the changes in epithelium during vitamin A deficiency usually lead to terminal bronchial pneumonia. Recovery among tuberculosis patients has been more rapid when the diet is high in vitamin A. Efforts to relate susceptibility to the common cold to vitamin A intake have shown no relationship, but those on diets high in vitamin A have had colds of shorter duration.

Changes in skin. Dry rough skin, especially in the area of the shoulders, may be an early sign of a vitamin A deficiency. The condition, known as **folliculosis,** in which there are small bumps near the base of the hair follicle that subsequently undergo keratinization, is used as an indication of possible vitamin A deficiency in many nutritional status studies.

Changes in gastrointestinal tract. Many disturbances in the gastrointestinal tract, such as diarrhea, have been linked by various investigators to the changes in epithelial tissue that takes place in the absence of vitamin A.

Failure of tooth enamel. The integrity of the enamel layer of teeth may reflect the ad-

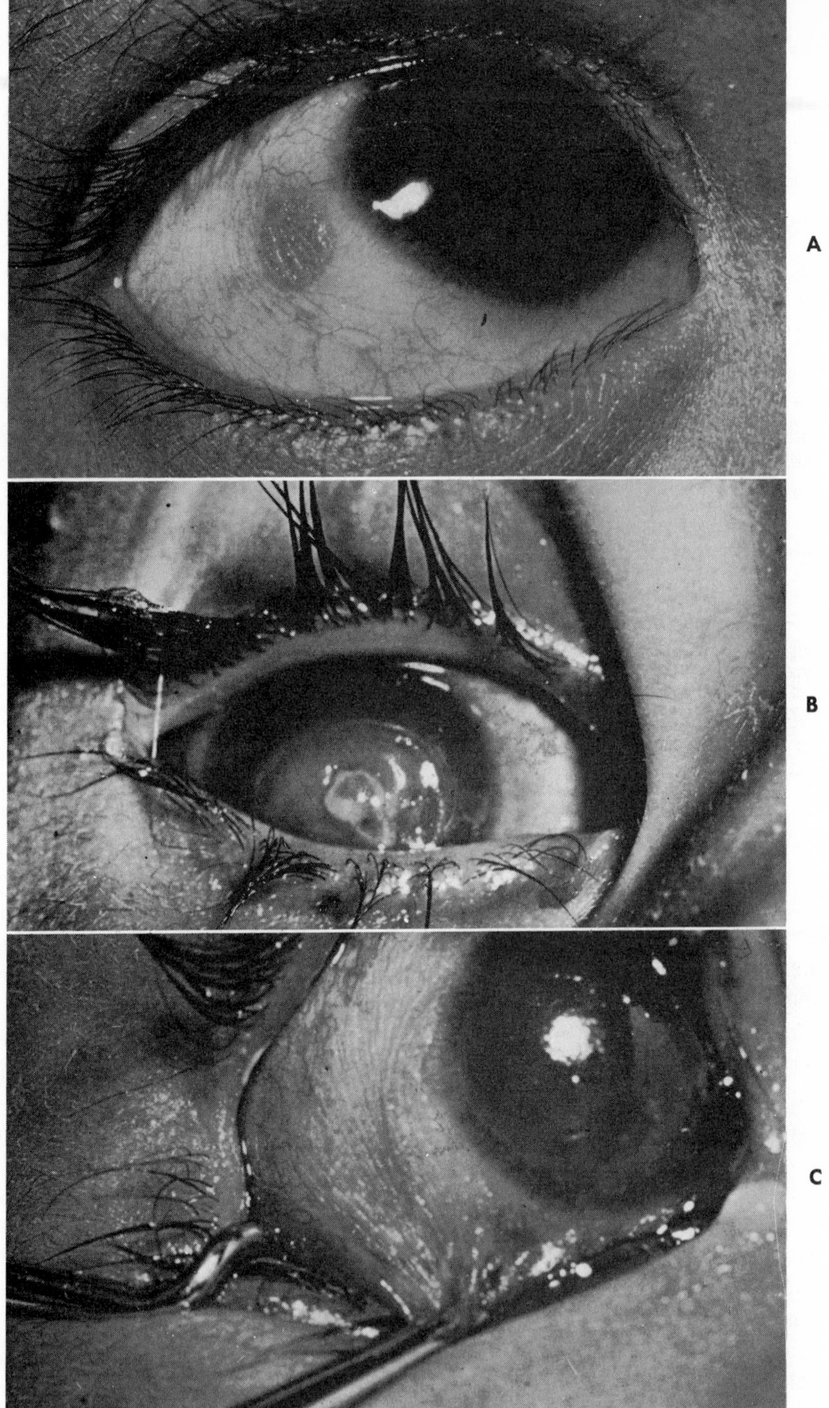

Fig. 11-10. Changes in the eyes characteristic of severe vitamin A deficiency. **A,** Early corneal xerosis, with infiltration in lower central cornea. **B,** Keratomalacia—softening and protrusion of whole central area of cornea. **C,** Generalized xerosis, with clearly demarcated Bitot's spots. (From McLaren, D. S., Shirajan, E., Tschalian, M., and Khoury, G.: Am. J. Clin. Nutr. **17:**117, 1965.)

equacy of vitamin A in the first five years of life. In vitamin A deprivation in animals the enamel layer of teeth is absent.

Other symptoms. Loss of sense of both taste and smell occur in vitamin A deficiency and may be partially responsible for growth failure related to decreased appetite and hence food intake. The increase in cerebrospinal fluid pressure has been explained on the basis of a failure of absorption of fluid from the deficient membranes or a decrease in the space for fluid due to the formation of thick bones in a vitamin A deficiency.

The extent of vitamin A deficiency in the United States is poorly documented. The Ten-State Survey showed that plasma vitamin A levels were low enough to be considered deficient in 33% of low-income children under 6 years of age.

Although there is little evidence of night blindness or other clinical signs of hypovitaminosis A, studies of vitamin A levels in the liver showed that they may be lower than expected. A third of the population has levels of 0 to 40 μg/g compared to normal values of 100 to 300 μg/g.

Evaluation of vitamin A status

The most sensitive indicator of vitamin A status is the measurement of vitamin A stores in the liver. However, since this method involves obtaining a sample of liver tissue by biopsy, it is of no practical significance. Since many factors such as an inadequate protein intake and possibly a zinc deficiency may prevent the release of vitamin A from the liver, the level of vitamin A in the blood does not correlate with clinical evidence of a deficiency and is a poor indicator of vitamin A reserves. In addition, values do not drop until reserves are depleted. Normal blood levels for vitamin A are 40 μg/dl. Any drop in plasma vitamin A levels below 20 μg/dl reflects a depletion of liver reserves, an inability to mobilize liver reserves, or prolonged diet deficiency. These reductions are associated with clinical symptoms such as follicular keratosis (hardening of the base of the hair follicle), impaired dark adaptation, or severe acne. Under experimental conditions it took 260 to 631 days on a deficient diet for evidence of clinical symptoms to appear. The measurement of retinol-binding protein levels necessary for the release of vitamin A from the liver, has been used, but this method has many of the same limitations as the use of plasma vitamin A values. The measurement of changes in the amount of vitamin A in the blood plasma following an oral dose of vitamin A shows promise as a more sensitive indicator. Blood carotene values reflect only the amount of unconverted dietary carotene and bear no direct relationship to nutritional status. Although night blindness represents an early symptom of more severe eye changes, its diagnosis in young children is difficult.

Clinical uses

Like most vitamins, vitamin A has been used as a therapeutic agent in attempts to control a wide variety of conditions. The use of high oral doses and topical applications in salves to control acne has had disappointing results. The topical use of retinoic acid, however, has proved somewhat successful in the treatment of acne and shows promise in the control of tumor growth.

Prophylactic doses have been used in India to reduce the incidence of blindness. Doses of 200,000 IU of vitamin A as tablets given to deficient children every six months cause only transient toxic symptoms and show promise as a short-term preventive measure.

In spite of the promise of desirable effects from the use of massive doses, the possibility of toxic reactions in sensitive individuals suggests that they be used under strict medical supervision.

Toxicity

The possibility that excessive amounts of vitamin A may produce detrimental rather than desirable results has been recognized only recently. Symptoms have appeared as a result of the use of polar bear liver, which has a vitamin A potency of up to 20,000 IU/g.

Symptoms have also appeared after treatment of a skin disorder in adolescents with daily doses of vitamin A of 50,000 to 100,000 IU, and after the use of large doses of vitamin A supplements for infants by overzealous mothers. The symptoms of vitamin A toxicity are many, ranging from headache, drowsiness, nausea, loss of hair, dry skin, and diarrhea in adults to a scaly dermatitis, weight loss, anorexia, and skeletal pain in infants. Loss of hemoglobin and potassium from red blood cells and cessation of menstruation occurs in young girls and women, and rapid resorption of bone occurs in adults. The period between the initiation of high intakes and the onset of symptoms varies from six to fifteen months. Wide individual differences in sensitivity to high levels seem to exist, some persons showing symptoms after long-term dosages of 50,000 IU daily and others exhibiting a reaction only at levels of 150,000 to 200,000 IU a day. Infants have shown bulging on the head, hydrocephalus, hyperirritability and increased intracranial pressure after dosages of 25,000 IU daily for thirty days.

Recovery is rapid and complete on withdrawal of excess intake, with symptoms subsiding in 72 hours in many cases. Toxic reactions can occur only from overconsumption of the preformed vitamin not of the precursor. Permanent effects of vitamin A toxicity are rare. Some workers are concerned that long-standing high intakes on the part of the mother, resulting in storage levels in the mother's liver of 1000 IU or more per gram, may have harmful effects on the fetus even if the mother has not exhibited a toxic reaction herself. In animals single injections of vitamin A in the pregnant female have produced cleft palate in the young.

Hypervitaminosis A can result in a decreased stability of membrane structure. This may account for the increase in fragile bones when excess intake is provided, since the resultant release of enzymes leads to degeneration or resorption of bone tissue. This, in turn, may be responsible for the simultaneous increase of calcium in both urine and blood.

Animal studies suggested that toxicity results only after the capacity to carry vitamin A in the retinol-binding protein has been exceeded, and free retinol rather than retinol in a RBP complex is made available to the cells.

The Food and Drug Administration has become sufficiently concerned to attempt to require that a ceiling of 10,000 IU be placed on the amount of vitamin A that can be included in a multivitamin preparation available without a prescription. The availability of vitamin A supplements of high potency at a low price had led some persons to oversupplement their diet. This, coupled with the widespread practice of enriching food products for trade advantages, increases the possibility of a person receiving a toxic dose. The chance of this occurring in a normal mixed diet is remote.

VITAMIN D

Although it has been known for over sixty years that the condition called rickets, characterized by defective bone formation, could be prevented or cured if infants were exposed to sunlight or received cod-liver oil, only in the last decade have scientists identified the way in which these two seemingly unrelated cures work. The active substance responsible was originally identified as vitamin D but now is offically designated as cholecalciferol (vitamin D_3) if it comes from animal sources and ergosterol (vitamin D_2) if it comes from vegetable sources. Vitamin D had been known previously as the *sunshine vitamin* because sunshine is one of its sources to the body, and as the *antirachitic factor,* or *rickets-preventive factor,* because of its effectiveness in curing rickets.

Since the precursor of vitamin D can be produced in the body, it is considered by some to be technically a hormone. However, when it is supplied by the diet, it is technically a vitamin. Regardless of whether this substance is a vitamin or a hormone the nutritionist is interested in assuring that adequate amounts are available for its role in promoting normal development of bones and teeth.

Vitamin D has been shown to be necessary for all animals with a bony skeleton, since it facilitates the absorption and utilization of calcium and phosphorus for bone formation.

Rickets

Rickets is a condition that has plagued infants in the temperate zone for centuries. It was so common in England that some writers referred to it as the *English disease.* Before a dietary factor was implicated as the causative agent, many environmental factors had been investigated. The fact that it occurred more frequently among people living in the crowded, smoky, industrial areas of cities where standards of sanitation were often poor suggested that rickets was a disease of bacterial origin. Dark-skinned persons moving from the tropics to the temperate zone were especially susceptible to rickets. Since they frequently lived in crowded housing, the environmental theory seemed to be supported. This theory, however, was called into question by the observation that children of the wealthy who were kept bundled in large amounts of clothing were more prone to rickets than the scantily clad children of the poor who were allowed to run freely outdoors. From time to time it was suggested that sunshine had a curative effect on rickets, but the relationship between sunshine and rickets was not established until the late 1920s, after the nature of vitamin D had been clarified.

Rickets is essentially a disease of defective

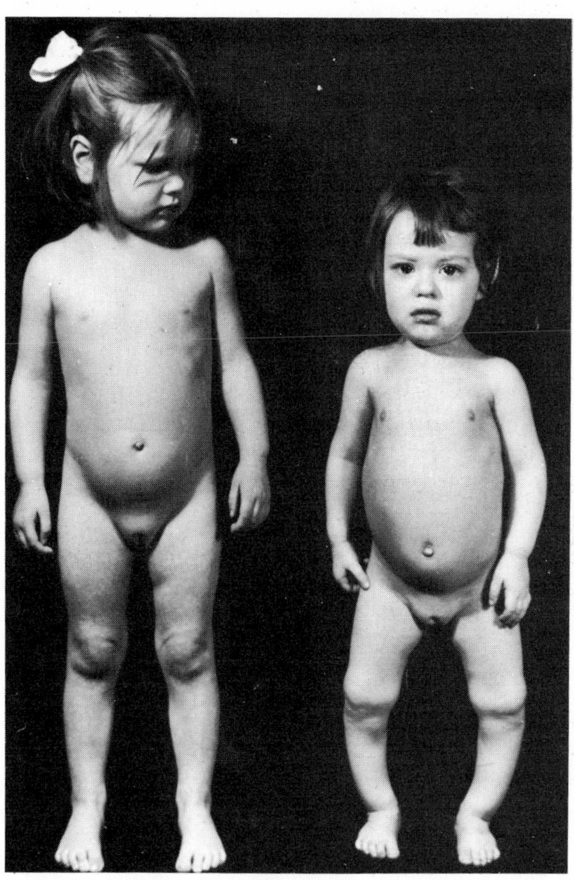

Fig. 11-11. Typical case of rickets (right) compared to normal child (left). (From Arneil, G. C.: World Rev. Nutr. Diet. **10:**239, 1969.)

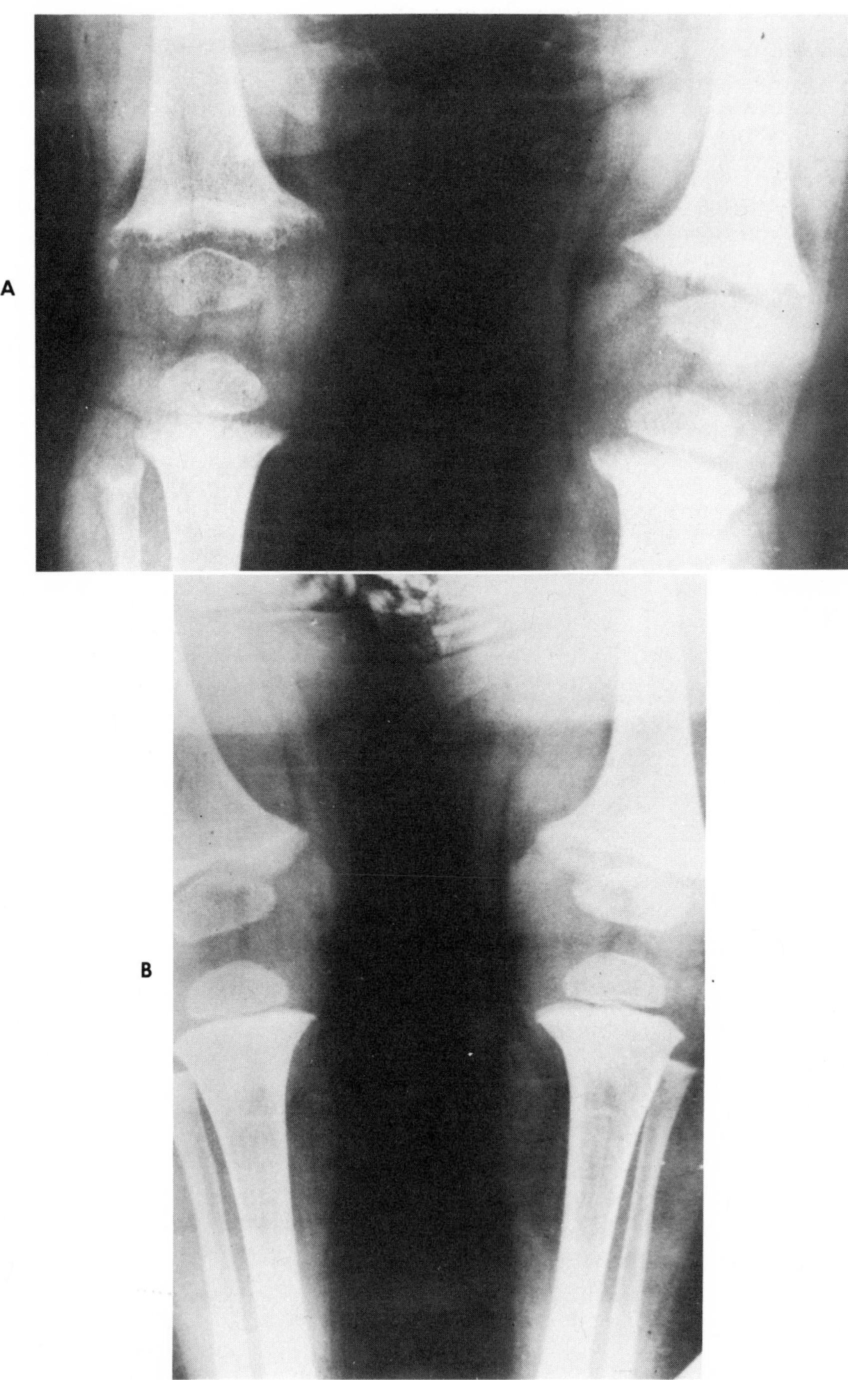

Fig. 11-12. X-ray film of bones of young child. **A,** At diagnosis of rickets. **B,** Three months after treatment. (Courtesy Dr. Johanna Dwyer, Boston.)

bone formation that manifests itself in many ways. Basically it results from an inadequate deposition of calcium and phosphorus in bone. The bones, normally poorly calcified at the time of birth, remain soft and pliable. Deformities develop when these poorly calcified bones are called on to perform functions for which they are not sufficiently strong. Bowing of legs occurs when a child starts to walk before the bones have become rigid enough to support the weight of the body. The ends of the long bones become enlarged, causing difficulties in movement. Knock-knees are a manifestation of this enlargement, which results from the flattening that occurs when the poorly calcified ends of the bones are subjected to the weight of the body. Deformities of the ribs result in a concave breast (pigeon breast) that causes crowding in the chest cavity. Ribs also develop irregularly spaced areas of swelling that take on the appearance of beading, which has led to the use of the term *rachitic rosary* to describe this syndrome. The failure of the fontanel, or opening in the skull, to close normally in early life allows rapid enlargement of the head, sometimes erroneously interpreted as a sign of health in a child.

Teeth erupt later, are less well formed than normal, and decay earlier. Growth is generally retarded, but the severity of the disease as measured by other symptoms is frequently greater in children who have undergone rapid growth.

Rickets is a condition that primarily affects children. The symptoms are very slowly reversible so that some symptoms produced during early childhood may remain throughout adulthood. The long-held belief that rickets does not develop in children over 2 years of age is no longer tenable. Many of the cases that were associated with the recurrence of rickets in the 1960s in both Great Britain and the United States were identified in children between age 2 and 4. They showed a growth retardation and the typical bowed legs. Such a case is shown in Fig. 11-11. The effects of vitamin D deficiency on bone structure is shown in Fig. 11-12.

The term *adult rickets* is sometimes applied to the disease osteomalacia, which reflects a defect in bone formation but not necessarily a vitamin D deficiency.

Although rickets was practically eradicated as a health problem, in the early 1960s there was a reappearance of the condition. In England 633 patients were diagnosed with rickets, which suggests that many more were suffering from subclinical rickets. Most of those affected were dark-skinned immigrants who undoubtedly did not receive enough radiation.

Discovery

The discovery of vitamin D followed by six years the identification of fat-soluble A. In 1918 a British nutritionist, Mellanby, presented the first evidence of a fat-soluble substance with antirachitic properties. By 1919 scientists had produced rickets experimentally by feeding animals diets in which vegetable or animal fats replaced cod-liver oil. By 1922 the antirachitic properties of cod-liver oil, which had been used as a folk remedy since early in the nineteenth century, were recognized. Because those properties were not destroyed by oxidation, as was the vitamin A value of cod-liver oil, it seemed likely that a second fat-soluble vitamin existed. It was soon identified as vitamin D, which occurred in plants as **ergosterol** and in the skin as 7-**dehydrocholesterol.**

The existence of provitamin D, which could be activated into vitamin D by the short ultraviolet rays of the sun, was discovered in 1922. This antirachitic factor was isolated in a crystalline form in 1930, twelve years after the first report of the substance. By 1937 its chemical structure had been elucidated. Most vitamin D used in supplements or in fortification of the food products has been obtained from irradiation of the precursors of vitamin D with ultraviolet light. Methods are now available for the synthesis of two derivatives of vitamin D that are even more effective than the naturally occurring vitamin in preventing several types of rickets.

Absorption

Dietary vitamin D is absorbed primarily in the jejunum and duodenum of the small intestine. Once absorbed it is incorporated into the small fat particles, the chylomicrons, and transported in the lymphatic system. Factors such as bile, which facilitate fat absorption, also enhance the absorption of vitamin D. Conversely, conditions such as steatorrhea (fatty stools) in which fat absorption is incomplete or obstructive jaundice in which the flow of bile is decreased are associated with decreased absorption of vitamin D. The way in which vitamin D, formed from the irradiation of precursors in the skin, is absorbed is not clear. One theory suggests that the precursor, 7-dehydrocholesterol, is secreted by the sebaceous glands to the surface, is irradiated, and absorbed. About 80% of the vitamin D in the body is obtained this way.

From the lymphatic system, vitamin D is removed from the chylomicrons and transported in the blood plasma attached to a protein carrier, alpha-globulin$_2$. Here it is indistinguishable from vitamin D formed from the irradiation of 7-dehydrocholesterol in the skin and is present at levels of 8 to 45 mg/dl. This vitamin D is removed from the blood to be stored in adipose tissue and muscle or metabolized directly to the active form.

Metabolism

Vitamin D is removed from the plasma by the liver and converted by a reaction called hydroxylation, which adds an OH group, into related metabolites (25-hydroxycholecalciferol or 25-hydroxyergocalciferol). As soon as enough is produced, a feedback mechanism cuts off production. These substances are then transported in the blood to the kidneys attached to the same or similar protein carrier that took their precursors to the liver. Here they are further hydroxylated to form 1,25-dihydroxycholecalciferol (1,25 DHCC), which differs from the ingested or skin precursors only in the presence of two hydroxyl (OH) groups in its structure.

The formation of these related compounds or metabolites is stimulated by the parathyroid hormone that is secreted when blood calcium levels drop. These substances have now been identified as the form of the vitamin responsible for the ability of vitamin D to regulate calcium and phosphorus metabolism and bone formation. When the level of calcium in the blood increases to a certain level, the thyroid gland secretes another substance, calcitonin, which causes a reduction in the production of 1,25 DHCC and diverts metabolism to another form, 24,25 DHCC. This substance (24,25 DHCC) can be converted further to 1,24,25-trihydroxy vitamin D with three hydroxy groups.

A synthetic analog of 1,25 DHCC is now available which can be quickly converted in many tissues of the body to the active form so that it is not necessary to involve the kidneys.

Similarly, low levels of phosphorus stimulate 1,25 DHCC production, and high levels stimulate 24,25 DHCC production. The mechanism by which phosphorus levels function in this role is not known.

Excretion

Most vitamin D is excreted in the bile in combination with glucuronic acid or as part of the bile acid.

Functions

Calcium metabolism. Vitamin D has long been recognized as a nutrient associated with the calcification of bone. In part it accomplishes this by assuring that calcium is available to be deposited in the bone matrix by enhancing the absorption of calcium from the intestine. There is convincing evidence that the active form of the vitamin stimulates the formation of messenger RNA in the nucleus of the intestinal mucosal cell, which in turn regulates the synthesis of a calcium-binding protein (CaBP). This protein must be available if calcium is to be taken up by the mucosal cells lining the intestinal tract, transported across the intestinal cells, and released by them into the blood.

Vitamin D also acts to raise blood calcium

levels by facilitating resorption of bone. This mechanism is stimulated by all forms of vitamin D, but especially by 1,25 DHCC produced in the kidneys from absorbed vitamin D. Several theories have been advanced to explain this effect. One suggests that vitamin D stimulates the production of an enzyme that speeds up the breakdown of the organic matrix of the bone. Another attributes its action to the production of citrate, which increases solubility of bone. Still another postulates a relationship with collagen metabolism. Regardless of the mechanism, the result is increased blood calcium levels.

Whether vitamin D acts to increase absorption of calcium or stimulates the release of calcium from the bone, whenever serum calcium drops a series of biochemical reactions is set up to counteract the drop. First, the parathyroid gland is stimulated to produce parathyroid hormone. This in turn stimulates the kidneys to produce 1,25-dihydroxycalciferol, which promotes the absorption of calcium from the intestine or its resorption from the bone. Once serum calcium levels increase again, the production of parathyroid hormone declines, shutting off the formation of the active form of vitamin D (1,25 DHCC) in the kidneys. At the same time the thyroid produces another hormone, calcitonin, which facilitates the deposition of calcium in the bone. The trihydroxy-

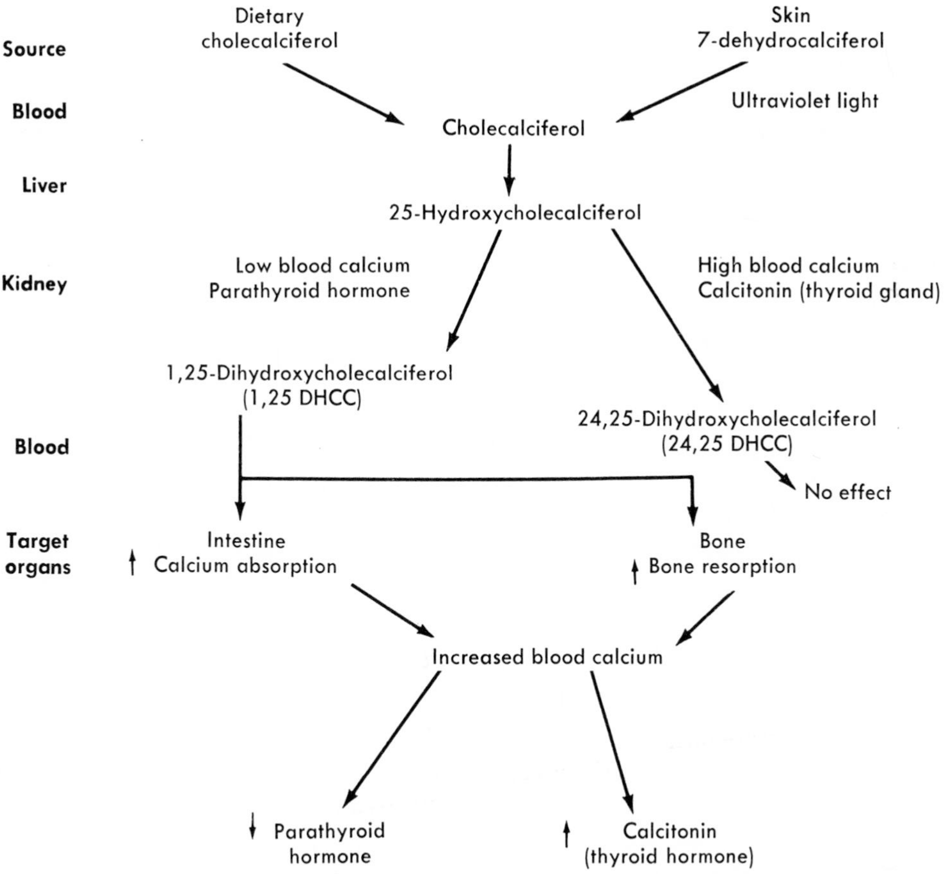

Fig. 11-13. Summary of metabolism and effects of vitamin D.

cholecalciferol produced by further addition of hydroxyl groups to the DHCC in the kidneys stimulates the transport of calcium in the intestine but does not affect calcium mobilization from the bone.

A summary of vitamin D metabolism and its effect on calcium metabolism is shown in Fig. 11-13.

Phosphorus metabolism. Failure of calcification of bone is more often caused by an inadequate supply of phosphate than of calcium, although the term *calcification* to describe the deposition of calcium phosphate crystals in the bone matrix implies that calcium is primarily involved. The addition of vitamin D to the diet increases the rate of absorption of phosphate. It is postulated that the same transport mechanism which facilitates calcium absorption facilitates phosphorus absorption but in a different segment of the intestine. Of greater importance is the fact that it increases the resorption of phosphate from the tubules of the kidneys. It is believed that 24,25 DHCC acts here. In the absence of vitamin D much phosphate is lost in urinary excretions, and the blood levels of phosphate drop. Alkaline phosphatase, which is produced in large amounts in the growing surfaces of bone, helps release inorganic phosphate into the blood from organic compounds, another method of increasing phosphorus available for calcification.

Other functions. Vitamin D influences the rate of resorption of amino acids in the kidney tubules. Evidence indicates that the level of amino acids in the urine (aminoaciduria) is a fairly sensitive indication of vitamin D status, increasing in a deficiency and decreasing when vitamin D restores the normal rate of resorption.

A discussion of the role of vitamin D would be incomplete without mention of the antagonistic relationship between vitamin D and hydrocortisone, a hormone secreted by the adrenal gland and used therapeutically in the treatment of many conditions. Hydrocortisone can depress the high blood levels of calcium associated with excessive intakes of vitamin D. It can also decrease the permeability of the intestinal membrane and hence calcium absorption when administered along with normal levels of vitamin D.

The rate of intestinal absorption of calcium is greatly increased in the presence of adequate dietary vitamin D; a rate of 10% absorption without vitamin D may be increased to 33% in the presence of the vitamin.

Requirements

Vitamin D is measured in International Units defined in terms of a biological response to the administration of the vitamin to a depleted animal. One International Unit of vitamin D weighs 0.025 μg, and 1 mg contains 40,000 IU. The units are both used in expressing the vitamin D content of foods.

Because of the two sources of vitamin D, the evaluation of minimum requirements is difficult. Indications are that 100 IU of vitamin D will protect against rickets and will promote growth when adequate amounts of calcium and phosphorus have been ingested. However, since intakes of 300 to 400 IU (7.5 to 10 mg) seem to promote better calcium absorption and some increase in growth, the Recommended Allowances have been set at 400 IU a day for infants, children, adolescents, and pregnant and lactating women. There are no recommendations for normal healthy adults, since their needs seem to be met through the action of sunlight on precursors in the skin. Intakes above 800 IU appear to provide no greater protection against rickets and at levels over 1800 IU may have detrimental effects, reversing the beneficial effects of lower levels.

Previous recommendations that breast-fed infants receive a supplement of 400 IU by 2 weeks of age may be changed with the recent discovery of a water-soluble analog of vitamin D in breast milk. This may account for the virtual absence of rickets among breast-fed children even though breast milk contained practically no vitamin D. If fortified milk or commercial infant formulas are used, it is not only unnecessary but also possibly undesirable to add a supplement, since they alone provide adequate amounts.

Premature infants whose calcium reserves

are much lower than those of full-term infants, in whom half the calcium is deposited in the last six weeks of fetal life, have a need for vitamin D to facilitate the absorption of the high level of calcium needed to meet the demands of rapid growth. Apparent ineffectiveness of dosages of 400 IU of vitamin D in breast-fed premature infants may be a function of the low-calcium content of breast milk rather than of an increased need for vitamin D.

During pregnancy and lactation an intake of 400 IU is deemed desirable, although these recommendations are not well documented. Otherwise, adults appear to obtain sufficient amounts if they are exposed to some degree of sunshine and have a varied diet. If occupational or clothing habits are such that exposure to sunlight is limited, a dietary source for adults is recommended.

In older children and adults who seldom develop rickets, who have a greater exposure to ultraviolet light and many other food sources, and whose growth rate is relatively slow, it is much more difficult to evaluate minimal needs, since no other criterion of adequacy of vitamin D has been established. It is only when exposure to sunlight is inadequate, dietary intake of vitamin D is restricted, and needs are relatively high that deficiency symptoms develop.

Sources

Irradiation of precursor in skin. Vitamin D is available to the body by two separate pathways. The skin normally contains a fat-related substance, 7-dehydrocholesterol, which constitutes 0.15% to 0.42% of the sterols in the skin and performs no biological function. However, when exposed to the short ultraviolet rays from 275 to 300 mμ in length from the sun or from mercury vapor sunlamps, it is converted into the biologically active substance vitamin D_3, or **cholecalciferol.** This is then absorbed from the skin into the general circulation. It is still not clear whether the conversion takes place in the epithelial cell of the skin or on the surface of the skin, but evidence seems to favor the latter. The amount of vitamin D available through irradiation of the precursor in the skin is influenced more by the amount of ultraviolet light to which the individual is exposed than by the amount of the precursor present. During the summer in the temperate zone ultraviolet rays may penetrate sufficiently far north for a maximum of 4 hours in the middle of the day. In winter this time may be reduced to less than an hour. Ultraviolet rays are incapable of penetrating fog, smog, clouds, smoke, ordinary window glass, window screening, clothing, or skin pigment. The presence of any or all of these reduces the potential vitamin D available through radiation. The pigment in the skin, which acts as a protection against overproduction of vitamin D in dark-skinned persons living in the tropics, reduces the benefits from the much smaller amount of irradiation available in the temperate zone. For this reason the incidence of rickets among dark-skinned infants in the temperate zone is much higher than among light-skinned infants and dark-skinned infants in the tropics. Some protection against overirradiation is necessary, since it can lead to the production of potentially toxic substances, such as tachysterol, toxisterol, and suprasterol.

A special window glass, mercury quartz, permits the transmission of ultraviolet rays. Its use in windows in hospital nurseries where infants are unable to be taken outdoors can hardly justify the cost, which is over ten times that of regular glass, when supplements are readily available.

Dietary intake. The other source of vitamin D, and in the temperate zone the major source, is ingested vitamin D. Some foods of animal origin, such as eggs, milk, butter, and fish-liver oils, constitute the major sources of the preformed vitamin, but they are characteristically poor and unreliable sources, the amount present varying with the diet and breed of the animal. Most diets contain cholecalciferol but some may contain 25 HCC, the metabolite formed in the liver. Vegetables are poor sources. Even when all potential dietary sources are included, it is possible to obtain only about 125 IU a day. This would include egg yolk, butter, and milk. As a result it is now customary to rely on foods fortified with vitamin D or nutritional supplements during periods of maximum need for vitamin D.

A study of the sources of vitamin D in the United States showed that 6-month-old babies received 400 IU from food and 400 IU from supplements for a total of 800 IU; 2-year-olds received 600 IU, and 8-year-olds received 800 IU. For those in each group who received more generous supplements, intakes were estimated at 1400, 2600, and 2900 IU, respectively.

Milk, a carrier of both calcium and phosphorus needed for calcification of bones, is the food most commonly fortified with vitamin D. Evaporated milk, irradiated to provide 400 IU/L of reconstituted milk, was the first food to be sold as an irradiated product. Now 95% of homogenized milk, practically all of nonfat milk and much of the dried nonfat milk solids have vitamin D added. Regular milk, in which a cream layer rises to the top, is not fortified because the fat-soluble vitamin D would concentrate in the cream layer. Most milk sold in the United States is fortified with vitamin D at a level that will permit maximum utilization of its calcium and phosphorus. It is anticipated that this may decrease if milk is subjected to full requirements of the nutrient labeling regulations. The cost of fortifying 380 liters (100 gallons) of milk is estimated at 4 cents.

Although milk is the only product that has been endorsed for fortification, vitamin D is being added to many other products, such as infant cereals, prepared breakfast cereals, milk flavorings, bread, and even some beverages. If a person consumed one serving of each of these along with 1 liter of fortified milk a day, the intake could readily reach 1000 IU daily! However, since processors are continually changing the amount added to foods and the foods to which they are adding it, assessing the amount of vitamin D in the diet is difficult without access to the labels on the products. For instance, in the United States, millers have the option of adding from 250 to 1000 IU of vitamin D per 0.45 kg of flour. Although the United States does not allow the addition of vitamin D to margarine, England requires 1300 to 1600 IU per 0.45 kg and Germany 135 IU.

In the temperate zone, where neither sunshine nor a diet of nonfortified products can be relied on to provide enough vitamin D for protection from rickets, it has become standard pediatric practice to introduce a supplementary source of vitamin D in infant diets. The use of cod-liver oil standardized to provide 85 IU/g or 3.40 IU/tsp, which had been traditional since the early 1920s, has been almost completely replaced by water-soluble preparations of vitamin D. This overcomes the problem of lipoid pneumonia in infants, caused by aspirating the oily cod-liver oil. The odor of the cod-liver oil was much more objectionable to mothers than to infants, as was the problem of oil-stained clothing. Water-miscible preparations traditionally contain vitamin A and also ascorbic acid. Most drug companies had voluntarily reduced the recommended dosage to provide only 400 IU of vitamin D per dose rather than the 800 IU previously suggested before the Food and Drug Administration made 400 IU mandatory in 1965. Labels usually carry warnings against excessive use of the supplement.

A solution of irradiated ergosterol (ergocalciferol) in a neutral oil is marketed as viosterol. The use of this very concentrated source of vitamin D increases the likelihood of an overdose.

The presence of calcium salts with vitamin D in therapeutic preparations may adversely effect the stability of vitamin D. Distributors of mineral-vitamin preparations are being discouraged from combining vitamin D with mineral supplements, even though it may seem logical.

In Europe, where the habit of using daily supplements of vitamin D or foods enriched with vitamin D has not been established, physicians have found that massive injections of 300,000 IU of vitamin D at intervals of six weeks to three months is an effective way to control rickets. Apparently no adverse effect result from such large doses, but in the

United States smaller daily doses are preferred.

Toxicity

Since the demonstration over sixty years ago that cod-liver oil was effective in preventing rickets, the disease has ceased to be a cause of concern to medical and public health authorities. Now the cause for concern lies at the other end of the continuum, with attention being directed toward the problem of overuse of vitamin D. In one of the earliest studies to assess the need for vitamin D, Jeans and Stearns showed that no extra benefit was derived from levels above 400 IU a day, and that levels of 1800 IU a day actually retarded linear growth. More recently, reports of hypercalcemia in infants, in which practically all tissues of the body are adversely affected, have focused attention on the possibility that high levels of vitamin D are causative. The withdrawal of all sources of vitamin D alleviated the high blood calcium levels with their rapid onset of loss of appetite, nausea, weight loss, and failure to thrive.

The level of vitamin D intake that precipitates hypercalcemia varies greatly from one individual to another. Adults receiving 100,000 IU of vitamin D for weeks or months will develop symptoms. An intake of 1000 to 3000 IU/kg of body weight in infants (10,000 to 30,000 IU per day) is usually toxic. Apparently some infants experience a hypersensitivity to vitamin D and exhibit symptoms at levels as low as 1000 IU a day, although the lower limit of toxicity is likely closer to 2000 to 3000 IU. Toxicity in children results from intakes varying from 10,000 IU a day for four months to 200,000 IU daily for two weeks. Most cases have involved intakes of 25,000 to 60,000 IU each day for one to four months.

All forms of vitamin D are potentially dangerous, and the effects of an overdose resemble those of toxisterol or suprasterol toxicity.

Because benefits did not increase from vitamin D intakes in excess of 400 IU a day and because of the possibility of detrimental effects for sensitive individuals at levels above 2000 IU, British authorities concerned about an increasing incidence of hypercalcemia persuaded processors of vitamin D–fortified products to reduce the level of fortification so that a person consuming the recommended amount of the food would be protected against rickets and yet would not be in danger of excessive intakes if he consumed all such fortified products. A report three years after the introduction of this policy, which reduced vitamin D intakes by a third to a half, indicated a decrease in the incidence of hypercalcemia and no increase in the incidence of rickets. It is generally recommended that the dose of vitamin D not exceed that shown to be safe for children most reactive to vitamin D.

Studies with pregnant rats showed that changes in the placenta and impaired maturation of osteoblasts, the bone-forming cells result in defective bone formation on high intakes of vitamin D. However, the effect of hypervitaminosis D in human pregnancy has not been established.

Large doses of vitamin A given concurrently with potentially toxic doses of vitamin D tend to reduce the incidence of toxic symptoms.

Interrelationship with drugs

The increases in the incidence of rickets and osteomalacia associated with anticonvulsant therapy in epilepsy and with the use of sedatives and tranquilizers have been attributed to the breakdown of the active forms of vitamin D to inactive forms.

Alcoholism predisposes to symptoms of vitamin D deficiency since it interferes with conversion of 25 HCC in the kidneys to the active 1,25 DHCC.

One theory to explain the antagonistic effect of strontium on calcium absorption is attributed to its ability to block the synthesis of the active form of vitamin D in the kidneys. This then results in a decreased synthesis of the calcium-binding protein needed for calcium absorption.

Clinical uses

Vitamin D therapy has been used in the treatment of osteoporosis, renal osteomalacia, sex-linked low levels of phosphate in the blood, and the decreased bone density associated with anticonvulsive therapy.

A number of bone diseases that had been resistant to treatment with vitamin D, especially those associated with the use of renal dialysis in treating kidney failure, are now being treated successfully with 1,25 DHCC or its less expensive synthetic analog. The intravenous use of this active form of the vitamin eliminates the need to have vitamin D changed first in the liver and then in the kidneys. Thus it is effective even if the functioning of these tissues is impaired.

Deficiency

Persons on low-fat diets and strict vegetarians are the most frequent victims of vitamin D deficiency. Premature infants and the elderly, both of whom have minimal exposure to sunlight, also develop problems. Deficiencies develop at any age when intake drops below 70 IU a day.

Osteopenia (osteomalacia and osteoporosis) occurs quite frequently after gastric surgery or in chronic obstructive jaundice, possibly the result of malabsorption of vitamin D. Chronic alcoholics also suffer from osteopenia.

Some forms of rickets, characterized by low blood levels of phosphorus, are resistant to treatment with vitamin D. These conditions are associated with failure to absorb both calcium and phosphorus and to resorb phosphorus from the kidney tubules. Since 25 HCC is effective in curing the condition, it appears to be caused by poor conversion of cholecalciferol to 25 HCC in the liver.

In North African countries reports indicate that from 45% to 60% of the children have some signs of rickets, and 3% to 18% have severe rickets.

VITAMIN E

Vitamin E, now known to be needed by twenty species, including humans, was first recognized as a dietary essential in 1922. At that time it was found to be necessary for normal reproduction in animals. Since a deficiency was shown to produce permanent sterility in male animals and a decrease in the ability of the female animals to conceive or to carry a fetus to term if conception did occur, vitamin E became known as the antisterility factor. Although it is now understood that a failure in normal reproduction in animals is only one of the results of a vitamin E deficiency and that human reproduction is unlikely to be affected, the use of this term has persisted.

Vitamin E deficiency states have been experimentally produced in many species, and several theories of its biochemical role have been advanced. Its role in human nutrition, however, is still poorly understood. The understanding of vitamin E is complicated by the fact that a variety of other nutrients are capable of performing some but not all of the functions of this nutrient, and in some but not all species. Vitamin E has been aptly described as "the vitamin in search of a disease." As research continues it is possible that an important clinical use of the vitamin will emerge.

Chemical forms

The term *vitamin E* is applied to a group of chemical compounds that have the biological activity of alpha-tocopherol. Alpha-tocopherol in turn represents a group of compounds called tocols in which the methyl (CH_3) group is essential. Eight related tocopherols have been identified as having vitamin E activity. Biochemically they differ only slightly, but physiologically marked differences exist in their effectiveness. Alpha-tocopherol, which accounts for 80% of the activity of the vitamin, is considered the biologically active form.

Functions

Since vitamin E deficiences have only recently been produced in humans, most of our knowledge of vitamin E functions has come from experimentation on animals such as chicks, rats, rabbits, and guinea pigs. From these it has become obvious that vitamin E affects different species in different ways.

Until recently there was no unifying theory to explain the mode of action of vitamin E in its apparently diverse roles. It is now postulated that vitamin E acts to stabilize polyunsaturated fatty acids in cell membranes and protect them against destruction due to oxidation. Some of the evidence for this antioxidant role is discussed here.

Antioxidant in both animal and plant tissue. By being readily oxidized or using oxygen itself, tocopherol reduces the amount of oxygen available to other substances that may otherwise be destroyed or changed undesirably by the uptake of oxygen. Thus fats containing vitamin E are less susceptible to oxidation and resulting rancidity than are those devoid of vitamin E. Vitamin A, unsaturated fatty acids, and vitamin C in foods are similarly protected against destruction when vitamin E is present. Tissue lipids are likewise less susceptible to excessive oxidation (peroxidation), which may modify structure of the tissue and hence its function.

Similarly, there is evidence that the antioxidant properties of vitamin E may prevent the formation of a lipofuscin pigment, also known as ceroid pigment, which accumulates in adipose tissue and in the uterus and may play a role in the fetal death and resorption observed in vitamin E deficiency. The accumulation of this same substance characterizes the aging process. Products of the oxidation of lipids, especially the polyunsaturated fatty acids, have been demonstrated to have the same damaging effect on proteins as that observed as the result of radiation. While adequate levels of vitamin E protect against the acceleration of these undesirable changes, there is no evidence that intakes in excess of recommended levels provide additional protection or delay aging.

Other evidence of the antioxidative role of vitamin E has been established. In fact, some investigators believe that no other biochemical function can be attributed to vitamin E and that a loss of this antioxidant property and the resultant lipid oxidation and damage of intercellular membranes, enzymes, and metabolites can provide an explanation for all manifestations of a vitamin E deficiency. Others dispute this on the basis that other antioxidants can substitute for or can spare vitamin E in some but not all of its metabolic roles.

Cellular respiration. Vitamin E plays an essential role in the final biochemical changes by which energy from glucose and fatty acids is finally released and water is formed. This function has not been completely clarified. The fact that it seems to be involved primarily in respiration in heart and skeletal muscles may provide a rationale for earlier but unsuccessful attempts to treat human heart diseases and muscular dystrophy with vitamin E.

Synthesis of other essential body compounds. In species capable of synthesizing vitamin C, tocopherol acts as a necessary cofactor. It also stimulates the synthesis of coenzyme Q, essential in the respiratory chain in which energy is released from carbohydrate, fat, or protein. Tocopherol also plays a regulatory role in the incorporation of pyrimidines into the nucleic acid structure. This seems to be especially true in the bone marrow, where red blood cells are manufactured. In a vitamin E deficiency, abnormally large red blood cells (macrocytes) are formed when vitamin E fails to regulate the formation of nucleic acids.

Heme synthesis. The synthesis of heme, an iron-containing compound that is an essential part of many proteins, is dependent on the presence of two enzymes whose synthesis, in turn, is regulated by vitamin E. One theory suggests that at least one heme-containing protein acts as a scavenger and counteracts the peroxides formed by the oxidation of unsaturated fatty acids in the absence of vitamin E or other antioxidants.

Membrane metabolism. It is well established that the membrane of the red blood cell is weakened in a vitamin E deficiency, resulting in rupture of the cell membrane (hemolysis). The theory that this was due to the oxidation of the lipid in the membrane in the absence of an antioxidant such as vitamin E has been questioned. Alternative theories are that vitamin E acts to inhibit the breakdown of fatty acids, which are part of the membrane structure, or that it is an integral part of the cell membrane, providing stability and strength to its structure. These resultant changes in membrane structure could explain the interference in amino acid absorption observed in a vitamin E deficiency.

Interrelationships with vitamin A

The long recognized interrelationship between vitamin A and vitamin E in which vitamin E appears to spare vitamin A has been attributed to (1) the protection of vitamin A from oxidation in the gut, (2) the increase in the absorption of vitamin A, or (3) the increased storage of vitamin A.

Absorption and metabolism

As a fat-soluble substance, vitamin E requires the presence of bile for absorption, either from oil solutions or aqueous emulsions. It is absorbed best in the presence of fat. Although some enters the portal vein, most is apparently absorbed unchanged into the lymph and is transported in the bloodstream as tocopherol attached to lipoproteins. At normal levels of intake only 20% to 30% of dietary vitamin E is absorbed. As intake increases the proportion decreases. Vitamin E is stored in various tissues, but adipose tissue, muscle, and liver are the major sites with the heart, uterus, testis, and adrenals also containing high amounts. Excess vitamin E can be conjugated and excreted in the urine or bile.

A newborn infant has approximately 20 mg of vitamin E stored in the body and an adult 3 to 4 g.

Requirement

Vitamin E requirements and food sources are expressed as International Units (IU) with 1 IU equivalent to 1 mg of alpha-tocopherol.

1968 was the first time the Food and Nutrition Board of the National Research Council believed that sufficient information existed on which to base recommended dietary allowances. It determined that desirable intake was related to a unit of metabolic body size (weight in $kg^{3/4}$) rather than to body weight or caloric intake and recommended that the diet provide 1.25 alpha-tocopherol equivalents per unit of metabolic body size. The 1974 revision placed recommended intakes for adult males at 15 IU of total vitamin E activity and for adult women at 12 IU, based on data of vitamin E content of American diet and lack of any clinical or biochemical evidence of vitamin E deficiency on these intakes. This assumes that 80% of intake is alpha-tocopherol and 20% other tocopherols. The requirement will increase with an increase in the level of polyunsaturated fatty acids in the diet at the usual level of fat intake—40% of the calories coming from fat.

The requirements for pregnancy and lactation have been set at 15 IU. It appears that vitamin E is transferred much more effectively through the milk than through the placenta to the infant.

Serum tocopherol levels are low at birth (0.25 mg/dl), although the mother's level increases to a high of 1.5 to 2 mg/dl at the end of pregnancy. These levels are associated with preparation for lactation. Human milk, which provides 2 to 5 IU/L or approximately 0.5 mg/kg of body weight of the infant is four times as high in vitamin E as cow's milk and results in a faster increase in serum tocopherol levels of breast-fed babies. All milk substitutes for infants must now contain adequate levels of vitamin E. Infants with defective fat absorption may need supplementary vitamin E. Since premature infants have low serum vitamin E values, reflecting the fact that most of the vitamin E is transferred to the fetus in the last two months of fetal life, supplements are recommended.

Food sources

Tocopherols occur in greatest concentration in vegetable oils. Wheat germ oil is the

Table 11-4. Tocopherol content of 100 g of various oils*

Food	mg/100 g
Wheat germ oil	260
Corn oil	
Unhydrogenated	100
Hydrogenated	105
Cottonseed oil	
Unhydrogenated	91
Hydrogenated	80
Soybean oil†	
Unhydrogenated	101
Hydrogenated	73
Safflower oil	
Stabilized	59
Unstabilized	36
Olive oil	10
Coconut oil	8

*From Bunnell, R. H., Keating, T., Quaresimo, A., and Parmin, G. K.: Alpha-tocopherol content of foods, Am. J. Clin. Nutr. **17**:1, 1965.
†The tocopherol in soybean oil is predominantly gamma-tocopherol, which is only 10% as active as alpha-tocopherol. However, since soybean oil is used in such large amounts in margarines and salad oils, most diets contain two to three times as much gamma- as alpha-tocopherol.

Table 11-5. Vitamin E content of 100 g of some representative foods*

Food	mg/100 g
Mayonnaise	50.0
Margarine (made with corn oil)	46.7
Yellow cornmeal	3.4
Whole wheat bread	2.2
Spinach	2.0
Beef liver, broiled	1.62
Egg	1.43
Broccoli	1.3
Fillet of haddock, broiled	1.20
Butter	1.0
Tomatoes, fresh	0.85
Green peas, frozen	0.65
Ground beef	0.63
Pork chops, pan-fried	0.60
Chicken breast	0.58
Cornflakes	0.43
Banana	0.42
White bread	0.23
Carrots	0.21
Orange juice, fresh	0.20
Potato, baked	0.055

*From Brunell, R. H., Keating, J., Quaresimo, A., and Parmin, G. K.: Alpha-tocopherol content of foods, Am. J. Clin. Nutr. **17**:1, 1965.

source from which vitamin E was first obtained. The vitamin E value of this and other vegetable oils is given in Table 11-4. Generally speaking, the amount of naturally occurring vitamin E in oils increases along with an increase in polyunsaturated fatty acids. Tocopherols are also present in a wide variety of other plant and animal tissue, as shown in Table 11-5.

One study of the vitamin E activity of typical meals showed that breakfasts ranged from 0.59 to 3.68 mg, lunches from 0.44 fo 5.37 mg, and dinners from 1.61 to 6.38 mg. Only by choosing the meals highest in tocopherol from each group was it possible to obtain 15 mg daily, which is believed to be an adequate level of intake. A range for three meals of 2.6 to 15.4 mg, with an average intake of 7.4 mg, was found. This was considered low in the light of increased consumption of polyunsaturated fatty acids, which increases the need for tocopherol. Approximately 0.6 mg of vitamin E/mg of PUFA is required.

There is little destruction of tocopherol during normal cooking except for deep-fat frying, but appreciable losses occur during freezing if temperatures are not sufficiently low to prevent oxidative destruction of the vitamin. Since an increasing number of foods are being stored frozen, this may be additional cause for concern about the observed intake. The heating of cooking oils destroys virtually all of the tocopherol present, but active esters of tocopherol such as tocopherol acetate are less than one fifth destroyed.

Fruits and vegetables are relatively poor

sources of tocopherol, but fresh and frozen vegetables retain much more than canned products. Little is lost in normal cooking procedures.

About 64% of dietary tocopherol comes from oils, shortening, and margarine; 11% from fruits and vegetables, primarily green leafy vegetables; and only 7% from grains. Up to 90% of the tocopherol of cereals is lost in processing.

Deficiency

In animals. A lack of vitamin E in animals is manifest in a wide variety of seemingly unrelated ways, with symptoms involving muscles, nervous system, reproductive organs, vascular system, and glandular system. In chicks vitamin E deficiency causes characteristic central nervous system changes, known as *encephalomalacia,* and *exudative diathesis,* in which large patches of fluid accumulation appear beneath the skin on the breast, legs, abdomen, and neck. In rats, liver degeneration occurs, along with reproductive failure, affecting both males and females. In male rats there is degeneration of the epithelium, resulting in permanent sterility; in females resorption of the fetus occurs by the eighth day of the 22-day gestation period. Fetuses can be salvaged if vitamin E is given by the fifth day, but if it is delayed until after the sixth day, many congenital abnormalities appear. Although all of these symptoms can be relieved by administration of tocopherol, in many instances other substances such as selenium, cystine, and ubichromenol are also effective.

Muscular dystrophy occurs in vitamin E deficiency in guinea pigs, rabbits, and monkeys. It is characterized by muscular weakness caused by fragmentation of muscle fibers, accumulation of fluid in interstitial spaces, and deterioration of hyaline membrane. The premature release of enzymes from the cell lysosome when the membrane becomes more susceptible to lipid peroxidation and accompanying breakdown has been suggested as a cause of muscular dystrophy. Vitamin E levels in humans suffering from muscular dystrophy are normal. Thus no relationship has been established between vitamin E nutrition and human muscular dystrophy, which is believed to be a hereditary condition causing extensive wasting of certain voluntary muscles, with an onset from birth to adulthood.

In humans. Except in premature infants and in persons suffering from malabsorption, vitamin E deficiency is rarely seen in humans. Certain biochemical changes have been associated with a low dietary intake coupled with either an increased need, as in a diet high in vegetable oils with a high polyunsaturated fatty acid content, or with conditions that interfere with fat absorption. Increased susceptibility of the membrane of the erythrocytes to hemolysis is the most easily detected evidence of vitamin E deficiency. Other indications of vitamin E inadequacy are a drop in the level of tocopherol in blood, an increase in urinary excretion of creatine, and a decrease in creatinine excretion.

Work done on induced vitamin E deficiencies in Illinois mental patients indicates that with 3 mg of tocopherol in the diet, plasma tocopherol levels drop below normal values of 1 mg/dl of blood. This drop is accompanied by an increased tendency to hemolysis in red blood cells, especially on intakes below 0.5 mg of tocopherol. When the lard (low in polyunsaturated fatty acids) in the diet was replaced by corn oil (high in polyunsaturated fatty acids), a further drop occurred in serum tocopherol levels. An already high rate of erythrocyte hemolysis was not increased further. Larger amounts of vitamin E were required to maintain normal blood tocopherol levels when corn oil was substituted for lard.

In premature infants with an impaired ability to absorb vitamin E, hemolytic anemia, which is exaggerated by the administration of large amounts of iron that promotes the oxidation or destruction of vitamin E, has been observed. The ability to absorb vitamin E develops only with gestational maturity; therefore, the premature infant with poor fat absorption may need other forms of vitamin E. The observation that infants who suffer sudden unexpected death (SUD) have blood levels of vitamin E similar to those of premature infants has led to suggestions that the respiratory stress to which SUD is attributed may be the result of low antioxidant protection of the membranes in early life.

Low serum levels of vitamin E have been associated with a macrocytic anemia in which the life span of the red blood cells is decreased and the synthesis of both DNA and RNA is increased. Children with both kwashiorkor and the vitamin A deficiency disease xerophthalmia have much lower serum tocopherol levels and a greatly reduced chance of responding to therapy than do children with kwashiorkor without xerophthalmia. Low blood levels of vitamin E, but no other symptoms that respond to vitamin E therapy, are found in children and young adults suffering from cystic fibrosis. These individuals have a defect in the ability to absorb fat and hence fat-soluble vitamins.

Substitutes

Much of the confusion over the role of vitamin E has risen because of the ability of many other chemically unrelated substances to substitute for some or all of the many biochemical functions of the tocopherols. The mineral selenium either replaces vitamin E as an antioxidant or spares it. However, the distribution of selenium in certain tissues may be low, thereby explaining its failure to protect against all vitamin E deficiencies. The distribution of selenium in the diet is unrelated to vitamin E.

Ubichromenol has been shown to have vitamin E activity and the chemical antioxidant DPPD (*N,N'*-diphenyl-*p*-phenylene) can replace vitamin E in preventing fetal resorptions in rats.

The presence of the sulfur-containing amino acid cystine also increases the antioxidative effectiveness of vitamin E and its substitutes.

Clinical uses

Since vitamin E is present in such a wide variety of foods, is stored in the body, and turns over very slowly, there have been few demonstrated clinical cases of vitamin E deficiency. However, because of the seemingly unrelated pathological changes in tocopherol deficiencies in animals there has been a temptation to use vitamin E in the treatment of over sixty different conditions. No relationship between vitamin E nutrition and either the cause or the cure of these conditions has been confirmed. It has been prescribed in large dosages, essentially as a drug, in the treatment of diseases of the circulatory, reproductive, and nervous systems and as protection against the effects of aging and air pollution. Some 2000 articles have appeared on the therapeutic uses of vitamin E. Contradictory reports on its effectiveness continue to appear, and in a few cases reasonable evidence of its therapeutic value exists.

Substantial evidence shows that the use of therapeutic dosages of 400 IU daily for three months were effective in relieving calf pain when walking, a condition technically known as intermittent claudication. Vitamin E in tissues provides some protection against the detrimental effect of pollutants in the air such as ozone and nitrogen dioxide. Some forms of ulcers have responded well to the use of vitamin E, but evidence is insufficient to support claims for its effectiveness in muscular dystrophy, male infertility, diabetes, complications of menopause, gangrene, and many others. Controlled studies have failed to demonstrate any benefits to performance of physical fitness from use of 400 mg of vitamin E a day for six weeks.

Perhaps the most controversial of all clinical applications of vitamin E has been its widely acclaimed usefulness in the treatment of various forms of heart disease. In no case have the results of controlled studies demonstrated any of the beneficial effects attributed to vitamin E, such as reduced blood clotting time, vasodilation, or oxygen sparing. Proponents of the use of the vitamin assert that the dosage given in the controlled studies was inadequate while the opponents point to use of other forms of medication along with vitamin E in the cases in which success has been claimed.

Almost as widespread as the use of vitamin

E in heart disease has been its use in treating women who have suffered repeated spontaneous abortions. Although there is some evidence to support this application of the vitamin, the results of most tests have been at best discouraging, even though vitamin E possibly enhances utilization of oxygen by the placenta. In spite of some evidence of beneficial effects from vitamin E in preventing male sterility or altering the outcome of pregnancy, most clinicians believe that it is of no benefit.

In light of the tremendous number of anecdotal claims for therapeutic uses of vitamin E, it seems desirable to subject at least the most plausible ones to scrutiny under controlled experimental conditions before dismissing them all as useless. Good evidence exists to support the therapeutic use of vitamin E when absorption of fat has been depressed, when the intake of polyunsaturated fatty acids has increased, or in severe protein deficiency.

Toxicity

The extent of self-medication with massive dosages of vitamin E has given rise to concern over the possibility of toxicity resulting.

Table 11-6. Interrelationship and properties of compounds with vitamin K activity

Naturally occurring (fat-soluble)	Synthetic		
	Fat-soluble	Water-soluble	Water-miscible
Form			
Phytylmenaquinone		Synkayvite	Mephyton
Green plants		Hykinone	Konakion
Multiprenylmenaquinone	Menaquinone		Mono-Kay
Bacterial synthesis	(Menadione)		
Mode of administration			
Orally (except for infants)	Subcutaneously		Orally
Intravenously	Intramuscularly		Intramuscularly
Subcutaneously			Subcutaneously
			Intravenously
Uses			
Orally several days before delivery	Obstructive jaundice		1 mg to newborn
To counteract anticoagulants	Woman in labor		
Gastrointestinal surgery	Newborn		
Special precautions			
No side effects	Small margin of safety		Wide margin of safety
	Safe after first few weeks		
	Large doses produce hemolytic anemia, hyperbilirubinemia, and kernicterus		

So far, the limited number of studies have shown that vitamin E is the least toxic of the fat-soluble vitamins, but the effects of long-term supplementation of the diet have not been assessed. There is considerable reason to believe that high intake of vitamin E increases the need for the other fat-soluble vitamins and that it reduces the amount of vitamin A formed and stored in the liver. In the absence of any evidence supporting the use of high levels, and with the possibility of adverse effects, there is no reason to encourage the use of supplements, especially at the levels currently available on the open market (100 to 800 mg). Aside from causing gastrointestinal distress in a few individuals, intakes of up to 300 mg appear innocuous but also unnecessary and of no known effectiveness.

Evaluation of vitamin E status

There is currently no good test for determining vitamin E status. Blood levels do not reflect either intake or storage levels. Plasma tocopherol levels may be meaningful if reported in relation to total plasma lipids. A ratio of 0.8 mg of tocopherol per gram of lipids is indicative of adequate vitamin E status. The widely used test of measuring the extent of hemolysis, or rupture of red blood cells, is considered a crude indicator. Hemolysis does not occur until blood levels of tocopherol drop below 0.5 mg.

VITAMIN K

Vitamin K was first discovered in 1934 by a Danish scientist who identified it as the fat-soluble factor necessary for the coagulation of the blood. Since the Danish word for the process is *Koagulation,* he designated this factor as vitamin K. The term *vitamin K* now is used to designate a group of substances belonging to a chemical group known as quinones. These include the naturally occurring fat-soluble vitamins phytylmenaquinone and multiprenylmenaquinone (found in animal foods), formerly known as vitamins K_1 and K_2, respectively, and the synthetic related substance menaquinone, formerly known as vitamin K_3 or menadione. Current evidence suggests that phytylmenaquinone is the biologically active form of the vitamin and that the cells are able to convert the other forms into it. This form of the vitamin occurs primarily in green leafy plants and was first isolated from alfalfa meal in 1939. Multiprenylmenaquinone has 35 carbons in its side chain and is produced by bacterial synthesis in the gastrointestinal tract. It has also been isolated from putrified fish meal.

In addition to the naturally occurring vitamin K and synthetic menaquinone, all of which are fat soluble, Hykinone and Synkayvite are water soluble, and Mephyton, Konakion, and Mono-Kay are water miscible. These latter forms have properties that make them especially suited to the treatment of vitamin K deficiencies when fat absorption is impaired. The relationship among these various forms is somewhat confusing. Table 11-6 attempts to clarify these interrelationships and tabulates the special properties of each.

The naturally occurring fat-soluble forms of the vitamin may be stored in the body, primarily in the liver.

Vitamin K is stable to heat and reducing agents but is destroyed by light, acid, alkali, oxidizing agents, and alcohol.

Functions

The only established function of vitamin K is in the synthesis of blood-clotting factors. The ability of the blood to coagulate is dependent on the presence of many factors, among which are prothrombin and factors IV, VII, IX, and X. Vitamin K appears to be necessary for the conversion of a protein precursor of prothrombin in the synthesis of prothrombin. This activation of the precursor, which involves a chemical process called carboxylation, occurs primarily in the liver. Similarly, vitamin K stimulates the conversion of the precursor of fibrinogen, another factor involved in blood coagulation, into fibrin and accelerates its release into the circulation.

Prothrombin levels in the blood determine

the rate at which the blood will clot, high levels indicating good coagulability and low levels a depressed rate of coagulation. There is some reason to believe that vitamin K is also required in bloodclotting.

Coenzyme Q, which is a link in the respiratory chain of reactions involved in the ultimate release of energy from fatty acids and glucose, is similar to vitamin K chemically. Vitamin K participates in cellular respiration in lower forms of animals.

Absorption

Since vitamin K is fat soluble, its absorption is regulated by the same factors that govern fat absorption. An obstruction of the bile duct limiting the secretion of fat-emulsifying bile salts, as occurs in obstructive jaundice, will reduce absorption, as will failure of the liver to secrete bile. The use of a nonutilizable oil such as mineral oil as a laxative will cause the excretion of vitamin K in the feces.

Vitamin K is absorbed in the upper part of the gastrointestinal tract, as are other fat-related factors. Studies using radioactively labeled isotopes of fat-soluble forms of vitamin K showed that it is excreted in both the bile and the urine, whereas water-soluble forms are excreted rapidly, primarily in the urine.

An anticoagulant, Dicumarol, which is similar chemically to vitamin K, stimulates the formation of vitamin K oxide in the liver. This substance then inhibits or interferes with the role of vitamin K in stimulating the conversion of prothrombin precursor to prothrombin. The widespread use of anticoagulant drugs in phlebitis and thrombosis has made the use of vitamin K therapy more important to control hemorrhaging.

Requirements

The National Research Council recognizes vitamin K as a dietary essential but has been unable to make any quantitative evaluation of needs because of its abundance in most diets.

Only for newborn infants is there any need for special attention to vitamin K. The American Academy of Pediatrics estimates that the newborn infant requires from 0.15 to 0.25 μg/kg daily. Assuming 10% absorption of orally administered vitamin K, a daily intake of 0.2 mg (200 μg) would appear adequate for the neonate. Similarly, adult requirements are estimated at 0.3 to 15.0 μg/kg.

Sources

For most individuals adequate levels of vitamin K are provided by green and yellow vegetables and from the synthesis of the vitamin by intestinal bacteria. The concentration of vitamin K in foods is highest in dark leafy green vegetables, with some being found in fruits, tubers, and seeds. It usually occurs in association with chlorophyll in the chloroplasts. Alfalfa is an especially rich source, but in spite of the efforts of health-food advocates, it is not an accepted item in the average diet. No evidence of adult dietary inadequacies exists to warrant suggestions that the diet be supplemented with such a rich source.

Since much of the intestinal synthesis occurs in the lower intestine, only a small portion of that synthesized may actually be absorbed. The amount synthesized will also be reduced when substances are taken that depress the growth of intestinal bacteria. Salicylic acid, an ingredient in most pain depressants of the aspirin type, and certain antibiotics and sulfonamides may act in this way.

Young infants are the ones most likely to suffer from a subnormal level of intestinal synthesis. During the first few days of life their relatively sterile intestinal tract does not contain the organisms that synthesize vitamin K. Little vitamin K passes the placental barrier from the maternal circulation to be stored in fetal tissue, although if vitamin K is given to the mother at delivery, a sufficient amount passes to stimulate prothrombin levels. Milk is low in vitamin K; therefore even those infants who receive nourishment in the first few days of life do not receive an appreciable amount of vitamin K. Breast-fed infants are at an even greater disadvantage than bottle-fed infants because mother's milk is often not produced in significant amounts for several days. It contains about a fourth of the amount of vitamin K as does cow's milk and there is less chance of vitamin K-synthesizing bacteria developing in the lower intestine where *Lactobacillus bifidus* is the predominant organism. As a result breast-fed infants have a prolonged blood clotting time compared to bottle-fed infants.

Older infants who are fed a meat-based or casein hydrolysate formula are more prone to vitamin K deficiency, since such a diet suppresses the activity of intestinal organisms. In cases of malabsorption, such as occurs in cystic fibrosis, diarrhea, starvation, and with the use of antibiotics, the amount of vitamin K available is reduced and the use of supplements is suggested.

Deficiency

A prolonged coagulation time and an increased incidence of hemorrhage are the only known symptoms of a vitamin K deficiency.

Because vitamin K can be synthesized and also is provided in adequate amounts in practically all diets, a deficiency in adults is invariably caused by a failure in absorption. Recent studies have linked the bruising and increased blood clotting time observed in over 50% of a group of elderly persons with vitamin K deficiency. The deficiency was attributed to liver disease, poor absorption, and use of salicylates (aspirin).

In infants, however, the lack of bacteria to synthesize vitamin K, the low stores of vitamin K in the infant at birth, and the small amount provided in milk characteristically lead to low prothrombin levels and a prolonged coagulation time. This occurs at a time when the incidence of hemorrhage is high. The association between vitamin K and blood coagulation times led to the routine administration of vitamin K either to the mother just prior to delivery or to the infant in the first few days of life to reduce neonatal deaths caused by hemorrhage. However, an increase in a hemolytic type of anemia, an accumulation of bilirubin in the blood, and a condition known as kernicterus, in which bile pigment accumulates in the gray matter of the central nervous system, were attributed to vitamin K toxicity from the uncontrolled use of synthetic vitamin K. An evaluation of vitamin K therapy in newborn infants has shown that it is desirable but that certain precautions should be observed to provide the greatest benefits and the greatest margin of safety.

Several studies have shown that the normal incidence of hemorrhage of the newborn of 1 in 400 infants is markedly reduced with vitamin K therapy and especially in babies who may get less than adequate oxygen at birth. Natural vitamin K is considered the most desirable form, as there have been no reports of toxicity from oral administration of 1 to 2 mg. Dosages of 0.5 to 1 mg of water-miscible preparation provide protection when given intravenously or intramuscularly to the infant. Synthetic vitamin K cannot be given orally, as it causes vomiting. A dose of 2 to 5 mg given to the mother usually transfers adequate protection to the infant, but larger doses may be hazardous to some infants. It is recommended that protection be provided by administering natural vitamin K to the infant after birth rather than to the mother, with larger doses recommended for an infant whose mother has been given anticoagulant therapy. It can be given orally, subcutaneously, intramuscularly, or intravenously. The Food and Drug Administration has prohibited the inclusion of vitamin K in prenatal supplements.

BIBLIOGRAPHY

Bieri, J. G.: Fat-soluble vitamins in the eighth revision of the Recommended Dietary Allowances, J. Am. Diet. Assoc. **64:**171, 1974.

Vitamin A

American Academy of Pediatrics: The use and abuse of vitamin A, Pediatrics **48:**655, 1971.

Ames, S. R.: Factors affecting absorption, transport,

and storage of vitamin A, Am. J. Clin. Nutr. **22**:934, 1969.

Bieri, J.: Effect of excessive vitamins C and E on vitamin A status, Am. J. Clin. Nutr. **26**:382, 1973.

Chopra, J. G., and Kevany, J.: Hypovitaminosis A in the Americas, Am. J. Clin. Nutr. **23**:231, 1970.

Dowling, J. E., and Wald, G.: Role of vitamin A acid, Vitam. Horm. **18**:515, 1960.

Editorial: Hypervitaminosis A.: its broadening spectrum, Am. J. Clin. Nutr. **6**:335, 1958.

Goodman. D. S., and Huang, H. S.: Biosynthesis of vitamin A with rat intestinal enzymes, Science **149**:879, 1965.

Greaves, J. P., and Tan. J.: Vitamin A and carotene in British and American diets, Br. J. Nutr. **20**:819, 1966.

Herbert, V.: Megavitamin therapy: facts and fictions, Food Nutr. News **47**(4):1976.

McLaren, D. S., Shirajan, R., Tchalian, M., and Khoury, G.: Xerophthalmia in Jordan, Am. J. Clin. Nutr. **17**:117, 1965.

McLaren, D. S., Tchalian, M., and Ajans, Z. A.: Biochemical and hematologic changes in the vitamin A-deficient rat, Am. J. Clin. Nutr. **17**:131, 1965.

Michaelsson, G., Juhlin, L., and Vahlquist, A.: Effects of oral zinc and vitamin A in acne, Arch. Dermatol. **113**:31, 1977.

Olson, J. A.: The alpha and omega of vitamin A metabolism, Am. J. Clin. Nutr. **22**:953, 1969.

Olson, J. A.: Metabolism and function of vitamin A, Fed. Proc. **28**:1670, 1969.

Owen, E. C.: Some aspects of the metabolism of vitamin A and carotene, World Rev. Nutr. Diet. **5**:132, 1965.

Rodrequez, M. S., and Irwin, M. I.: A conspectus of research on vitamin A requirements of man, J. Nutr. **102**:909, 1972.

Smith, J. E., and Goodman, D. S.: Vitamin A metabolism and transport. In Sipple, H., and McNutt, K., editors: Present knowledge of nutrition, ed. 3, New York, 1976, Nutrition Foundation, Inc.

Underwood, B. A., Siegel, H., Weisell, R. C., and Dolinski, M.: Liver stores of vitamin A in a normal population dying suddenly or rapidly from unnatural causes in New York City, Am. J. Clin. Nutr. **23**:1037, 1970.

Wolf, G.: International symposium on metabolic function of vitamin A, Am. J. Clin. Nutr. **22**:903, 1969.

Wolf, G.: Some thoughts on the metabolic role of Vitamin A, Nutr. Rev. **20**:161, 1962.

Vitamin D

Avioli, L. V., and Haddad, J. G.: Vitamin D: current concepts, Metabolism **22**:507, 1973.

Bronner, F.: Recent advances in vitamin D: clinical implications, Am. J. Clin. Nutr. **29**:1253, 1976.

Bronner, F.: Vitamin D deficiency and rickets, Am. J. Clin. Nutr. **29**:1307, 1976.

Committee on Nutrition: The prophylactic requirement and toxicity of vitamin D, Pediatrics **31**:512, 1963.

Committee on Nutrition: Vitamin D intake and the hypercalcemic syndrome, Pediatrics **35**:1022, 1965.

DeLuca, H. F.: Metabolism of vitamin D: current status, Am. J. Clin. Nutr. **29**:1258, 1976.

DeLuca, H. F.: Vitamin D: the vitamin and the hormone, Fed. Proc. **33**:2211, 1974.

Ebel, J. G., Taylor, A. N., and Wasserman, R. H.: Vitamin D-induced calcium-binding protein of intestinal mucosa, Am. J. Clin. Nutr. **22**:431, 1969.

Food and Nutrition Board: Hazards of overuse of vitamin D, Nutr. Rev. **33**:61, 1975.

Harris, F., Hoffenberg, R., and Blach, E.: Calcium kinetics in vitamin D deficiency rickets, Metabolism **14**:1101, 1965.

Harrison, H. E.: Vitamin D and permeability of intestinal mucosa to calcium, Am. J. Physiol. **208**:370, 1965.

Haussler, M. R.: Vitamin D: mode of action and biomedical applications Nutr. Rev. **32**:257, 1974.

Kimberg, D. V.: Effect of vitamin D and steroid hormones on the active transport of calcium by the intestine, N. Engl. J. Med. **280**:396, 1969.

Lukert, B. P., and Adams, J. S.: Vitamin D metabolism in man, Arch. Intern. Med. **136**:1241, 1976.

Norman, A. W.: Actinomycin D and the response to vitamin D, Science **149**:184, 1965.

Omdahl, J. L., and DeLuca, H. F.: Regulation of vitamin D; metabolism and function, Physiol. Rev. **53**:327, 1973.

Stamp, T. C. B.: Vitamin D metabolism, Arch. Dis. Child. **48**:2, 1973.

Vitamin E

Bieri, J.: Vitamin E, Nutr. Rev. **33**:161, 1975.

Booth, V. H., and Bradford, M. P.: Tocopherol content of fruits and vegetables, Br. J. Nutr. **17**:575, 1963.

Bunnell, R. H., Keating, J., Quaresimo, A., and Parman, G. K.: Alpha-tocopherol content of foods, Am. J. Clin. Nutr. **17**:1, 1965.

Farrel, P. M., and Bieri, J. G.: Megavitamin E supplementation in man, Am. J. Clin. Nutr. **28**:1381, 1975.

Green, J., and Bunyan, J.: Vitamin E and the biological antioxidant theory, Nutr. Abstr. Rev. **39**:321, 1969.

Haeger, K.: Long-time treatment of intermittent claudication with vitamin E, Am. J. Clin. Nutr. **27**:1179, 1974.

Herting, D. C.: Perspectives on vitamin E, Am. J. Clin. Nutr. **19**:210, 1966.

Hodges, R. E.: Vitamin E and coronary heart disease, J. Am. Diet. Assoc. **62**:638, 1973.

Horwitt, M. K.: Vitamin E: a reexamination, Am. J. Clin. Nutr. **29**:569, 1976.

Horwitt, M. K.: Vitamin E: biochemistry, nutritional requirements, and clinical studies, Symposium, Am. J. Clin. Nutr. **27**:939, 1974.

Institute of Food Technologists: Vitamin E, Nutr. Rev. **35**:57, 1977.

Olsen, R. E.: Vitamin E and its relation to heart disease, Circulation **48**:179, 1973.

Parman, G. K.: Alpha-tocopherol content of foods, Am. J. Clin. Nutr. **17:**1, 1965.

Supplementation of human diets with vitamin E, Nutr. Rev. **31:**327, 1973.

Suttee, J. W.: Vitamin K and prothrombin synthesis, Nutr. Rev. **31:**105, 1973.

Tappel, A. L.: Will antioxidant nutrients slow aging processes? Geriatrics **23:**97, 1968.

Wasserman, R. H., and Taylor, A. N.: Metabolic roles of fat-soluble vitamins D, E and K, Ann. Rev. Biochem. **41:**179, 1972.

Vitamin K

Committee on Nutrition: Vitamin K compounds and the water-soluble analogues, Pediatrics **28:**501, 1961.

Goldman, H. I., and Amades, P.: Vitamin K deficiency after the newborn period, Pediatrics **44:**745, 1969.

Johnson, B. C.: Dietary factors and vitamin K, Nutr. Rev. **22:**225, 1964.

Olson, R.: Present knowledge of vitamin K. In Sipple, H., and McNutt, K., editors: Present knowledge of nutrition, ed. 3, New York, 1976, Nutrition Foundation, Inc.

Owen, G. M., Nelson, C. E., Baker, G. L., Connor, W. E., and Jacobs, J. P.: Use of vitamin K_1 in pregnancy, Am. J. Obstet. Gynecol. **99:**368, 1967.

Vitamin K and prothrombin structure, Nutr. Rev. **32:**279, 1974.

Wefring, K. W.: Hemorrhage in the newborn and vitamin K prophylaxis, J. Pediatr. **63:**663, 1963.

12

Water-soluble vitamins

Each of the water-soluble vitamins, vitamin C and members of the B complex, plays a unique role in body metabolism. Although there are some interactions among these nutrients, each must be treated individually in considering its role in diets. Intakes moderately in excess of needs are readily excreted in the urine. Intakes at several times normal requirements, however, must be considered as pharmacological doses with the possible harmful side effects.

ASCORBIC ACID

Vitamin C, cevitamic acid, hexuronic acid, and ascorbic acid are names that at one time or another have been applied to the antiscorbutic (scurvy-preventive) substance isolated from lemon juice in 1932 by King and Waugh. Almost simultaneously, Szent-Györgyi found it in the suprarenal gland, located near the kidneys, and in oranges and cabbage.

Descriptions of scurvy can be found in a papyrus from 1500 BC found at Thebes, in the writings of Hippocrates in 400 BC and in other early recorded history. It had been known for almost 400 years that scurvy could be controlled by dietary means and since 1906 that it was a deficiency disease, but the search for the effective agent ended only with the isolation of the relatively simple white crystals of vitamin C in 1932.

The conquest of scurvy, in which the symptoms are dramatic and clear-cut, is of special historical interest because it was in an effort to cure this "scourge of the Navy" that the first carefully conceived nutrition experiment was conducted with humans. Seamen who embarked on long sea voyages without an opportunity to replenish supplies for long periods did so knowing that a large portion of the crew would die or be incapacitated by scurvy. For instance, Magellan lost many of the 196 men who started around Cape Horn with him in 1520, and in 1497 Vasco da Gama lost 100 of 150 men. In 1775 Captain Cook's crew was spared by his insistence that they eat a thick soup he called "sour krout." Cartier's vivid description of the disease as it affected his men at Quebec in 1536 is classic.

"Legs became swollen and puffed up while the sinews contracted and turned coal-black and, in some cases, all blotched with drops of purplish blood. Gums were so decayed that the flesh peeled off down to the roots of the teeth while the latter almost all fell out . . . by February out of our group of 110 there were not ten left in good health . . . already eight were dead, and over fifty more were given up for lost."*

In 1747 Lind, a British physician, hypothesized that various "acidic principles" might have antiscorbutic properties. To test his theory he assigned twelve sailors suffering from scurvy into six groups of two each and fed them the ship's basic diet plus one of five potential cures—oil of vitriol (sulfuric acid) in water three times a day, 2 teaspoonsful of vinegar three times a day, ½ pint of seawater

*From Jacques Cartier's journal as cited in Anderson, T. W.: New horizons for vitamin C, Nutr. Today **12:**6, 1977.

a day, and two oranges, or one lemon, a day. The results of his experiment are now legendary—both oranges and lemons had miraculous curative powers; the sailors assigned to this treatment were restored to active duty within six days, whereas those on other treatments showed no progress. Not only did Lind prove that scurvy could be cured, but he laid the foundation for the theory that lack of an essential food element could cause illness. Others had advanced similar theories even a century earlier, but their observations had gone virtually unnoticed.

It was fifty years before the British Navy recognized Lind's work to the point of requiring that all ships leaving British ports carry sufficient lime juice to have it available for its crew throughout the whole voyage. The routine use of lime juice led to the term "limey" to refer to a British seaman, a term that now has extended to all British servicemen.

Although the British Navy was the first to take steps to prevent scurvy, many other groups had suffered from it and in some cases had found a cure. Crusaders believed that those who could survive the pain that attacked feet and legs and the changes in their gums until spring would usually be cured by warm temperatures, a time that coincides with the availability of fresh fruit and vegetables. Cartier's expedition, which was forced to spend a winter in Canada in 1536, was spared when the Indians taught his group to use the bark of a pine tree, the ameda, which contains only small amounts of vitamin C, to cure scurvy. French and Spanish sailors were saved because of the quantities of onions and leeks they consumed. Sailors in the Mediterranean were seldom away long enough to deplete their tissue reserves of vitamin C. Scurvy had been known to occur in the late spring in European cities but not in rural areas. By this time, city dwellers had been reduced to a diet of meat and bread, whereas their counterparts in the country still had some cabbage, onions, and potatoes left in storage. After failure of the potato crop even rural populations experienced scurvy outbreaks. Spaniards landing after long sea voyages in California in 1602, 1603, and again in 1769 lost many of their numbers, and their first task after landing was the search for an herb or plant to cure scurvy. As late as 1846 Mormons making their way west to Utah were forced to winter in Nebraska on a diet of mush. Many of them succumbed to scurvy as did troops in the Civil War.

Medical authorities who have considered scurvy a disease of the past were appalled by some reports of infantile scurvy in the 1960s and 1970s. Infantile scurvy (Fig. 12-1) was first reported in the late nineteenth century

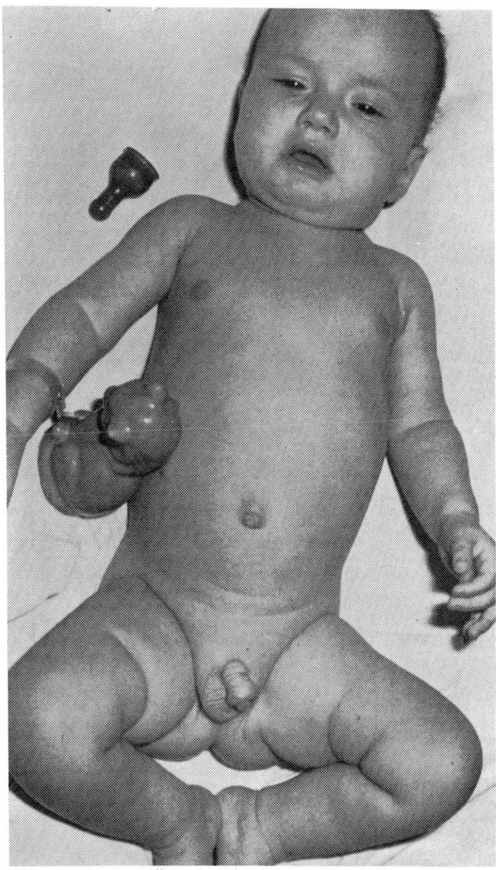

Fig. 12-1. Infant with scurvy. Note frog position of legs and apprehension of infant in anticipation of handling of tender limbs. (From Grewar, D.: Clin. Pediatr. [Phila.] **4**:82, 1965.)

and paralleled the change from wet nurses to the use of preserved milk. It increased again when pasturization of milk became mandatory. Again, it seemed to be occurring among bottle-fed infants whose formula had been subjected to prolonged heat treatment and who received no fruit juice or vitamin C concentrate.

Similarly, infants born to mothers taking megadoses of vitamin C during pregnancy have a conditioned need for more vitamin C than usually provided in milk or formula, and adults who suddenly stop taking large amounts also develop symptoms of scurvy.

The enrichment of infant formula, use of vitamin supplements, and encouragement of breast-feeding are among the most effective methods of assuring a vitamin C intake sufficient to prevent scurvy. A typical case of infantile scurvy is shown in Fig. 12-1.

Chemical properties

Chemically, ascorbic acid is a simple 6-carbon compound closely related to the monosaccharides. It is stable to acid but easily destroyed by oxidation, alkali, and heat. The synthetic form of the vitamin, first produced in 1933, is derived from the monosaccharides—glucose or galactose. Since the body cannot discriminate between natural and synthetic forms, they can be used interchangeably.

Synthetic vitamin C is used to enrich food products and in nutrient supplements, including the majority of those labeled "from natural acerola or rose hips." The extent to which synthetic vitamin C is used in the United States is evident from an announcement of the opening of a plant by one pharmaceutical company capable of producing 2.7 metric tons of the vitamin every day.

Vitamin C, with the formula $C_6H_8O_6$, is known as reduced ascorbic acid and is susceptible to oxidation. It has now been established that the first product of the oxidation of this biologically active compound, **dehydroascorbic acid** ($C_6H_6O_6$), which has 2 fewer hydrogens, can be used equally as well by the body. Some evidence exists that reduced ascorbic acid is changed in kidney cells to dehydroascorbic acid, a form in which it is more readily transported to the tissues. It also penetrates into the cell more easily in this oxidized form. It is apparently reduced again to the active form by the body before taking part in biological reactions. Further oxidation of dehydroascorbic acid produces a substance, diketogulonic acid, with no antiscorbutic properties. The oxidative process is irreversible. The changes are shown schematically in Fig. 12-2.

Another related compound, D-araboascorbic acid (isoascorbic acid) is less well absorbed. It has antiscorbutic properties, although it cannot fulfill the growth-promoting function of L-ascorbic acid.

Ascorbic acid sulfate also has **antiscorbutic** properties. It is not known, however, whether it is hydrolyzed to ascorbic acid with the removal of the sulfate before being absorbed.

Most animals have the ability to synthesize ascorbic acid and therefore need no dietary supply of it. This synthesis takes place primarily in the microsomes of the cell, especially liver cells. A few species lack the enzyme necessary to complete the conversion of glucose or galactose to ascorbic acid. Humans, monkeys, guinea pigs, Indian fruit bats, red-vented bulbul birds, carp, and trout are known to rely on a dietary source of ascorbic acid. Of these the guinea pig is used most extensively in research, but fish are proving useful in studies of the role of ascorbic acid in collagen formation.

In plants ascorbic acid is accumulated dur-

Ascorbic acid $\underset{\text{Reduction}}{\overset{\text{Oxidation}}{\rightleftharpoons}}$ Dehydroascorbic acid $\xrightarrow{\text{Oxidation}}$ Diketogulonic acid*

Fig. 12-2. Relationship of various chemical forms of ascorbic acid. *Biologically inactive form.

ing the ripening process, presumably synthesized in the plant cells from the natural glucose in fruit.

D-Ascorbic acid, structurally related to the biologically active L-ascorbic acid, is not utilized by humans unless it is given in small doses throughout the day. It is being used extensively as a preservative in processing meat. To avoid possible confusion and any implication that D-ascorbic acid is a vitamin, it has been recommended that the term *erythrobic acid* be applied to this compound.

Other reducing compounds have been found that can replace ascorbic acid in some of its biological roles, but none is effective in curing scurvy.

Functions

Although ascorbic acid is a relatively simple compound that has been available in a purified form at reasonable cost for over forty-five years, biochemists, nutritionists, and physiologists have been unable to shed much light on the nature of its biochemical role. It appears to be essential to the normal functioning of both plant and animal cells. In contrast to most water-soluble vitamins, it has no clear-cut role as a catalyst, nor is it part of any enzyme or structure. Fragments of knowledge that will eventually form the total picture suggest some of its potential roles, but the same general terms are still applied to ascorbic acid deficiency now as were used over fifty years ago. Following are some of the more widely accepted roles.

Collagen formation. The primary defect in vitamin C deficiency is the failure of collagen formation in the fibroblasts in connective tissue. Collagen, the protein substance that binds the cells together in much the same way that mortar binds bricks, is characterized by the amino acids hydroxyproline and hydroxylysine. Hydroxyproline, which constitutes a third of the amino acid composition of collagen, and hydroxylysine are not available from food. They are formed by hydroxylation, or the addition of a chemical unit (OH), once they have been incorporated in the amino acid chain of the collagen molecule. These reactions are catalyzed by ascorbic acid. Thus, in an ascorbic acid deficiency the basic building material for collagen is not formed and the unhydroxylated collagen fibers are then degraded and excreted. A failure in collagen synthesis is observed primarily in tissues subjected to stress. Most collagen is inert metabolically and once laid down does not require vitamin C for maintenance, but certain fractions of collagen in some tissues such as scar tissue are highly active and subject to rapid breakdown in ascorbic acid deficiency.

When the collagen is not formed or maintained in a scorbutic animal, the failure shows up in many ways. The need for ascorbic acid in healing of wounds is great. Here, new connective tissue, which is primarily collagen, must be formed. The high concentration of ascorbic acid found in scar tissue and the drops in blood level of the vitamin that occur during healing indicate that it is mobilized to the site of the healing. Immediately following an injury, fibroblast cells migrate to the wound area, multiply, and begin to synthesize short collagen units of the amino acids glycine, proline, and lysine. If vitamin C is not present, the proline cannot be changed to hydroxypoline. If it is available, these short units are excreted from the fibroblasts into the extracellular spaces, where they are united to form larger collagen fibers which bind the cells together, increase the strength of the scar tissue, and support the capillaries that accumulate in the wound area. Once a wound has healed, there is constant remodelling of the collagen with synthesis and destruction taking place alternately. High levels of vitamin C are maintained after the scar tissue has been completely formed, reflecting a need for maintenance of scar tissue. If there is a lack of vitamin C, the faster loss of collagen results in a weakening and breaking of the scar tissue.

Ascorbic acid may also be involved in maintaining the health of connective tissue through its role in transferring sulfate in the synthesis of the ground substance present between connective tissue cells.

There is some controversy regarding the need for increasing the dietary intake preoperatively and postoperatively for individuals whose tissues are apparently saturated with vitamin C. Some authorities recommend intakes of 100 to 300 mg daily to ensure rapid and complete healing, whereas others believe this is unnecessary. However, since no evidence of adverse effects from higher levels exists, there is little reason to forego possible benefits from larger intakes.

Small pinpoint hemorrhages occur with a lack of vitamin C due to weakness in the membranes that line the capillaries and in the fibers that join the cells together under the surface of the skin. Both of these tissues are composed of collagen, which is defective or absent when vitamin C is not available. Blood then escapes into the enlarged intercellular spaces, accounting for the capillary bleeding associated with scurvy. These subcutaneous hemorrhages show up most often in areas subjected to mechanical stress, such as the gums, which often become soft, spongy, and hemorrhage easily, and the ends of the long bones.

The matrix, which makes up a fifth of the weight of the bone shaft, is primarily collagen. If it is defective when collagen formation fails, it is less capable of holding calcium and phosphorus during bone calcification, resulting in weakened bone structure. The intercellular spaces do calcify, however. Sometimes bones are displaced when the supporting cartilage, which is also primarily collagen, is weakened as a result of a lack of vitamin C for maintenance. Characteristic bone changes in scurvy are shown in Fig. 12-3 and gum changes in Fig. 12-4.

Dentin formation. Changes in tooth structure have been related to ascorbic acid status during a critical period in tooth formation. The dentin layer, arising from a group of cells known as odontoblasts, does not form nor-

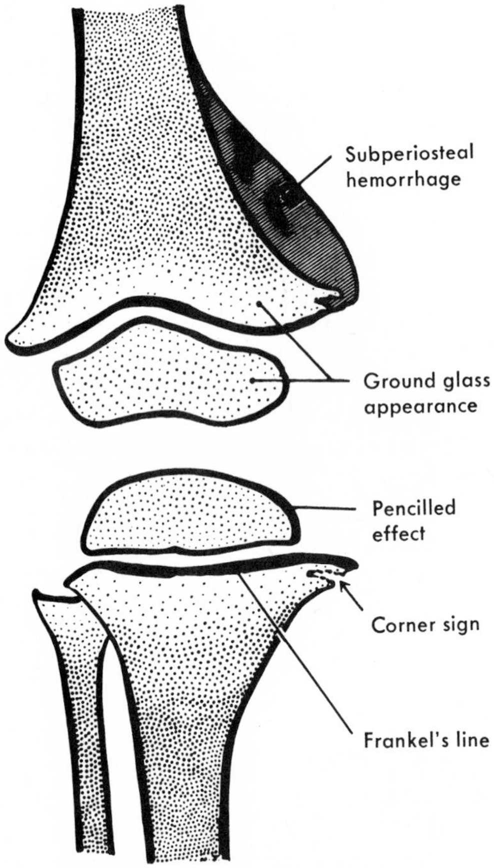

Fig. 12-3. Radiographic signs of scurvy in ends of long bones. (From Grewar, D.: Clin. Pediatr. [Phila.] **4:**82, 1965.)

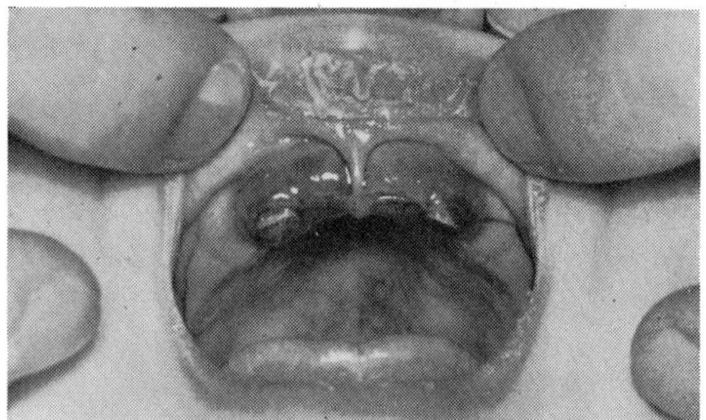

Fig. 12-4. Gum hemorrhage in scorbutic infant. Note occurrence only where teeth have erupted; it does not occur in edentulous gum. (From Grewar, D.: Clin. Pediatr. [Phila.] **4:**82, 1965.)

mally in scorbutic animals, apparently because of the degeneration of the odontoblasts at the time calcification of the dentin layer should occur. This, of course, produces a tooth with a structural weakness that is less able to resist mechanical injury or decay once it is initiated.

Tyrosine metabolism. Although it has been clearly demonstrated that vitamin C is necessary for the synthesis of the enzymes needed for the normal oxidation of large amounts of the amino acid tyrosine, it does not appear necessary to metabolize the amount of tyrosine present in the usual diet. Ascorbic acid may be needed, however, by premature infants on a relatively high-protein diet.

Synthesis of neurotransmitters. Two of the neurotransmitters, or substances needed to transfer nerve impulses from one cell to another, in the brain can be produced only if adequate vitamin C is available. It is needed to convert dopamine to the neurotransmitter norepinephrine and the amino acid tryptophan to the precursor of the neurotransmitter serotonin, which also plays a role in regulating blood pressure. Failure to produce these essential compounds may be responsible for the fatigue and weaknesss experienced by persons with scurvy.

Utilization of iron and calcium. The absorption of iron from the intestinal tract is facilitated by the presence of vitamin C. It is effective as a reducing agent by keeping ferrous iron in the reduced form in which it is most readily absorbed. Ascorbic acid also aids in the transfer of iron from the carrier transferrin to ferritin, the storage form of iron. The interrelationship with iron is also evident in that vitamin C activates some iron-containing enzymes. The role of ascorbic acid in facilitating calcium absorption may involve preventing its precipitation as an insoluble complex by creating an acid medium in the stomach.

Utilization of folic acid. The conversion of the inactive form of the vitamin folic acid to the active form, the citrovorum factor, is catalyzed by ascorbic acid. It may be in this way that vitamin C is effective in preventing the megaloblastic anemia of infancy.

Other functions. Many other functions have been attributed to ascorbic acid. In some cases the evidence indicates a strong possibility of a relationship, but no explanation of the biochemical mechanism involved has been found.

It is reasonable to assume that the high levels of ascorbic acid in the adrenal gland reflect a need for the vitamin in either the synthesis or secretion of steroid hormones in response to stress. However, so far, no acceptable explanation of a biochemical role has been identified.

It is possible that through its role in lipid metabolism ascorbic acid may be involved in the prevention of atherosclerosis. It may mobilize cholesterol from the arterial wall, stimulate the conversion of cholesterol to bile acids, or decrease the release of fat from storage depots into the blood, keeping blood lipid levels low. In heart disease it is proposed that vitamin C helps maintain heart muscles so that they are less susceptible to lack of blood.

A preventive role for ascorbic acid in cancer control is highly speculative. As a reducing agent it could prevent the oxidation of harmless precursors to carcinogens or promote the synthesis of mucopolysaccharides (ground substance), which inhibit the growth of cancerous cells; alternatively it may provide protection against the stress of surgery, chemotherapy, or radiotherapy.

Evidence that ascorbic acid acts to detoxify histamine, which is increased under conditions of stress, may explain its apparent effect in alleviating symptoms of many conditions such as hay fever or frostbite. Ascorbic acid blood levels drop with smoking, although there is no biochemical explanation of this observation.

The presence of ascorbic acid sulfate in many tissues has suggested a role in the transfer of sulfate molecules necessary for the formation of many essential body compounds such as chondroitin and mucopolysaccharide, components of skin, nails, and mucous secretions. It is also proposed that ascorbic acid sulfate is the form in which ascorbic acid crosses the blood-brain barrier, accounting for the concentration in the brain tissue. The sulfation of cholesterol may result in its mobilization from tissues and its eventual excretion in the urine as a water-soluble compound, accounting for the lowering of blood cholesterol levels observed on the administration of ascorbic acid. A similar effect has been attributed to the role of ascorbic acid in the conversion of cholesterol to bile acids, the form in which much cholesterol is excreted.

Studies in guinea pigs have demonstrated a synergistic relation between ascorbic acid and the amino acid methionine in protecting against the adverse effects of nitrites.

The low blood levels of ascorbic acid reported in infections such as tuberculosis may be caused by a shift of the vitamin to the infected tissue. Much the same mechanism seems to operate during stress, with the mobilization of ascorbic acid from tissues of the body to be concentrated in traumatized areas.

In the case of burns, skin grafts heal more quickly when ascorbic acid is present.

Large doses of ascorbic acid (525 mg a day) have been demonstrated as beneficial in exposure to low environmental temperatures. The subjects maintained skin temperature more readily and experienced fewer and less severe symptoms of frostbitten feet. It is postulated that vitamin C accelerates the metabolism of the amino acids tyrosine and phenylalanine, precursors of the hormones thyroxin and epinephrine which may stimulate basal metabolic rate and hence heat production.

Ascorbic acid has been effective in the treatment of such conditions as poisoning, hay fever, arsenic sensitivity, cadmium toxicity, and muscular pains.

Biochemically, evidence exists that ascorbic acid has a sparing action in relation to several vitamins of the B complex group—thiamin, riboflavin, niacin, pantothenic acid, pyridoxine, biotin, and folic acid. In some cases it appears to replace them; in others it prevents their destruction.

Dehydroascorbic acid may function in the regulation of cell division by controlling the release of the enzymes that initiate mitosis, or cell division.

Absorption and metabolism

Ascorbic acid is absorbed by humans in the upper part of the intestine, either by simple diffusion or a sodium-dependent active transport mechanism and is circulated in the blood.

The level of ascorbic acid in the serum reflects the usual intake of the vitamin, reaching a maximum of about 12 mg/L on an intake of 100 mg/day and dropping to a level of 1 to 2 mg when the intake is less than 10 mg/day. Intakes above 100 mg do not result in any further increase in ascorbic acid levels. However, immediately following ingestion of vitamin C the amount in the serum is temporarily elevated until the excess is either picked up by the tissues able to store it or excreted in the urine. The highest concentration (60 mg/100 g) is found in the adrenal gland, but because of its small size, the total amount stored there is less than in the larger brain and liver, where the concentration is 46 and 14 mg/100 g, respectively. Although tissues such as the adrenal gland and the liquid in the eye have concentrations up to fifty times that in the serum, others such as the kidneys, spleen, and liver have levels in equilibrium with those of the blood. The amount in muscle is relatively small (2 mg/100 g) but because of its mass, as much as 600 mg may be held in the muscles of a 70 kg man. Before it can be picked up from the blood for storage in the tissues, reduced ascorbic acid must be changed in the kidneys to the oxidized form, dehydroascorbic acid. In either form, energy is required for the nutrient to enter the cell.

The total pool of ascorbic acid in the body has been estimated to be from 1500 to 4000 mg, sufficient to prevent the onset of scurvy for ninety days on a vitamin C–free diet. The pool declines at a rate of about 3% a day until it reaches 300 mg and signs of scurvy begin to appear. After that the rate at which vitamin C stores are depleted declines noticeably.

Ascorbic acid is excreted primarily in the urine. As the vitamin passes through the kidneys, enough is reabsorbed to maintain a plasma concentration of 12 to 14 mg/100 g. Once that level is reached, little ascorbic acid is retained, and any excess is lost in the urine. Most of that lost in the urine has been changed to other metabolites of ascorbic acid, such as oxalic acid and threonic acid. The ability to excrete an excess means there is little likelihood of toxicity developing on high intakes. However, excessive doses may result in an accumulation of oxalic acid in the kidneys, which has potentially harmful effects in promoting the formation of kidney stones. A small portion, about 2%, of the vitamin C intake is broken down to carbon dioxide and water and expired through the lungs.

For women taking contraceptive pills it is difficult to maintain normal tissue levels. These orally administered sex hormones may stimulate the metabolism of ascorbic acid or increase its excretion.

Requirements

In the case of ascorbic acid there has been considerable controversy as to what criteria should be used in establishing recommended allowances. Some scientists base their estimates on the amount capable of preventing scurvy and maintaining a high level of health. Others recommend a higher amount that will permit tissue saturation and still not introduce any potential hazard.

Adults. Current standards reflect consideration of recent information that an intake leading to saturation of vitamin C reserves in the tissues is the most desirable. As a result, recommended levels are many times those known to prevent frank signs of scurvy. It has long been recognized that intakes as low as 6.5 mg a day are sufficient to prevent scurvy. (Lind provided 20 to 30 mg of ascorbic acid in the dosage he prescribed for the British Navy.) Some research suggests that minimum requirements may be even lower. In adults 10 mg has been shown to prevent scurvy for a year and to cure it in ten to fourteen weeks. However, the level for maintenance of optimal health is undoubtedly higher.

Recommended allowance for adults is based on the assumption that 30 mg is needed to replenish losses. This should allow for maintenance of an optimal level of health, optimal resistance to physiological and pathological stress, and maintenance of healthy gums. Saturation of adult tissues can be achieved at intakes of slightly over 80 mg in five weeks. No increase in benefits occurs with a large dose of 340 to 400 mg. No evidence exists to indicate that needs increase with age, although high levels may improve iron absorption in older persons whose level of hydrochloric acid secretion may be low. Storage of ascorbic acid declines with age.

Pregnancy. American standards for ascorbic acid intake in pregnancy are increased. This is based on studies indicating a drop in blood serum levels and a decreased urinary excretion during pregnancy. It has been established that the developing fetus is parasitic on the mother in respect to vitamin C. Plasma levels in the fetus remain high (two to four times as high as maternal levels), and a high concentration is also found in the placenta. The placenta may act as a barrier for the return of the vitamin to maternal circulation. Too high an intake by the mother during pregnancy may condition the infant to a rich supply so that he is much more susceptible to deficiency symptoms on restricted intakes.

Lactation. The ascorbic acid content of mother's milk reflects to a certain extent the dietary intake of the mother and usually varies from 4 to 8 mg/dl of milk. An intake of 80 mg a day by the mother should result in optimal levels in her milk.

The lack of agreement regarding what constitutes a desirable level of intake of ascorbic acid is evident from Table 12-1, which compares recommendations prevailing in various countries. Even when the different philoso-

Table 12-1. Comparison of dietary standards for ascorbic acid for selected age groups (in milligrams)*

		U.S. NRC	U.S.S.R.	Canada	Japan	Great Britain	Australia	Norway	FAO
Children	1-2 yr	40	40	30	15	—	30	20	20
	4-6 yr	40	50	20	40	20	30	30	20
Boys	12-14 yr	45	70	30	80	25	30	50	20
Men		45	70	30	65	30	30	30	30
Women		45	70	30	60	30	30	30	30
Pregnancy		60	100	50	100	60	80	50	50
Lactation		80	120	60	150	60	100	75	50

*Modified from Young, E.G.: Dietary standards. In Beaton, G., and McHenry, E. W.: Nutrition, II. New York, 1964, Academic Press, Inc.

phies on which the standards are based are considered, some obvious discrepancies still remain.

Infants. Based on the amount of ascorbic acid found in mother's milk (average, 4 to 8 mg/dl) it is believed that a breast-fed infant receives 15 to 50 mg daily. This leads to plasma ascorbic acid levels of 0.5 to 1.5 mg/dl. Cow's milk provides only 4 to 6 mg/dl and maintains much lower blood levels. It is recommended that 35 mg be a minimum level of supplementation and that premature infants receive double this dosage. Ascorbic acid supplementation should be started within the first ten days of life for bottle-fed infants not receiving a vitamin C–enriched formula. Orange juice diluted with water has been satisfactory for most children, but the fact that some developed allergic reactions when a portion of the oils from the rind were extracted along with the juice has resulted in more reliance on synthetic preparations, especially as provided in multivitamins, for early feeding of vitamin C. Fruit juices other than citrus juices do not provide enough vitamin C to make them effective in the diet of infants. For children the National Research Council recommendations increase from 40 mg for those 1 to 3 years of age to a high of 45 mg for both males and females over 11 years. Research on which recommended allowances are based presents discrepant findings. Long-term studies show that children with an adequate supply of ascorbic acid have a better general condition in regard to growth and resistance to infection.

Food sources

Vitamin C is found almost exclusively in foods of plant origin. Aside from liver, no other animal food is considered a significant source. The amount present in a plant tissue depends on many factors.

Part and type of plant. The head of broccoli was shown to have 158 mg of vitamin C per 100 g of vegetable compared to 115 mg per 100 g stem. But stems retained 82% during a 10-minute cooking period, whereas heads retained only 60%. In general, thin-stemmed vegetables contain more vitamin C than do thick-stemmed ones. Vegetables that wilt lose much more vitamin C than do those that do not wilt. Kale loses 1.5% of its total vitamin C per hour at room temperature, whereas cabbage loses much less. Roots lose vitamin C slowly, but the loss is accelerated at higher temperatures.

Stage of maturity. Since the vitamin accumulates throughout the ripening process from the setting of the fruit, the longer the fruit remains on the vine or tree before harvesting, the higher the ascorbic acid content up to peak maturity.

In contrast, immature seeds, such as peas and beans, contain some ascorbic acid but lose it all at maturity. Sprouting of peas or beans results in a vegetable with an appreciable amount of vitamin C, however.

Conditions of storage. Storing of vegetables at refrigerator temperatures in high humidity with a minimum of air movement will reduce ascorbic acid losses. The amount present in fresh vegetables bought in the temperate zone in the winter months is a function of the storage conditions during harvesting, shipping, and display in stores previous to selling. Losses are minimized at low temperatures and minimum exposure to air.

Losses vary with the vegetable. One study showed losses of 88% of ascorbic acid in green beans and none in broccoli after six days at 2.2° C.

Season of year. A study of the ascorbic acid content of broccoli showed wide fluctuations, with low values reported in May and peak values in December.

Method of processing. Any method of food processing that involves the application of heat is likely to result in a reduced ascorbic acid content. If processing is done in the absence of air, losses will be much lower. In frozen and canned foods that are picked at the peak of maturity and are processed immediately under optimal conditions, the resulting product may have a higher vitamin C value than does the fresh product for which the period between harvesting and consumption may be long and characterized by poor storage conditions.

Blanching of vegetables prior to freezing is necessary to destroy certain enzymes that otherwise would catalyze the destruction of ascorbic acid. In home-frozen vegetables the vitamin C content is likely to be less than that in commercially frozen vegetables that have been picked at the peak of maturity and processed immediately.

Irradiation of potatoes results in no immediate decrease in ascorbic acid values but a 50% loss occurs after 1 week. Freeze drying of fruit results in little or no loss.

Method of cooking. Many of the best sources of ascorbic acid are normally consumed raw. For those usually cooked, however, the effect of cooking method assumes much importance.

In most cooking the greater part of the losses occur in the early stages. For instance, broccoli heads lose 40% of their ascorbic acid value in the first 10 minutes. In the case of broccoli most of the loss is represented by leaching into the cooking water. On the other hand, cabbage, with a lower initial amount, loses more by heat destruction of ascorbic acid than by leaching. The amount of water used has a greater effect on losses than does the total cooking time. Steaming was found to lead to higher retentions (69% versus 45%) than did boiling when tested on five vegetables. Steaming had no advantage over pressure-cooking.

Microwave cooking caused less destruction of ascorbic acid than did either pressure-cooking or boiling. In the case of broccoli, retentions of 85%, 80% and 45%, respectively, were reported. For cabbage comparable values were 80%, 70%, and 38%.

Method of preparation. Any method that reduces the surface area exposed to air or water minimizes losses. Thus finely shredded cabbage loses more ascorbic acid than cabbage wedges. In the case of cabbage, however, the practice of serving it in vinegar, as in coleslaw, helps counteract the losses from exposure on the surface. Potatoes peeled, cut into smaller pieces, and cooked lose more than those cooked whole in their skins. The use of a dull knife in cutting fruit and vegetables may mash the cells, resulting in increased losses. The practice of crisping vegetables in cold water is undesirable, since it

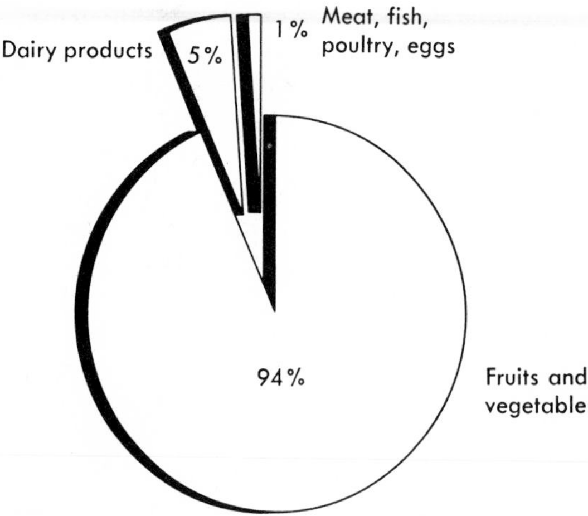

Fig. 12-5. Contribution of various food groups to ascorbic acid content of American food supply. (Based on Contribution of major food groups to nutrient supplies available for civilian consumption. National Food Review NFR-1, Washington, D.C., 1978, Economic Research Service.)

results in the leaching of ascorbic acid into the water. Holding hot vegetables causes considerable loss of ascorbic acid. Losses from reheating are even greater, however.

In Fig. 12-5, which shows the contribution of various food groups to the ascorbic acid in the American diet, it is seen that fruits and vegetables provide 94% of the ascorbic acid. The remaining 6% comes from meat, fish, poultry, eggs, and dairy products. Cereal products contribute none. Although one would have expected an increase in the total amount of vitamin C in the diet in recent years with the greater use of frozen vegetables and the increased availability of fresh produce the year round, dietary studies indicate that the ascorbic acid in the American diet was lower in 1959 than in either 1947 to 1949 or 1935 to 1939. A shift from rich toward poorer sources has taken place in both vegetables and fruit juices.

The change in the sources of ascorbic acid

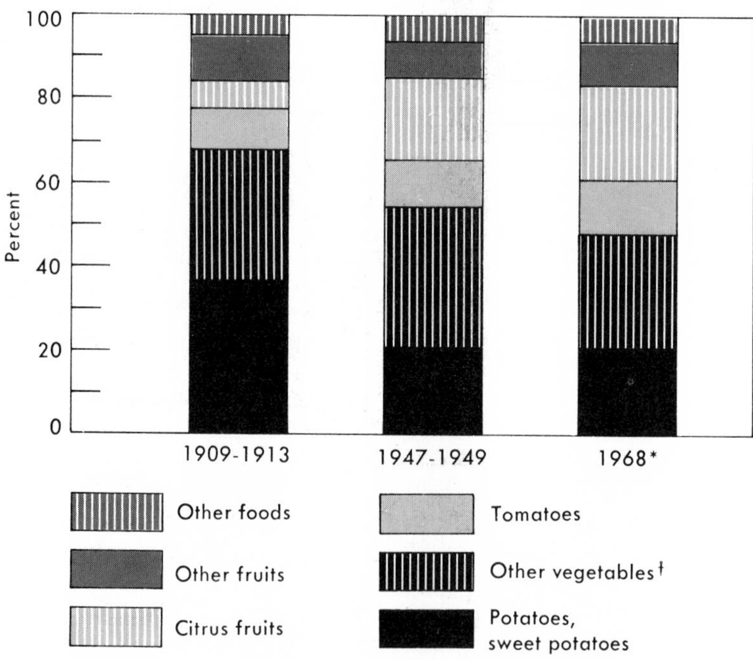

Fig. 12-6. Sources of ascorbic acid in food supply from 1909 to 1968. *Includes fortification, data preliminary; †excluding tomatoes, potatoes, and sweet potatoes. (From Agricultural Research Service, U.S. Department of Agriculture, 1969.)

in the American diet between 1909 and 1968 is depicted in Fig. 12-6. Fig. 12-7 shows the adequacy of the dietary intake as reported in two nutrition surveys in the United States.

Tables of food composition continue to record only the reduced ascorbic acid content of fruits and vegetables, although considerable evidence exists that the body utilizes both reduced and dehydroascorbic acid. In spite of the fact that values representing total ascorbic acid would be more meaningful, the food composition table in Appendix G is based on reduced ascorbic acid except for frozen fruits and vegetables, for which total values are provided. The ascorbic acid content of 100 g and 100 kcal portions of some representative foods is presented graphically in Fig. 12-8. Table 12-2 give both reduced, dehydroascorbic, and total ascorbic acid values for some representative foods for which data is available and Table 12-3 the INQ for ascorbic acid for some representative foods.

Aside from the more frequently used sources of vitamin C, such as citrus fruits and juices, broccoli, spinach, strawberries, and

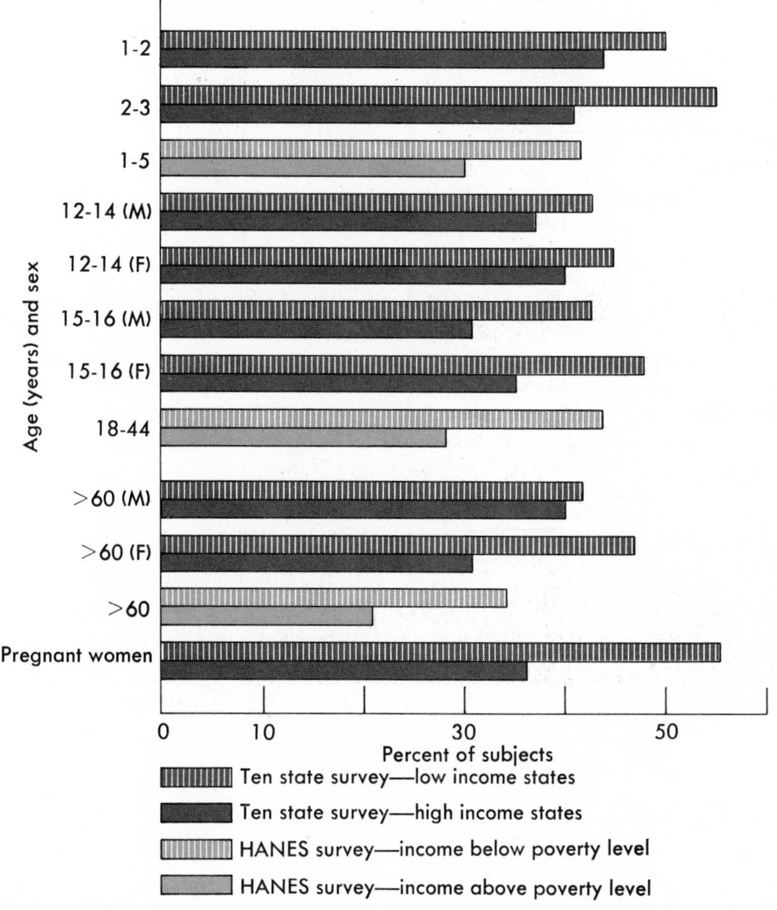

Fig. 12-7. The percentage of persons with dietary vitamin C intake below two-thirds RDA by age, sex, and income level. Data based on results of Ten-State Nutrition Survey (1968-1970) and preliminary findings of first Health and Nutrition Examination Survey (HANES) (1971-1972).

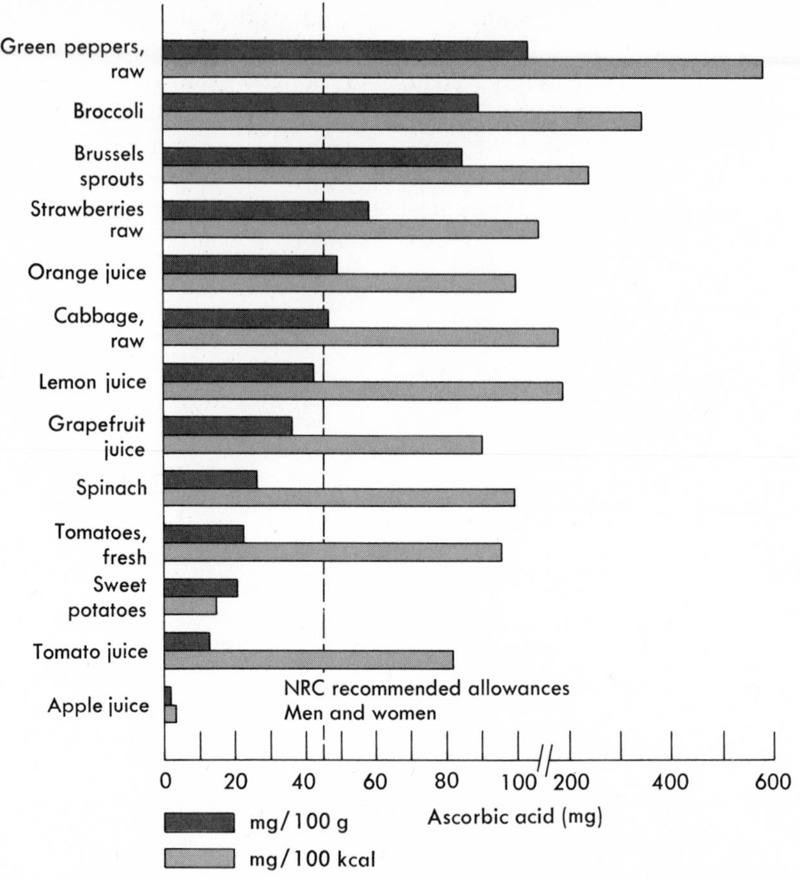

Fig. 12-8. Ascorbic acid content of 100 g and 100 kcal portions of some representative foods. (Based on Watt, B. K., and Merrill, A. L.: Composition of foods—raw, processed and prepared, Handbook No. 8, Washington, D.C., 1963, U.S. Department of Agriculture.)

melon in season, several other sources are rich. Parsley has a high content (per 100 g) but is consumed in such small quantities that it is not an important source. Many of the early concentrates of vitamin C before synthetic vitamin C was readily available were made from rose hips gathered mostly by Indians in northern Alberta. The acerola cherry, native to the tropics, has been identified as an extremely rich source (1500 mg/100 g), and although unpalatable alone, it is being used to fortify juices less rich in ascorbic acid, especially for infant feeding. Camu-camu, a fruit native to South America, averages even more with 2000 mg/100 g.

In the food industry, especially among processors of fruit juices and fruit juice mixtures, the trend is to add vitamin C at a level of about 30 mg per 120 ml serving to give them a better chance of competing with citrus juices. For consumption by persons who do not recognize the difference in ascorbic acid values of various juices, this is a commendable practice, although evidence exists that many times analyzed values vary considerably (usually higher) from that on label, indicating a need for greater quality control. In keeping with the policy of recommending the enrichment of food products only when there is evidence of a lack of the particular

Table 12-2. Reduced, dehydroascorbic, and total ascorbic acid in 100 g of some representative foods (in milligrams)*

Food	Reduced ascorbic acid	Dehydroascorbic acid	Total ascorbic acid
Asparagus	7.9	26.9	34.8
Broccoli	48.2	9.8	58.0
Brussels sprouts	60.9	4.4	65.3
Cabbage, raw	54.4	22.3	76.7
Cantaloupe	15.5	18.2	33.7
Green pepper	41.0	4.8	45.8
Strawberries	53.8	12.9	66.7
Sweet potatoes	18.8	8.1	26.9
Tomato juice	15.2	2.3	17.5

*From Davey, B. L., Dodds, M. L., Fisher, K. H., Schuck, C., and Shih, D. C.: Utilization of ascorbic acid in fruits and vegetables. 1. Plan of study and ascorbic acid content of 24 foods, J. Am. Diet. Assoc. **32:**1064, 1956.

nutrient in a significant segment of the population, it is difficult to rationalize such a practice. However, in Canada the enrichment of apple juice with ascorbic acid has the approval of government agencies, since it conceivably puts a native product in a better place competitively with an imported one. The addition of ascorbic acid to dehydrated potatoes is a questionable practice because of the likelihood of its being destroyed by heat and oxidation in preparation. The enrichment of milk or carbonated beverages with ascorbic acid has not been endorsed in the United States. In the processing of frozen fruits, such as peaches and apples, ascorbic acid is frequently added because of its reducing properties that help prevent discoloration of the fruit.

Ascorbic acid is used as a preservative in jams and jellies, a color stabilizer in fruit cocktail, a dough conditioner in white flour, an acidulant in frozen deserts, and in wine and beer to prevent darkening of color and deterioration of flavor. In jams and jellies ascorbic acid is used at a level of 15 mg per serving; in meat 2000 mg per 0.45 kg may be

Table 12-3. INQ for selected sources of vitamin C providing at least 15% of the U.S. RDA per serving

Food	INQ
Sweet peppers	178.9
Broccoli	134.2
Cauliflower	101.2
Kale	86.9
Lemon	74.8
Strawberries	61.3
Papayas	55.9
Asparagus	48.6
Spinach	48.0
Cantaloupe	40.3
Oranges	39.0
Orange juice	38.3
Grapefruit	33.7
Tomato juice	33.2
Snap beans	19.2
Pineapple	12.3
Peas	11.0
Onions	10.5
Potatoes, boiled	9.6
Raspberries	8.2
Sweet potatoes	5.6

used in fixing color. These additions represent a significant intake. In other cases the levels of 150 to 700 ppm result in only 3 to 4 mg per 0.45 kg. At least one study has shown that synthetic L-ascorbic acid is more available than the natural vitamin C in orange juice.

Evaluation of nutritional status

In spite of the fact that the biochemistry of ascorbic acid in the cell is less well understood than is that of other nutrients, the assessment of nutritional status in regard to ascorbic acid is more satisfactory.

Several methods have been used to assess the nutritional status of vitamin C in the body. Since no one method alone is completely satisfactory, a more accurate assessment is possible by a combination of several methods. By these methods it is possible to detect a difference between optimal and less than optimal nutrition.

Serum ascorbic acid levels have been widely used but do not bear a direct relationship to either dietary intake or white blood cell levels, which are believed to reflect the state of tissue saturation. When serum values fall below 0.4 mg/dl, they parallel white blood cell levels, but correlation for individuals is low. When tissues are less than 50% saturated, serum levels are too low to measure, making this determination virtually useless in discriminating between low and scorbutic levels of tissue saturation. When tissues are saturated, serum levels are close to 1 mg/dl of blood.

The white blood cell, or leukocyte, level of ascorbic acid is a much more sensitive test of ascorbic acid nutrition. When tissues are completely saturated, leukocyte values are between 27 and 30 mg/dl of blood. The fall in white blood cell level parallels the degree of saturation of the tissues; therefore a fall in these levels is indicative of depletion of body reserves. Scurvy does not develop until tissues are less than 20% saturated. This will not occur unless levels of intake fall below 10 mg a day.

A measure of the amount of a test dose excreted in the urine within a short period after its administration has been the basis of the urinary excretion test for vitamin C status. The theory behind this test is that a depleted tissue will take up more of a test dose than will saturated tissues. Thus, when the intake has been adequate, the percentage of a test dose recovered in the urine will be high. When tissues are depleted, the amount appearing in the urine decreases, showing that more has been retained in the body. Table 12-4 shows the levels of these measurements under varying degrees of saturation.

Table 12-4. Comparison of biochemical data on ascorbic acid at different levels of saturation in the tissues

	Saturated	Less saturated	50% saturation	25% saturation
White blood cell levels of ascorbic acid	27-30 mg/dl			20 mg/dl
Serum levels of ascorbic acid	1 mg/dl	0.4-1 mg/dl	Too low to measure	
Urinary excretion; percent of test dose	60%-80%	20%-60%	Very low	
Dietary intake	>100 mg	40-100 mg	10-15 mg	5-7 mg

Deficiency

Scurvy represents the most severe form of ascorbic acid deficiency but is relatively rare, especially in adults, now that its cause and cure are known. When it does develop, however, the early symptoms are relatively nonspecific, such as listlessness, fatigue, weakness, shortness of breath, muscle cramps, aching bones, joints and muscles, and loss of appetite. The skin becomes dry, feverish, and rough and is covered by reddish-blue spots. Hemorrhaging of the gums often predisposes to secondary infection.

In a study of experimental scurvy in men it was found that clinical symptoms of scurvy, such as enlargement, or hypertrophy, of the cornea, congestion of follicles or ducts, swollen joints, bleeding gums, muscular aches and pains, fatigue, difficulty in breathing, and pinpoint hemorrhages, developed when the normal ascorbic acid reserves of 1500 mg dropped to 300 mg or less. The first symptoms of petechial, or pinpoint, hemorrhages began to appear after twenty-nine days on a deficient diet at which time urinary excretion had dropped to zero. By ninety days all subjects were showing many and severe symptoms of scurvy. These changes occurred as whole blood ascorbic acid levels measured 0.3 mg/dl and plasma ascorbic acid measured 0.13 to 0.24 mg/dl. Intakes of 6.5, 66.5, and 130 mg of ascorbic acid were all effective in reversing the symptoms of scurvy and repleting the body reserves.

Associated with the depletion of ascorbic acid were a depressed glucose tolerance and a decrease in blood cholesterol level, impaired physical performance involving the use of the legs, and personality changes characterized by hypochondriasis, depression, and hysteria.

Infantile scurvy, illustrated in Figs. 12-1 and 12-4, is most likely to occur in the period of rapid growth between 5 and 24 months of age. Breast-fed infants never have scurvy, but bottle-fed infants whose diets are not varied by 6 months of age develop symptoms of scurvy such as irritability, anorexia, growth failure, tenderness of hips, and anemia. The onset is extremely rapid, and unless treated promptly, the condition may result in rapid death. If treated, the recovery is equally as dramatic.

Delayed or incomplete wound healing is a frequent manifestation of ascorbic acid deficiency, and anemia invariably occurs after two months of restricted intake. A drop in white blood cell levels is frequent.

Common cold and flu

The publication of a popular book promoting large (1 g or more) doses of ascorbic acid in the prevention and cure of both the common cold and flu has led many people to follow this regimen and academicians to conduct studies to test the validity of this claim. The lay public has shown little concern for possible harmful effects of such large doses. Scientists, on the other hand, although they have somewhat conflicting test results, still recommend an intake of 45 mg as adequate to meet adult needs, and well above the level necessary to prevent scurvy.

A double-blind clinical study in which 1000 volunteers received either 1000 mg of ascorbic acid or a placebo daily for fourteen weeks and 4 g during the first three days of any illness was conducted at the University of Toronto. Results showed a 7% decrease in the number of illnesses, a 12% decrease in the number of days on which symptoms were recorded, and a 30% decline in the number of days subjects were confined to the house. Although only the latter change was statistically significant, the results did indicate that vitamin C had reduced the severity of the symptoms. A subsequent study on 3500 volunteers showed that the effect was not due to the regular use of 250, 1000, or 2000 mg daily but to the increased dosage at the time of the illness. A concurrent study of children in Arizona did show a reduction in symptoms in children given 1 to 2 g daily without an extra therapeutic amount at the time of illness. The contradictory findings may have been due to differences in vitamin C status at the beginning of the studies.

Thus at this time there is reason to believe

that the course of the common cold may be modified by the ingestion of ascorbic acid. However, there still is no precise information concerning what level will provide benefits and minimize the risk of side effects. The possibility that continued use of pharmacological dosages of over 1 g, representing over twenty times the recommended intake, may lead to as yet unidentified metabolic changes suggests the need for caution.

Megavitamin therapy

The availability of synthetic ascorbic acid at very reasonable cost (less than $7 per kilogram) has made it possible for the public to obtain the vitamin at pharmacological levels of 2000 to 4000 mg, many times the requirement. Although scientists are still assessing the possible benefits of such therapy, they are at the same time becoming aware of the possible risks. The conversion of excess ascorbic acid to oxalic acid before it is excreted increased the possibility of the formation of kidney stones. The development of a vitamin C dependency in adults or infants of women who have ingested large amounts of ascorbic acid over extended periods during pregnancy has caused deficiency symptoms when intakes dropped to normal levels. Other problems associated with megadoses of ascorbic acid include destruction of vitamin B_{12}, a decrease in copper absorption, an increase in plasma cholesterol, interference with anticoagulants, destruction of red blood cells, and reproductive failure. Those individuals who find that high intakes, especially before meals, cause diarrhea, nausea, and stomach cramps usually withdraw from the use of large amounts.

THIAMIN*

The discovery of the chemical structure of thiamin and its synthesis by Williams in 1936 marked the end of a long and tedious search on the part of German, English, and American scientists to identify the substance in ric bran responsible for the cure of **beriberi** (' can't, I can't"). As early as 1855 Takaki ha cured beriberi in the Japanese Navy by usin meat and milk to supplement the regular die of the seamen, among whom over 30% wer usually afflicted with the disease.

In 1890 Eijkman, a Dutch physician, wa able to cure the paralytic **polyneuritis** tha had developed in chickens fed scraps of polished rice by feeding unhusked rice or ric polishings. He also showed that he coul cure human beriberi by a similar treatment His method of treatment was successful although his explanation that beriberi was du to a toxin in rice starch has since been prove to be erroneous.

By 1910 Vedder in the Phillipines had recognized that an active factor present in a ric bran extract, *tikitiki* was capable of curin polyneuritis in chicks and beriberi in humans. By 1926 Dutch scientists had produce 5 g of thiamin crystals from 0.9 metric ton o bran, but another ten years elapsed befor they were chemically identified and synthesized. By 1937 both Swiss and America firms were producing thiamin and Britai was formulating plans to use it to enric bread. By 1961 thiamin production in th United States had risen to 180 metric tons. I 1977 it had reached 300 metric tons. Compulsory enrichment of bread and flour in th United States began in 1941.

Beriberi

Although it had been described by the Chinese as early as 2600 BC, beriberi was virtually unknown until the middle of the nineteenth century. With the increasing use o more highly refined cereals with increase storage life but low in thiamin, beriberi became a major health problem. This was especially true in countries where a staple foo item such as rice provided as much as 80% o the calories in the diet. The cause of beriber was not identified at first as a dietary deficiency resulting from the removal of th outer layers of cereal grains. Various othe theories were advanced. One suggested th

*Use of the terms thiamin and thiamine in referring to vitamin B_1 is still being debated. We have chosen to use thiamin, although thiamine is considered equally acceptable.

presence of a toxic substance in the starch of rice for which there was an antidote in rice bran. Others proposed the presence of a microbe, the absence of nitrogen in the diet, or the production of a toxic substance in the stomach from the use of rice. None of these theories withstood scrutiny, and eventually the search narrowed to one for the active substance in a rice bran extract that had almost magical curative properties in beriberi, especially infantile beriberi. It was identified as a water-soluble substance easily destroyed by heat and alkali.

In spite of knowledge of food sources of thiamin and the ready production of synthetic thiamin at reasonable prices, beriberi is still a problem in many parts of the world. The Philippines still reports an incidence of infantile beriberi deaths of 75 per 100,000 births. There, beriberi is listed as the fourth leading cause of death and led to 15,200 infant deaths and 6130 adult deaths in the peiod of 1954 to 1958. In addition, it is estimated that at least 1.5 million persons suffer from some manifestation of the disease, either clinically or subclinically. The incidence of beriberi can be attributed to the fact that the small rice mills, which have taken over all but 5% of the milling, are producing a highly polished rice and with few exceptions are failing to comply with government regulations regarding enrichment even at a cost of a fifth of a cent per 0.5 kg. The practice of repeatedly washing the milled rice to remove the dust that accumulates during marketing in open bins causes a further loss of thiamin. It is estimated that after milling, washing, and cooking losses are considered, the average consumption of less than 0.5 kg of rice daily provides only 0.27 mg of thiamin. On the basis of the Food and Agricultural Organization criterion of 0.27 mg of thiamin per 1000 nonfat kcal in the diet, this level of intake will not protect against beriberi. Low calcium intakes increase the likelihood of beriberi developing in a thiamin-deficient diet. Tea drinkers are at even greater risk.

Infantile beriberi occurs most frequency from 2 to 5 months of age. It has a very rapid onset, and unless treated within a matter of hours often results in death. Beriberi occurs more often in breast-fed than bottle-fed infants, reflecting the fact that the lactating mother's dietary intake of thiamin is too low to produce a milk with sufficient thiamin to protect her infant. Human milk normally contains less than half as much thiamin as cow's milk, but the level in the milk of a woman on a thiamin-deficient diet is much lower. The situation may be complicated by the transfer of methyl glyoxal (pyruvic aldehyde), a product of metabolism that accumulates in the body in thiamin deficiency, to the mother's milk. Milk from mothers suffering from beriberi has been found to contain about half as much thiamin as that from normal mothers.

A baby with beriberi very rapidly develops such symptoms as cyanosis (too much carbon dioxide in blood, causing a bluish color), tachycardia (a very fast heartbeat), and a characteristic cry changing from a loud piercing one to a thin, weak, almost inaudible one, sometimes accompanied by vomiting and convulsions. Once thiamin is made available, symptoms are dramatically relieved within a matter of hours.

In adults, beriberi is a different condition and takes two distinct forms. In wet (edematous) beriberi the victim suffers from swelling of the limbs, usually starting at the feet and progressing upward throughout the body until the accumulation of fluid in heart muscle leads to eventual heart failure and death. The victim has difficulty walking and suffers from wristdrop and ankledrop.

In dry (wasting) beriberi a gradual loss of body tissue occurs, with the patient becoming thin and emaciated. In both forms, symptoms are numbness in the legs, irritability, vague uneasiness, disorderly thinking, and nausea, all suggesting an involvement of the nervous system.

The heart failure associated with thiamin deficiency has been attributed to the increased work necessary to get a greater amount of blood to tissues deprived of thiamin.

The disease continues to be a problem in areas of the world where polished rice is a staple in the diet and where the milling of rice has shifted from the home to the mill. In the United States, alcoholics are almost the only group in which the disease ever occurs. This deficiency is caused not only by the low thiamin intake but also by a reduction in absorption due to a concurrent deficiency of another vitamin, folic acid, and a lack of a coenzyme for thiamin. However, considerable evidence exists of subclinial thiamin deficiency, especially among persons who eliminate bread and cereal products from their diets, often in an effort to lose weight. The incidence of beriberi is greater when low intakes of cereal and bread occur in conjunction with the use of foods such as tea leaves and raw fish, which contain a thiamin antagonist that interferes with its utilization.

Early work in the study of beriberi was facilitated by the availability of chickens for research purposes. When fed the beriberi-producing diet these animals developed polyneuritis (inflammation of nerves). They also showed loss of neuromuscular coordination, had a poor sense of balance, and died within a short time of onset of the symptoms.

Chemical properties

Thiamin, which is available as the biologically active but more stable thiamin hydrochloride, is a white crystalline substance, soluble in water, and easily destroyed by heat or oxidation, especially in the presence of alkali. The term *thiamin* indicates that it is a sulfur-containing substance (thio) and is also amine or nitrogen containing. It has also been known as a neurin and the antineuritic factor, indicative of its role in preventing symptoms involving nerves.

Functions

Vitamin B_1 is known to be a part of the coenzyme thiamin pyrophosphate (TPP) or thiamin diphosphate (TDP). This is thiamin with two molecules of phosphate attached to it, which was formerly known as cocarboxylase, required in metabolism of carbohydrate. There are three stages in the metabolism of carbohydrates at which the absence of thiamin as part of this coenzyme leads to a slowing or complete blocking of the chemical changes. The accumulation of the intermediary products of metabolism in the absence of the necessary thiamin-containing enzyme is believed to cause typical thiamin deficiency symptoms. As TPP, thiamin is the coenzyme necessary for the decarboxylation (removal of carbon dioxide) from pyruvic acid as it is prepared to enter the citric acid cycle (Appendix to Part I). When thiamin is lacking, pyruvic acid tends to accumulate.

A similar role for TPP in oxidative decarboxylation exists at the stage in the metabolic cycle at which another intermediary product of both fat and carbohydrate metabolism, alpha-ketoglutaric acid, is decarboxylated to succinic acid.

A third enzymatic role of thiamin is in activating transketolase, an enzyme necessary in the direct oxidative pathway for metabolism of glucose that can occur in all cells except skeletal cells. Even though this pathway involves less than 10% of all glucose, it is vital, since it is the only way the body can produce either ribose, the sugar needed for the synthesis of RNA so essential in cell reproduction, or an intermediary product needed for the synthesis of fatty acids. The effect of TPP in increasing the activity of transketolase found in the red blood cells has been shown to be a sensitive indicator of thiamin status.

Attempts to explain the neurological symptoms associated with thiamin deficiency have led to the identification of thiamin triphosphate in the nerve cell membrane. Thiamin apparently acts in the transmission of high frequency impulses at the nerve synapse either through the production or release of the neurotransmitter substance acetylcholine or the formation of complexes with other neurotransmitters. Thiamin also plays a role in the conversion of the amino acid tryptophan to niacin.

Absorption

The absorption of thiamin occurs primarily in the duodenum of the small intestine, reaching a maximum at intakes of 2.5 to 5 mg a day. Thiamin in small amounts is absorbed in an active process requiring energy and sodium. Large amounts are absorbed by passive diffusion. Any thiamin synthesized in the lower gastrointestinal tract appears as TPP which cannot be absorbed at this point, therefore intestinal synthesis in humans appears to have no significance. Once it has entered the mucosal cell thiamin reacts with phosphate to form thiamin phosphate; it is transported to the liver in this form.

A substance in onion oil and garlic oil, alliin, combines with thiamin to form alliithiamine, a form in which the vitamin is more readily absorbed. The widespread use of onions and garlic in oriental diets with marginal amounts of thiamin may thus help to alleviate thiamin deficiencies. Another thiamin compound, thiamin disulfide, is absorbed more freely than thiamin hydrochloride.

Since thiamin pyrophosphate (TPP) is too large a molecule to pass through the cell membrane, it becomes clear that this coenzyme is produced in the cell as needed and that the thiamin existing in either animal or plant foods as TPP must be split before being absorbed. With the aid of enzymes it is then rejoined to phosphates as needed in individual cells to produce TPP.

The decrease in gastric acidity that occurs in thiamin deficiency decreases the release of thiamin from thiamin complexes in the gastrointestinal tract, inhibiting its absorption and accentuating the deficiency symptoms.

Metabolism

The adult human contains from 30 to 70 mg of thiamin, about 80% of which is TPP. Half of body thiamin is distributed in muscle. Although there is no storage site for the vitamin, it has been observed that normal levels of 2 to 3 μg/g of heart muscle, 1 μg/g of brain, liver, and kidneys, and 0.5 μg/g of skeletal muscle double after thiamin therapy and rapidly drop to half these values in thiamin depletion.

It is known that thiamin in excess of body needs is excreted in the urine. A measure of urinary thiamin in relation to dietary thiamin has been the basis for balance studies to assess the adequacy of intake. When thiamin excretion is low, a larger portion of the test dose is retained, indicating a tissue need for the vitamin. A high excretion, on the other hand, indicates tissue saturation. On low intakes excretion drops to zero. The level of excretion of thiamin is related to weight and daily intake. A radioactive dose of thiamin appears in the urine as thiamin and over twenty-four other degradation products, which account for half the thiamin in the urine.

Requirements

Efforts to determine the minimal needs and optimal intakes for humans of thiamin have involved balance studies in which the relationship between dietary intake and urinary excretion has been determined. A level of intake that leads to minimal but not zero excretion is believed to represent minimal needs but provides no protection against further reduction in thiamin intake.

Recommendations for all age groups assume a relationship between caloric intake and thiamin need. The assumption is based on the fact that thiamin is part of the coenzyme needed in at least three places in the metabolism of carbohydrate. As caloric intake varies with age, size, physical activity, environmental temperature, or physical state of the animal, carbohydrate intake changes, and an increased carbohydrate intake creates an increased need for thiamin. The current recommendations of the National Research Council based on a level of 0.5 mg of thiamin per 1000 kcal are presented in Table 12-5. These figures represent optimal intakes, which for the most part are about 100% above minimal requirements. This is in keeping with the philosophy of setting recommendations at a level compatible with the potential of the nation's food supply to provide it and sufficiently high to provide a margin of safety to take into account practically all individual variations in need and efficiency of absorption and normal losses in food preparation. These levels protect against deficiency symptoms and provide a

Table 12-5. Recommended daily intake of thiamin (in milligrams)

		United States*	Great Britain†	Canada‡	FAO/WHO§
Children	2-3 yr	0.7	0.6	0.7	0.5
	6-9 yr	1.2	0.8	0.9	0.9
Boys	12-15 yr	1.4	1.1	1.4	1.2
Girls	12-15 yr	1.2	0.9	1.1	1.0
Men	18-35 yr	1.5	1.1	1.5	1.2
	35-55 yr	1.5	1.0	1.4	1.2
Women	18-35 yr	1.0	0.9	1.1	0.9
	35-55 yr	1.0	0.8	1.0	0.9

*Food and Nutrition Board: Recommended dietary allowances, ed. 8, Washington D.C., 1974, National Academy of Sciences-National Research Council.
†Department of Health and Social Security: Recommended intakes of nutrients for the United Kingdom Reports on Public Health and Medical Subjects, No. 120, London, 1969, Her Majesty's Stationery Office.
‡Dietary Standards for Canada, Canadian Bulletin on Nutrition 6, No. 1, 1964; Revised, 1975.
§FAO/WHO: Handbook on human nutritional requirements, Rome, 1974, Food and Agriculture Organization.

buffer against zero intakes of thiamin. There is no evidence of benefits to be derived from intakes in excess of these levels. Since thiamin is water-soluble and the body has limited capacity to store it, excesses are excreted. There is no indication of toxicity from its use. In the last trimester of pregnancy, the recommendation increases to 0.6 mg/1000 kcal.

Studies of older individuals show that their needs are relatively high. They excrete less at all levels of intake, they experience a faster reaction to moderate depletion, and they respond more slowly to the addition of thiamin to the diet.

The need for thiamin increases with an increased consumption of alcohol. This accounts for the reported incidence of beriberi among alcoholics in the United States. It appears that the vitamin is necessary for the metabolism of acetaldehyde, an intermediary product in alcohol metabolism. Thiamin absorption decreases in alcoholics due to changes in the intestinal wall.

The amount of fat in the diet, especially medium-chain fatty acids, bears an inverse relationship to the need for thiamin, and fat has frequently been referred to as a "thiamin sparer." Since only one of the reactions for which thiamin is needed is involved in the metabolism of fatty acids, it follows that when fat calories replace carbohydrate calories, less thiamin will be required. Thus thiamin intakes that are suboptimal in a high-carbohydrate diet prove adequate when fat replaces some of the carbohydrate. It is suggested that a toxic product, presumably methyl glyoxal, arises from carbohydrate metabolism but not from fat metabolism in the absence of thiamin. Fatty acids play a role in regulation of enzymes needed for glucose metabolism. Another possibility is that fat protects thiamin from loss or destruction in the body.

Considerable evidence exists that the need for thiamin decreases when some sulfonamides and other antibiotics are given. Sev-

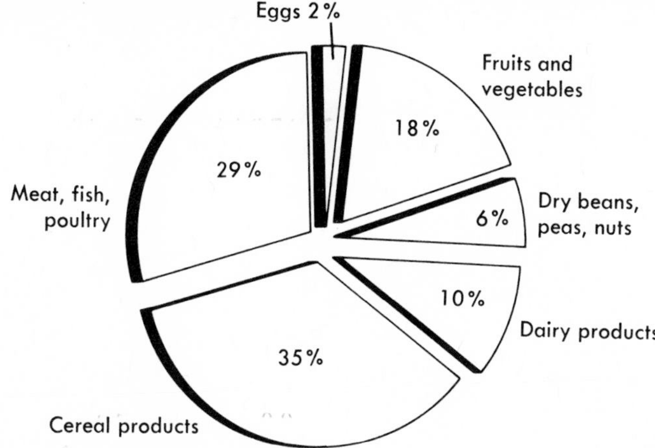

Fig. 12-9. Contribution of various food groups to the thiamin content of the American food supply. (Based on Contribution of major food groups to nutrient supplies available for civilian consumption, National Food Review NFR-1, Washington, D.C., 1978, Economic Research Service.)

ral theories have been suggested to explain his effect, but no clear-cut evidence has een established to support any one of hem.

ood sources

As shown in Fig. 12-9, cereal products proide about a third of the available dietary hiamin; meat, fish, and poultry, about a ourth; and dairy products, about a tenth of hat available to the American public.

Fig. 12-10 shows the thiamin content of 00 g and 100 kcal portions of some of the nore dependable sources of thiamin in the verage American diet. Foods with an INQ of .5 or more for thiamin are shown in Table 2-6. Thiamin in vegetables is in nonphoshorylated form, whereas that in meat ocurs primarily as cocarboxylase or diphoshate, from which it must be released before t is absorbed.

The richest sources of the vitamin are pork roducts. For that segment of the population who eats pork frequently, it presents a deendable source of thiamin. Those whose reigious beliefs prohibit consumption of pork an, however, obtain adequate amounts rom other sources.

Table 12-6. INQ for selected sources of thiamin providing at least 15% of the U.S. RDA per serving

Food	INQ
Yeast	76.7
Peas	5.9
Pork	3.9
Orange juice	2.9
Lima beans	2.5
Pecans	1.9
Whole wheat bread	1.9
Macaroni	1.9
Rice	1.9
White bread	1.5

Peas and other legumes are good sources. As will be noted from a comparison of fresh and dried peas, the amount of thiamin increases with increasing maturity of the seed. The amount of the nutrient actually obtained from dried legumes will be reduced if they are soaked for a long period in water, which is discarded, or if baking soda is used to hasten the cooking time by softening the cellulose. The U.S. Department of Agriculture suggests that the use of minute amounts of

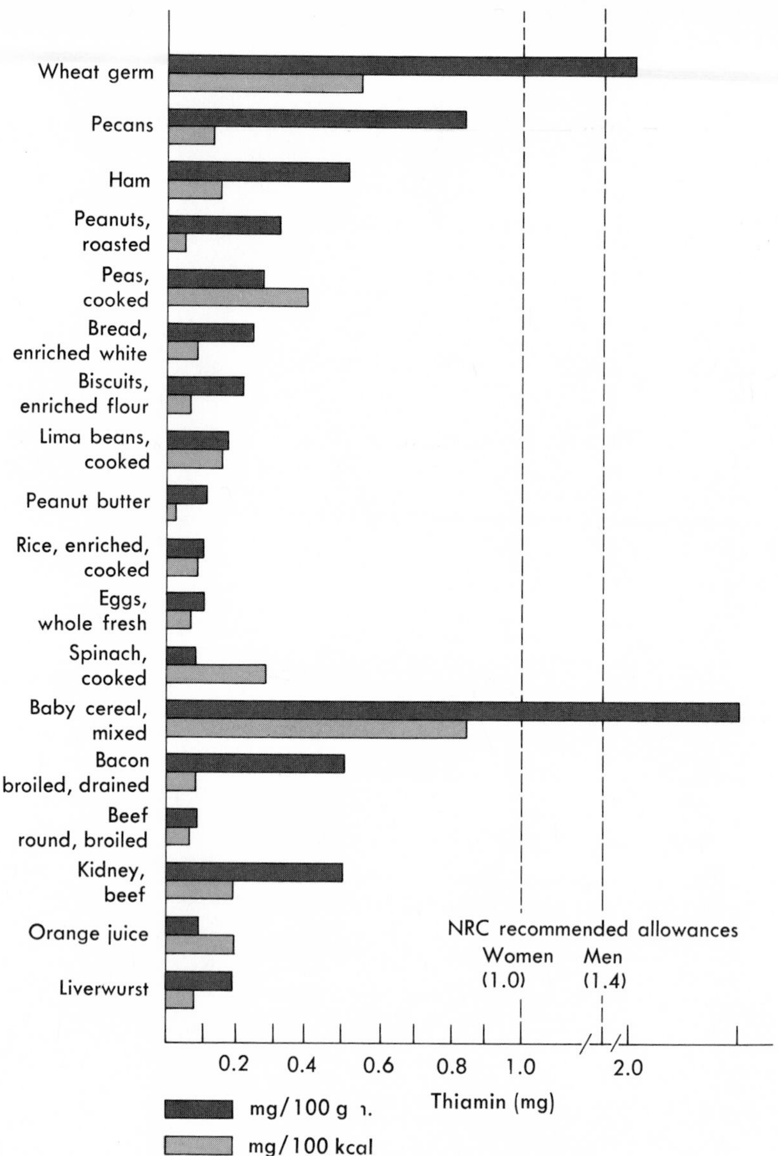

Fig. 12-10. Thiamin content of 100 g and 100 kcal portions of some representative foods. (Based on Watt, B. K., and Merrill, A. L.: Composition of foods—raw, processed and prepared, Handbook No. 8, Washington, D.C., 1963, U.S. Department of Agriculture.)

baking soda (1/16 teaspoon per cup of beans) is satisfactory, since reduced cooking time reduces thiamin losses sufficiently to compensate for increased losses resulting from the addition of an alkali.

Whole-grain cereals contain 94% of their thiamin in their outer husks, the part that is removed in the milling process.

Enriched and whole wheat bread may at first appear as an insignificant source, but in the amounts consumed, especially by low-income families, the use of bread products

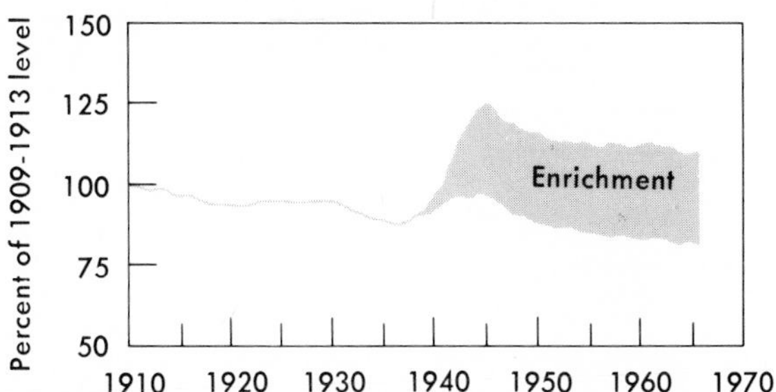

Fig. 12-11. Effect of enrichment program on thiamin content of American diet from 1910 to 1966. Thiamin per capita consumption, five-year moving average. (From Agricultural Research Service, U.S. Department of Agriculture, 1969.)

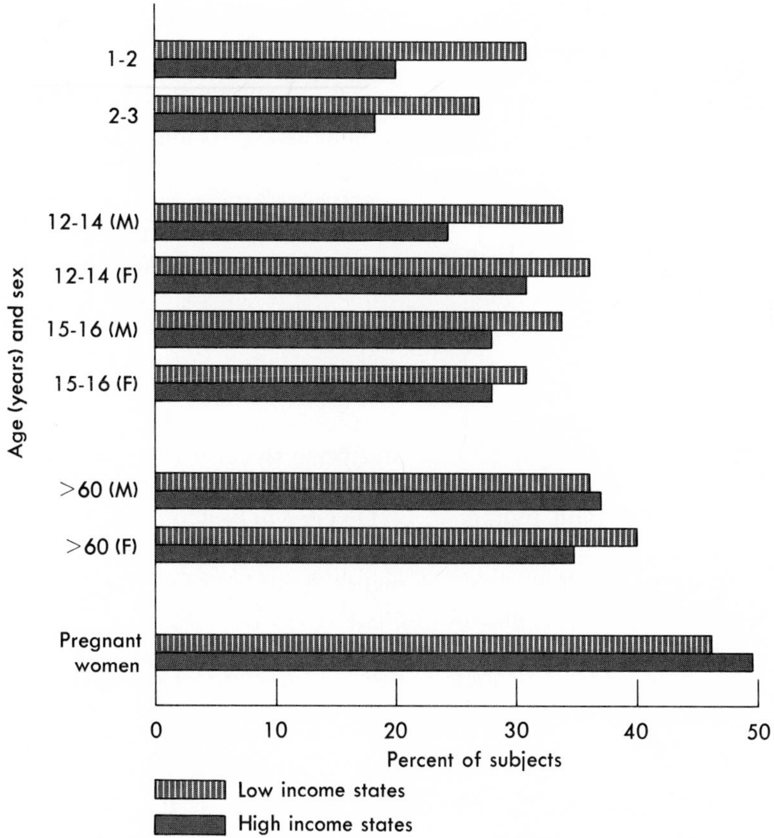

Fig. 12-12. The percentage of persons with dietary thiamin intake below two-thirds RDA by age, sex, and income level. Data based on results of Ten-State Nutrition Survey (1968-1970).

provides enough thiamin to ensure an adequate intake in diets that would otherwise be marginal. The use of enriched bread, the result of mandatory enrichment laws in thirty-five states, has been credited with decreasing the incidence of beriberi among alcoholics, many of whom eat bread or bread products—one of the cheaper sources of calories. Of bread and flour marketed in the United States 90% is now enriched at a cost of approximately 4 cents per 50 kg. The effect of the enrichment program on the thiamin content of the American diet is evident from Fig. 12-11.

Dried brewer's yeast and wheat germ, both rich in thiamin, assume little importance in the American diet because of the infrequency of their use. Live yeast, found in compressed yeast cakes, is high in thiamin but it has been established that these same yeast cells deprived the body of thiamin and may precipitate thiamin-deficiency symptoms. Cooking kills the yeast cells; thus it is only when live yeast is taken, as was once recommended as a therapeutic agent in certain skin conditions, that a problem occurs.

The enrichment of other cereal products, such as rice, macaroni, corn grits, and flour, assumes practical importance, depending on the extent to which these items are a staple food item in a diet.

The U.S. Department of Agriculture reports that the American food supply provides about 1.8 mg per person per day, which is not much above the daily adult requirement. The results of the Ten-State Nutrition Survey of low-income families showed that from 20% to 50% of persons in certain age and sex categories had thiamin intakes below two thirds of the 1968 Recommended Dietary Allowances (Fig. 12-12). On the other hand, results of the HANES (Health and Nutrition Examination Survey) with samples from all economic groups showed that the intake was at least 0.4 mg/1000 kcal for all age, sex, economic, and racial groups. Biochemical evidence of thiamin deficiency suggests that 25% of the general population fall below adequate levels.

Certain freshwater fish, a few saltwater fish, bracken ferns, tea, and some shellfish, such as clams, shrimp, and mussels, contain a thiamin-splitting enzyme, thiaminase. Fortunately, this enzyme is heat labile (its coenzyme is heat stable); therefore only in circumstances in which raw fish is regularly consumed or large amounts of tea are used is the presence of this enzyme detrimental to human nutrition.

Effect of food preparation

The extent to which foods lose thiamin in preparation is a function of the physical and chemical properties of the vitamin.

Loss in solution. Since thiamin is water soluble, it will leach out of a product in proportion to the amount of water available, the extent to which it is agitated, and the surface area of the food exposed to the water. Any method of preparation that minimizes the length of time a food is in contact with water and the amount of surface area will decrease thiamin losses. As much as 18% of the thiamin in rice is reportedly lost in the Oriental method of washing the rice several times before cooking. Modern marketing procedures, which protect the food from contamination from the air, eliminate the necessity for preliminary washing of rice. In fact, most packages warn the consumer not to wash rice and to cook it in a minimum of water to reduce cooking losses. This is especially important when the rice is fortified by coating it with an enrichment mixture.

Loss due to heat. Thiamin is destroyed by heat at temperatures above 100° C. The higher the heat, the greater the loss. Roasting pork at 163° C allows a retention of 75% to 100% of the original thiamin whereas higher temperatures give lower yields. Destruction appears no greater in cooking in microwave ovens than in conventional ones. Thiamin in food is less susceptible to heat destruction than is the free form. Also, a difference is found in rate of heat destruction between various foods. For example, that in spinach, heart, liver, and lamb is more susceptible to heat destruction than that in peas, beans, pork, and carrots.

Loss due to oxidation. Cooking procedures that increase the amount of oxygen in contact with the food, especially under conditions of moist heat, speed up the destruction of thiamin. The use of rapidly boiling water in cooking vegetables is an example of this.

Loss due to alkali. The destruction of thiamin is greatest in the presence of alkali. The addition of baking soda, an alkali, to cooking water is sometimes suggested as a means of preserving the bright green color of fresh vegetables. Its use for such purposes cannot be recommended because of the destructive effect it has on both thiamin and vitamin C. Baking soda used as a leavening agent in baked products has no detrimental effect on thiamin.

Loss due to processing. The thiamin content of pork is virtually destroyed by the irradiation procedures sometimes used in food preservation. Thiaminase is also destroyed. The use of sulfite as a preservative, especially in ground meat, leads to a reduction in thiamin activity.

Evaluation of nutritional status

The most sensitive test available for the determination of thiamin status is effect of TPP on the red blood cell transketolase activity. These values reflect changes in dietary intake before any other signs of thiamin inadequacy are detectable. In animals, growth response is considered a fairly sensitive indicator of thiamin intake but is not as specific to thiamin as is transketolase activity, which was shown to drop 30% at one week and 51% at two weeks in rats who continued to grow during this period of thiamin deficiency.

Another promising indicator of thiamin status of an individual is the carbohydrate index, which is a function of pyruvic acid, lactic acid, and glucose in the blood after the administration of glucose and a standard exercise test. Of course, it is useful only for persons able to exercise.

The urinary excretion test for thiamin involves measuring the amount of thiamin excreted in the urine following a test dose. Persons with low levels of saturation in the tissues will retain more and excrete less than will persons whose intake has been more adequate, but since so many other factors influence excretion, load tests are not considered reliable.

Deficiency

Thiamin deficiency may result from a low dietary intake or when the diet is very low in calories or limited in variety. It may also result from failure of absorption (usually caused by some abnormality in the gastrointestinal tract, possibly as a result of a folic acid deficiency), the inability of tissues to accumulate adequate stores of the vitamin, failure to utilize available thiamin or an increased requirement such as occurs in a diet high in carbohydrate or alcohol. At the moment there is no clear-cut indication of the relationship between clinical symptoms and biochemical changes that occur in a thiamin deficiency. Several explanations have been considered—that a lack of thiamin causes a failure to provide energy for the cell; that in thiamin deficiency some product essential for metabolism in heart or muscle cells is not formed; that neurotransmitters needed to transmit nerve impulses are not formed; and that some toxic product accumulates.

Since thiamin deficiency in humans usually occurs along with symptoms of deficiencies of other vitamins of the B complex, it is difficult to attribute symptoms specifically to lack of thiamin. The condition is often complicated by symptoms brought on by concurrent infection and varies with degree of deficiency and presence of stress situations such as pregnancy. However, in cases in which thiamin has been effective in relieving particular symptoms, it is customary to consider them specific to thiamin deficiency. The following have been associated with a lack of thiamin, although similar symptoms may occur as a result of other dietary inadequacies, especially those of B complex vitamins.

Loss of appetite. Loss of appetite, or anorexia, has been clearly demonstrated in experimental animals and has been related in many cases to thiamin inadequacy in humans, especially when transketolase levels drop. Anorexia accompanied by vomiting was the first sign of deficiency shown by a group of normal men subjected to an induced thiamin deficiency. Even at intakes of 0.2 mg/1000 kcal, which did not cause any other symptoms, loss of appetite, nausea, and constipation occurred. Although increased intake of thiamin will restore a depressed appetite to normal levels, it is ineffective in stimulating the appetite beyond that level.

Decreased muscle tonus. The tonus, or elasticity, of the wall of the lower gastrointestinal tract drops in thiamin deficiency to the point that normal gastric motility is decreased, the colon becomes distended, and constipation results. Thiamin has been used with varying degrees of success in treating constipation in older individuals in whom gastrointestinal motility is frequently subnormal.

Depression. Mental depression and confusion sometimes alleviated by the administration of thiamin has led to the somewhat misleading designation of thiamin as the "morale vitamin." Persons on low thiamin intakes show pronounced mood changes, vague feelings of uneasiness, fear, disorderly thinking, and other signs of mental depression. Mental changes associated with inadequate thiamin respond readily to thiamin supplements. This is well illustrated in a study of 10 older women (52 to 72 years of age) limited to 0.33 mg of thiamin a day. They all showed increasing irritability, complained of fatigue and headache, and voluntarily restricted their social engagements. Urinary excretion of thiamin dropped progressively. Immediate improvement was observed when they were given 1.4 mg for one day. Similarly, the restoration of thiamin to the diets of men who had been on a restricted thiamin intake led to the restoration of normal attitudes. Reports demonstrating that the use of thiamin supplements with children was effective in raising their IQ and intellec-

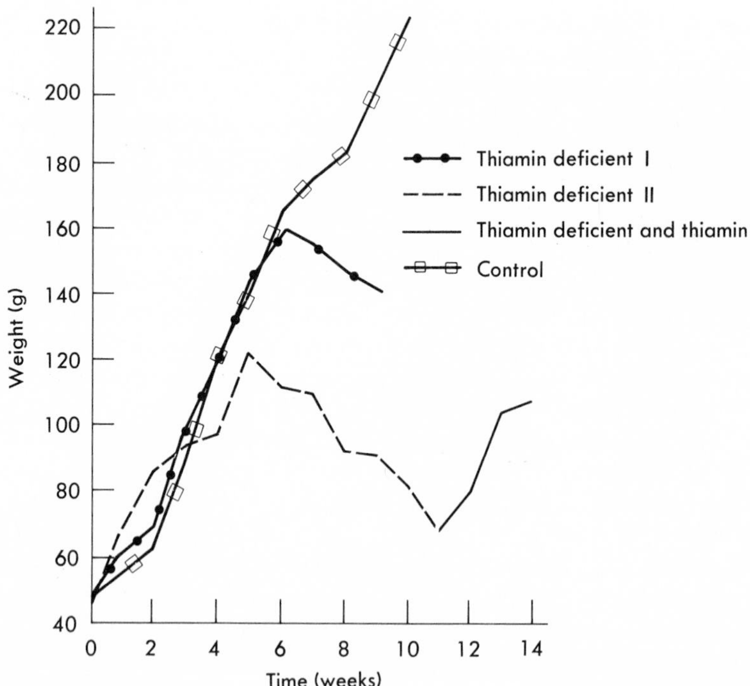

Fig. 12-13. Growth pattern of weanling albino rats with and without thiamin.

tual performance have subsequently been discredited. In beriberi the most acute symptom is mental confusion leading to coma.

Neurological changes. Nystagmus caused by a weakness in the sixth cranial nerve is known as Wernicke's syndrome. This symptom, a manifestation of changes occurring in the central nervous system, is easily reversed by thiamin administration. Levels of thiamin in the brain can be reduced by 50% without any noticeable clinical signs; further reduction to 30% of normal leads to slow and unsteady gait, and at 20% severe disturbance of posture of equilibrium occurs.

Peripheral neuritis, in which the nerves that control the extremities fail to function properly, shows up in a variety of ways in humans, usually affecting the legs first.

Neuromuscular coordination is affected in persons on low thiamin intake, resulting in decreased work output and mechanical efficiency. Motor speed, eye-hand coordination, and body and manual steadiness reactions that had deteriorated on an intake of 0.05 mg of thiamin per 1000 kcal were quickly restored with thiamin supplementation. Other signs of peripheral nervous system involvement are loss of ankle and knee jerk, painful calf muscles, and general atrophy of leg muscles manifest as difficulty in walking.

Beriberi. Beriberi, the final form of thiamin deficiency, has been mentioned earlier.

Deficiencies in animals. In experimental thiamin deficiency in rats complete deprivation lead to death in three to six weeks, with no specific clinical symptoms; when small amounts are provided, death was delayed to eight to twelve weeks. Rats developed spasticity of muscles and usually died in convulsive seizures complicated by heart lesions unless treated promptly.

Growth retardation accompanying a dietary lack of thiamin is readily demonstrated in animals. Typical growth patterns of rats with and without thiamin are shown in Fig. 12-13.

In birds, polyneuritis occurred on thiamin deprivation. Birds lost their sense of balance and had depressed appetites and a chronic state of head retraction. All symptoms were relieved with thiamin intake.

Clinical uses

Thiamin has been used in the medical treatment of a wide variety of conditions other than beriberi. One survey of the literature showed that it had been tried in 230 different conditions. In the period from 1936 to 1945 these included neuritis, neuralgia, pains of various origins, diseases of the central nervous system, and cardiovascular symptoms. A renewed interest in thiamin therapy occurred from 1951 to 1960. It was used in acidosis, diabetic coma, pyruvemia (accumulation of pyruvic acid in the blood), and toxemia of pregnancy. In addition, it is widely used as a supplement to stimulate a poor appetite. The possibility of observing beneficial results are greatest when malnutrition, nutritional imbalance, or impaired intestinal absorption have precipitated the symptoms.

RIBOFLAVIN

Riboflavin, which has also been known as vitamin B_2, vitamin G, and the yellow enzyme, was recognized in 1917 when it became clear that vitamin B retained some growth-promoting properties after its antiberiberi properties had been destroyed by heat. To differentiate the heat-labile component from this heat-stable fraction, the two components were designated vitamin B_1 and vitamin B_2, respectively. Riboflavin is known to be essential for growth and tissue repair in all animals from microorganisms to humans, but so far no readily identifiable deficiency syndrome has been associated with it.

At the time of discovery of riboflavin in 1925, reports appeared almost simultaneously announcing the isolation of four substances necessary for growth—hepatoflavin, lactoflavin, ovoflavin, and verdoflavin. These investigators, obviously isolating their factors from liver, milk, eggs, and grass, respectively, had agreed that they were flavin compounds—substances that produce an intense yellow-green fluorescence in water. These substances had been concentrated from natural foods in 1925 and isolated in 1932, at which time it became evident that the active factor was composed of a protein plus a pigment, the flavin. With the synthesis of riboflavin in 1935 it soon became clear that the 5-carbon sugar ribose was common to all forms, which were then designated riboflavine. Shortly afterward the final *e* was dropped but was added in 1961 to the official spelling in Britain, although other countries have retained the new spelling.

Chemical properties

Riboflavin is a relatively stable vitamin; it is resistant to the effects of acid, heat, and oxidation. It is unstable in the presenc of alkali and light. Since it is slightly soluble in water, some losses occur when riboflavin-containing vegetables cut in small pieces are cooked in large amounts of water for long periods of time. The major loss of riboflavin in food (up to 70% in 4 hours) is due to the action of either the ultraviolet or visible rays of sunlight on milk, a significant source of riboflavin in the American diet. The almost universal use of opaque wax-lined cardboard or plastic containers is reducing the problem. Another successful effort has been the provision of covered insulated boxes that protect the milk from exposure to sunlight after home deliveries.

Functions

Riboflavin is a part of several enzymes and coenzymes in which it contributes to their capacity to accept and transfer hydrogen atoms, or positive charges. These reactions are essential for the release of energy from glucose and fatty acids within the cell mitochondrion. The two coenzymes flavin mononucleotide (FMN, or riboflavin monophosphate) and flavin adenine dinucleotide (FAD), which is FMN with an ATP group, are attached to a variety of proteins and are known as flavoproteins. Riboflavin is also an integral part of other enzymes specifically involved in the transfer of hydrogen atoms in protein metabolism. Through its role in activating vitamin B_6, riboflavin is necessary before the amino acid tryptophan can be converted into the active form of the vitamin niacin. It is also involved in the conversion of folic acid to its coenzymes and their subsequent storage in the body. Since these are needed for DNA synthesis, riboflavin has an indirect effect on cell proliferation and hence on growth.

Among other biochemical roles in which riboflavin is believed to participate are the production of corticosteroids in the adrenal cortex, the formation of red blood cells in bone marrow, the synthesis of glycogen (glycogenesis), fatty acid catabolism, and the effectiveness of the thyroid in regulating enzyme activity.

Some substances chemically related to riboflavin can replace riboflavin completely; others are effective for a short time, apparently replacing the reserves of riboflavin but leading to death as soon as the original reserves are depleted; and still others act as riboflavin antagonists. These antagonists replace riboflavin in enzyme systems in which they cannot function as riboflavin does and in so doing prevent any available vitamin from functioning. In humans riboflavin deficiencies have been produced experimentally by the use of the riboflavin antagonist galactoflavin, in which the 5-carbon ribose is replaced by a 6-carbon sugar, galactose.

Absorption

The absorption of riboflavin occurs primarily in the upper portion of the gastrointestinal tract. Absorption is regulated by a specific transport system that determines how much will be taken up into the cells lining the intestinal mucosa. There appears to be an upper limit to the amount that can be taken up. More riboflavin (60% compared to 15%) is absorbed when it is taken with meals than when taken separately. Older persons absorb more than do younger and those on thyroid medication absorb less than others.

t is possible that the slower passage through he intestinal tract allows more contact with he absorbing surface, or there may be an ıcrease in sites for absorption.

Within the intestinal cells much riboflavin s linked with a phosphate molecule (phos›horylated) to form the coenzyme flavin nononucleotide (FMN). Once absorbed, oth riboflavin and FMN are transported atached to albumin in the blood. It is readily eleased from the blood to the tissues, prinipally the liver, where it is converted into nother coenzyme (FAD) by the addition of ATP. In the tissues it is stored as FMN and FAD ather than as free riboflavin. With higher ntakes the amount in the liver will not inrease beyond a certain level. Conversely, in deficiency, liver reserves do not drop below 0% of saturation levels. The presence of the hyroid hormone appears to stimulate the bsorption and storage of riboflavin.

Riboflavin is excreted primarily in the rine after the kidneys have allowed the eabsorption of sufficient vitamin to mainain tissue saturation within established up›er and lower levels. Riboflavin excreted in he feces is either unabsorbed dietary ribolavin or some of the riboflavin secreted in he bile which is not reabsorbed. A small mount of this riboflavin is broken down by ntestinal microorganisms into different end ›roducts. There is relatively little storage of iboflavin in the body although the liver with 16 μg/g and kidneys with 25 μg/g contain higher concentrations than do other tissues, such as muscle with 2 to 3 μg/g.

Requirements

Although in previous editions of *Recommended Dietary Allowances* by the Food and Nutrition Board of the National Research Council riboflavin requirements had been based alternatively on caloric intake, protein allowances, and metabolic body size (weight in kg$^{3/4}$) as a criterion, current standards are related to energy allowances. For all ages 0.6 mg of riboflavin per 1000 kcal is recommended to ensure tissue saturation with the vitamin. This estimate was based on data from studies of excretion relative to intake when intake was above normal. During pregnancy an additional 0.3 mg is recommended and during lactation an additional 0.5 mg.

The FAO/WHO committee has continued to base its recommendations on caloric intake and has set 0.55 mg/1000 kcal as a practical goal. During pregnancy a 0.3 mg increase in intake beyond the needs of an adult woman is recommended. An increase of 0.5 mg is recommended for lactation.

Food sources

Riboflavin is widely distributed in both animal and vegetable foods. The amount present in 100 g and 100 kcal portions or representative foods is presented graphically in Fig. 12-14. Fig. 12-15 shows the relative contributions of the major food groups.

The riboflavin content of protein-rich foods contributes about a third of the vitamin in the American diet and is little effected by the usual methods of food preparation.

About 60% to 90% of the vitamin in fruits and vegetables is retained in cooking. On the other hand, the milling of cereal causes up to 60% loss of riboflavin. Because the yellow color of riboflavin may make an enriched product unacceptable, it is often not used in fortifying cereals such as rice, although it is always added to enrich flour and bread at a level above that found in whole wheat products. Originally the high standards were the result of errors in determining the amount of riboflavin present in whole wheat, but the standards have been retained because of the relative deficiency of riboflavin in some segments of the population.

Milk makes a significant contribution, with 1 liter providing all the recommended intake suggested for all ages and 2 cups providing a sufficient amount for minimal needs. This assumes that adequate precautions are taken to minimize exposure to sunlight, which drastically reduces the amount of riboflavin available. Cheese retains about a fourth the amount in the milk from which it was made.

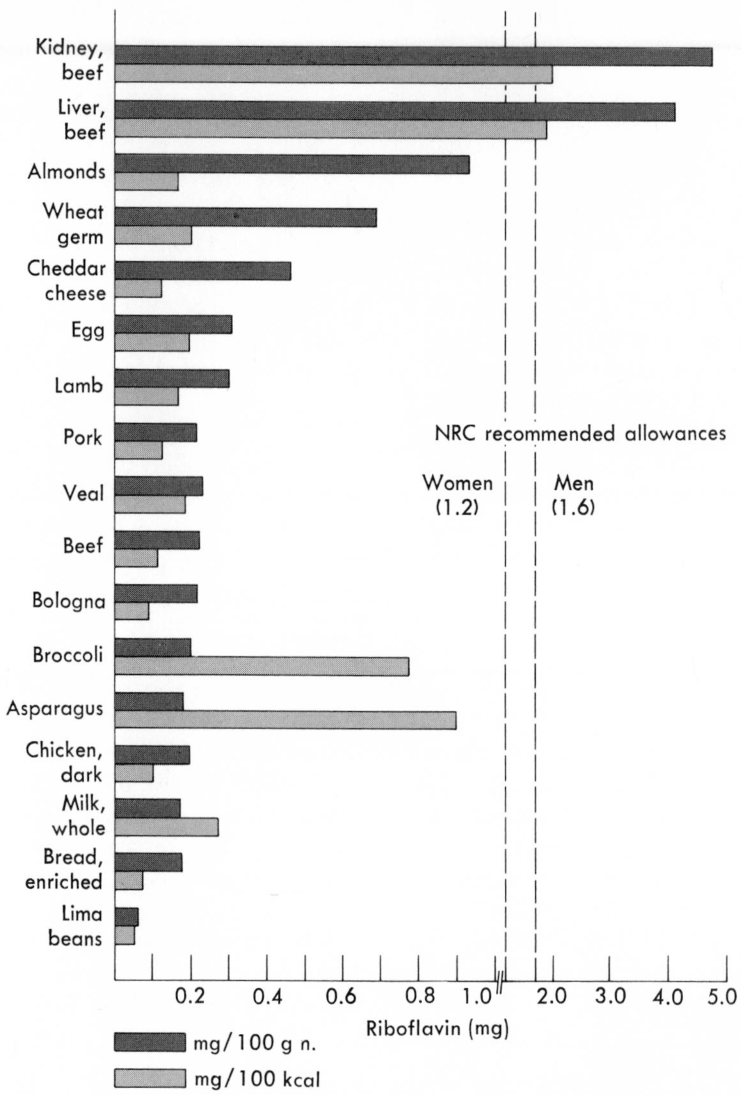

Fig. 12-14. Riboflavin content of 100 g and 100 kcal portions of representative foods. (Based on Watt, B. K., and Merrill, A. L.: Composition of foods—raw, processed and prepared, Handbook No. 8, Washington, D.C., 1963, U.S. Department of Agriculture.)

Cereals are low in riboflavin except after germination. Enriched cereals have about twice as much riboflavin as do whole-grain cereals but still contribute only a seventh of the intake. Neera, a palm juice used in India, has been found to be high in riboflavin and accounts for a positive improvement in health when it is in season. The INQ for riboflavin for representative foods is shown in Table 12-7.

Evidence exists that riboflavin is synthesized by bacteria in the gastrointestinal tract, but there is little indication that a significant amount is absorbed by humans except when the diet is high in starch. A diet high in starch, cellulose, and lactose stimulates ribo-

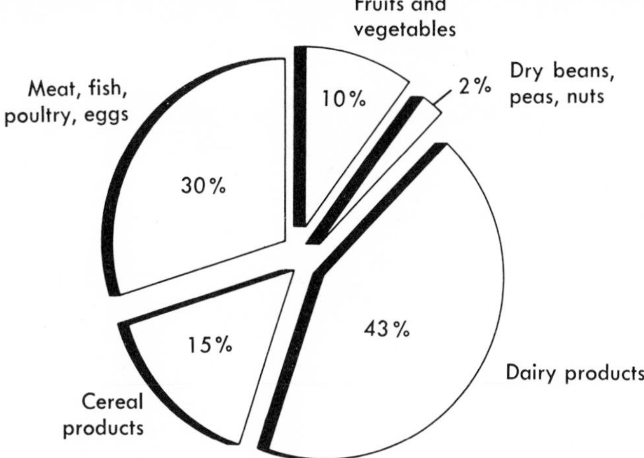

Fig. 12-15. Contribution of various food groups to the riboflavin content of American food supply. (Based on Contribution of major food groups to nutrient supplies available for civilian consumption, National Food Situation NSF-159, Washington, D.C., 1977, Economic Research Service.)

Table 12-7. INQ for selected sources of riboflavin providing at least 15% of the U.S. RDA per serving

Yeast	25.7
Liver	24.7
Broccoli	10.5
Beef heart	8.8
Yogurt (partially skim milk)	4.8
Milk, whole	3.4
Cheese	3.2
Almonds	2.1

flavin synthesis in the intestines, whereas fat and protein have an inhibitory effect.

Evaluation of nutritional status

Although the measurement of urinary and red blood cell levels of riboflavin has been frequently used in the assessment of riboflavin status, these values are not considered sensitive indicators, since they tend to reflect the immediate past intake by decreasing soon after dietary levels are reduced. In addition, urinary riboflavin is influenced by many other factors such as exercise, stress, and temperature; the red blood cell level also increases in a pyridoxine deficiency; excretion increases ten to fifteen times normal during starvation. The measurement of the activation of the enzyme erythrocyte glutathione reductase to which riboflavin is closely bound in red blood cells is now being used as a sensitive indicator of riboflavin status.

Deficiency

Considerable evidence is accumulating to suggest that riboflavin deficiency is more common than previously suspected.

A study of the riboflavin status of 431 high school students showed that about 16% of the girls and 6% of the boys had glutathione reductase activity coefficients indicative of inadequate riboflavin intakes. This evidence of deficiency was eliminated by riboflavin supplementation with 0.5 mg a day for one week. Other studies have demonstrated a high incidence of riboflavin deficiency among chronic alcoholics.

In an experimentally induced severe riboflavin deficiency (less than 0.07 mg of riboflavin for thirty-nine to fifty-six days) six adult males showed measurable personality shifts toward hypochondriasis, depression and hysteria and reduced strength in hand grip. In this study changes in the red blood cell glutathione reductase activity coefficient were found to be a more sensitive indicator of riboflavin status than was urinary riboflavin excretion.

The lack of riboflavin manifests itself in a wide variety of ways that can be assessed clinically. In humans an early form of ariboflavinosis (a lack of riboflavin) is a condition known as **cheilosis,** in which cracks appear at the corners of the mouth and the lips become inflamed. The tongue becomes smooth and takes on a characteristic purplish red color in a condition described as *glossitis.* These are the signs used most frequently in nutrition surveys as indicative of low riboflavin intakes, although the intake must be low for several months before these symptoms manifest themselves. Changes in the skin, causing dryness and scaliness, have been associated with low riboflavin intakes but are not specific to this vitamin.

As is true in a deficiency of all vitamins, growth retardation occurs with a lack of riboflavin. Reproductive capacity is also reduced when riboflavin is lacking, and if conception does take place, certain congenital malformations such as harelip and cataracts have been associated with a deficiency at a crucial stage in early (embryonic) development. This effect has been clearly demonstrated in animal experiments, but the relationship is much more difficult to establish in human pregnancy.

Other effects of a lack of riboflavin in the diet of animals for which no counterpart symptoms have been established in humans are loss of hair (alopecia) and infiltration of blood vessels into the cornea of the eye (corneal vascularization), which may eventually form cataracts. By preventing or slowing the breakdown of riboflavin by microorganisms in the intestine antibiotics tend to decrease the need for riboflavin.

Toxicity

No reports of riboflavin toxicity have appeared even though amounts as high as 10 g/kg have been given to animals. Neither is there evidence of toxicity in humans.

NIACIN (NICOTINIC ACID)

Niacin, formerly known as nicotinic acid, was originally obtained from the oxidation of nicotine in 1867. By 1912 it had been associated with antiberiberi substance in rice polishings and isolated in a crystalline form. It was not, however, until 1937 that it was recognized as the pellagra-preventive factor, a vitamin capable of curing the disease pellagra in humans and blacktongue in dogs. An amide (NH_2), nicotinamide, formed from nicotinic acid, is the state most active in metabolic reactions. The term niacin is now used to include nicotinic acid, nicotinamide, and other related compounds.

History

The disease known as *pellagra* in Italy and *mal del sol* or *mal de la rosa* in Spain was first described in the eighteenth century when it occurred mainly among the poor, for whom corn introduced from the New World was the dietary staple. Although there was evidence that the disease could be cured by changing the diet, it was only in 1917 that it was associated with the absence of a dietary factor.

The association of **pellagra** with diets monotonously high in highly refined maize, or corn, led to the theory that it was caused by a mold or a toxic or infectious substance in spoiled corn. A lack of nitrogen was implicated, and later the absence of lysine, tryptophan, or cysteine in conjunction with high leucine content in corn diets suggested that an amino acid imbalance was the cause. The skin symptoms associated with pellagra were aggravated by exposure to sunlight, leading to the belief that the disease was the result of sun poisoning (mal del sol). Since the pellagragenic corn diets, in which molasses and salt pork were often the only other foods, were consumed by persons on limited incomes often living in crowded unsanitary surroundings, theories suggesting an infectious or parasitic nature for the disease received further support. The fact that several members of the same family often developed pellagra seemed reason to look for a hereditary factor.

Only in 1817 when Goldberger, a physician working with the United States Public Health Service, confirmed his theory by producing pellagra through dietary restriction was progress made in controlling the disease. His experiment with a group of prisoners who were promised reprieve if they would switch from the prison diet to one typical of

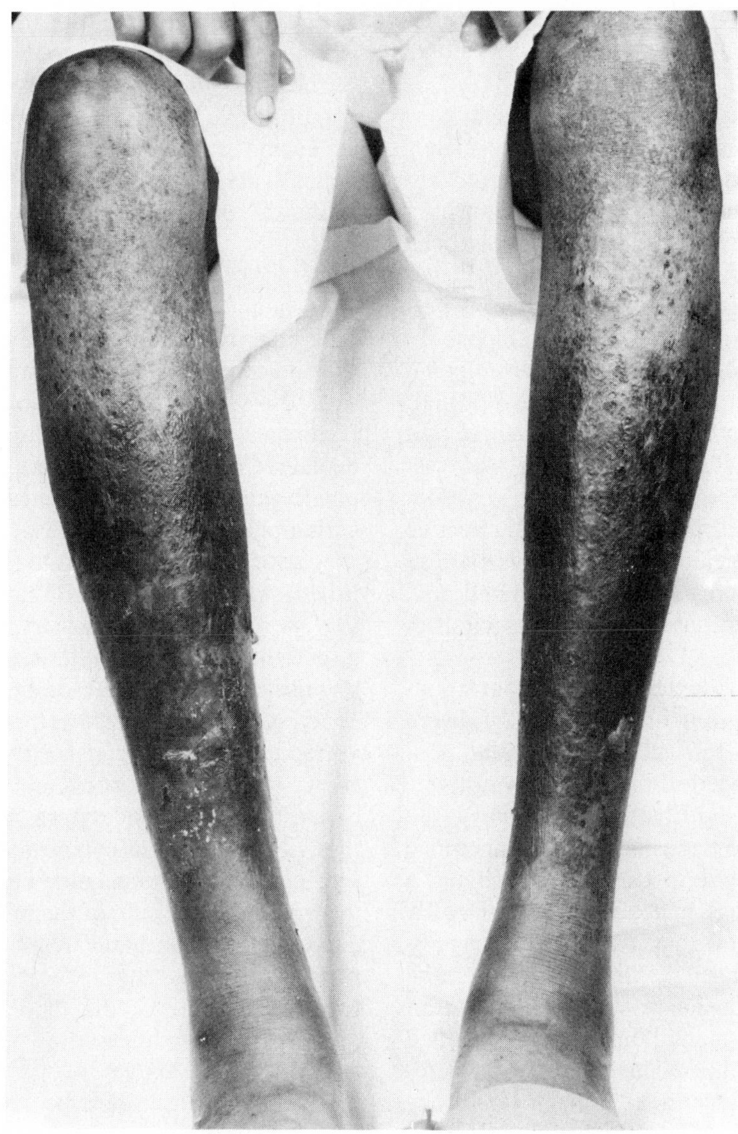

Fig. 12-16. Severe dermatitis of legs in patient suffering from pellagra. (Courtesy Dr. J. L. Spivak, The John Hopkins University School of Medicine.)

the villages in which pellagra was prevalent is now classic. Since this diet in many cases was the one most familiar to the prisoners, they were willing subjects. After about five months, however, these men began to develop the classic symptoms of pellagra—dermatitis, diarrhea, and depression—whereas those on regular prison fare remained healthy. This fairly well refuted the theory that pellagra was an infectious condition and established the theory that the dietary factor was involved. It took researchers an additional twenty years to identify the nutritional factor.

Pellagra, first reported in the state of New York in 1875, is the only vitamin-deficiency disease that has ever been considered endemic to the United States and a major public health problem. Its incidence has been fairly well confined to the small mill villages of the southern states where the diet is predominantly corn, molasses, and salt pork. In 1918 an estimated 10,000 deaths from pellagra and another 100,000 cases were reported, primarily in cotton-growing areas. At that time, when a dietary deficiency was suspected but the identity of the lacking nutrient had not been established, the most effective means of controlling the disease was to encourage the increased use of meat and milk products by promoting home production of food.

Efforts to isolate the dietary factor responsible for preventing or curing pellagra were complicated by the fact that many other deficiencies produced similar skin symptoms. Not until 1937 did Elvehjem, working at the University of Wisconsin, show that nicotinic acid was effective in curing blacktongue, a condition in dogs analogous to human pellagra. The use of nicotinic acid in treating human pellagra brought dramatic results and the census of pellagra victims in southern hospitals and mental institutions dropped precipitously. There have been several recent reports indicating that niacin deficiency is still prevalent in some areas, usually associated with alcoholism or an infection in the pancreas. Fig. 12-16 depicts the skin changes associated with a diet inadequate in niacin and protein.

Pellagra is still found in corn-eating countries such as Romania, Yugoslavia, and some parts of Egypt and in sorghum-eating areas in India. The fact that it is not found in Central America, where corn provides 80% of the calories, can be attributed to the use of alkalis (usually soda lime) in its preparation. This helps to liberate the niacin bound in the cereal.

The pellagragenic nature of a diet of sorghum has been attributed to the high content of the amino acid leucine. The fact that the condition can be corrected by the addition of isoleucine suggest that leucine-isoleucine balance may be an important factor in the incidence of pellagra.

Tryptophan-niacin relationship

A chemical analysis of some foods such as milk effective in curing or preventing pellagra indicated a low niacin content. Moreover, diets low in niacin were not always pellagragenic. This apparent discrepancy was explained in 1945 with the discovery that the amino acid tryptophan was also effective in curing pellagra. The role of tryptophan as a precursor of niacin has since been well established. Although for a while some investigators were convinced that tryptophan promoted the intestinal synthesis of niacin, with the use of radioactive isotopes it was unequivocally proved that tyrptophan was converted to niacin in the cells. It has now been shown that under most circumstances 60 mg of tryptophan will yield 1 mg of niacin. Although current food composition tables do not record the nicotinamide equivalent values for foods, the sum of the preformed niacin and the niacin equivalent of the tryptophan more accurately reflects the pellagra-preventive value of the food. Dietary requirements are expressed as niacin equivalents.

A comparison of dietary intake of niacin based on calculations from tables of food composition with recommended intakes underestimates the value of the diet in meeting requirements, which are expressed as niacin equivalents.

Tryptophan needed for synthesis of body protein will not be available for conversion to niacin, although it has not been clearly defined which need has priority. The conversion of tryptophan to niacin requires the presence of at least three other vitamins—thiamin, pyridoxine, and riboflavin and possibly biotin. Since vitamin B_6 (pyridoxine) is involved in the formation of niacin, it has not been surprising to find symptoms of pellagra appearing when isonicotinic acid hydrazide (INH, or isoniazid), a vitamin B_6 antagonist used in the treatment of tuberculosis, is administered in high doses. Only the L form of tryptophan can be converted; D-isomers are biologically inactive. The conversion of tryptophan to niacin may be more efficient during pregnancy than at other times.

Chemical properties

Niacin is extremely stable to heat, light, acid, alkali, and oxidation. Because of its stability, little of the nutrient is lost in normal procedures of food processing and preparation. It is active either as the acid or as the amide nicotinamide. The amide is preferred for therapeutic doses, since the use of large amounts of acid, which acts as a vasodilator, may lead to flushing of the skin and tingling sensations.

Functions

Niacin is required by all living cells, where it plays a vital role in the release of energy from all three energy-building nutrients—carbohydrate, fat, and protein—and is involved in the synthesis of protein, fat and pentoses needed for nucleic acid (DNA) formation. It is part of the coenzymes nicotinamide adenine dinucleotide (NAD) and nicotinamide adenine dinucleotide phosphate (NADP), both of which can accept or release hydrogen atoms readily. Because of this, they are effective in assisting a group of enzymes known as dehydrogenases in removing hydrogen in many biological reactions. They have previously been known as coenzymes I and II and as DPN and TPN (di- and triphosphopyridine nucleotide), and the use of these terms still persists in some literature. No other biochemical role for niacin has been established yet, but the central role it plays as a part of these coenzymes means that without it the body is unable to utilize carbohydrate, fat, or protein or synthesize fat.

Evidence exists that doses of 1 to 2 g three times a day of niacin (but not of nicotinamide) may result in lowered blood cholesterol levels. The way in which it works is still subject to debate, but it has been suggested that it may interfere with cholesterol or lipoprotein (lipid carrier in the blood) synthesis; or it may stimulate the synthesis of lipoprotein lipase, the enzyme which causes the breakdown of lipoprotein. Studies on human subjects have shown that large doses of niacin prevent the heart muscle from using free fatty acids, its usual source of energy, and forces it to rely on glycogen and stored fat instead. These observations raise the question of the desirability of the use of large doses of niacin by athletes, especially since it is known that niacin reduces the ability of exercising subjects to mobilize fatty acids.

At the same time that niacin causes a lowering of blood lipids it causes an increase in the amount of uric acid in the blood and aggravates diabetes.

The use of large doses (4 to 5 g daily) in the treatment of schizophrenia is the subject of much controversy. At the moment, the bulk of the evidence seems to question its value.

Absorption and metabolism

Niacin is readily absorbed and is stored to a limited extent. Any excess niacin is methylated and excreted in the urine either as *N*-methyl nicotinamide or as the pyridone of *N*-methyl nicotinamide. The observation that animals excrete some radioactively labeled vitamin as carbon dioxide through the lungs has not been tested in humans. About two thirds of the niacin metabolized by adults may come from tryptophan.

Requirements

In establishing the recommended dietary allowances, the National Research Council has defined a niacin equivalent as 1 mg of niacin or 60 mg of tryptophan. Estimates of niacin requirements are based on the amount needed to prevent pellagra to which allowances for individual variations have been added.

Since niacin is intimately involved in the release of energy from food, it is not surprising to find that the recommended allowance for niacin is based on the caloric intake. The minimum need has been established at 4.4 mg of niacin per 1000 kcal, to which a 50% margin of safety has been added in the recommended allowances of 6.6 mg of niacin per 1000 kcal. It is also suggested that a minimum intake of 9 to 13 mg be maintained regardless of caloric intake, since this appears to be a level needed to prevent pellagra. Recommendations of FAO and WHO are essentially the same.

The amount required is influenced by factors other than caloric intake. In an amino acid imbalance (especially high leucine as found in the cereal millet) the need for niacin increases. The type of carbohydrate may also have some effect, as data show that carbohydrates containing fructose increase the need for niacin. During starvation, tryptophan from the breakdown of protein serves as a source of niacin.

During the second and third trimesters of pregnancy an increase of 2 mg over normal needs is indicated. For lactation, when human milk contains 0.15 to 0.17 mg/dl or 70 kcal, the maternal diet should provide 6 mg more than that needed under normal circumstances. This will provide the breast-fed infant with 8 mg/day, of which two thirds comes from tryptophan. Bottle-fed infants almost always have a higher intake.

Most American diets that are adequate in protein supply sufficient niacin. Animal protein contains 1.4% tryptophan and vegetable protein, 1%. Thus a diet with 60 g of protein provides a minimum of 600 mg of tryptophan, which can be converted into 10 mg of niacin. Any tryptophan needed for the synthesis of body protein would not be available for niacin formation. However, once the growth process is completed, much more tryptophan can be diverted for niacin synthesis.

Most diets contain a sufficient surplus of tryptophan to result in 8 to 14 mg of niacin. An additional 8 to 17 mg of preformed niacin in the diet makes a total of 16 to 33 mg, an amount sufficient for practically all adult needs. Only when the diet is low in protein and relatively high in a tryptophan-poor cereal is a deficiency likely to occur. Gelatin is one protein completely devoid of tryptophan. In general, the niacin equivalent of American diets is considered to be 50% above the niacin content.

Food sources

The major sources of niacin are shown in Table 12-8. Liver, meat, poultry, peanut butter, and legumes are the richest sources. Milk and eggs, although low in preformed niacin, contain high amounts of tryptophan and as such have a high niacin equivalent. Fig. 12-17 shows the relative contribution of different food groups to dietary niacin. These values are based on niacin content and not niacin equivalents. The vitamin is present in plants as nicotinic acid and in animal foods as nicotinamide.

Evidence shows that much of the niacin in cereals such as rice and corn occurs as niacinogen, a peptide of at least seventeen amino acids. For this reason the niacin in these foods has low biological value and contributes little to the body's requirement for the vitamin unless prepared with alkali, as in the preparation of corn tortillas. The alkali aids in separating the vitamin into a form available to the body. In wheat bran niacin occurs as niacytin, a complex of either peptides or 5- or 6-carbon sugars and is likely not available at all. Niacytin is excreted in the urine as a substance known as trigonelline (methylated derivative).

As much as 90% of the niacin of cereals is in the outer husk and is removed in the mill-

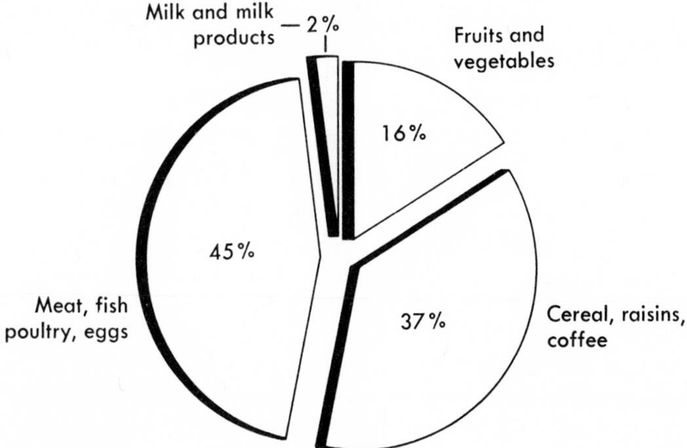

Fig. 12-17. Contribution of various food groups to the niacin content of American food supply. (Based on Contribution of major food groups to nutrient supplies available for civilian consumption, National Food Review NFR-1, Washington, D.C., 1978, Economic Research Service.)

Table 12-8. Niacin, tryptophan, and niacin equivalents of some representative foods (mg/100 g of food)

Food	Niacin*	Tryptophan†	Niacin equivalent of tryptophan‡	Total niacin
Beef liver	16.5	296	4.9	21.4
Peanut butter	15.7	330	5.5	21.2
Chicken, cooked	7.4	250	4.1	11.5
Beef, round	5.6	203	3.4	9.0
Bread, enriched	2.3	91	1.5	3.8
Orange juice	0.4	3	0.05	0.45
Spinach	0.3	37	0.6	0.9
Cottage cheese	0.2	179	2.9	3.1
Whole milk	0.1	49	0.8	0.9
Eggs	0.1	221	3.5	3.6

*From Watt, B. K., and Merrill, A. L.: Composition of foods—raw, processed and prepared, U.S. Department of Agriculture Handbook No. 8, Washington, D.C., 1963, U.S. Department of Agriculture.

†From Amino acid content of foods, Home Economics Research Report No. 4, Washington, D.C., 1957, U.S. Department of Agriculture.

‡Since 60 mg of tryptophan can be converted into 1 mg of niacin, niacin equivalent = $\frac{\text{mg tryptophan}}{60}$.

Table 12-9. INQ for selected sources of niacin providing at least 15% of the U.S. RDA

Food	INQ
Liver	8.3
Chicken breast	8.3
Fish and shellfish (tuna)	6.8
Beef heart	4.7
Peas	3.7
Peanuts	3.4
Veal	3.3
Ground beef	3.2
Pork	1.7
Lamb chop	1.6

ing process. The addition of niacin in enriched cereal products has done much to compensate for this loss at a very low cost. The INQ for niacin for representative foods is given in Table 12-9.

Evaluation of nutritional status

Since there is little storage of this water-soluble vitamin in the body, much has been learned about it by studying the forms and the amounts in which it is excreted in the urine after a test dose. When the dietary intake is adequate, a large percentage of the test dose is excreted, and most is in the form of methylated end products of niacin metabolism. When the dietary intake of both tryptophan and niacin has been low, less of the test dose is excreted, indicating that the body needs to retain more. About a fourth is excreted as methyl nicotinamide and the rest as a derivative known as pyridine. The latter disappears several weeks before clinical signs appear and the former at the time clinical signs of pellagra develop. The use of a ratio of urinary excretion of pyridone to urinary excretion of *N*-methyl nicotinamide per gram of creatinine (indicative of muscle mass of the body) has provided a criterion on which to evaluate nutritional status of population groups with respect to niacin adequacy. A ratio of less than 1:1 is considered indicative of pellagra, whereas a ratio between 1:1 and 1.3:1 is considered borderline. Values up to 4:0:1 are considered normal. There is no good blood test for niacin status.

Deficiency

In pellagra the skin, gastrointestinal tract, and central nervous system are affected. The symptoms progress through *dermatitis, diarrhea,* and *depression* preceding *death* in what has been characterized as the four Ds of pellagra. The dermatitis of pellagra is often complicated by symptoms of other B vitamin deficiencies, but when a niacin deficiency occurs, the character of the skin inflammation is specific. It occurs almost exclusively on areas of the skin exposed to sunlight and in a symmetrical pattern on both sides of the body. There is a clearly demarcated line between the afflicted and healthy areas of the skin.

As the mucous linings of the gastrointestinal tract become involved, the patient suffers from diarrhea and other manifestations of infection. The hydrochloric acid secretion normally present in the gastric juice may be absent, and this may reduce the bactericidal function of the gastric juice and allow the growth of infection-producing organisms. These changes in the gastrointestinal tract usually precede the degenerative changes that occur in the mental outlook of the patient. The irritability, headaches, and sleeplessness of early stages is soon followed by more severe mental symptoms, such as loss of memory, hallucinations, delusions of persecution, and finally a severe depression that almost inevitably precedes death.

Megavitamin therapy

Large doses of niacin have been used therapeutically in attempts to reduce blood cholesterol levels, a known risk factor in coronary heart disease, and to treat schizophrenia.

Massive doses of 3 g of nicotinic acid but not nicotinamide result in lower serum cholesterol and lipoprotein levels. A study involving 1100 patients did show a reduction in nonfatal heart attacks, but also showed an increase in side effects such as gastrointestinal problems and an increase in serum uric acid and plasma glucose levels. It failed, however, to establish a decreased mortality from coronary heart disease over a five-year-period. Subjects mobilized fewer fatty acids from fat stores and used more muscle glycogen as a source of energy.

In treating psychiatric problems, not only niacin but other vitamins have been used in extremely large amounts in what is known as orthomolecular therapy. So far there is no scientific evidence of its effectiveness.

PYRIDOXINE (VITAMIN B_6)

The terms vitamin B_6 and pyridoxine are used to denote at least three chemically, metabolically, and functionally related substances—pyridoxol, pyridoxal, and pyridoxamine—all of which are biologically active for all animals studied so far. Pyridoxine was first identified in 1934 as vitamin B_6 or *adermin*, a substance capable of curing a characteristic dermatitis in rats that did not respond to any of the three factors then known in the B complex. This was followed by its isolation in 1938 and the elucidation of its structure and its synthesis in 1939. The same year, György suggested the name pyridoxine. Since then many scientists have been involved in attempts to elucidate its role in metabolism.

Vitamin B_6 is found widely distributed in nature. In plants it occurs as pyridoxine, the alcohol form (formerly known as pyridoxol) bound to protein, a state in which it is not readily absorbed. Pyridoxamine and pyridoxal, the most prevalent forms in animal tissues, are more easily absorbed. Vitamin B_6 is relatively stable to heat but is destroyed by oxidation and ultraviolet light. Pyridoxal is labile to alkali, but all three forms are stable to acid. The broad distribution of vitamin B_6 in food coupled with a relatively small need for the vitamin makes it difficult to induce a human deficiency sufficiently severe to produce characteristic symptoms. However, certain undesirable biochemical changes do occur on a diet containing suboptimal amounts of vitamin B_6, although no physical changes may be observed. The antagonist deoxypyridoxine in conjunction with diet low in vitamin B_6 has been used to study some aspects of pyridoxine deficiency even though it does not have exactly the same effects as the deficiency alone.

Functions

Vitamin B_6 in the form of pyridoxal phosphate (PLP) functions as a coenzyme for many biological reactions. Zinc or magnesium catalyzes the formation of this active coenzyme in both the liver and red blood cells. In contrast to thiamin, riboflavin, and niacin, which act primarily as coenzymes for energy metabolism, vitamin B_6 plays no direct role in energy metabolism. Instead, it is involved primarily with reactions occurring in protein metabolism, being necessary in the synthesis and catabolism of all amino acids.

Pyridoxine is necessary for the process of transamination, in which the characteristic amino (NH_2) group from one amino acid is transferred to another substance to produce a different amino acid. Similarly, deamination, the removal of the amino group from some amino acids to form a nitrogen-free remnant to be excreted, is dependent on enzymes containing vitamin B_6–deaminases. This process of deamination must take place before protein in excess of needs for growth can be used as a source of energy. In addition, the removal of the carboxyl (COOH) group from certain amino acids in the process called decarboxylation also requires pyridoxal phosphate. This decarboxylation is a necessary step in the synthesis of the vital body regulators serotonin from tryptophan, norepinephrine from tyrosine, and histamine from histidine.

The decarboxylation of glutamic acid in the brain is dependent on vitamin B_6, which also functions in the removal of sulfur from sulfur-containing amino acids such as cysteine.

Pyridoxal phosphate plays a role in hemoglobin synthesis as a cofactor in the formation of a precursor of heme, an essential part of the hemoglobin molecule.

The most intensively studied role of vitamin B_6 in protein metabolism is in the conversion of the amino acid tryptophan into the vitamin niacin. This conversion involves several biochemical steps, in one of which an intermediary product, kynurenine, is formed. Kynurenine in turn is changed to niacin in a series of reactions; one step is catalyzed by pyridoxal phosphate.

If large amounts (from 5 to 10 g) of tryptophan are fed in what is known as a tryptophan load test, a person whose diet is low in pyridoxine does not produce enough pyridoxal phosphate to allow the conversion of all the kynurenine produced from tryptophan to niacin. Instead, xanthurenic acid, a substance that is not utilized by the body, is produced from kynurenine. It is excreted in the urine, and a determination of xanthurenic acid in the urine is used as an indication of the availability of pyridoxine. High urinary xanthurenic acid levels occur when available pyridoxine is limited, and low levels occur when available vitamin B_6 is sufficient to allow more complete conversion of tryptophan to niacin.

Vitamin B_6 is essential for the production of antibodies, as evidenced by the reduced production as available pyridoxine drops. This is believed to be due to a reduced incorporation of amino acids into protein and a deficient production of messenger RNA necessary to direct protein synthesis in the cells that normally produce antibodies. Skin grafts take longer to heal in the absence of pyridoxine, apparently because of delayed hypersensitivity.

Further evidence of a relationship between the availability of pyridoxine and protein metabolism is provided in the fact that when pyridoxine is increased, the availability of the D form of the amino acids methionine, tryptophan, and valine, not normally used by the body, is increased 100%, 50%, and 33%, respectively.

In other aspects of protein metabolism, pyridoxine is a cofactor for the enzym amino oxidase, which is essential for the syr thesis of a substance involved in the forma tion of essential cross linkages in the protei elastin, an important intercellular consti uent. Vitamin B_6 is known to be essential i the production of one of the precursors c nucleic acids.

Vitamin B_6 is also involved, at least ind rectly, in several aspects of lipid metabolism It appears to be required for the conversio of the essential fatty acid linoleic acid t arachidonic acid. There is also evidence fro rat studies that both the synthesis and tur over of cholesterol is enhanced in vitamin F deficiency with the result that there is littl change in blood cholesterol levels. The fo mation of some of the lipids, especiall sphingolipids necessary for the developme of the myelin sheath surrounding all nerv fibers, depends on adequate levels of vitami B_6.

In carbohydrate metabolism, vitamin B as part of the enzyme glycogen phosphor lase, is essential for the release of glycoge from the liver and muscle as glucose-pho phate. This must occur before any store carbohydrate can be available to the cells glucose to be used as a source of energy. Ha of the pyridoxine stored in the body is in th form of this enzyme in the muscle. Eviden indicates that pyridoxine may be needed fo the formation of other enzymes involved carbohydrate metabolism. Low blood gl cose levels, low glucose tolerance tests, and sensitivity to insulin in a pyridoxine de ciency provide additional evidence of a rel tionship with carbohydrate metabolism.

The role of pyridoxine in the metabolis of the central nervous system is the conce of many workers. In mild pyridoxine de ciency there are changes in electroenceph lograms, and in severe deficiency convulsi seizures take place. In addition, the role pyridoxine in the synthesis of the substan serotonin in the brain will influence beha ior.

The interrelationship between pyridoxi and hormones has been studied for son

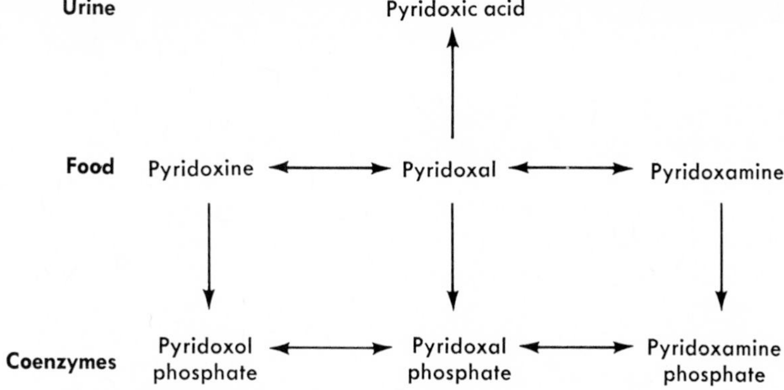

Fig. 12-18. Relationship of various chemical forms of pyridoxine.

time. For example, an excessive level of thyroxin results in depressed levels of the enzymes dependent on pyridoxine, and a deficiency of vitamin B_6 results in decreased levels of insulin and growth hormone.

Metabolism

Vitamin B_6 is active as pyridoxal phosphate, which can be formed in the body from any one of the three forms found in food—**pyridoxine, pyridoxal,** and **pyridoxamine**, which circulate in the blood attached to the protein albumin. The pathways by which these substances can form pyridoxal phosphate are shown in Fig. 12-18. The maximum amount of pyridoxine that can be converted to the coenzyme form is 7 mg a day.

Since pyridoxine is a water-soluble vitamin, virtually no storage of it occurs in the body. From 40% to 50% of dietary vitamin B_6 for males and from 22% to 35% for females is oxidized to pyridoxic acid, a metabolically inert substance, and excreted in the urine in amounts ranging from 0.5 to 1.3 mg a day. Pyridoxal, pyridoxamine, and pyridoxal phosphate also appear in the urine and have been measured in attempts to assess vitamin B_6 status. Some pyridoxine (from 0.7 to 0.9 mg a day) is excreted in the feces, but it arises primarily from synthesis by intestinal microorganisms and does not indicate loss of ingested pyridoxine.

Requirements

Estimates of the requirement for vitamin B_6 are based on information on the production and cure of clinical symptoms, data on the tryptophan load test, the measurement of vitamin B_6 dependent enzymes in the blood, and the excretion of the inactive form of the vitamin, pyridoxic acid.

Since pyridoxine is necessary for practically all aspects of protein metabolism, the requirement for the vitamin varies directly with the protein content of the diet, the requirement of which in turn is a function of body size.

Not until 1968 did the National Research Council believe adequate data existed on which to base recommendations for the dietary intake of vitamin B_6. After evaluating evidence indicating that the need for vitamin B_6 was a function of the amount of protein in the diet and relatively independent of the caloric content of the diet, it recommended an intake of 2 mg a day, which it postulated would be adequate to allow for the metabolism of 100 g of protein. For the pregnant woman, who transfers sufficient pyridoxine to the fetus to maintain a level of the vitamin in fetal blood five times that in the maternal blood, an additional intake of 0.5 mg is recommended. This is based on evidence that the stress of pregnancy increases the need for pyridoxine, as the body is then less able to handle large amounts of tryptophan. Although 2 to 10 mg of supplemental vitamin B_6 should be given during the third trimester of pregnancy, larger supplements should be avoided because of the danger of conditioning the infant to a higher requirement. A similar intake of 2.5 mg is the level recommended to provide for the needs of lactation when 0.1 mg/L is transferred to human milk.

Since vitamin B_6 is involved in many aspects of protein metabolism, when the diet contains very high amounts of protein, as do some of the currently popular (although nutritionally questionable) high protein–no carbohydrate diets, supplementary vitamin B_6 may be needed.

The recommended intake for infants is based on the observation that both human and cow's milk contain approximately 0.015 mg/g of protein, or 0.04 mg/100 kcal, levels which allow for adequate metabolism of protein. For the older infant and child from 0.5 to 1.2 mg are suggested, and for the adolescent from 1.4 to 2 mg appear desirable.

Older persons may have increased needs for the vitamin. They have a lower level of the enzyme transaminase in the plasma, have less pyridoxal kinase in the brain, and excrete more xanthurenic acid after a tryptophan load test.

Table 12-10. Pyridoxine content of average servings of some representative foods*

Food	μg per serving
Beef liver	840
Bananas	510
Round steak	435
Ham	400
Egg yolk	300
Canned salmon	300
Cabbage	160
Lima beans, frozen	150
Spinach	150
Egg	110
Potatoes	91
Cheddar cheese	80
Strawberries	55
Milk, whole	40
Grapefruit	34
Orange juice, frozen	28

*From Orr, M. L.: Pantothenic acid, vitamin B_6 and vitamin B_{12} in foods, Home Economics Research Report No. 36, Agricultural Research Service, Washington, D.C., 1969, U.S. Department of Agriculture.

Food sources

To satisfy nutrient needs, a diet should provide 2 ppm pyridoxine. Few foods can be considered poor sources of vitamin B_6. Among the richest, however, are muscle meats, liver, vegetables, whole-grain cereals, and egg yolks.

Since the pyridoxine in vegetable sources is more resistant to losses during processing and storage than are the pyridoxal and pyridoxamine found in animal sources, vegetable sources make a more significant contribution to the total dietary intake.

Before the vitamin B_6 content of foods was listed in any standard tables of food composition, the U.S. Department of Agriculture prepared a separate table of food composition with the pyridoxine content of food. This information is more frequently provided in standard tables now. The pyridoxine content of some representative foods is shown in Table 12-10.

Freezing of vegetables causes a 25% reduction of the amount present, and milling of cereals leads to losses as high as 90% of the original values. At the present time, the addition of pyridoxine to enriched bread and cereals is not mandatory under enrichment laws, although adequate justification might be found for such a practice on the basis of data suggesting that the intake of pyridoxine is marginal in many American diets. However, until there is a sensitive test for vitamin B_6 status to provide biochemical evidence of the extent of deficiency states in this country,

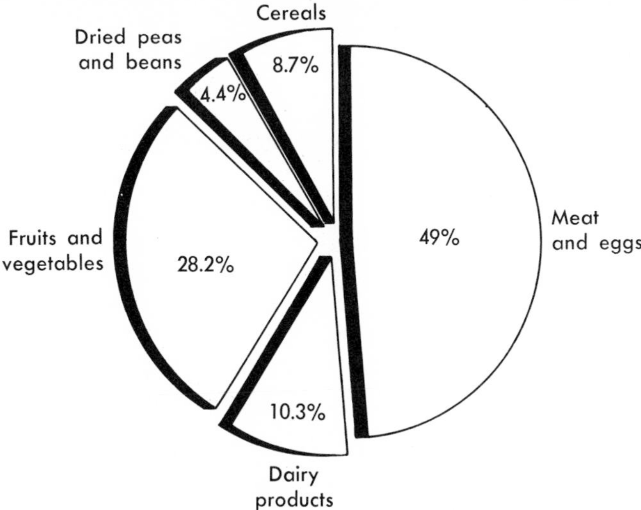

Fig. 12-19. Contribution of various food groups to pyridoxine (vitamin B_6) content of the American diet. (Based on National Food Review NFR-1, Washington, D.C., 1978, Economic Research Service.)

such action might not be justified. It is added to many of the cereals for which a standard of identity has not been established, but which are fortified by the processor with the added nutrient declared on the label. Contribution of various food groups to the pyridoxine content of the diet is shown in Fig. 12-19.

Evaluation of nutritional status

Although no specific nutritional deficiency disease can be attributed to a lack of vitamin B_6, evidence exists that certain biochemical changes do occur when the intake is low or the needs of the individual are above normal.

Since vitamin B_6 catalyzes the conversion of tryptophan to niacin, a pyridoxine deficiency can be detected by measuring the amount of xanthurenic acid (an intermediary that accumulates in a vitamin B_6 deficiency) excreted after a test dose of 10 g of tryptophan. In another test, requiring only one sample of blood, the amount of pyridoxal phosphate in the blood following an oral dose of 100 mg of pyridoxine is determined. This indicates relative tissue saturation.

Since most pyridoxine is converted into pyridoxic acid before it is excreted in the urine, the determination of the level of this metabolite in the urine is a useful indicator of vitamin B_6 status. The excretion of 0.1 to 0.2 mg of pyridoxic acid is considered indicative of a state of vitamin B_6 depletion, and excretion of less than 1 mg in 24 hours suggests that the adequacy of the intake should be questioned. This is especially true if blood levels of the vitamin are low. In severe deprivation, pyridoxic acid disappears from the urine entirely.

Measurement of the vitamin B_6–dependent enzyme aminotransferase in red blood cells is also considered a sensitive indicator of vitamin B_6 status. In spite of some technical difficulties a number of investigators are proposing the use of plasma pyridoxal phosphate levels as a possible indicator of nutritional status. Another proposed test is based on the fact that vitamin B_6 is necessary for the biochemical changes involved in the conversion of the amino acid methionine to cysteine. In a deficiency there is increased urinary excretion of cystathionine, an intermediary product that accumulates in the absence of the vitamin B_6–dependent enzyme necessary to continue the conversion to cysteine. Thus measurement of the amount of cystathionine in the urine may prove a sensitive indicator of vitamin B_6 status.

Developing a simple test to assess vitamin B_6 status is necessary to determine if there is a deficiency of this vitamin in the American diet. Only then will it be possible to decide on a rational basis if the enrichment of foods with vitamin B_6 is either desirable or to be recommended.

The range of circumstances that may lead to a vitamin B_6 deficiency are presented in Table 12-11.

In recent years it has become evident that the use of oral contraceptives may lead to metabolic changes that result in an increased need for vitamin B_6. This is demonstrated by the elevated urinary levels of intermediary products of tryptophan metabolism in women taking the estrogen-containing pills and the relief of the symptoms after administration of vitamin B_6. Estrogen may either activate tryptophan metabolism, inhibit an enzyme needed in tryptophan metabolism, interfere with the activation of the coenzyme, or stimulate metabolism of amino acids for which vitamin B_6 is required. Since the formation of urinary stones is associated with vitamin B_6 deficiency, the possibility of an increased incidence in women taking oral contraceptives should be considered. Depression associated with the use of oral contraceptives has been attributed to a failure to convert tryptophan to serotonin, a neurotransmitter substance in the brain. Although 75% of the women tested corrected tryptophan metabolism with 10 mg of pyridoxine, as much as 30 mg may be needed to compensate for the increased need due to use of contraceptives. Since there is no evidence of adverse effects from this level of supplementation, it may be desirable. Higher dosages may be associated with an imbalance among B vitamins.

Table 12-11. Factors that may lead to vitamin B_6 deficiency or dependency

- Inadequate dietary intake
- Impaired delivery of vitamin (intake adequate)
  - Defective intestinal absorption
  - Defective cellular and intracellular transport
  - Impaired oxidation of pyridoxine
  - Impaired phosphorylation to form active coenzyme
- Excessive loss of vitamin
  - Through kidneys
  - Through oxidation
  - Inactivation by drugs
- Relative deficiency (primary intake inadequate relative to demand)
  - Increased metabolic activity (pregnancy, fever, etc.)
  - Increased protein intake
- Metabolic defects that alter utilization

Clinical uses

Vitamin B_6, which is available in an inexpensive synthetic form, has been used in the treatment of many conditions. When isoniazid (isonicotinic acid hydrazide), which is chemically related to pyridoxine, is used in the treatment of tuberculosis, patients develop many of the symptoms of a vitamin B_6 deficiency, including an increase in xanthurenic acid in the urine and peripheral neuritis. These symptoms are readily counteracted with the use of higher than normal amounts of pyridoxine. Apparently isoniazid combines with pyridoxal phosphate and inactivates the enzyme involved in decarboxylation of amino acids. Penicillamine therapy used in treating Wilson's disease, cystinuria, and rheumatoid arthritis may also increase the requirement for vitamin B_6. Although serum B_6 levels are low in many persons suffering from rheumatoid arthritis, the use of B_6 to raise the blood levels does not result in a relief of symptoms.

Pyridoxine has been used in doses of 50 mg

per day in the treatment of the nausea of pregnancy with at least some success. Pyridoxine-containing lozenges sucked three times a day during pregnancy significantly reduce the incidence of new cavities, possibly because of an inhibitory effect on the growth of microorganisms that favor caries development. A similar reduction in tooth decay was observed in 10- to 15-year-olds who were given lozenges with 3 mg of B_6 three times a day.

Some types of anemia have responded to treatment with large (50 mg) doses of pyridoxine, which may be necessary for the synthesis of the heme in iron-containing portions (protoporphyrin) of the hemoglobin molecule. Pyridoxine applied topically is beneficial in treating sicca-type dermatitis.

There are several genetic errors of metabolism associated with abnormalities of pyridoxine metabolism that require an increased intake of the vitamin. One involves the synthesis of a compound needed in brain metabolism, another the development of anemia associated with high levels of iron in the blood, and a third the formation of excessive xanthurenic acid or cystathionine in the urine. Others are manifest in mental symptoms.

Megavitamin therapy at levels of 1.5 g have been shown to produce alterations in metabolism in adult males. Although these changes have not been thoroughly investigated, the potential harmful effects of such large doses should not be overlooked.

Deficiency

Deficiencies in both animals and humans result in a large number of abnormalities in amino acid and protein metabolism with clinical signs such as poor growth, convulsions, anemia, decreased antibody formation, and skin lesions.

In 1951 it was first observed that infants who were inadvertantly given a formula providing less than 0.1 mg of vitamin B_6 showed signs of hyperirritability and convulsions. These symptoms disappeared on the administration of the vitamin.

In adults the only symptom that has been attributed to lack of pyridoxine is a microcytic hypochromic anemia in association with high serum iron. Other less specific symptoms, such as weakness, nervousness, irritability, insomnia, and difficulty in walking, have been associated with inadequate intakes of vitamin B_6. Efforts to induce a deficiency state by dietary deficiency in humans produced only symptoms of irritability after fifty-four days. When the vitamin antagonist deoxypyridoxine was fed, skin changes (glossitis, cheilosis, and stomatitis) different from those of a riboflavin or niacin deficiency occurred.

Changes in urinary components occur in a pyridoxine deficiency. The amount of oxalate increases and the amount of urinary citrate decreases. Since citrate favors the solubility of oxalates, it is possible that the formation of urinary calculi (kidney stones), which occurs in pyridoxine deficiencies, reflects decreased solubility of the oxalate. This may also be explained by the low levels of the transaminases necessary to convert oxalic acid to the nonessential amino acid glycine. However, when both magnesium and pyridoxine levels are low, urinary calculi are not formed.

PANTOTHENIC ACID

Discovery

Pantothenic acid, identified first as vitamin B_3, was so named to designate its widespread occurrence in foods (from the Greek word *pantos,* everywhere). As knowledge of its role in biological reactions has developed its central role in the metabolism of carbohydrate, fat, and protein has been recognized. A newly recognized form of pantothenic acid, acyl carrier protein (ACP), has recently been identified.

Pantothenate had been recognized as a growth factor for yeast and as a cure or prevention for dermatitis in chicks and graying of hair in rats before it was finally isolated in 1938 and synthesized in 1940. A yellow viscous oil, pantothenic acid has never been crystallized, although its synthetic calcium

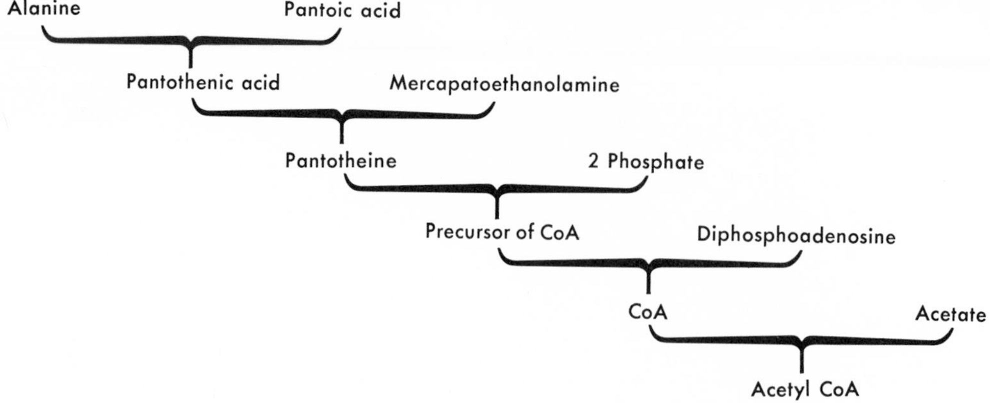

Fig. 12-20. Relationship between pantothenic acid and CoA.

salt, calcium pantothenate, has been available in crystalline form for some time. It is in this form that it is incorporated into most nutritional supplements. The alcohol form, pantothenol, is used in supplements and cosmetics.

Chemical properties

Pantothenic acid is a water-soluble vitamin that is stable in moist heat in neutral solution but is readily destroyed by dry heat. In acid or alkali it is relatively unstable. There is little loss in cooking at normal temperatures.

Chemically, pantothenic acid is a relatively simple compound containing the amino acid alanine. Before it participates in biological reactions, it unites with a sulfur-containing compound to form pantotheine, which in turn adds phosphate and an adenine molecule to form coenzyme A (also called CoA). Coenzyme A is the form in which most pantothenic acid is found in microorganisms and in animal tissues and in which it participates in a central role in most biological reactions. The activation of CoA involves the addition of the 2-carbon acetate compound to form acetyl coenzyme A, or acetyl CoA. These acetate molecules are readily accepted and are transferred from the CoA molecule.

The relationship between pantothenic acid and activated CoA is shown in Fig. 12-20.

Since CoA appears within the cell but not in the blood, it must by synthesized within the cell and can pass the cell membrane with difficulty, if at all. In red blood cells it exists bound to a protein. CoA appears in highest concentration in the liver, adrenal gland, kidneys, brain, and heart, all of which are tissues characterized by high metabolic activity.

Functions

As part of CoA, pantothenic acid participates in the release of energy from all three energy-yielding nutrients—carbohydrate, fat, and protein. Products in the oxidation of each of these eventually react with CoA in the Krebs cycle before all their energy is released. In addition, CoA—and hence pantothenic acid—is necessary for the synthesis of fat. Besides functioning in the transfer of acetate groups to the Krebs cycle, CoA is involved as a source or acceptor of acetate groups for amino acids, vitamins, and sulfonamides. It provides acetyl groups for the formation of acetylcholine needed in the transmission of nerve impulses and for the detoxification of certain drugs. It is essential for the formation of porphyrin (a part of the hemoglobin molecule), for the stimulation of antibody response, and for the synthesis of cholesterol and some of the steroids produced by the adrenal glands. In essence, because of its central role in energy metabolism, it can be considered vital to all energy-requiring processes within the body.

In addition to its functions related to its role in CoA, pantothenic acid functions as part of a glucose-carrier system to facilitate absorption through the intestinal mucosa.

Requirements

It is well established that humans and practically all other animals and microorganisms have a need for pantothenic acid. The amount needed has not been estimated with any certainty but is generally believed to be from 5 to 10 mg, or ten times the thiamin requirement. A 3000 kcal diet will usually provide from 13 to 19 mg of total pantothenic acid, of which 5 to 10 mg will occur as free pantothenic acid. From 7 to 10 mg is excreted daily in the urine. One study of both pregnant and nonpregnant teenagers, however, showed intakes of 4.7 mg, well below the recommended 10 mg. The wide range of intakes, blood values, and urinary excretion levels that appear in individuals with no evidence of deficiency make it difficult to determine a minimum intake. Except for periods of stress such as pregnancy, when needs may be relatively high, most diets will provide adequate amounts of pantothenic acid. Protein exerts a sparing effect on pantothenic acid.

Table 12-12. Food sources of pantothenic acid*

Food	mg/100 g
Beef liver	7.70
Egg yolk	4.40
Beef kidney	3.85
Wheat bran	2.90
Whole egg	1.60
Broccoli, frozen	1.45
Lima beans, frozen	1.24
Beef, round	0.62
Cornmeal	0.59
Cheddar cheese	0.50
Milk, nonfat	0.37
Milk, whole	0.34
Bananas	0.26
Almonds	0.25
Yellow corn, canned	0.22

*From Orr, M. L.: Pantothenic acid, vitamin B_6 and vitamin B_{12} in foods, Home Economics Research Report No. 36, Agricultural Research Service, Washington, D.C., 1969, U.S. Department of Agriculture.

Food sources

The amount of pantothenic acid in foods representative of the main food groups is given in Table 12-12. Pantothenic acid is a component of all living matter. Although organ meats, most fish, and whole-grain cereals are the richest sources, all food groups make a significant contribution to the dietary intake. The richest sources so far determined have been royal jelly from the queen bee and fish ovaries prior to spawning.

Of 507 foods analyzed for pantothenic acid, 47% had over 5 ppm, a level that should provide an overall dietary intake of 5 to 10 mg.

Foods processed in dry heat are relatively poor sources of pantothenic acid. In canning from 20% to 35% of the pantothenic acid is lost from animal foods and from 46% to 78% is lost in vegetable foods. About 50% is lost in the refining of wheat.

Deficiency

The wide variety of reactions for which pantothenic acid is necessary is paralleled by an equally wide variety of deficiency symptoms. Chicks show a characteristic dermatitis around the eyes, a degeneration of the spinal cord, changes in the thymus gland, and fatty degeneration of the liver. Ducks experience anemia; rats experience growth failure, the accumulation of the reddish pigment porphyrin in their whiskers, and hemorrhaging in the adrenal gland; and pigs experience changes in the sensory nerves. Biochemically, an increase in copper in the skin has occurred in a pantothenic acid deficiency.

Although humans apparently do not experience pantothenic acid deficiencies of sufficient magnitude to precipitate deficiency symptoms in most mixed diets, low intakes may slow down many metabolic processes, resulting in a wide variety of subclinical symptoms. Lowered resistance to infection is well documented. When human volunteers were fed a pantothenic acid antagonist along with a diet low in pantothenic acid, the list of symptoms reportedly reversed by the vitamin was rather extensive. It included irritability, restlessness, burning feet, muscle cramps, impaired muscular coordination, sensitivity to insulin, decreased antibody formation, easy fatigue, mental depression, gastrointestinal disturbances, and upper respiratory infections. This list likely reflects impaired health of cells in many tissues. The site at which the symptoms first appear may be a function of some particular metabolic stress factors. High levels seem to improve the ability to withstand stress.

Pantothenic acid neither prevents nor cures graying of hair in humans in spite of any claims to the contrary by vendors of food supplements.

Clinical uses

Pantothenic acid in the form of its calcium salt has been used successfully in treating the paralysis of the gastrointestinal tract after surgery, which causes the accumulation of gas and severe abdominal pain. It appears to stimulate gastrointestinal motility. High levels (from 10 to 20 g), however, cause diarrhea.

FOLACIN

Discovery

Folacin was discovered in the course of the search for the factor in liver responsible for its effectiveness in curing pernicious anemia, a fatal condition characterized by large red blood cells, megaloblastic anemia, and degeneration of nervous tissue. Although folacin (earlier known as folic acid) does not have the antipernicious anemia properties attributed to it in 1945, it has been established as a dietary essential for man, many animals, and microorganisms. It has been isolated from spinach, yeast, and liver, occurs in a wide variety of foods, and participates in many biological reactions.

The many names by which folacin has been known gives some indication of the various paths by which the substance was identified. As early as 1930 the Wills factor, now believed to be folacin, was identified in yeast and crude liver extracts and was found to be effective in curing a tropical macrocytic anemia. In 1938 the term vitamin M was applied to a growth factor for monkeys; in 1939 factor U and vitamin B_c were used to identify growth factors for chicks; and by 1940 the *Lactobacillus casei* factor or norit eluate factor was found to be essential for the growth of that microorganism. As the chemical nature of all these substances became known, it was learned that the effectiveness of all these was due to the presence of pteroylglutamic acid (PGA). Since this substance could be extracted from green leafy vegetables such as spinach, it was designated in 1941 as *folic acid* (from the Latin, *folium,* leaf). The term has now been officially changed to *folacin* in keeping with current practices in nomenclature. Since many substances are now known to give rise to folacin in the body, the use of the term has been restricted to pteroylmonoglutamate, the form from which the active coenzymes are directly derived. The term *folate* is applied to the broader group of substances that give rise to folacin in the body.

Substances with folic acid activity are synthesized by plants, in animal tissues, and by microorganisms in the intestinal tract. By 1945 scientists knew the chemical structure of pteroylglutamic acid and had succeeded in isolating and synthesizing it inexpensively. Folic acid has been established as a dietary essential for chicks, hamsters, monkeys, and humans, but it is not needed by rats, dogs, and rabbits.

Chemical composition

Folacin (or folic acid) is a complex substance made up of the combination of the chemical compounds pterin and para-aminobenzoic acid together known as pteroic acid. To this is attached 1 molecule of glutamic acid, a nonessential amino acid. This vitamin occurs in food, however, with from 1 to 7 (but primarily with 1, 3, or 7) glutamic acid molecules attached. Before folacin can be used as the vitamin, the extra glutamic acid units must be removed. This is accomplished in the gastrointestinal tract through the action of specific enzymes and vitamin B_{12}. Folacin, or PGA with one unit of glutamic acid, is then changed (reduced) in the presence of ascorbic acid and a niacin containing coenzyme NADPH to a substance known as tetrahydrofolic acid. This compound is relatively unstable and reacts quickly with a single carbon unit that can be obtained from many sources to form one of several biologically active substances. This conversion of folacin to its biologically active forms, generally referred to as folates, must occur before the vitamin can perform its role as part of a coenzyme. Anything that blocks the addition of these single carbon units prevents folacin from functioning as a vitamin. Minor changes in the structure of these active forms leads to the formation of the coenzymes responsible for many of the roles played by folic acid.

A synthetic form of folic acid (5, formyl THFA) known as the citrovorum factor, or leucovorin, is metabolically inactive except for a role in histidine metabolism. The relationship among the various forms of the vitamin is shown in Fig. 12-21.

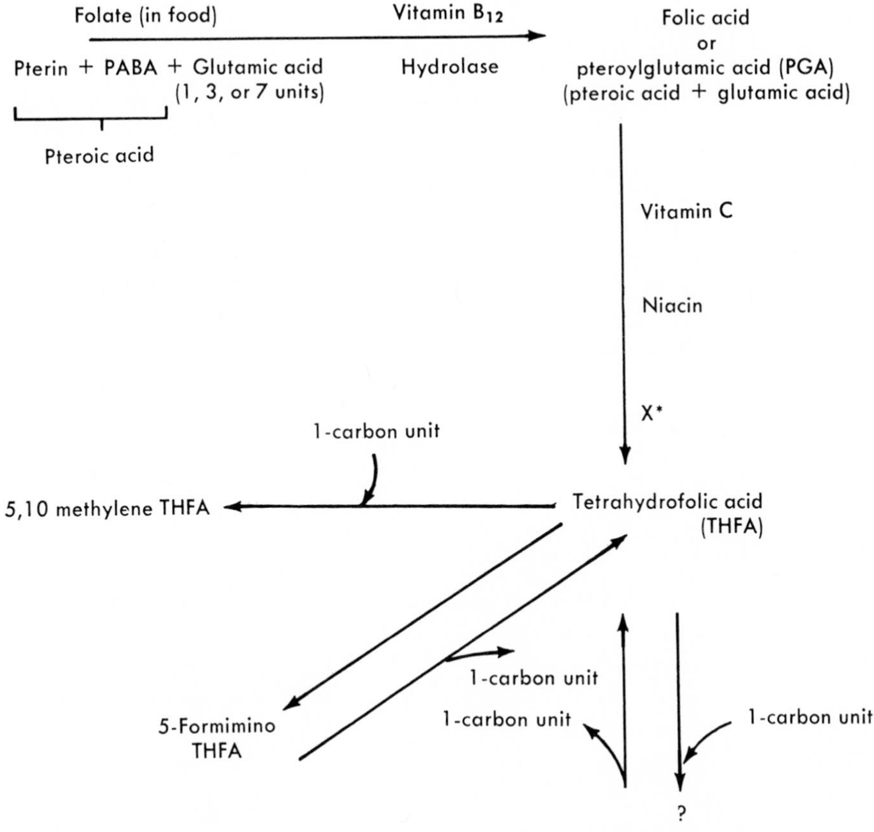

Fig. 12-21. Relationship among various chemical forms of folacin. (PABA = para-aminobenzoic acid.) *Most common block in conversion of folic acid to active form.

Folic acid antagonists such as aminopterin and amethropterin, which are chemically related to folic acid, block the action of folacin by interfering with its conversion to THFA. This explains why the active factor has been effective in overcoming the effect of the antagonist, whereas folate has not.

Absorption and metabolism

Folic acid is absorbed in the upper part of the intestine by both active transport and diffusion. About 80% of a therapeutic oral dose and 30% to 50% of dietary folate is absorbed. Its absorption is facilitated by ascorbic acid and by some antibiotics. The extra glutamic acid molecules, which occur in 80% of dietary folate, are split off by enzymes in either the pancreatic juice or within the cells of the intestinal wall. Absorbed folacin is removed rapidly from the serum into the tissues, which apparently have a protein that actively binds folacin. Within the cell folacin may recombine with additional glutamic acid molecules to form large polyglutamate molecules. These large molecules can leave the cell only with difficulty; this may constitute a method of retaining folates. As a result, little folic acid is excreted. The liver is the major storage site with reserves of 10 mg, which last four to five months.

The absorption of folic acid is reduced in nontropical sprue, a condition in which structural and functional abnormalities occur as a result of the degenerative changes in the jejunum portion of the small intestine. These changes may also occur in alcoholics and in persons taking anticonvulsive drugs or oral contraceptives. Thus symptoms of folacin deficiency occur under all these conditions.

Functions

It was determined shortly after the discovery of folacin in 1945 that although it cured macrocytic anemia by stimulating the regeneration of both red blood cells and hemoglobin, folacin was not the antipernicious anemia factor for which scientists were searching, since it was ineffective in relieving the neurological symptoms. It did, however, play several essential roles in metabolism, especially in rapidly proliferating cells, such as red blood cells, white blood cells (leukocytes), or cells of the intestinal mucosa. Of the biochemical roles that have been clearly established, several are closely involved in blood formation.

Folacin functions in all biological reactions involving the transfer of single-carbon units, such as methyl (CH_3) groups, from one substance to another. In this role it appears to act as an intermediary, accepting the single-carbon group from one compound and passing it on to the next. Examples of this function are the formation of the amino acid methionine from one of its precursors, homocysteine; the formation of the 3-carbon amino acid serine from the 2-carbon amino acid glycine; the formation of the vitamin choline from its precursor ethanolamine; and the synthesis of the amino acid histidine. The conversion of nicotinic acid to *N*-methyl nicotinamide, the form in which it is excreted, depends on the addition of a methyl (single-carbon) unit obtained from folacin.

The synthesis of the purines, adenine and guanine, and pyrimidine and thymine, all part of the nucleic acids DNA and RNA, is dependent on folic acid coenzymes. Because of this role in nucleic acid synthesis, folic acid is especially important in conditions in which rapid cell division is occurring. The formation of each new cell requires the synthesis of DNA to carry the genetic information in it. Since nucleic acids control protein synthesis, folic acid exerts an indirect effect on the synthesis of enzymes and other essential protein compounds.

The conversion or oxidation of the essential amino acid phenylalanine to tyrosine also requires folacin, as do the oxidation and decarboxylation of tyrosine, the formation of part of the structure of hemoglobin (the porphyrin group), and the metabolism of long-chain fatty acids in the brain.

Requirements

The need for folate has not been clearly established. It is believed that the minimum need for adults is approximately 50 μ or 0.05 mg. The National Research Council, assuming 25% absorption and allowing a wide margin of safety for differences in availability from various food sources, has set the recommended dietary allowances for adolescents and adults at 0.4 mg (or 400 μg). Some investigators believe that this might reasonably be reduced to 300 μg or even 250 μg without any health risks. After a deficiency this level of folic acid will stimulate normal red cell production and normal bone marrow tissue but will not immediately cause an increase in serum folic acid levels or any storage of the vitamin. The minimum level may also be influenced by body size and metabolic rate. Additionally, the amount of folic acid in food to provide this level is variable because of uncertainty about how much is destroyed in cooking and processing and the extent to which it is absorbed, which varies greatly with the source. The requirement for folic acid increases with the increased consumption of alcohol, which interferes with absorption, and in any condition having a marked increase in the metabolism of single-carbon units associated with rapid cell growth, such as pregnancy, hyperthyroidism, and hemolytic anemia, and with the use of many drugs. Synthetic folic acid is much more completely utilized, with 0.1 mg protecting against folic acid deficiency.

On the basis of weight the need for infants of 4 μg/kg of body weight or 50 μg is four to ten times as high as that for adults because of the rapid rate of growth. Recommendations for children increase from 50 to 400 μg from 1 to 10 years of age. A comparison of the daily recommended allowance of the World Health Organization and the National Research Council (Table 12-13) shows fairly close agreement for most ages.

Table 12-13. Recommended daily intake of folate

Age	WHO (μg/day)	NRC (μg/day)
0-6 mo	40-50	50
7-12 mo	120	50
1-12 yr	200	100-400
13 yr	400	400
Pregnancy	800	800
Lactation	600	600

During pregnancy, when folacin needs are markedly increased to meet the needs of the rapidly growing fetus, an additional 400 μg for a total of 800 μg, is recommended. In lactation 600 μg will allow the secretion of adequate milk with a folacin content of 5 μg /dl of milk, assuming again that 25% of dietary folate is absorbed.

Food sources

Recent analytical data on the folacin content of food has made feasible more accurate estimates of folacin content of diets than was possible earlier. A comparison of calculations based on data from food composition tables and analytical values show very close agreement. Estimates of daily intakes range from 0.03 to 1.6 mg with higher amounts being found in high-cost diets. Most diets provide from 200 to 240 μg, which is considerably less than the current recommended allowances.

Data on the folacin content of representative foods are shown in Table 12-14. Wheat germ with 178 μg/100 g is one of the most concentrated sources. Liver, kidney, yeast, and mushrooms are also rich sources but since they play a relatively insignificant role in most diets, fruits and vegetables make a much more important contribution to the dietary intake. Oranges and orange juice with 25 to 30 μg/100 g are dependable sources. In addition, the acidity helps protect the folic acid from destruction.

The addition of yeast in preparing bread enhances its folate value even though about a third is lost in the heat of baking. Among vegetables, asparagus, broccoli, lima beans, and spinach rank highest; lemons, bananas, strawberries, and cantaloupes are rich fruit sources. Although milk contains little folacin, 60% of it is in the monoglutamate form.

Table 12-14. Folacin content of representative food (total folacin/100 g)*

Liver	145.0
Asparagus	64.0
Whole wheat bread	54.5
Potato chips	42.0
White bread	36.5
Cabbage, raw	30.2
Orange juice	30.0
Rice	28.8
Cucumber	24.0
Peas	22.4
Eggs	21.1
Bananas	20.4
Carrots	18.0
Onions	16.0
Potatoes, baked	14.1
Cottage cheese	12.1
Hamburger	7.7
Ice cream	5.1
Milk	5.0

*Modified from Folic acid: biochemistry and physiology in relation to the human nutrition requirement, Washington, D.C., 1977, National Academy of Sciences.

Fig. 12-22 shows the contribution of various food groups to the total intake in the American diet.

An analysis of the form in which folacin occurs in food shows that 35% in orange juice, 53% in soybeans, and 60% in milk occurs as the monoglutamate, which can be absorbed without the release of the extra glutamic acid molecules. The availability of folate varies greatly from one food to another and may be due to the inhibition of the enzymes needed to split off extra glutamate molecules at different levels of acidity or pH. The availability of folate from various sources is shown in Fig. 12-22.

Losses of folic acid in processing and in cooking may range as high as 50% to 90%, and even 100% when high temperatures and large volumes of water are used. For strained baby foods losses are high in fruits and vegetables but minimal in meats.

Free folacin activity of frozen dinners is reduced by 22% on reheating, while total folacin activity is unaffected. Most dinners studied contained 12 μg/100 kcal the majority of which was contributed by the vegetable component.

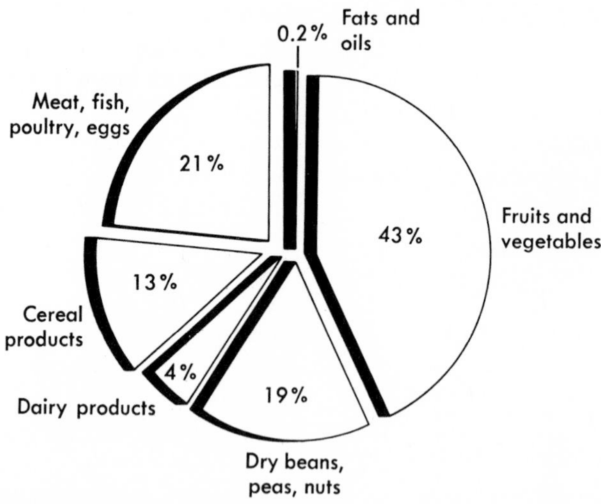

Fig. 12-22. Contribution of various food groups to total intake of folacin in American food supply. (Based on Contribution of major food groups to nutrient supplies available for civilian consumption, National Food Review NFR-1, Washington, D.C., 1978, Economic Research Service.)

Exposure to light also causes loss of folate. A high percentage of folacin in liver, yeast, and eggs is absorbed, but for other foods as little as 10% may be available. All these factors make estimations of folic acid intake of reduced value.

Evaluation of nutritional status

Since folacin is involved in normal blood formation, an analysis of components of the blood of humans has proved the most logical method of detecting an inadequacy of the nutrient.

In human folacin deficiency abnormally large red blood cells, known as megaloblasts, develop when the newly formed immature red blood cells (reticulocytes) fail to mature and to lose their nuclei. (These are easily identified by microscopic examination.) Under these conditions the number of red blood cells decreases, but the amount of hemoglobin does not decrease. These changes show up as a high color index (>1), in which the percentage of normal hemoglobin level is compared to the percentage of normal red blood cell count. Normally, the color index is approximately 1. However, since these same changes in red blood cells occur in a vitamin B_{12} deficiency, this test does not distinguish between a folic acid and a vitamin B_{12} deficiency.

Determination of folate levels in blood serum provides a sensitive indicator of folate status long before clinical symptoms of deficiency develop. Normal values of 6 to 20 ng/L drop to less than 3 ng/L in about one week on diets very low in folacin. In contrast, red cell folate levels provide a better guide to folate stores. Low values indicate a severe deficiency and are associated with megaloblastic changes in the bone marrow and depress DNA synthesis.

An analysis of the urine to determine the presence of the substance formiminoglutamic acid (FIGLU), which accumulates when folate is deficient, shows promise as a method of evaluating the folacin status of an individual. The metabolism of the amino acid histidine involves its conversion to glutamic acid. If folic acid is lacking, the complete change does not occur, and an intermediary product, formiminoglutamic acid, accumulates because there is no way to remove the formyl (single-carbon group) from the molecule. If folic acid is present, it removes the single carbon to form the active folic acid coenzyme. If folacin levels are inadequate, coenzymes are not formed, and the single-carbon unit (formimino) is not removed from the formiminoglutamic acid. This is then excreted in the urine.

Deficiency

Folic acid deficiency symptoms may result from inadequate intake, impaired absorption, excessive demands, metabolic derangements, or increased losses. They tend to occur in tissues with a high rate of cell proliferation and hence with greater need. In animals folate deficiency alone results in changes in the structure of the intestinal mucosa (lining). In humans this seems to occur only when folate deficiency is associated with excessive use of alcohol or with tropical sprue, both of which result in malabsorption of folate.

With increasing knowledge of folate metabolism has come an increasing number of reported folate deficiencies. A deficiency of the vitamin has been implicated in conditions ranging from toxemia of pregnancy (20% of pregnant women found to be deficient) to parasitic infestation, infections, scurvy and rheumatoid arthritis.

Although the exact mechanisms have yet to be identified, the use of oral contraceptives results in a decreased utilization of folacin, but the decrease does not appear to be sufficient to cause megaloblastic anemia. In rare individuals with other disorders of folate metabolism, the use of oral contraceptive hormones may aggravate the problem.

The high incidence of deficiency among pregnant women had led the Food and Nutrition Board to recommend an additional 400 μg per day, which should be provided as a supplement available only by prescription.

They suggest that it first be established that the woman does not have pernicious anemia because folic acid, by correcting the megaloblastic anemia, eliminates the possibility of diagnosing pernicious anemia, which itself usually prevents conception. Deficient intakes of folic acid have been associated with fetal damage and severe depletion of maternal reserves. The extent of the problem is illustrated in Fig. 12-23 based on data on 114 pregnant teenage girls.

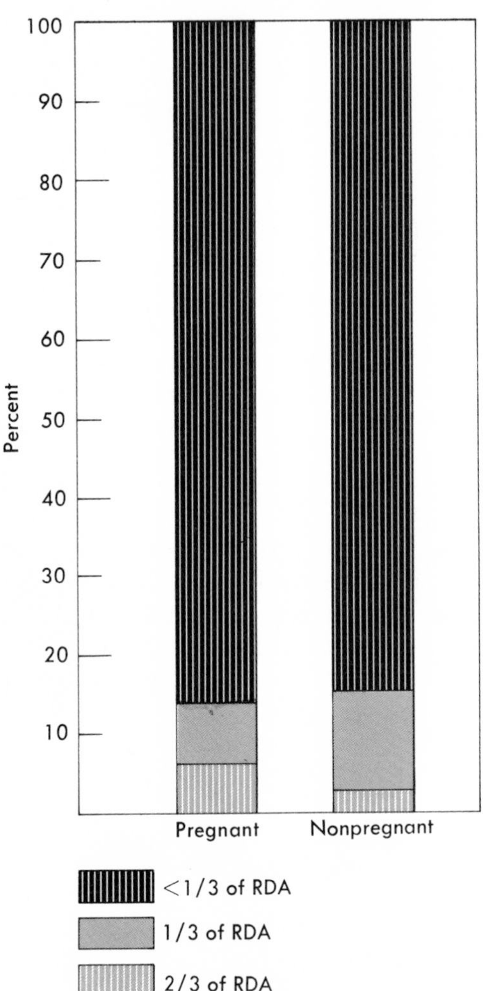

Fig. 12-23. Percentage of pregnant and nonpregnant girls meeting the recommended allowance for folic acid. (From Vandermark, M. S., and Wright, A. C.: J. Am. Diet. Assoc. **61:**514, 1972.)

In lactating women blood folate levels drop constantly, reflecting the stress imposed by maintaining folate content of breast milk at approximately 50 μg per day.

Infants and adolescents, who experience a rapid rate of cell multiplication associated with growth and the related need for DNA, are also especially vulnerable to a folate deficiency. Similarly the role of folacin in DNA synthesis implicates folate deficiency in cases of decreased cell immunity.

In addition to oral contraceptives other drugs such as antitumor agents and anticonvulsants interfere with folate utilization, resulting in increased needs and evidence of a deficiency.

About 50% of all hospital admissions in poor communities and 20% to 30% in other communities show evidence of folate deficiency. It tends to occur more frequently among the old, the lonely, and the poor. An incidence of 50% is reported among alcoholics and chronic invalids. Low levels among alcoholics are attributed to poor diet, malabsorption, liver damage, poor storage, excessive losses, and possibly a direct effect of alcohol on folate metabolism.

It has been suggested that as the relationship between folate deficiency and biochemical disorders is clarified, it may be apparent that folate deficiency is the most prevalent of all vitamin deficiencies. Almost all symptoms can be attributed to a failure to metabolize single-carbon units.

In experimental deficiency conditions it took adults about five months to develop symptoms of megaloblastic anemia. Infants with low reserves and higher needs for growth developed symptoms in eight weeks. Inadequate folate levels may reduce the production of leukocytes (white blood cells) and hence the ability of the body to produce antibodies.

In folic acid deficiencies the blood is affected differently in various animals. In monkeys a reduced number of white blood cells (leukopenia) occurs, with a reduced resistance to intestinal infection and an increase in enlarged red blood cells (macrocytes). Chicks also show macrocytic anemia, low hemoglobin levels and hematocrit ratios, and slow growth.

Clinical uses

Folacin is effective in treating nutritional megaloblastic anemia caused by folate deficiency, the megaloblastic anemia of pregnancy and infancy, and some other anemias that fail to respond to vitamin B_{12}. In addition, it is effective in relieving some of the symptoms that occur in tropical sprue, such as anemia, glossitis, and gastrointestinal disturbance.

Although folacin does relieve the anemia and glossitis associated with pernicious anemia, it not only fails to alleviate the degeneration of nervous tissue but also accentuates the changes. Thus, in addition to failing to provide a complete cure for pernicious anemia, the use of folic acid may be potentially dangerous in allowing the irreversible nervous system symptoms to develop.

Concern over the possibility that a dose of folacin, curing the megaloblastic anemia of pernicious anemia, may eliminate the most effective means of diagnosing the disease has led the Food and Drug Administration to set a limit of 0.1 mg of folic acid as the amount that is permissible for use in vitamin supplements available without prescription. This would be sufficient to protect against a folacin deficiency without curing megaloblastic symptoms of pernicious anemia. If the megaloblastic anemia has been primarily caused by vitamin B_{12} deficiency but has responded to folic acid therapy, the anemia is likely to recur.

The use of a folic acid antagonist such as aminopterin to interfere with the formation of the active coenzyme necessary for the production of white blood cells (leukocytes) has been effective in decreasing the rate of leukocyte formation in leukemia, a fatal condition characterized by overproduction of white blood cells. Unfortunately, such treatment also resists the growth of other cells; therefore it can be used only intermittently and provides only temporary relief.

Toxicity

There appear to be no toxic reactions to folic acid, since up to 15 mg may be taken daily for one month with no adverse effects.

Abnormalities of metabolism

Some individuals are born with metabolic defects that make them unable to utilize ingested folate. The effect of this shows up as mental retardation.

VITAMIN B_{12}

Discovery

Until 1926 pernicious anemia was a fatal disease of unknown origin with no known cure. In 1926 Minot and Murphy established that the condition could be cured if the patient was fed large amounts of raw liver (at least 0.3 kg each day). In 1934, together with Whipple, they were awarded the Nobel Prize in medicine for this treatment of pernicious anemia.

Also in 1926 Castle noted that pernicious anemia patients had an abnormal gastric secretion. He postulated that the antipernicious anemia substance was formed by the combination of an **extrinsic factor** in food, especially liver, and an **intrinsic factor** in the normal gastric secretion. Both the extrinsic and intrinsic factors were considered necessary for the prevention or cure of the disease. Castle's theory was held during succeeding years while scientists attempted to isolate and identify the active substance in food. The story of this search is the story of the discovery of vitamin B_{12}, now recognized as Castle's extrinsic factor.

The attempts to identify the active principle in liver were hampered by the fact that no animal other than humans had exhibited a need for the substance. Thus all clinical evaluations of new liver concentrates had to be made on human subjects suffering from pernicious anemia. Medical investigators were able to isolate progressively more concentrated extracts of liver that showed antipernicious anemia potency, but the progress was discouragingly slow in spite of the fact that with each advance pernicious anemia patients benefited. Only with the discovery that the microorganism *Lactobacillus lactis* also needed the antipernicious anemia factor for growth could more extensive experimental work be attempted and the final isolation of the effective principle become possible.

Clinical tests, which showed that an injected dose of the liver extract was much more effective than the same amount ingested, began to cast doubt on Castle's theory that intrinsic and extrinsic factor combined to form an antipernicious anemia substance. They eventually led to the conclusion that Castle's extrinsic factor in food was indeed the antipernicious anemia factor and that the intrinsic factor secreted by the parietal cells of the gastric mucosa was responsible and necessary for the active absorption of the substance. The favorable results that had been obtained when large amounts of liver were fed by mouth were explained on the basis that when such large amounts of vitamin B_{12} were available, from 1% to 3% was absorbed by diffusion rather than by active transport across the intestinal membrane, which required the intrinsic factor. This small amount was adequate to prevent the disease.

Chemical composition

By 1948, two years after folic acid had been discovered and determined *not* to be the sought-after antipernicious anemia factor, workers in Britain and the United States almost simultaneously succeeded in isolating small red crystals with high antipernicious anemia potency from liver extracts. This substance was soon identified chemically as one containing about 4% of its weight as the mineral cobalt, previously known to be essential only in the diets of sheep and cattle. The cobalt was present in the center of a large complex molecule known as a corrinoid, which resembles hemoglobin or chlorophyll. This compound is known as cobalamin. In addition to containing cobalt, one active form of the vitamin known as cyanocobalamin was found to possess a cyanide group closely bound in the molecule. It is now known that a form of the vitamin in which cyanide is replaced by a hydroxyl group (hydroxocobalamin) is also common. Commercial vitamin B_{12} is primarily cyanocobalamin obtained by bacterial synthesis. In food much of the vitamin B_{12} occurs as a coenzyme in which the hydroxyl or cyanide part of the molecule is replaced by a compound called adenosine. Since it still contains cobalt, it has vitamin B_{12} activity.

Although in a strict sense the term vitamin B_{12} should only be used to refer to cyanocobalamin, it is generally applied to this whole group of substances that are capable of performing the functions of the vitamin. Hydroxocobalamin, cyanocobalamin, nitritocobalamin, and thiocyanate cobalamin are among the forms known to exhibit vitamin effects, although others have been identified. While both cyanocobalamin and hydroxocobalamin, which can be converted in the body to the active coenzyme, are used in the treatment of vitamin B_{12} deficiency, hydroxocobalamin is now the preferred form. Because it binds more tightly to plasma and tissue proteins it is retained three times better and needs to be injected less frequently in the treatment of pernicious anemia patients.

The animal protein factor (APF) known to stimulate growth in animals has been found to be identical with vitamin B_{12}. It appears to promote the retention of nitrogen and hence to raise the biological value of the protein of the diet, leading to more rapid growth per unit of food. The apparent beneficial effects of the antibiotics aureomycin and penicillin in stimulating growth in animals is now attributed to the fact that they inhibit the growth of organisms that destroy vitamin B_{12}. Their use, then, essentially increases the vitamin B_{12} available and indirectly enhances growth. The usefulness of vitamin B_{12} as a growth factor for children has been investigated. Although results are inconclusive, they suggest that it is effective only in underweight children and only if the general nature of the diet improves.

The antipernicious anemia factor now identified as vitamin B_{12} was synthesized in 1973, twenty-five years after it had been discovered. Prior to this, concentrates of vitamin B_{12} to be used in the treatment of pernicious anemia and in supplements were obtained from the growth of microorganisms and fungi.

Once vitamin B_{12} was isolated and chemically identified and became available in a concentrated form, its role in biological reactions was more easily studied. In contrast to other vitamins, a deficiency of this vitamin is primarily the result of a defect in the mechanism by which it is absorbed rather than a dietary deficit.

Absorption

The absorption of vitamin B_{12} is governed by the intrinsic factor, a heat-labile mucoprotein secreted from specific cells known as parietal cells of the wall of the stomach as a normal part of gastric juice. As food passes through the digestive tract, vitamin B_{12} is released from the protein complex in which it occurs in food. The intrinsic factor, which is different for each species, then binds itself to vitamin B_{12} and helps attach the vitamin to a receptor in the cells lining the ileum or upper portion of the intestine, in a reaction catalyzed by the mineral calcium. Vitamin B_{12} is released from the intrinsic factor to the mucosa or absorbing cells in the intestinal wall by the action of intestinal enzymes, which also are different in each species. A failure in any stage in the absorption can render dietary vitamin B_{12} unavailable.

The percentage of the intake that is absorbed decreases as the actual amount in the diet increases. On an average intake of 16 μg, from 3 to 5 μg are absorbed. However, in minimal intakes of 0.5 μg as much as 70% is absorbed.

If the gastric juice of a person lacks the intrinsic factor necessary for absorption of vitamin B_{12}, there is no uptake of the vitamin at all from the amounts normally provided in food. However, if amounts about a thousand times the normal dosage are given, as in oral doses of liver extract, sufficient amounts to meet the needs of an individual may pass through the intestinal wall by diffusion. Since the intrinsic factor in the hog's stomach is similar to that from the human gastric mucosa, it has been possible to administer a concentrate of hog's stomach to facilitate the absorption of vitamin B_{12} from either food or therapeutic preparations. It is most effective if injected intramuscularly to bypass the defective absorptive mechanism.

The efficiency of absorption appears to diminish with increase in age, with a pyridoxine deficiency due to a decreased synthesis of intrinsic factor, with an iron inadequacy, and in hypothyroidism. It increases during pregnancy and when an intrinsic factor concentrate is fed along with vitamin B_{12}.

Malabsorption occurs in gastritis and with the use of some anticonvulsants and antibiotics, but the effect is usually not sufficiently great to cause deficiency symptoms.

The use of sorbitol, a derivative of carbohydrate now used as a sweetening agent, has improved cobalamin absorption, especially among older persons with depressed gastric secretions. Currently there is concern that the use of megadoses of ascorbic acid cause as much as 50% destruction of vitamin B_{12} in food.

The administration of a radioactive dose of cyanocobalamin and measurement of its excretion gives an indication of the effectiveness of absorption. Normal subjects usually absorb 30% of the test dose and excrete most of it in the urine. Persons with pernicious anemia absorb and excrete only 2% of the test dose.

Metabolism

Once cobalamin is absorbed, it passes into the bloodstream, where it is bound again to one of three transport proteins known as transcobalamins, the form in which it circulates to various tissues. The combination of a small molecule such as vitamin B_{12} with a larger protein molecule prevents it from passing through the kidneys to be lost in the urine. When sufficient transport protein is produced, the body is able to hold on tenaciously to the absorbed protein-bound vitamin and loses little. In the case of vitamin B_{12} any excess is stored in the liver primarily in the form of a protein-bound B_{12} enzyme. The liver is able to store up to 1 to 2 μg of the enzyme per gram or 2000 μg of tissue sufficient to last six years. There is considerable evidence that in humans the amount of serum vitamin B_{12} is a sensitive indicator of body stores of the vitamin.

Functions

Vitamin B_{12} is necessary for normal growth, for maintenance of healthy nervous tissue, and for normal blood formation. The exact biochemical role of the vitamin in maintaining all these functions has not been determined, but some aspects have been identified.

The functional form of the vitamin is a coenzyme that has many forms but is generally referred to as a cobamide coenzyme. The conversion of the vitamin to this active form involves many nutrients, including niacin, riboflavin, and manganese.

In the bone marrow where erythroblasts, the forerunners of red blood cells, are formed, vitamin B_{12} coenzymes are necessary to provide the methyl groups for synthesis of DNA. If DNA is not produced, the cells cannot divide but instead continue to produce RNA and to synthesize protein, increasing in size to become the large cells called megaloblasts. The red blood cells produced by these megaloblasts are large and immature macrocytes that are characteristic of the blood of pernicious anemia patients and differ from the smaller mature erythrocytes (red blood cells) in normal blood. Once cobalamin is available, the megaloblasts are no longer formed, and the erythroblasts produce normal mature red blood cells, the erythrocytes. The role of vitamin B_{12} in nucleic acid synthesis is important in all body cells, but its effect is more pronounced in erythrocytes, which develop at a rate of at least 200 million per minute.

The way in which cobalamin affects the nervous system is not clear. However, it is known that vitamin B_{12} keeps glutathione, an integral part of several enzymes involved in carbohydrate metabolism, in the reduced state in which it is biologically active. Since the nervous system relies almost entirely on carbohydrate as its source of fuel, anything that disrupts carbohydrate metabolism will deprive nervous tissue of its energy source and hence will interfere with its normal functioning. Since the nervous system has a limited range of pathways by which it can handle carbohydrate, it may be dependent on vitamin B_{12}. Levels of pyruvic acid and lactic acid, intermediary products in carbohydrate metabolism, increase from 50% to 100% in a vitamin B_{12} deficiency, suggesting a block in glucose metabolism.

Like folate, vitamin B_{12} is concerned with metabolism that involves single-carbon units such as methyl groups. This is especially evident in the conversion of homocysteine to the amino acid methionine and in the formation of an intermediary in folic acid metabolism (tetrahydrofolic acid). The interaction between folate and vitamin B_{12} becomes evident from the effect of vitamin B_{12} in regulating the amount of folate in the liver.

Unlike folate, which aids the transfer of these single-carbon units from one substance to another, vitamin B_{12} is necessary for the synthesis or formation of these units, which in turn are vital in the formation of many essential body compounds.

In the metabolism of folic acid, vitamin B_{12} catalyzes the release of folic acid with one glutamic acid molecule from folic acid conjugates of three or seven glutamic acid molecules that occur in foods. In addition, it facilitates the formation of the folic acid coenzymes.

Besides its direct role in folic acid and nucleic acid metabolism and its more indirect role in carbohydrate metabolism, the vitamin appears to play a role in fat and protein metabolism, but the mechanisms have not been clarified.

The nervous system damage in vitamin B_{12} deficiency has been attributed to damaged myelin, the sheath of lipoprotein surrounding nerve fibers. This is further evidence of a role in either lipid or protein metabolism.

Table 12-15. Cobalamin content of some representative foods*

Food	μg/100 g
Beef liver	80.0
Oysters	18.0
Lamb	2.2
Egg, whole	2.0
Salami	1.4
Frankfurters	1.3
Haddock	1.3
Cheddar cheese	1.0
Shrimp	0.9
Pork	0.7
Chicken	0.5
Milk, whole	0.4

*From Orr, M. L.: Pantothenic acid, vitamin B_6 and vitamin B_{12} in foods, Home Economics Research Report No. 36, Agricultural Research Service, Washington, D.C., 1969, U.S. Department of Agriculture.

Food sources

All vitamin B_{12} found in nature has been synthesized by microorganisms except for a minute amount produced by bacteria in the nodules on roots.

Since plants are unable to synthesize it, vitamin B_{12} is found only in foods of animal origin. Animals absorb the vitamin after it has been synthesized by bacteria in their rumen from the plant foods they eat, provided sufficient cobalt is available. Any excess is stored in their tissues. Microorganisms in the gastrointestinal tract of humans are also able to synthesize the vitamin, but the site of synthesis is too far down in the colon to permit absorption.

The contribution of various food groups to

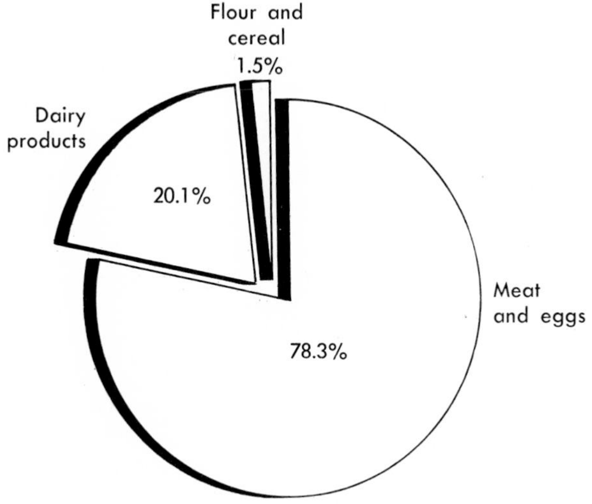

Fig. 12-24. Contribution of various food groups to vitamin B_{12} content of the American diet. (Based on National Food Review NFR-1, Washington, D.C., 1978, Economic Research Service.)

the vitamin B_{12} content of the diet is shown in Fig. 12-24.

The best sources of vitamin B_{12} are the animal foods—liver (containing about 1 ppm), kidney, milk, and meat, in all of which it occurs in a protein complex (Table 12-15). In diets of everyone except strict vegetarians, who make absolutely no use of animal products, the intake is always adequate. Deficiency symptoms result from failure in the absorptive mechanisms rather than any lack of the nutrient. Most methods of cooking do not destroy or damage vitamin B_{12}.

Over half the vitamin B_{12} in food is in the form of a coenzyme that is very unstable and destroyed by processing and methods of home production.

Cyanocobalamin is stable to acid and oxidation but is destroyed by alkali. About 70% is normally retained in cooking.

Requirements

The need for cobalamin is extremely small and has been difficult to determine. It is now recommended that a diet containing 3 μg a day, from which 1 to 1.5 μg is absorbed, will satisfy the need of most adults. (A typical Western diet provides from 7 to 30 μg.) On the other hand, studies of the whole body turnover of the vitamin suggest a need ranging from 0.5 to 2.5 μg.

Deficiency

Although body stores of approximately 2 to 4 mg are small, they are sufficient to last up to six years before symptoms would be expected to develop in a diet devoid of the vitamin.

As indicated earlier, virtually no evidence is found of a deficiency state from a lack of dietary source of the nutrient except among strict vegetarians, who develop neurological symptoms but no changes in their blood pattern. Pernicious anemia, the major manifestation of an inadequate amount of the nutrient, results from a lack of the intrinsic factor secreted by the glands of the stomach, from partial or complete removal of the stomach, from a lack of the protein in the blood that binds absorbed cobalamin, or from a lack of the substance that releases it from the mucosal cells to the blood. Intestinal infestation with a fish tapeworm that avidly absorbs any available vitamin also produces an induced deficiency state. Diagnosis of vitamin B_{12} deficiency can be made on the basis of blood levels of the vitamin, which are determined by microbiological techniques. Normal levels of 100 to 1000 μg/ml fall below 100 in pernicious anemia, and changes in the nature of red blood cells from small nonnucleated cells to larger nucleated ones confirm the diagnosis.

Pernicious anemia can now be readily controlled by injections of cobalamin. About 1000 μg are given twice in the first week, followed by 250 μg a week until the blood pattern has returned to normal. A dose of 250 μg every three weeks is usually sufficient to protect against recurrence of the condition. The most crucial aspect of pernicious anemia therapy is early diagnosis so that treatment can be begun before neural degeneration has become irreversible. In contrast to the victim of pernicious anemia prior to 1925, who faced almost certain death, or after 1926, who was forced to eat large amounts of liver daily, today's patient can be treated relatively simply and inexpensively.

Clinical uses of vitamin B_{12}

Although vitamin B_{12} has been promoted for use in a wide range of conditions from night blindness to psoriasis to warts to menopausal problems to general malaise, there is no clinical evidence that these problems are the result of a lack of the vitamin or that they can be prevented or cured through its use. Fortunately, there is no reason to believe that the levels being given, usually by injection, have any harmful or detrimental effects, other than economic waste. It is possible, however, if the widespread use of vitamin B_{12} therapy continues that scientists will begin to see evidence of adverse effects.

Currently the only legitimate use for vitamin B_{12} therapy is when there is evidence of a metabolic defect in absorption.

Crystals of cobalamin are bright red, which resulted in its being designated as the *red vitamin* in popular literature.

BIOTIN

Discovery

Recognition of biotin as a dietary essential occurred in 1924 when it was identified as bios II, one of three factors necessary for the growth of microorganisms. Between 1924 and the time of its synthesis in 1943, various scientists had sought to elucidate the nature of substances they had named vitamin H and coenyzme R. Once the chemical nature of this sulfur-containing nutrient was determined, it was clear, as had been the case in the study of many other nutrients, that all three were the same substance, now identified as biotin.

Symptoms of biotin deficiency occur in animals only after the ingestion of a diet low in biotin and high in raw egg white. Raw egg white includes a carbohydrate-containing protein, *avidin,* which binds biotin in a complex too big to be absorbed but which the body cannot break to release the biotin. Experimentally, it was found that in humans the diet had to provide 30% of its calories from raw egg white to induce a biotin deficiency. Since this represents approximately twenty-seven egg whites in a 3000 kcal diet it is obvious that the ingestion of the occasional raw egg white is not going to precipitate a deficiency state. Cooking denatures avidin; thus it no longer has the ability to bind biotin.

Chemical properties

Biotin has been isolated in at least five active forms from food. One of these, biocytin, is a combination of biotin and the amino acid lysine. Other forms are biotin sulfone, which is a potent antagonist, and biotinal, which can be oxidized to an active form.

In animal tissues the protein-bound biotin is fat soluble, whereas the free biotin found in plants and excreted in the urine is water soluble.

Biotin is stable to heat but labile to alkali and oxidation. As a water-soluble vitamin some will be lost in cooking water.

Functions

Biotin is an active substance participating in many biological reactions. In animal cells it occurs bound to protein where it acts as an enzyme.

The best established role of biotin coenzymes is in carboxylation, which involves the transfer of carbon dioxide in various reactions. Since these reactions are common in nature, biotin is found involved in both the synthesis and oxidation of fatty acids and the oxidation of carbohydrate. It also stimulates protein synthesis in the microsomes of the cell. Its role in deamination, which must occur before amino acids can be used as a source of energy, has been established for at least three amino acids—aspartic acid, threonine, and serine. It is necessary for the synthesis of nicotinic acid, but the mode of action is not clear. The synthesis of the digestive enzyme pancreatic amylase is another biotin-dependent reaction as is antibody formation.

Biotin plays an important role in carbohydrate metabolism. It acts to stimulate the synthesis of the enzyme responsible for the addition of phosphate to the glucose molecule so that it can enter the liver cell. This is necessary before it can be stored or released again into the bloodstream. Some results of animal studies suggest that biotin may influence carbohydrate metabolism by controlling either the synthesis or release of insulin.

Failure of some of these functions shows up in an impaired utilization of glucose, a decrease in the incorporation of amino acids into protein, and up to 30% reduction in fat caused by failure in the synthesis of fatty acids. There appears to be a metabolic interrelationship between zinc and biotin.

Requirements

For the first time, the 1979 revision of the Recommended Dietary Allowances will include provisional allowances for biotin requirements.

Food sources

Biotin is present in almost all foods. Most occurs bound to protein from which it can readily be liberated. Liver, kidney, milk, egg yolk, and yeast have been shown by biological assay to be the richest food sources, followed by some vegetables, such as cauliflower, nuts, and legumes. In general, all other meats, dairy products, and cereals are considered poor sources. Human milk has only a tenth the amount of biotin of cow's milk.

Most diets contain from 150 to 300 μg of biotin, which is supplemented by the intestinal synthesis of biotin by bacteria that is stimulated on a sucrose-containing diet.

Conditions that reduce the number of microorganisms in the intestine may reduce the amount of biotin synthesized. Sulfonamides and oxytetracycline are known to reduce the number of biotin-synthesizing organisms. Some of the symptoms that develop with the use of sulfonamides may be evidence of biotin deficiency, since biotin administration seems to counteract them.

No evidence exists on which to justify the inclusion of biotin in the formula for a multivitamin supplement.

Deficiency

The effects of a biotin-deficient diet in animals are many and varied but seem to be characterized by early changes in the skin. Dermatitis, characterized by either scaliness or hardening, which frequently starts in the region of the eye, is common. This is often followed by loss of hair and evidence of muscular atrophy.

In a study in which four human subjects became deficient on a diet devoid of biotin and high in avidin, the symptoms observed were similar to those of a thiamin deficiency and included dermatitis, loss of appetite, nausea, muscle pains, and high blood cholesterol levels, among many other symptoms. In both deficiencies a derangement of the metabolic enzyme system occurs. There is some evidence that a biotin deficiency results in high blood levels of both cholesterol and glucose.

Although no evidence exists of a natural biotin deficiency in human adults, evidence has suggested that two types of dermatitis that occur in infants—Leiner's disease and seborrheic dermatitis—may be caused by a lack of biotin. They respond rather dramatically to biotin therapy, although similar conditions in adults are not responsive.

BIBLIOGRAPHY

Ascorbic acid

Andersen, T. W., Reed, D. B., and Beaten, G. H.: Vitamin C and the common cold: a double blind trial, Can. Med. Assoc. **107:**503, 1972.

Anderson, T. W.: New horizons for vitamin C, Nutr. Today, **12:**6, 1977.

Baker, E. M.: Vitamin C requirements in stress, Am. J. Clin. Nutr. **20:**583, 1967.

Cook, J. D., and Monsen, E. R.: Vitamin C, the common cold, and iron absorption, Am. J. Clin. Nutr. **30:**235, 1977.

Coulehan, J. L., Reisinger, K. S., Rogers, K. D., and Bradley, D. W.: Vitamin C prophylaxis in a boarding school, N. Engl. J. Med. **290:**6, 1974.

Grewar, D: Infantile scurvy, Clin. Pediatr. (Phila.) **4:**28, 1965.

Hodges, R. E., Baker, E. M., Hood, J. Sauberlich, H. E., and March, S. C.: Experimental scurvy in man, Am. J. Clin. Nutr. **22:**535, 1969.

Hodges, R. E., Hood J., Canham, J. E., and others: Clinical manifestations of ascorbic acid deficiency in man, Am. J. Clin. Nutr. **24:**432, 1971.

Horowitz, I., Fabry, E. M., and Gerson, C. D.: Bioavailability of ascorbic acid in orange juice, J.A.M.A. **235:**2624, 1976.

Lorenz, A. J.: The conquest of scurvy, J. Am. Diet. Assoc. **30:**665, 1954.

New roles for ascorbic acid, Nutr. Rev. **32:**53, 1974.

Ossofsky, H. J.: Infantile scurvy, Am. J. Dis. Child. **109:**173, 1965.

Pauling, L.: Ascorbic acid and the common cold, Am. J. Clin. Nutr. **24:**1294, 1971.

Pelletier, O., and Keith, M. O.: Bioavailability of synthetic and natural ascorbic acid, J. Am. Diet. Assoc. **64:**271, 1974.

Preshaw, R. M.: Vitamin C and the common cold, Can. Med. Assoc. J. 107**:479**, 1972.

Schwartz, F. W.: Ascorbic acid in wound healing—a review, J. Am. Diet. Assoc. **56:**497, 1970.

Shaffer, C. F.: Ascorbic acid and atherosclerosis, Am. J. Clin. Nutr. **23:**27, 1970.

Sherlock, P., and Rothchild, E. O.: Zen diets and scurvy, J.A.M.A. **199:**794, 1967.

Szent-Györgyi, A.: Lost in the twentieth century, Ann. Rev. Biochem. **32:**1, 1963.

Udenfriend, S.: Formation of hydroxyproline in collagen, Science **152:**1335, 1966.

Uhl, E.: Ascorbic acid requirements of adults: 30 mg or 75 mg? Am. J. Clin. Nutr. **6:**146, 1958.

Thiamin

Bradley, W. B.: Thiamine enrichment in the United States, Ann. N.Y. Acad. Sci. **98:**602, 1962.

Brin, M.: Thiamine deficiency and erthyrocyte metabolism, Am. J. Clin. Nutr. **12:**107, 1963.

Brozek, J.: Phsychologic effects of thiamine restriction and deprivation in normal young men, Am. J. Clin. Nutr. **5:**109, 1957.

Dreyfus, R. M., and Victor, M.: Effects of thiamine deficiency on the central nervous system, Am. J. Clin. Nutr. **9:**414, 1961.

Gubler, C. J., Fujiwara, M., and Dreyfus, P. M.: Thiamine, New York, 1976, John Wiley & Sons.

Lipmann, F.: The biochemical function of B vitamins, Perspect. Biol. Med. **13:**1, 1969.

Requirements of vitamin A, thiamine, riboflavin and niacin, Report of Joint FAO/WHO Expert Group, Techn. Rep. Ser. No. 362, 1967.

Rindi, J., and Ventura, U.: Thiamine intestinal transport, Physiol. Rev. **52:**821, 1972.

Salcedo, J.: Experience in the etiology and prevention of thiamine deficiency in the Philippine Islands, Ann. N.Y. Acad. Sci. **98:**568, 1962.

Sauberlich, H. E.: Biochemical alterations in thiamine deficiency—their interpretation, Am. J. Clin. Nutr. **20:**528, 1967.

Tandhaichitir, V.: Thiamin. In Sipple, H., and McNutt, K., editors: Present knowledge of nutrition, ed. 3, New York, 1976, Nutrition Foundation, Inc.

Wurst, H. M.: The history of thiamine, Ann. N.Y. Acad. Sci. **98:**385, 1962.

Riboflavin

Foy, H., Kondi, A., and Verjee, Z. H. M.: Relation of riboflavin deficiency to corticosteroid metabolism and red cell hypoplasia in baboons, J. Nutr. **102:**571, 1972.

Lane, M., Alfrey, C. P., Mengel, C. E., Doherty, M. A., and Doherty, J.: The rapid induction of human riboflavin deficiency with galactoflavin, J. Clin. Invest. **43:**357, 1964.

Mayersohn, M., Feldman, S., and Gebaldi, M.: Bile salt enhancement of riboflavin and flavin mononucleotide absorption in man, J. Nutr. **98:**288, 1969.

McCormick, D. B.: The fate of riboflavin in the mammal, Nutr. Rev. **30:**75, 1972.

Rivlin, R. S.: Riboflavin metabolism, N. Engl. J. Med. **13:**626, 1970.

Sauberlich, H. E., Judd, J. H., Nichoalds, G. E., and others: Application of the erythrocyte glutathione reductase assay in evaluating nutritional status in a high school student population, Am. J. Clin. Nutr. **25:**756, 1972.

Sterner, R. T., and Price, W. R.: Restricted riboflavin: Within-subject behavioral effects in humans, Am. J. Clin. Nutr. **26:**150, 1973.

Niacin

Darby, W., McNutt, K., and Todhunter, E. N.: Niacin. In Sipple, H., and McNutt, K., editors: Present knowledge of nutrition, ed. 3, New York, 1976, Nutrition Foundation, Inc.

DeLange, D. J.: Assessment of nicotinic acid status of population groups, Am. J. Clin. Nutr. **15:**169, 1964.

Goldsmith, G. A.: Niacin-tryptophane relationship in man and niacin requirement, Am. J. Clin. Nutr. **6:**479, 1958.

Goldsmith, G. A.: Niacin, antipellagra factor; hypocholesterolemic agent, J.A.M.A. **194:**167, 1965.

Snydenstricker, V. P.: History of pellagra; its recognition as a disorder of nutrition and its conquest, Am. J. Clin. Nutr. **6:**409, 1958.

Pyridoxine

Baker, E. M., Canham, J. E., Nunes, W. T., Sauberlich, H. E., and McDowell, M. E.: Vitamin B_6 requirement for adult men, Am. J. Clin. Nutr. **15:**59, 1964.

Brown, R. R.: Normal and pathological conditions which may alter the human requirement for vitamin B_6, J. Agric. Food Chem. **20:**498, 1972.

Bunnell, R. H.: Vitamin B_6, Science **146:**674, 1964.

Committee on Nutrition, American Academy of Pediatrics: Vitamin B_6 requirements in man, Pediatrics **38:**75, 1966.

Coursin, D. B.: Vitamin B_6 requirements, J.A.M.A. **189:**27, 1964.

Donald, E. A., McBean, L. D., Simpson, M. H. W., Sun, M. F., and Aly, H. E.: Vitamin B_6 requirement of young adult women, Am. J. Clin. Nutr. **24:**1028, 1971.

Drenick, E. J., Vinyard, E., and Swendseid, M. E.: Vitamin B_6 requirements in starving obese males, Am. J. Clin. Nutr. **22:**10, 1969.

Food and Nutrition Board: Human vitamin B_6 requirements, Washington, D.C., 1978, National Academy of Sciences.

Frimpter, G. W., Andelman, R. J., and George, W. F.: Vitamin B_6-dependency syndromes: new horizons in nutrition, Am. J. Clin. Nutr. **22:**794, 1969.

Gershoff, S.: Vitamin B_6. In Sipple, H., and McNutt, K., editors: Present knowledge of nutrition, ed. 3, New York, 1976, The Nutrition Foundation, Inc.

Gyorgy, P.: Developments leading to the metabolic role of vitamin B_6, Am. J. Clin. Nutr. **24:**1250, 1971.

Gyorgy, P.: Reminiscences on the discovery and significance of some of the B vitamins, Nutr. Rev. **34:**141, 1977.

Linkswiler, H.: Biochemical and physiological changes in vitamin B_6 deficiency, Am. J. Clin. Nutr. **20:**547, 1967.

Lumeng, L., Cleary, R. E., Wagner, R., Yu, P. L., and Li, T. K.: Adequacy of vitamin B_6 supplementation during pregnancy: a prospective study, Am. J. Clin. Nutr. **29:**1376, 1976.

Orr, M. L.: Pantothenic acid, vitamin B_6 and vitamin B_{12} in foods, Home Economics Research Report No. 36, Agricultural Research Service, Washington, D.C., 1969, U.S. Department of Agriculture.

Polansky, M. M., and Murphy, E. W.: Vitamin B_6 in fruits and nuts, J. Am. Diet. Assoc. **48:**109, 1966.

Polansky, M. M., Murphy, E. W., and Toepfer, E. W.: Components of vitamin B_6 in grains and cereal products, J. Assoc. Agric. Chem. **47:**750, 1964.

Pyridoxine and dental caries-human studies, Nutr. Rev. **21:**143, 1963.

Sauberlich, H. E., Canhan, J. E., Baker, E. M., Raica, N., and Herman, Y. F.: Biochemical assessment of the nutritional status of vitamin B_6 in the human, Am. J. Clin. Nutr. **25:**629, 1972.

Shriver, C. R., and Hutchison, J. H.: The vitamin B_6 deficiency syndrome in human infancy: biochemical and clinical observations, Pediatrics **31:**240, 1963.

West, K. D., and Kirksey, A.: Influence of vitamin B_6 intake on the content of the vitamin in human milk, Am. J. Clin. Nutr. **29:**961, 1976.

Pantothenic acid

Nelson, R. A.: Intestinal transport, coenzyme A and colitis in pantothenic acid deficiency, Am. J. Clin. Nutr. **21:**495, 1968.

Wright, L. D.: Pantothenic acid. In Sipple, H., and McNutt, K., editors: Present knowledge of nutrition, ed. 3, New York, 1976, The Nutrition Foundation, Inc.

Zook, E. G., MacArthur, M. S., and Toepfer, E. W.: Pantothenic acid in foods, Agricultural Handbook No. 97, Washington, D.C., 1956, U.S. Department of Agriculture.

Folacin

Babu, S., and Srikantia, S. G.: Availability of folates from some foods, Am. J. Clin. Nutr. **29:**276, 1976.

Daniel, W., Jr., Daniel, W. A., Gaines, E. G., and Bennett, D. L.: Dietary intakes and plasma concentrations of folate in healthy adolescents, Am. J. Clin. Nutr. **28:**363, 1975.

Folic acid: biochemistry and physiology in relation to the human nutrition requirement, Washington, D.C., 1977, National Academy of Sciences.

Folic acid metabolism in vitamin B_{12} deficiency, Nutr. Rev. **33:**118, 1975.

Girdwood, R. H.: Abnormalities of vitamin B_{12} and folic acid metabolism—their influence on the nervous system, Nutr. Soc. Proc. **27:**101, 1968.

Herbert, V.: Biochemical and hematologic lesions in folic acid deficiency, Am. J. Clin. Nutr. **20:**562, 1967.

Herbert, V.: Folic acid deficiency. A symposium, Am. J. Clin. Nutr. **23:**841, 1970.

Hoffbrand, A. V.: The role of malabsorption in the development of folate deficiency, Clin. Med. **79:**19, 1972.

Hoppner, K., Lampl, B., and Perrin, D. E.: Folacin activity of frozen convenience foods, J. Am. Diet. Assoc. **63:**536, 1973.

Krundrieck, C. L.: Folic acid. In Sipple, H., and McNutt, K., editors: Present knowledge of nutrition, ed. 3, New York, 1976, The Nutrition Foundation, Inc.

Nixon, P. F., and Bertino, J. R.: Interrelationships of vitamin B_{12} and folate in man, Am. J. Med. **98:**555, 1970.

Perloff, B. P., and Butrum, R. R.: Folacin in selected foods, J. Am. Diet. Assoc. **70:**161, 1977.

Reed, B., Weir, D., and Scott, J.: The fate of folate polyglutamates in meat during storage and processing, Am. J. Clin. Nutr. **29:**1393, 1976.

Rosenberg, I. H., Streiff, R. R., Godwin, H. A., and Castle, W. B.: Absorption of polyglutamic folate: participation of deconjugating enzymes of the intestinal mucosa, N. Engl. J. Med. **280:**985, 1969.

Santini, R., Brewster, C., and Butterworth, C. E.: The distribution of folic acid active compounds in individual foods, Am. J. Clin. Nutr. **14:**205, 1964.

Streiff, R. R.: Folic acid deficiency anemia, Semin. Hematol. **7:**23, 1970.

Streiff, R. R., and Little, A. B.: Folic acid deficiency in pregnancy, N. Engl. J. Med. **276:**776, 1967.

Vilter, R. W., Will, J. J., Wright, T., and Rullman, D.: Interrelationships of vitamin B_{12}, folic acid and ascorbic acid in the megaloblastic anemias, Am. J. Clin. Nutr. **12:**130, 1963.

Cobalamin

Armstrong, B. K.: Absorption of vitamin B_{12} from the human colon, Am. J. Clin. Nutr. **21:**298, 1968.

Baker, S. J.: Human vitamin B_{12} deficiency, World Rev. Nutr. Diet. **8:**63, 1967.

Bernstein, L., and Herbert, V.: The role of pancreatic exocrine secretions in the absorption of vitamin B_{12} and iron, Am. J. Clin. Nutr. **26:**340, 1973.

Chow, B. F.: Nutritional significance of vitamin B_{12}, World Rev. Nutr. Diet. **1:**127, 1960.

Halstead, C. H.: The small intestine in vitamin B_{12} and folate deficiency, Nutr. Rev. **33:**33, 1975.

Herbert, V.: Nutritional requirements for vitamin B_{12} and folic acid, Am. J. Clin. Nutr. **21:**743, 1968.

Heyssel, R. M., Bozian, R. C., Darby, W. J., and Bell, M. C.: Vitamin B_{12} turnover in man, Am. J. Clin. Nutr. **18:**176, 1966.

Herbert, V.: Vitamin B_{12}. In Sipple, H., and McNutt, K., editors: Present knowledge of nutrition, ed. 3, New York, 1976, The Nutrition Foundation, Inc.

Newmark, H. L., Scheiner, J., Marcus, M., and Prabhudesai, M.: Stability of vitamin B_{12} in the presence of ascorbic acid, Am. J. Clin. Nutr. **29:**645, 1976.
Shinton, N. K.: Vitamin B_{12} and folate metabolism, Br. Med. J. **98**(57):556, 1972.
Stokstad, E. L. R.: Vitamin B_{12} and folic acid. In Sipple, H., and McNutt, K., editors: Present knowledge of nutrition, ed. 3, New York, 1976, Nutrition Foundation, Inc.
Sullivan, L. W., and Victor, H.: Studies on the minimum daily requirement for vitamin B_{12}, N. Engl. J. Med. **272:**340, 1965.
Wilson, T. H.: Intrinsic factor and B_{12} absorption—a problem in cell physiology, Nutr. Rev. **23:**33, 1965.

Biotin

Baugh, C. M., Malone, J. H., and Butterworth, C. E., Jr.: Human biotin deficiency. A case history of biotin deficiency induced by raw egg consumption in a cirrhotic patient, Am. J. Clin. Nutr. **21:**173, 1968.
Belnave, D: Clinical symptoms of biotin deficiency in animals, Am. J. Clin. Nutr. **30:**1408, 1977.
McCormick, D. B.: Biotin, Nutr. Rev. **33:**97, 1975.

13

Other nutrient factors

Although the last vitamin was discovered in 1948, there are many other factors in food that from time to time are promoted as essential nutrients. It is possible that some will eventually be designated as vitamins. In the meantime it is important that the student of nutrition be aware of the factors in food that are in this category and the roles that are being attributed to them.

In addition to the nutrients that have already been definitely established as vitamins there are several other vitamin-like substances that have some properties of vitamins but fail to meet all the criteria necessary to be classed as vitamins. In some cases they are present in larger amounts than vitamins; in others the body can synthesize sufficient amounts to meet body needs if precursors are present; and for still others it has been impossible to determine any essential biological role.

Because these dietary factors are sometimes given vitamin status, a brief discussion of present knowledge of their status is warranted here. Undoubtedly, in the future some will be established definitely as vitamins, whereas others will definitely be dropped from this classification.

MYOINOSITOL

Myoinositol, which is also known as muscle sugar, inositol, and mesoinositol, is one of nine 6-carbon compounds closely related chemically to glucose. Of these nine, only inositol is biologically active. It was first recognized in 1928 as a growth-promoting factor for yeast and as a cure for alopecia, or loss of hair, in mice.

It is present in practically all plant and animal tissues in concentrations higher than those normally associated with vitamins. In animal cells it occurs primarily as a phospholipid, which is sometimes referred to as lipositol. In grains it is present as a more complex water-soluble compound, phytic acid, the organic acid that binds both calcium and iron in an insoluble complex and prevents their absorption. It also occurs in nucleated erythrocytes. In soybeans it occurs in a free form, and in other plant and animal tissues it occurs as an unidentified complex. Some evidence exists that sharks and certain other fishes store carbohydrate as inositol rather than as glycogen.

Methods of analyzing for iositol are tedious and relatively inaccurate, but from available data it appears that heart muscle, brain, and skeletal muscle contain more inositol than do other tissues. Fruits, meat, milk, nuts, vegetables, and whole-grain cereals are the best food sources.

The biological significance of inositol in human nutrition is unknown, although it is widely distributed in the body. It may act as an intermediary product between carbohydrate and related compounds. It is believed to lead to a decrease in RNA synthesis, but none of these roles has been clearly established. It has, however, been found essential for the growth of liver and bone marrow cells and helps alleviate fatty livers.

Humans apparently consume about 1 g of inositol a day in food. In addition, the body is able to synthesize sufficient amounts to meet its needs from glucose. Synthesis occurs within the individual cell rather than by intestinal organisms. The amount excreted in the urine is small and variable, averaging 37 mg a day with a range from 8 to 144 mg. Diabetics excrete much more. Normal blood levels range from 0.37 to 0.67 mg/dl.

CHOLINE

Choline was identified in 1937 as a dietary factor that prevented the accumulation of fat in the liver of dogs. Since then it has been determined that the effectiveness of choline is due to three methyl (CH_3) groups present in its molecule, which are available to other biological compounds. As a methyl donor, choline provides one of the substances necessary to mobilize fat from the liver to be transported in the bloodstream to other cells in the body. Methyl groups are exchanged in a wide variety of biological reactions, and as a source of these, choline facilitates many reactions.

Choline can be readily synthesized in the body from the amino acid glycine, provided another source of the methyl group is available. These methyl groups may be provided by another amino acid, methionine; they can be synthesized in the presence of adequate folic acid or cobalamin; or they may be obtained from a variety of other sources. Thus it appears that choline cannot be considered a vitamin, since the human is not solely dependent on a dietary source of either choline or a direct precursor. In animals such as the guinea pig or fowl choline is a dietary essential, since it cannot be synthesized at a sufficient rate to meet their needs.

In the body choline occurs as a constituent of the fat-related substances lecithin, a form in which much fat is transported, and sphingomyelin, which occurs in nerve tissue. As such, it is a structural part of fat and nerve tissue and does not catalyze any reactions or act as part of a coenzyme. In addition, choline reacts with acetyl CoA to form an acetylcholine that is responsible for transmitting nerve impulses from one nerve ending to the next.

Choline is widely distributed in food, being present in relatively large amounts in all foods that contain fat, as shown in Table 13-1. With the exception of legumes, fruits and vegetables contain virtually no choline. The average diet provides from 500 to 900 mg daily.

Table 13-1. Choline content of representative foods

Food	Choline content (g/100 g)
Egg yolk	1.7
Beef liver	0.6
Soybeans	0.2
Fish	0.2
Cereal	0.1

The need for dietary choline has not been established since it is small or nonexistent when the diet contains sufficient methionine to provide methyl groups for the synthesis of choline or adequate amounts of folacin and cobalamin to stimulate the synthesis of methyl groups.

Choline is not associated with any specific deficiency disease in humans. It does, however, exert a protective action in cirrhosis of the liver among alcoholics. In rats and dogs the symptoms associated with choline deficiency are aggravated by a pyridoxine deficiency, whereas in chickens and turkeys the porosis induced by choline deficiency can be cured by administration of folic acid or manganese as well as choline.

COENZYME Q (UBIQUINONE)*

Coenzyme Q is a lipidlike substance that is somewhat similar in its chemical makeup to

*In a review "Survey of the Vitamin Aspects of Coenzyme Q" (Int. Z. Vitaminforsch. **39:**334 1969) Folkers suggests that the definition of a vitamin be modified to include substances produced by intestinal biosynthesis in mammalian cells. Since coenzyme Q synthesis depends on the availability of the amino acids tyrosine and phenylalanine and the vitamins niacin, folic acid, cobalamin, pyridoxine, and pantothenic acid, Folkers suggests that coenzyme Q should be considered a vitamin.

both vitamin K and vitamin E. It was recognized simultaneously by two different groups, one studying vitamin A and the other studying electron transport in the cell mitochondrion. It belongs to a group of compounds known as ubiquinones, and the forms that appear to be biologically important have from 30 to 50 carbon atoms in a side chain attached to the basic quinone structure. The 50-carbon side chain occurs exclusively in higher animals.

Coenzyme Q is found in practically all living cells and appears to be concentrated in the mitochondria. Here it apparently operates as an essential link in the respiratory chain in which energy is released from energy-yielding nutrients as the high-energy compound ATP. It appears to be reversibly oxidized and reduced readily. Without this substance one would anticipate incomplete release of energy.

The ubiquinones are likely to be synthesized readily in the body, the ring structure from amino acids such as phenylalanine and the side chain from acetate available as an intermediary in carbohydrate and fat metabolism. A pantothenic acid deficiency has been shown to depress coenzyme Q synthesis by 50%, likely because of decreased availability of acetate. Ubiquinones therefore are of little dietary significance and cannot be truly classed as vitamins. In contrast to other fat-soluble vitamins, they can be excreted in the urine.

Ubichromenol, which is similar to vitamin E in structure and biological activity, can be formed from ubiquinone. Both vitamin E and selenium operate to maintain high tissue concentration of coenzyme Q.

Coenzyme Q-type compounds are widely distributed in food. They are found in soybeans, vegetable oils, and a great variety of animal tissues.

BIOFLAVONOIDS

The bioflavonoids were first suggested as dietary factors in 1936 when it was observed that extracts of both red pepper and lemon increased the antiscorbutic effect of ascorbic acid. A wide range of chemical substances, mostly belonging to the flavine and flavonoid compounds, were believed to exert a favorable influence in reducing capillary bleeding caused by the increased permeability of the cell membrane. For a while these compounds, of which *hesperidin* was one of the most active, were designated vitamin P, but the use of this term was dropped in 1950. It has recently been established that the bioflavinoid rutin does not enhance the utilization of synthetic vitamin C.

So far, scientists have been unable to ascertain any specific biological role for this group of compounds, although it is agreed that they may have some pharmacological effects. In addition, no proof has been found of clinical usefulness of the compounds that have been advocated at various times as therapeutic agents in the treatment of a range of unrelated conditions, such as cerebral vascular accidents, arthritis, spontaneous abortions, common colds, and retinal hemorrhages. Many suggestions have been made regarding the mode of action of the bioflavonoids, but none have been substantiated.

Bioflavonoids occur in highest concentration in the peel and juice of citrus fruit, in tobacco leaves, in buckwheat, and in some other fruits and vegetables. No evidence exists at the present time of a dietary need for bioflavinoids, and certainly there is no justification for their inclusion in nutritional supplements; nor is there a justification in the promotion of certain foods on the basis of a high concentration of the substances. Several bioflavonoids are being investigated as potential low-calorie sweetening agents.

LIPOIC ACID

Lipoic acid is known to be essential for the growth of several microorganisms. It has been isolated from liver and yeast, and several aspects of its biochemical role have been elucidated. At the present time there is some question whether it should be considered a vitamin for humans, since no evidence has yet been established that humans or other mammals require a dietary source of the substance. Although it does participate in biochemical reactions in mammalian tissues, the amounts needed to meet these needs are likely synthesized in the body.

Lipoic acid is now identified in five distinct forms; three forms are fat soluble; one is a water-soluble complex; and one, which is bound to protein, has been known as factor 11 and 11A, pyruvic oxidation factor, thioctic acid, and protogen. Lipoic acid, the official name, and thioctic acid, indicative of the sulfur found in the molecule, are the names most frequently used now. The fat-soluble lipoic acid can be reversibly oxidized to the water-soluble beta-lipoic acid.

Function

Lipoic acid is essential along with the thiamin-containing enzyme pyrophosphatase for the reactions in carbohydrate metabolism that convert pyruvic acid to acetyl CoA. This is the point at which it joins the intermediary products of protein and fat metabolism in the Krebs cycle for the reactions involved in liberating energy from these nutrients. In its active form, lipoic acid is bound to a protein in a reaction requiring energy in the form of ATP and a metal ion, such as calcium or magnesium. In plant cells it may be involved in catalyzing some of the reactions of photosynthesis.

Several attempts have been made to relate lipoic acid nutrition to metabolic disorders in animals and humans, but most of the results have been contradictory. Some evidence showed that lipoic acid limited the plasma lipid formation on cholesterolgenic diets in rabbits; other evidence showed that it stimulated tumor growth; and still other evidence indicates that it led to a reduction in voluntary alcohol consumption. But none of the evidence is clear cut. In humans lipoic acid has been beneficial in the liver disease hepatic coma.

NONNUTRIENTS

The substances discussed in this section are included not because they have been established as vitamins or as essential nutrients but because they have *not*, yet they are frequently promoted as vitamins or vitamin-like substances.

Laetrile (vitamin B_{17})

This cyanide-containing, potentially toxic substance was first promoted in 1952 and belongs to a group of chemicals called amygdalin. It is derived from the pits of apricots, peaches, and bitter almonds and from apple seeds. Laetrile has been widely promoted as a preventive medication and a cure for cancer. Since there is absolutely no evidence of its effectiveness, the Food and Drug Administration has prohibited its promotion as a cancer-curing drug. Its proponents have tried to circumvent this restriction by offering it for sale as a food under such names as bitter food tablets or Seventeen and by not making claims for its role in cancer therapy. In spite of their argument that patients should have freedom of choice in treatment, so far they have only been able to legalize laetrile in 16 states, and it still cannot be sold through interstate trade or in Canada. Those promoting laetrile claim either that the substance seeks out cancer cells and releases hydrocyanic acid, which in turn kills the cells, or that cancer is caused by a deficiency of vitamin B_{17}. Currently there is no scientific evidence that laetrile is either a vitamin or a cancer cure.

Pangamic acid (Vitamin B_{15})

Pangamic acid has been recently (1978) introduced to the public as vitamin B_{15}, reportedly helpful in alleviating such diverse problems as indigestion, alcoholism, hepatitis, heart disease, and schizophrenia. Although pangamic acid, isolated from apricot pits, was patented in 1949, there has been no evidence in scientific literature that it has any physiological function or that a lack of the substance results in any adverse effects. It is being marketed in the United States under a wide range of names and in a great variety of forms. Although the majority of these products contain dichloroacetate and calcium gluconate, a derivative of the amino acid glycine, the FDA has ruled that it is an unidentifiable substance. The Canadian government, after concluding that there is no proof of it being an identifiable substance that is safe for human use or of it having any therapeutic benefit, has prohibited its sale.

In the absence of anything but anecdotal evidence to the contrary, pangamic acid is considered nutritionally worthless and deceptively labelled as a vitamin.

Caffeine, theophylline, and theobromine

Caffeine, a component of tea, coffee, and cocoa, common dietary items, has no nutritional significance, but since its use does have physiological significance, it is appropriate to discuss it as a dietary component. The caffeine content of common beverages ranges from 60 to 85 mg in a 150 ml cup of coffee, 30 to 50 mg for tea, 6 to 142 mg for cocoa, and 32 to 65 mg per 350 ml (12 oz) of a cola drink. In addition to its well-known role as a central nervous system stimulant, caffeine acts as a diuretic, increasing urine production, a relaxant of smooth muscles, and a stimulant for the heart muscle and gastric acid secretion. It also increases free fatty acid and glucose levels in the plasma and oxygen consumption. Caffeine is absorbed completely and quickly and is distributed in the water component of various tissues. It is excreted as xanthines and uric acid. Intakes of 65 to 130 mg have beneficial effects on motor and mental performance, whereas intakes of 400 mg cause insomnia and poor performance.

Of two related compounds, theophylline, which is found in tea, is also a central nervous system stimulant, and theobromine, which is found in cocoa, has no effect.

BIBLIOGRAPHY

Kulsis, A., and Mookerjea, S.: Choline, Nutr. Rev. **36:**201, 1978.

Stephenson, P. E.: Physiologic and psychotropic effects of caffeine on man, J. Am. Diet. Assoc. **71:**240, 1977.

APPENDIX TO PART ONE

Metabolism

In Chapters 2 to 4, the digestion and metabolism of carbohydrates, lipids, and proteins are considered. Chapters 7 and 8 deal with the functions of minerals, including their roles as cofactors in biological reactions and as parts of enzymes (metalloenzymes). In those chapters, frequent references are made to the roles of minerals in (1) facilitating the catabolism (breakdown) of carbohydrates, lipids, and proteins to provide energy, (2) facilitating the transport of nutrients across the cell membranes, and (3) the synthesis of essential body compounds. The role of vitamins as parts of the nonprotein coenzymes involved in catalyzing many of these same reactions is discussed in Chapters 11 and 12.

The purpose of this Appendix is to summarize, first, the interrelationships that exist in the metabolism of each of these nutrients and, second, the roles of vitamins and minerals in facilitating the biochemical changes involved. It may be helpful for the reader to refer back to this Appendix from time to time when studying applied aspects of nutrition in later chapters.

Digestion and absorption

As summarized in Table 1, each of the energy-yielding nutrients provided in food must be changed in the digestive tract into its simplest component parts or into sufficiently small particles that they can enter the epithelial cells lining the lumen, or inner surface, of the digestive tract. There they may be further broken down by enzymes within the cell before being released into the blood. Monosaccharides (the products of carbohydrate digestion), amino acids (the product of protein digestion), short-chain fatty acids and glycerol (from fat digestion), minerals, and water-soluble vitamins are transported across the cells that line the digestive tract.

Absorption takes place either by diffusion, in which these materials flow easily across the intestinal membrane, or by active transport, a process that not only uses energy but also requires that a particular carrier protein be available inside the mucosal cells lining the tract. These substances are then released on the serosal side of the membrane into the blood, in which they are carried through the portal vein to the liver.

In the intestinal cells the medium- and long-chain fatty acids (with more than 12 carbon atoms) are recombined with glycerol to form lipids. These lipids are absorbed into the lymphatic system and carried to the general circulation from which they are removed by the liver. From the liver, glucose (formed from all carbohydrates), amino acids, fatty acids, and glycerol are released into the general circulation, as are the recombined lipids. The lipids have been further combined with protein to form lipoproteins, a form in which they are more soluble in the aqueous medium of the blood. The end products are taken up by the cells that can utilize them as sources of energy, as building material for growth, or in the formation of essential body compounds.

Catabolism

Glycolysis. Figs. 1 and 2 show the general relationships among the three nutrients during their catabolism as energy sources. Glu-

Table 1. Summary of digestion and metabolism of energy-yielding nutrients

Nutrient in food	End product of digestion*	End products of metabolism†	
		Anabolism	Catabolism
Carbohydrate→	Monosaccharides→ Glucose Fructose Galactose	Glycogen (muscle, liver) Fat	CO_2 H_2O Energy (ATP)
Lipid→	Fatty acids→ Glycerol→ Monoglycerides→	Fat	CO_2 H_2O Energy (ATP)
Protein→	Amino acids→	Tissue protein Enzymes Hormones Fat	CO_2 H_2O Energy (ATP) Urea

*Changes occur within lumen digestive tract or in cells lining tract.
†Changes occur within individual body cells.

cose is first converted through a series of biochemical changes from a 6-carbon molecule to two- 3-carbon molecules of pyruvate (pyruvic acid). These steps, called glycolysis, occur in the cytoplasm, or filling, of the individual body cells and are anaerobic, that is, they do not require the presence of oxygen. ATP serves as a "chemical trap" for energy within the cell, assuring that there will be a continual supply of energy available as needed. Each molecule of ATP represents 7 kcal. Glycolysis does require an initial input of 2 molecules of adenosine triphosphate (ATP), the high-energy compound but results in the later generation of 4 ATP molecules, for a net gain of 2. These 2 molecules of ATP are only a small portion of the energy available in 1 molecule of glucose, but glycolysis provides a mechanism for production of ATP when the need is great and the amount of available oxygen is limited (such as during strenuous physical activity, when oxygen cannot get to the individual cells fast enough to allow complete release of the energy in glucose).

All the steps in glycolysis can be reversed to form glucose in a process known as *glucogenesis*. An additional step in glycolysis, the conversion of pyruvic acid to lactic acid, may occur when the need for energy exceeds oxygen availability. This lactic acid production, by preventing an accumulation of pyruvic acid, allows the continued production of ATP by glycolysis. The lactic acid diffuses into the blood and is then picked up by the liver to be reconverted into glucose (less glucose than it came from because glucogenesis is an energy-consuming process and because some had been converted into ATP).

All further changes involved in releasing energy from glucose, glycerol, fatty acids, and amino acids occur in a special organelle of the cell called the mitochondrion. The number of mitochondria within any one cell varies from one to as many as 2000 in a liver cell, which is very active metabolically. The location of the mitochondria within the cell is related to the need for energy. In a cell synthesizing protein they will be located near the protein-synthesizing organelle, the ribosome. In a cell needing energy to transport

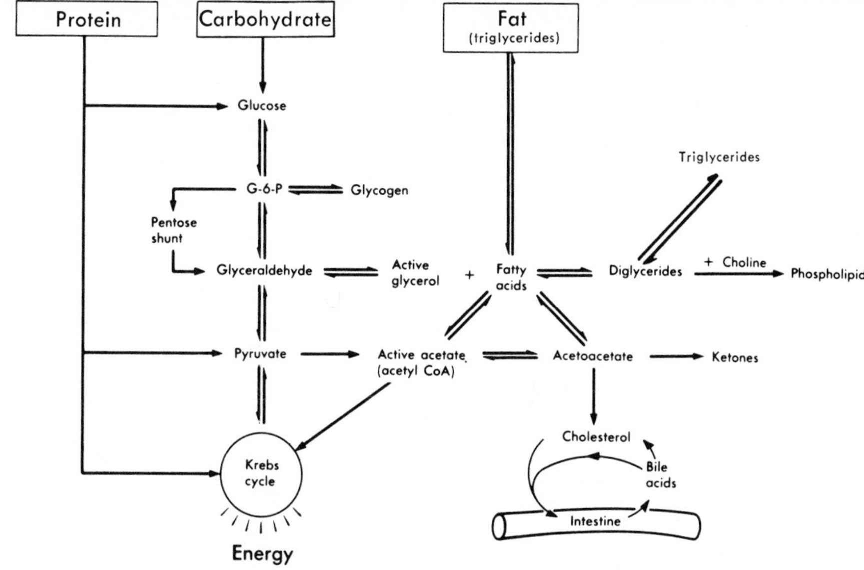

Fig. 1. Summary diagram of metabolism of the nutrients. Note metabolic interrelationships of carbohydrate, protein, and fat. (From Williams, S. R.: Nutrition and diet therapy, ed. 2, St. Louis, 1973, The C. V. Mosby Co.)

nutrients they will be located near the cell wall.

Energy-yielding nutrients enter the cell mitochondria as pyruvic acid, fatty acids, or amino acids. Once within the mitochondrion, pyruvic acid undergoes oxidative decarboxylation. In this series of reactions, 1 carbon atom is oxidized to carbon dioxide, and 2 hydrogen atoms are removed, leaving the 2-carbon compound, acetic acid. This change requires three vitamins, thiamin, riboflavin, and niacin, and the mineral magnesium. The 2-carbon compound quickly unites with coenzymes A, a compound containing the vitamin pantothenic acid, to form acetyl CoA. Acetyl CoA is a key compound in further metabolic changes.

Fatty acids also undergo stepwise degradation with the release of 2-carbon fragments, each of which combines with CoA to form acetyl CoA. The conversion of one 18-carbon fatty acid to nine 2-carbon fragments of acetyl CoA involves forty-five different reactions, the vitamins biotin, niacin, and riboflavin, and the minerals magnesium, copper or iron, and potassium. The glycerol component from the digestion of fat can be converted to glyceraldehyde-3-phosphate, one of the intermediate compounds in the glycolysis sequence of reactions. From this point, glycerol follows the same pathways as the same compound (glyceraldehyde-3-phosphate) derived from glucose.

Some amino acids are also converted to acetyl CoA by several different pathways. The glucogenic amino acids alanine, serine, glycine, cysteine, methionine, and tryptophan are converted to pyruvic acid after being deaminated by the coenzyme pyridoxine (vitamin B_6). Then they may undergo either decarboxylation to acetic acid or glucogenesis to form glucose or glycogen. After deamination to remove the characteristic NH_2 group, ketogenic amino acids, such as phenylalanine, tyrosine, leucine, and isoleucine, undergo the same changes as fatty acids, and are eventually converted to acetyl CoA. These latter amino acids can be used as a source of energy through the same pathway as fatty acids; they also provide the basis for

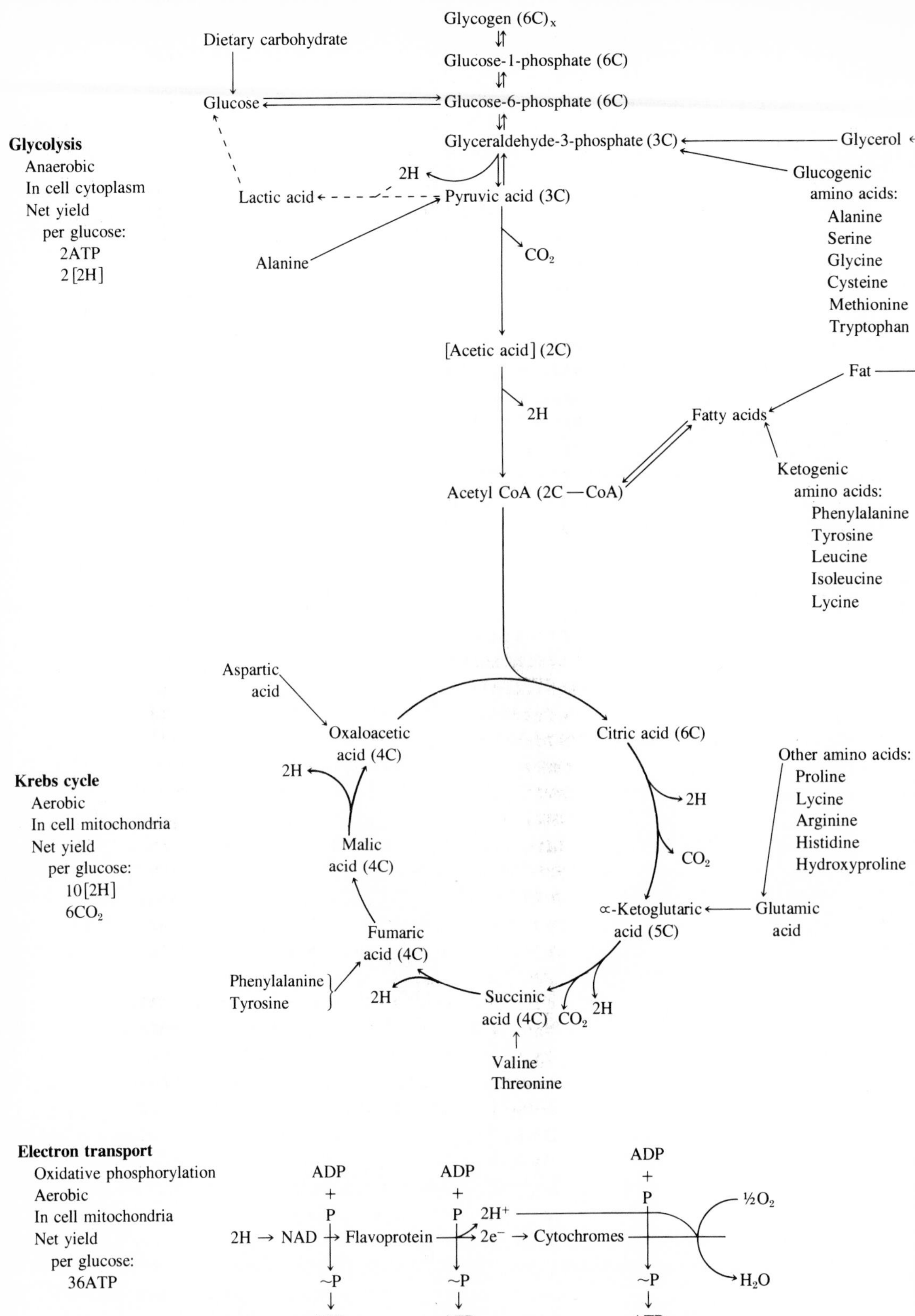

Fig. 2. Simplified version of the metabolism of carbohydrates, lipids, and proteins to demonstrate the interactions in the metabolism of each of these. ~P represents a high-energy form of phosphate.

the synthesis of fats or other fat-related compounds. Other amino acids enter the common energy cycle at later points (Fig. 2).

Fig. 2 shows that within the cell cytoplasm, carbohydrate, fat, and protein are metabolized independently at first.

Krebs citric acid cycle. After glucose, fatty acids, glycerol, and some amino acids have been converted into acetyl CoA, they are all handled in the same series of metaoblic changes. This process is known by several names—Krebs cycle, named after the scientist who discovered it; tricarboxylic acid (TCA) cycle, because it involves acids with three carboxyl (COOH) groups; and the citric acid cycle, because citric acid with 6 carbons, is the first substance formed after the entrance into the cycle of the 2-carbon fragment attached to CoA (acetyl CoA). This series of reactions is identified as a cycle because it is a circle of changes. To begin the cycle, acetyl CoA condenses with 1 molecule of the 4-carbon compound, oxaloacetate. This represents the last substance formed from the previous cycle, or it may be derived from the amino acid aspartic acid. The citric acid (6-carbon) resulting from this condensation then undergoes a series of biochemical changes in which the major intermediate products formed are α-ketoglutaric acid (5-carbon), succinic acid (4-carbon), fumaric acid (4-carbon), malic acid (4-carbon), and oxaloacetic acid (4-carbon).

During these changes, 2 molecules of carbon dioxide are released and 8 hydrogen atoms are removed by the niacin-containing coenzyme NAD to form NADH or by the riboflavin-containing coenzyme flavoprotein to form a reduced flavoprotein. In the course of this cycle of reactions, it is possible for some deaminated amino acids to enter the metabolic pathway. Some, such as proline, lysine, arginine, histidine, and hydroxyproline are first changed into glutamic acid and then to the 5-carbon α-ketoglutaric acid; aspartic acid is converted to oxalacetate and phenylalanine and tyrosine to fumaric acid. Oxalacetic acid can also be converted to pyruvic acid; therefore these amino acids can become potential precursors of glucose through glucogenesis.

Once these products of deamination are in the cycle, they are treated the same as the molecules that entered first as acetyl CoA, and their full energy potential is released. Thus, after this point, the cell cannot distinguish whether the original source was carbohydrate, lipid, or protein, or even whether it was of dietary origin or from the catabolism of a body tissue.

Electron transport system. Once the hydrogen atoms have been removed from Krebs cycle intermediates by niacin- and riboflavin-containing enzymes to form NADH and reduced flavoprotein, they enter into another series of reactions known as the electron transport system, which takes place in the membranes of the mitochondria. This system is responsible for a process known as oxidative phosphorylation. At the end of this sequence, the hydrogens combine with molecular oxygen (O_2) to form water. This overall reaction is catalyzed by a series of iron-containing cytochromes, which are compounds very much like hemoglobin. The electrons from the hydrogen atoms pass from one of these electron carriers (cytochromes) to another and eventually to oxygen. Some energy is released at each transfer reaction; thus the final product, water, has the lowest energy content of all. At three of these transfers enough energy is released to drive the addition of phosphate to adenosine diphosphate (ADP) to form the high-energy compound adenosine triphosphate (ATP).

If the hydrogen were transferred directly to the oxygen without going through the electron transport system involving the cytochromes, a great deal of energy would be lost as heat. This would not only be wasteful but would also mean that the body would need to have alternative ways of releasing the heat to prevent the body temperature from rising.

ATP is the form in which energy is stored until it is needed for the energy-requiring processes of the body. These many processes include mechanical work such as muscle contraction and chemical processes such as synthesis of essential body compounds, the transport of nutrients across cell membranes, and the secretion of hormones. About 40% of the potential energy of the dietary nutrients is extracted and stored as ATP; the remainder is converted to heat. Some heat is required to maintain body temperature; the rest is released through evaporation of moisture from the skin or by direct heat loss.

The processes described above are summarized in Fig. 2. The system is much more complex than this presentation suggests, but the illustration demonstrates how all three major dietary nutrients interact in the energy-releasing process. In addition, it shows how each nutrient can be used for the synthesis of fat. Of the end products, carbon dioxide is excreted through the lungs and water is lost through the skin, lungs, and kidneys. Urea, produced from amino groups, is an additional end product of protein catabolism and is released through the kidneys.

Thus far this discussion has focused on the interrelationships in the catabolism of carbohydrates, fats, and proteins as they provide energy for vital body processes. Anabolism, the synthesis of body components, is the other major aspect of metabolism.

Anabolism

Glucose in excess of the immediate energy needs of the cells is converted by the liver to the complex carbohydrate glycogen. Glucose is stored in this form in the liver and muscle. That stored in the muscle is used in the muscle; that in the liver may be released as a source of blood glucose for use by all body cells. In addition, the 3-carbon compound glycerol, one of the products of lipid digestion, can be converted into a 3-carbon intermediary product of glycolysis. Like pyruvic acid, from here it can either enter the Krebs cycle or be converted back to glucose and/or glycogen. Similarly, the glucogenic amino acids, which are converted to pyruvic acid after deamination, can be used to synthesize glucose and glycogen.

Thus glycerol and the glucogenic amino acids provide an alternative source of glucose, which is the major energy substrate utilized by nerve cells and red blood cells. This means that in periods of starvation or when a carbohydrate-free diet is consumed, the nerve cells are able to function on the energy from glucose that has been derived from glycerol and amino acids. These are available from the breakdown of body fat reserves and from the constant catabolism and anabolism of tissue protein.

The synthesis of fat starts with acetyl CoA. Since all amino acids, carbohydrates, fatty acids, and glycerol can be converted directly or indirectly into acetyl CoA, they all represent potential sources of lipid synthesis. The only energy source that does not involve acetyl CoA is alcohol. Since alcohol can be used directly as a source of energy after being dehydrogenated in the liver, it spares the other sources of energy, which will then be converted to energy-storage forms—glycogen or fat—rather than metabolized as sources of energy. Thus indirectly alcohol is also a source of body fat.

Most body tissue is protein and can be formed only from amino acids. Further, the intracellular processes necessary for protein synthesis on the cell ribosomes require energy. This energy must be derived from the ATP produced in the mitochondria as a result of operation of the citric acid cycle and the electron transport mechanism.

There is considerable evidence that the constituents of the body are in a constant dynamic state with the interchange of products of anabolism and catabolism of both dietary and body sources interacting in myriad ways. The exact nature of the interactions at any one point is determined by a complex of factors, including hormones, enzymes, and availability of vital tissue substances.

Role of minerals and vitamins

The changes necessary to convert food nutrients into energy can proceed only when minerals and vitamins are available for roles as catalysts of the reaction, either in conjunction with or as part of the enzymes involved. In the absence of any of these, the metabolic

Table 2. Requirements of vitamins and minerals in catalyzing the digestion, absorption, and metabolism of energy-yielding nutrients

Process	Vitamin	Mineral
Digestion		Chloride Zinc*
Absorption		Sodium
Catabolism		
Glycogenesis	Riboflavin Niacin Pyridoxine	Magnesium, manganese, or cobalt
Glycolysis	Niacin Lipoic acid Thiamin Pantothenic acid	Potassium Magnesium
Krebs cycle	Pantothenic acid Niacin Lipoic acid Thiamin Riboflavin	Manganese Iron Magnesium
Electron transport	Niacin Riboflavin	Iron* Copper

*Functions as an essential part of the enzyme.

pathway may be blocked, resulting in the accumulation of the intermediary product. Depending on the point at which such blockage occurs, the intermediate may be shifted to an alternative pathway, or it may continue to accumulate.

The accumulation of an intermediary product almost always interferes with cellular functioning and always results in a failure to produce the normal end product of metabolism. For instance, thiamin is a necessary part of the enzyme decarboxylase, which is needed to change pyruvic acid to acetic acid. A lack of thiamin thus inhibits the entrance of glucose into Krebs cycle, resulting in an accumulation of pyruvic acid in the blood.

There are a great number of such reactions in the human body; Table 2 indicates some of the vital roles that vitamins and minerals play in the metabolism of the three major energy-yielding nutrients.

Although many of the terms and concepts used throughout the text have been identified in this chapter, a glossary of terms to help the student in interpreting other concepts is included in Appendix A. For students with a high degree of curiosity and a desire for a more in-depth understanding of the physiology of the body, an elementary physiology text or a high school biology text may prove helpful.

PART TWO

Applied nutrition

14

Selection of an adequate diet, dietary standards, and tables of food composition

The first section of this book provides information on the functions, metabolism, sources, requirements, and results of deficiencies of the more than forty nutrients now believed to be required for adequate nutrition. This study makes it amply clear that although there are still many unanswered questions, there is a great deal of information on which to base recommendations for achieving an adequate intake of most of these nutrients. Results of surveys of nutritional status indicate that nutritionists still face a challenge in encouraging the consumption of a diet compatible with a high level of health. There is an increasing interest on the part of the public and legislators in the role of nutrition in preventive health care with its potential for substantially reducing the cost of medical care in the United States. This section on applied nutrition deals with the application of the basic principles of nutrition to the issues and concerns related to achieving an acceptable level of nutritional adequacy at various stages in the life cycle.

SELECTION OF AN ADEQUATE DIET

The Recommended Dietary Allowances (RDA), which have been mentioned in the discussion of most nutrients, provide a useful guide for nutritionists, dietitians, and agricultural experts in planning and evaluating diets of population groups and in deciding on food production and agricultural policies and programs. They are, however, of little usefulness to the average individual, who does not have access to food composition tables and who will seldom be motivated to carry out the extensive calculations necessary to use the RDA effectively. In addition, the many different units—milligrams, retinol equivalents, international units, etc.—in which both the allowances and food composition data are recorded are confusing.

It thus becomes the challenge of the nutrition educator to find an effective way(s) to interpret the knowledge of the nutrition scientist about nutrient requirements and food composition in terms that are meaningful and useful in helping the average person make rational food choices. Any guide must be sufficiently simple to allow it to be used within the framework of accepted socially and culturally determined food habits. At the same time it must be sufficiently detailed to keep it consistent with scientific facts.

The Food and Nutrition Board, which is responsible for establishing dietary standards, emphasizes that it is possible to achieve the level of nutrition it advocates through a well-chosen diet of natural foods readily available in all supermarkets. It also points out that it is possible to achieve this optimal nutrition through an unlimited number of combinations of foods—the choice of which may be determined by the availability of foods in the local market, socioeconomic status of the family, and the cultural background, physical condition, and food preferences of the individual.

A sound nutrition program involves ascertaining the nutritive value of available foods and their potential in meeting nutritional needs, and educating and motivating the public to make the appropriate choice of foods. As methods of processing change, as needs for additional nutrients are identified, and as fabricated foods appear on the market, this process of nutrition education becomes increasingly more complex. In general, educational approaches have been either food based or nutrient based. It seems evident that neither will meet the needs of everyone and that they should both be promoted and evaluated simultaneously.

The first attempt to translate scientific knowledge of nutrient needs into food guides to help families select an adequate diet was made in 1916. At that time knowledge that humans needed the five nutrient classes—protein, starch and similar carbohydrate, fat, mineral substances, and organic acids and sugars—was interpreted in the recommendation that the public have the five food groups represented in their daily diet. These groups are shown in Table 14-1. It was believed that by including these foods, a diet would provide not only the materials needed for body fuel and building and repair but also the "unknown" essentials.

Following this period, as nutritionists identified essential minerals and vitamins, the emphasis in food selection guides shifted from providing adequate calories to providing the necessary vitamins, minerals, and

Table 14-1. Comparison of United States food guides—1916, 1943, and 1956

Five food groups 1916	Basic Seven 1943*	Basic Four 1956*
Milk, meat, fish, poultry, eggs, and meat substitutes	Milk and milk products (2) Meat, fish, etc. (2), eggs (4 per week)	Milk and milk products (2) Meat, fish, poultry, eggs (2)
Vegetables and fruits	Green and yellow vegetables (1) Citrus fruit and raw cabbage (1) Potatoes, other fruit and vegetables (2)	Fruits and vegetables (4)
Bread and other cereal foods	Bread, flour, cereal enriched or whole grain (3)	Bread, flour, cereal (enriched or whole grain) (4)
Butter and wholesome fats	Equivalent of 2 tablespoons butter or fortified margarine	
Simple sugars		

*Number of servings per day in parentheses.

protein. This led to the designation of some foods as "protective." By 1941 the United States recognized the importance of good nutrition in protecting the nation's health and through the National Research Council published the first Recommended Dietary Allowances. To guide the public, which had no scientific knowledge of nutrients and food composition, in selecting a diet that would meet these standards, the Bureau of Home Economics published a food guide in which they recommended that certain classes of foods be included in the diet in specified amounts. Their recommendations formed the basis for the *Basic Seven,* promoted as part of the National Wartime Nutrition Program of the Food Distribution Administration of the Department of Agriculture in 1943. This familiar guide, presented in Table 14-1, was the basis of practically all nutrition education programs from 1943 until its revision in 1956. Other plans, differing only in minor details, had been promoted by both government and special trade groups, but the Basic Seven became and remained the standard. It served a major purpose in providing a guide that would lead to the consumption of a diet adequate in most nutritional factors, since each food group makes a unique nutritional contribution. This was accomplished through the use of the so-called protective foods—foods that provided a larger proportion of the needs for two or more nutrients than for energy. At that time there was limited data on the trace element composition of foods. The recommendation that a variety of both animal and vegetable foods be included was thought to satisfy the needs for these nutrients because they are widely distributed in foods.

However, the complexity of a seven-group plan coupled with the lack of specificity about what constituted a serving was thought to limit its effectiveness in many nutrition education situations.

While the United States was promoting the seven-group plan, many other countries were developing plans that were designed to accomplish the same educational objective but which involved three, four, or five groups, based on their particular food patterns.

Basic Four food groups

In 1956 the United States Department of Agriculture recommended that the complex seven-group plan be replaced by a simpler, less detailed four-group plan, which it termed Essentials of an Adequate Diet. This plan, shown in Table 14-1, differed from the Basic Seven only in that the three fruit and vegetable categories were grouped as one and the fat group was eliminated entirely. The elimination of the fat group was justified on the grounds that the consumption of foods from the other groups usually led to the use of fat to improve the flavor and palatability of the food. In addition, the change was made at a time when there was concern about the increase in fat consumption by the American public and its possible role in the development of atherosclerosis. The Department of Agriculture did not want to find itself encouraging the consumption of a food that might later be proved to be the villian in a degenerative disease. However, it now appears that some emphasis on fats and oils is justified on the basis of their contribution of vitamin E.

This four-group plan overcame some of the obstacles to the effectiveness of the seven-group plan but suffered from some of the same limitations. Most of the problems have become evident only as knowledge has increased concerning the need for specific nutrients and the contribution of specific foods in satisfying this need. It is now known that some key nutrients are removed in processing and are not returned under current enrichment programs. In other cases the addition of nutrients to some foods either for their nutritional or food processing value (for example, phosphorus used in soft drinks and polyunsaturated fats in margarine) may result in nutrient imbalances that are equally as serious as nutrient deficiencies. In addition, many nutrients such as iodine, vitamin B_{12}, and magnesium were not considered in formulating the four-food group plan. It is entirely possible that a person will select foods within these guidelines that will provide adequate amounts of these nutrients, but is equally possible he will not. There is growing concern that we develop a food plan that gives the homemaker more guidance in selecting foods to more adequately meet needs for all nutrients, not merely the key nutrients, which were the matter of concern when food plans were first developed.

Reports that a significant portion of the United States public consumes inadequate amounts of one or more nutrients in their diets have led many critics to question the effectiveness of food guides in nutrition education. These critics, however, fail to consider the possibility that even more frequent and severe inadequacies might have been found had these food guides not been promoted.

Food plans

As an aid to persons with a specified amount of money to spend on food, the Department of Agriculture publishes food plans

Table 14-2. Low-cost food plan (amounts of food for a week)*†

Family member	Milk, cheese, ice cream‡ (qt)	Meat poultry, fish§ (lb)	Eggs (no)	Dry beans and peas, nuts ‖ (lb)	Dark-green, deep-yellow vegetables (lb)	Citrus fruit, tomatoes (lb)
Child						
7 mo-1 yr	5.70	0.56	2.1	0.15	0.35	0.42
1-2 yr	3.57	1.26	3.6	0.16	0.23	1.01
3-5 yr	3.91	1.52	2.7	0.25	0.25	1.20
6-8 yr	4.74	2.03	2.9	0.39	0.31	1.58
9-11 yr	5.46	2.57	3.9	0.44	0.38	2.13
Male						
12-14 yr	5.74	2.98	4.0	0.56	0.40	1.99
15-19 yr	5.49	3.74	4.0	0.34	0.39	2.20
20-54 yr	2.74	4.56	4.0	0.33	0.48	2.32
55 yr and over	2.61	3.63	4.0	0.21	0.61	2.38
Female						
12-19 yr	5.63	2.55	4.0	0.24	0.46	2.17
20-54 yr	3.02	3.21	4.0	0.19	0.55	2.34
55 yr and over	3.01	2.45	4.0	0.15	0.62	2.54
Pregnant	5.25	3.68	4.0	0.29	0.67	2.80
Nursing	5.25	4.16	4.0	0.26	0.66	2.99

*From Family Economic Review, p. 4, Winter 1975.

†Amounts are for food as purchased or brought into the kitchen from garden or farm. Amounts allow for places to allow for greater accuracy, especially in estimating rations for large groups of people and for lo a pound.

‡Fluid milk and beverage made from dry or evaporated milk. Cheese and ice cream may replace some mi ice cream, 1½ quarts.

§Bacon or salt pork should not exceed ⅓ pound for each 5 pounds of this group.

‖Weight in terms of dry beans and peas, shelled nuts, and peanut butter. Count 1 pound of cann

#Includes coffee, tea, cocoa, punches, ades, soft drinks, leavenings, and seasonings. The use of iodiz

**Cereal fortified with iron is recommended.

indicating the amounts of eleven types of food to purchase per week for each member of the family. The three plans are based on different income levels—low, moderate, and liberal cost. When followed, they help to ensure a satisfactory level of nutrition for the whole family, assuming reasonably good practices in food preparation. The distribution of food to various family members is, however, the responsibility of the homemaker. The Department of Agriculture periodically publishes information on the actual costs of foods in these plans. Estimated costs for food for a family of four (March, 1978) are $54.20, $67.90, and $80.90 per week for these three economic levels. An example of a food plan is shown in Table 14-2.

NUTRITIVE CONTRIBUTION OF FOOD GROUPS

Each of the four food groups in the Essentials of an Adequate Diet is chosen because of a unique contribution it makes to the nutritive value of the diet. The contribution of each of the groups is shown graphically in Figs. 14-1, 14-2, 14-4, and 14-6. The values

Potatoes (lb)	Other vegetables, fruit (lb)	Cereal (lb)	Flour (lb)	Bread (lb)	Other bakery products (lb)	Fats, oils (lb)	Sugar, sweets (lb)	Accessories# (lb)
0.06	3.43	0.71**	0.02	0.06	0.05	0.05	0.18	0.06
0.60	2.88	0.99**	0.27	0.76	0.33	0.12	0.36	0.68
0.85	2.95	0.90	0.30	0.91	0.57	0.38	0.71	1.02
1.10	3.67	1.11	0.45	1.27	0.84	0.52	0.90	1.43
1.41	4.81	1.24	0.62	1.65	1.20	0.61	1.15	1.89
1.50	3.90	1.15	0.67	1.88	1.25	0.77	1.15	2.61
1.87	4.50	0.90	0.75	2.10	1.55	1.05	1.04	3.09
1.87	4.81	0.93	0.71	2.10	1.47	0.91	0.81	2.11
1.72	4.92	1.02	0.62	1.73	1.23	0.77	0.90	1.16
1.17	4.57	0.75	0.63	1.44	1.05	0.53	0.88	2.44
1.40	4.17	0.71	0.55	1.31	0.94	0.59	0.72	2.13
1.22	4.57	0.97	0.58	1.24	0.86	0.38	0.64	1.11
1.65	4.99	0.95	0.66	1.52	1.06	0.55	0.78	2.56
1.67	5.33	0.78	0.61	1.55	1.16	0.76	0.91	2.70

card of about one tenth of the *edible* food as plate waste, spoilage, etc. Amounts of food are shown to two decimal riods of time. For general use, amounts of food groups for a family may be rounded to the nearest tenth or quarter of

unt as equivalent to a quart of fluid milk: Natural or processed Cheddar-type cheese, 6 oz; cottage cheese, 2½ lb;

beans—pork and beans, kidney beans, etc.—as ⅓ pound.
is recommended.

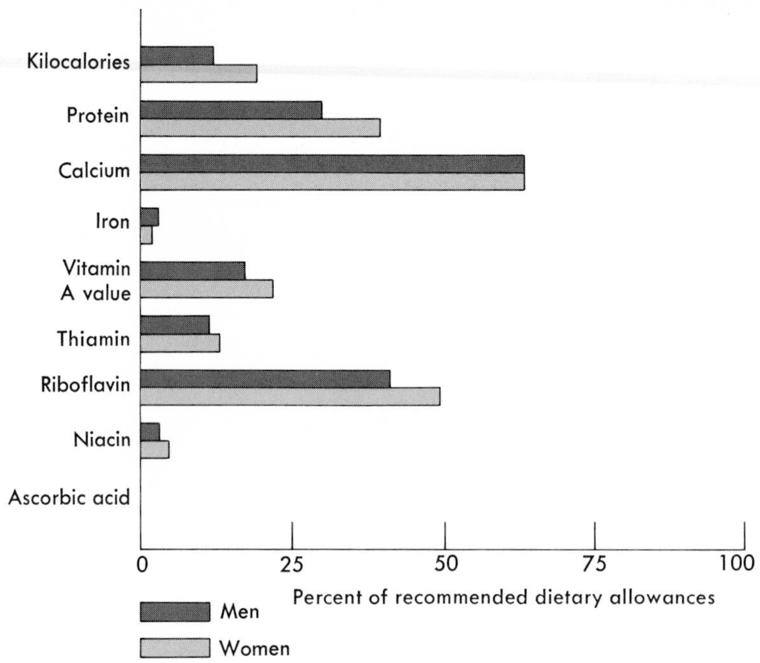

Fig. 14-1. Nutritive contribution of 2 cups of milk to diet of an adult.

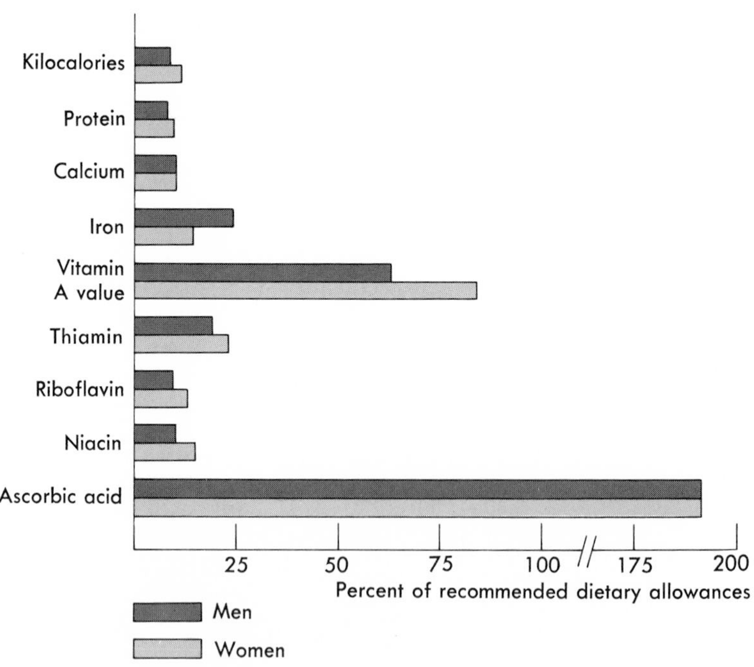

Fig. 14-2. Nutritive contribution of four servings of fruit or vegetables to diet of an adult.

shown in the graphs represent a typical selection of foods within each category. It must be recognized that by differing the choices within the framework of the guide, wide variations in the nutritive quality of the diet may result, not only in regard to the nutrients considered here but also with regard to many others. For instance, the choice of foods presented in the graphs represent approximately 1400 kcal. It is possible to stay within the framework of the plan and to choose foods ranging in caloric value from 800 to 1800. Likewise, the choice of vegetables may result in a diet providing less than 1000 or more than 10,000 IU of vitamin A. Magnesium and folacin values would vary at the same time.

Milk and milk products

As shown in Fig. 14-1, the major contributions of the milk group are high-quality protein of which 80% is present as casein and lactalbumin, containing all nine essential amino acids; calcium, which is difficult to obtain in sufficient amounts from other sources alone; and riboflavin.

Milk protein is readily digested and has a relatively high concentration of lysine, which is limiting in both rice and wheat. Thus milk is especially effective in supplementing these cereal proteins.

The contribution of various dairy products to the intake of calcium is shown in Fig. 7-8. The riboflavin available from milk depends on the conditions under which it is stored. Although exposure to sunlight may reduce the riboflavin content by as much as 50%, the use of opaque plastic containers and paper cartons helps to reduce this loss.

The significant nutritional contribution of milk is evident from data showing that in 1976 dairy foods contributed 11.2% of the energy in the United States diet compared to 75% of the calcium, 39% of the riboflavin, 22% of protein and magnesium, 20% of vitamin B_{12}, 13% of vitamin A value, 10% of pyridoxine, 9% of thiamin, and practically all of the vitamin D. The INQ for calcium, protein, vitamin A, thiamin, riboflavin, niacin, and vitamin B_{12} is greater than 1, indicating that if milk were the sole source of energy in the diet it would also provide the recommended intake of these nutrients.

Although the nutritive content of cow's milk varies with the breed, nutritional status and feed of the cow, stage of lactation, and environmental temperature, most dairy products on the market are blends of milk from many sources, thus these differences tend to balance out.

The recommendation that the equivalent of 2 cups of milk be used by an adult can be satisfied in many ways, as shown by the list of equivalents in Table 14-3. The use of nonfat

Table 14-3. Amount of milk substitutes needed to provide the amounts of calcium and protein in 1 cup of whole milk

	Amount required to provide 280 mg calcium			Amount required to provide 9 g protein		
	g	kcal	measure	g	kcal	measure
Nonfat milk	250	90	1 cup	250	90	1 cup
Cheddar cheese	36	150	1⅓ ounces	36	150	1⅓ ounces
Cottage cheese	298	220	1⅓ cups	66	55	⅓ cup
Ice cream (10% fat)	220	380	1½ cups	220	380	1½ cups
Cream cheese	451	1500	30 tbs	113	410	9 tbs

milk, with less than 0.5% fat, in place of whole milk, with at least 3.2% fat, will reduce the energy value by half but eliminate the vitamin A and the essential fatty acids altogether. Neither of these is necessarily undesirable. Most persons have no difficulty in obtaining sufficient calories, and the vitamin A in one serving of a vegetable such as carrots will make up for the loss of vitamin A in 20 cups of nonfat milk. In addition, an increasing proportion of the nonfat milk and nonfat dried milk solids reaching the market is being fortified with both vitamins A and D. Thus nonfat milk can be used to restrict calories while providing the same nutritive value as whole milk. Chocolate milk has a higher caloric value but otherwise has the same nutritive value as whole milk; chocolate drink has the same value as nonfat milk.

Cottage cheese may be a poor substitute for whole milk, since calcium will be reduced if the cheese has been prepared by acid coagulation rather than rennin coagulation. It is a good source of protein in either case, but water-soluble vitamins are often lost in the whey.

The limiting nutritional factors in milk are iron, manganese, and copper, and ascorbic acid. All of these are present in small amounts in a form that is available, but it has been well established that a milk diet alone is incapable of providing adequate iron to regenerate hemoglobin in infants after 6 months of age. The small amount of ascorbic acid normally found in milk is reduced still further by the process of pasteurization; therefore it is an undependable source of the vitamin.

Ice cream is a good substitute for milk as a source of calcium on the basis of weight but contains only half as much calcium on the basis of calories. Cheese is a popular substitute for milk. It has a nutritive value comparable to the milk from which it is made depending on processing, which influences what nutrients are lost in whey. As in the case of milk, the protein, calcium, and riboflavin content decreases, and the energy content increases proportionately as the fat content increases. For lactose-intolerant individuals, cheese in which lactose has been changed to lactic acid has advantages.

Milk is available to the consumer in many forms at widely varying prices determined primarily by the perishability of the product rather than by nutritive considerations. The relative costs of various forms of milk of essentially equal nutritive value are presented in Table 14-4. By choosing the least expensive form that meets a particular need, it is possible to reduce the cost of milk in the diet by an appreciable sum. In any case, milk is a relatively inexpensive source of protein. Commercially prepared yogurt often has the fat that was removed replaced by nonfat milk giving a product with a high (20%) galactose content. Conversely, yogurt with fruit may have up to 50% of the milk replaced by the fruit and sugar.

The per capita consumption of dairy products has been declining slowly but steadily since 1960, in spite of an increase in the sales of yogurt, sour cream, low-fat milk, and cheese. The decline has been attributed to concern about obesity and blood cholesterol levels, lack of understanding of the nutritive value of milk, competition from other bever-

Table 14-4. Relative costs of other forms of milk compared to fresh whole milk

Form	Relative cost*
Fresh whole milk	$1.00
Fresh 2% milk	$1.00
Fresh homogenized chocolate milk	$1.30
Fresh nonfat milk	$0.96
Evaporated whole milk	$0.80
Evaporated nonfat milk	$0.78
Dried whole milk	$1.12
Dried nonfat milk	$0.75-0.85
Yogurt	$3.50

*Based on prices in northeastern United States, Summer, 1978.

ages, and the development of dairy substitutes.

For the 10% to 20% of the adult population who are lactose intolerant due to a lack or insufficient secretion of the intestinal enzyme lactase, the only dairy products that are well tolerated are fermented milk products such as cheese, yogurt, or buttermilk. In these products the disaccharide lactose has been fermented to form lactic acid, which does not require lactase. Many individuals who are lactose intolerant at relatively high intakes are not totally milk intolerant and can drink up to 1 liter of milk if taken in divided portions. For those who experience allergic symptoms a tolerance can be built up by taking increasingly larger amounts until no symptom are evident.

Fruits and vegetables

The U.S. Department of Agriculture in *Essentials of an Adequate Diet* recommends that the diet contain four servings of fruits and vegetables but does not include suggestions regarding the choice to be made within this group. Since foods in this group are so diverse in nutritional value, persons who use this guide as a basis for a nutrition education program urge the consumption of one serving of a citrus fruit or another fruit or vegetable high in ascorbic acid every day and a serving of dark green, yellow, or orange vegetable as a source of vitamin A every other day. In this way the major contribution of this group in providing vitamin C and A and iron will be satisfied, as shown in Fig. 14-3. Because of the low caloric content of this group of foods, the INQ for all these nutrients exceeds 1. In addition, valuable amounts of folacin, magnesium, and calcium will be contributed. Fig. 14-3 shows the pattern of vegetable and fruit consumption in the United States.

Table 14-5. Comparison of ascorbic acid content of different fruit juices*

Juice	mg of ascorbic acid per ½ cup
Orange, fresh	62
Orange, frozen	60
Grapefruit, canned	42
Tomato, canned	19.5
Pineapple, canned	11.5
Apple, canned	1
Prune, canned	2.5
Grape, canned	Trace
Commercially enriched juices	30

*Based on Adams, C. F.: Nutritive value of American foods. Handbook No. 456, Washington, D.C., 1975, U.S. Department of Agriculture.

A 4-ounce serving of fruit juice is considered an average serving. Citrus juices are generally rich sources, but other fruit juices provide varying amounts of ascorbic acids, as shown in Table 14-5. In using the guide, emphasis should be placed on those juices that provide at least 30 mg of vitamin C in a 4-ounce portion, especially if the diet contains no other rich source. Many juices naturally low in vitamin C are now enriched at this level. An analysis of samples of fruit juices with ascorbic acid shows a wide variation in the amount present, usually above the amount declared on the label. Fortification with acerola, a vitamin C–rich tropical fruit, has no merit over fortification with synthetic ascorbic acid.

In other fruits and vegetables the amount of vitamin C present varies with the variety, the degree of maturity, the season, climatic conditions, the length and conditions of storage, and the part of the plant used. In freshly picked apples, for instance, ascorbic acid values range from 5 to 19 mg/100 g, depending on the variety, and these values fall to almost half after several months of storage. The loss of nutrients that occurs in fruits and vegetables begins right after harvest and may be rapid in the first few hours. In addition to biochemical losses due to oxidation further loss is attributable to the removal of parts of the plant during preparation to make the product more palatable. The wilted outer

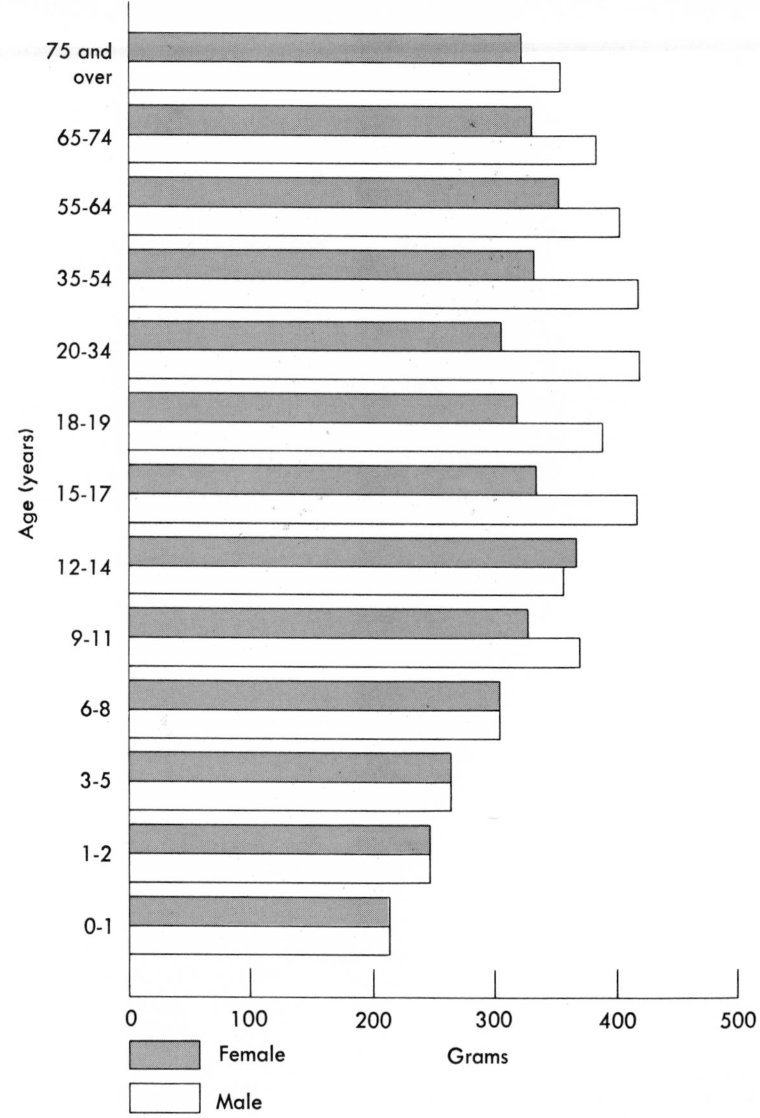

Fig. 14-3. Consumption of fruits and vegetables (quantity per person per day) related to age in the United States—spring, 1965; 28 g = 1 oz. (From Agricultural Research Service, U.S. Department of Agriculture, 1969.)

leaves of lettuce, the leaves of broccoli, the skin on potatoes, and the bitter dark green leaves of endive, all of which are often discarded in preparation, have higher concentrations of some nutrients than do the parts consumed. The fact that ascorbic acid is a relatively unstable nutrient, being readily destroyed by heat, oxidation, and alkali, suggests the use of methods of preparation and harvesting that minimize the loss of nutrients. These include limiting exposure to air, especially at high temperatures, cooking in a minimum amount of water for the shortest period of time, keeping the period of storage to a minimum, and serving immediately after cooking.

Other seasonal fruits rich in ascorbic acid are strawberries, cantaloupe, and cherries; among vegetables, broccoli, asparagus, spinach, and cabbage are important sources, especially when they are served raw or prepared in a way that minimizes losses.

Since relatively few of the dark green or yellow fruits and vegetables that are rich sources of carotene are popular items in the diet, a realistic approach to a food guide suggests the use of these every other day. This is additionally justified because of the stability of vitamin A and carotene and the fact that those foods that are rich sources usually provide more than the day's allowance in one serving, which means that the excess will be stored for future use. Thus a daily intake of foods high in vitamin A value is not absolutely necessary, although it may be desirable. The vitamin A value of some typical dark green and yellow vegetables is given in Table 14-6, where the relationship between degree of pigmentation and vitamin A values become apparent. The practice of using butter, margarine, or salad oil to enhance flavor of vegetables is desirable since carotene is more readily absorbed in the presence of fat.

Table 14-6. Vitamin A content of representative vegetables*

Vegetable	Vitamin A per ½ cup (IU)
Sweet potatoes, cooked	10,075
Carrots, cooked	7615
Spinach, cooked	7290
Kale	4565
Winter squash, baked	4305
Mustard greens	4060
Endive	825
Asparagus, cooked	810
Leaf lettuce	525
Peas, cooked	430
Green beans, cooked	340
Yellow corn, cooked	330
Lima beans, cooked	240
Celery, raw	160
Head lettuce	125

*Based on Adams, C. F.: Nutritive value of American foods, Handbook No. 456, Washington, D.C., 1975, U.S. Department of Agriculture.

Aside from the unique contributions of carotene and ascorbic acid, the fruit and vegetable group contributes about 25% of the day's intake of iron. The amount varies with the foods and parts chosen, iron content being higher in leaves than in stems, fruit, or underground portions. The absorption of iron from fruits and vegetables is very low (less than 5%) due primarily to the high cellulose and phytic acid found in most vegetables. The simultaneous consumption of foods containing heme iron (present in the hemoglobin and myoglobin of animal tissue) greatly enhances the absorption of the nonheme iron of vegetables.

The trace element content of fruits and vegetables is an important factor. The content is dependent in the amount present in the soil in which the plant was grown, but generally it will not vary appreciably.

Calcium intake from this group is small compared to that from the milk group but will assume more importance if milk intake is low. The low phosphorus is a desirable factor. If peas or beans are chosen, a rich source of thiamin is provided, and if dark green leafy vegetables such as spinach are used, riboflavin will be high.

Generally, fruits and vegetables are poor sources of protein and that present is of low biological value because of a lack of some essential amino acids. Roots and tubers contain 2% protein and 20% carbohydrate, whereas legumes such as peas and beans have 4% protein and 13% carbohydrate. Of the latter group, soybeans have protein of a relatively high biological value. They have been promoted extensively in underdeveloped countries as a source of protein, but the production of soybean oil and textured vegetable protein for meat substitutes are the major uses of the product in the United

States. The energy contribution of the fruit and vegetable group is generally low because of the high proportion of cellulose and water and low fat content. Immature seeds such as peas and beans and starchy tubers such as potatoes contribute two to eight times as many calories per serving as do celery, carrots, spinach, and cabbage, which are high in cellulose and water but low in starch. One must remember, however, that the caloric contribution of a fruit or vegetable dish may be double or triple that of the food alone, depending on the way it is served or the type of product in which it is incorporated, as shown in Table 5-4.

The introduction of synthetic citrus beverages made from sucrose, glucose, fructose and citric acid and fortified with ascorbic acid have provided a low-cost, uniform product which, unfortunately, is inferior to the natural product in that it lacks the trace elements and other nutrients of the natural juices.

Another important nutritional benefit from the use of fruits and vegetables is attributed to the bulk provided by cellulose. This promotes normal gastrointestinal mobility and greatly facilitates the passage of food through the digestive tract, helping to prevent constipation. Recent evidence that low dietary fiber may be responsible for the increasing incidence of diverticulosis and associated with cancer of the colon is further reason to use fruits and vegetables.

One should not overlook the value of many fruits in stimulating the appetite. They also serve as sources of an organic acid in the stomach and facilitate calcium and iron absorption in persons with a reduced secretion of hydrochloric acid. If fruits, sometimes described as "detergent foods," are eaten at the end of a meal they help remove carbohydrate that may have adhered to the tooth surface, thus having a beneficial effect on dental health.

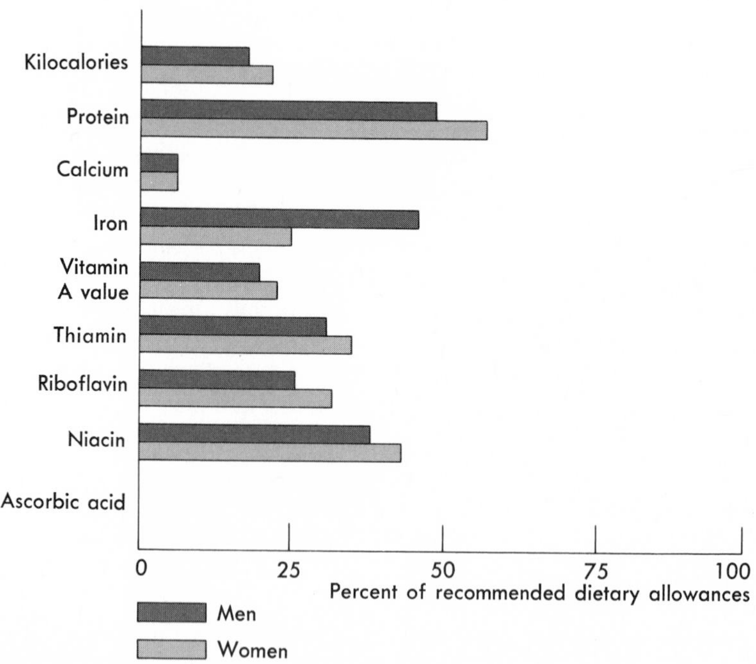

Fig. 14-4. Nutritive contribution of two servings of meat or meat substitute to diet of an adult.

Protein-rich foods

The inclusion of meat, fish, and poultry as a separate group is justified on the basis of the amount of high-quality protein they provide. As shown in Fig. 14-4, this group contributes over 50% of the protein recommended in the diet as well as from 25% to 50% of the iron and 35% of the niacin. One average 3- to 4-ounce serving provides at least 20 g of protein, but the amount will vary slightly with the type of meat. Table 14-7 expresses the approximate composition of different meats, and Table 14-8 shows the amount needed to provide 20 g of protein. Meat substitutes, such as eggs, cheese, peas, beans, and peanut butter, may contain somewhat less per average serving. However, since they are usually consumed in combination with cereal protein, as in cheese or peanut butter sandwiches, macaroni and cheese, or eggs on toast, the combined protein values will approach that of a meat and will usually cost less. The quantity of meat, fish, and poultry consumed in the United States in 1965 is shown in Fig. 14-5.

The lipid content of meat is variable, ranging from 1% to 40%; it depends on the type of animal and its diet, its condition at the time of slaughter, the cut, the extent to which the meat is trimmed, and the method of preparation. The higher the grade of meat, the more fat marbled throughout the muscle fiber and the higher the caloric value. Prime grade beef may have 25% lipid compared to 16% in standard grade and even less in utility grade. Animal nutritionists are able to change fatty acid composition of meat of some animals by manipulating the fat and carbohydrate in the animal's diet. Fish and shellfish are relatively low (1% to 7%) in lipid content and good sources of iodine and other trace elements and contain high-quality, easily digested protein.

Dried peas and beans, with a protein content ranging as high as 35%, and nuts, with 15% protein, are frequent substitutes in the meat group, but as seen from Fig. 4-12 have less protein per 100 kcal. Since most legumes provide protein with limiting amounts of one or more amino acids, they are most effective is used in combination with cereal protein or as extenders of animal protein. Two or three eggs, with 6 g of protein each, are also a good substitute for meat.

The amount of iron depends on the meat chosen, being low in chicken and fish but

Table 14-7. Approximate composition of meat, fish, poultry, and eggs

Food	Moisture (%)	Protein (%)	Fat (%)	kcal/100 g
Beef	60.3	18.5	21.0	263
Pork (medium fat)	48.5	12.7	38.5	401
Veal	68.0	19.1	12.0	190
Lamb	56.0	13.4	27.1	310
Chicken	63.8	31.6	3.4	166
Egg (whole)	73.7	12.9	11.5	163
Salmon	63.4	27.0	7.4	182
Cod	64.6	28.5	5.3	170
Lobster	76.8	18.5	1.5	95
Scallops	73.1	23.2	1.4	112
Sardines	70.7	19.2	8.6	160

high in glandular organs. Pork liver is the richest source of iron and also one of the least expensive. Muscle meats high in both hemoglobin and myoglobin plus liberal amounts of iron-containing enzymes are good iron sources.

Meat is also a major source of zinc in the American diet.

Since phosphorus is a component of most proteins, meat is one of the best sources of phosphorus in the diet.

The vitamin content of the general classes of meat is shown in Table 14-9. If pork is chosen, the meat group becomes the major source of thiamin.

Because of its high protein and hence tryp-

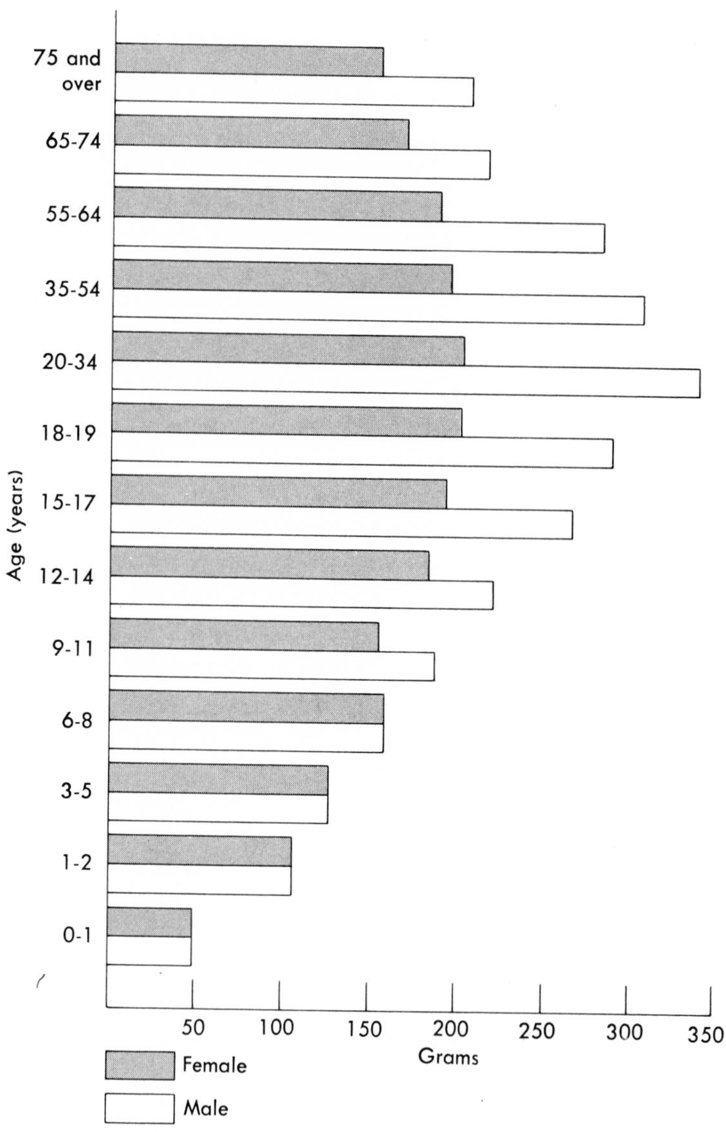

Fig. 14-5. Consumption of meat, fish, and poultry (quantity per person per day) as related to age in the United States—spring, 1965; 28 g = 1 oz. (From Agricultural Research Service, U.S. Department of Agriculture, 1969.)

tophan content, the meat group becomes a major contributor of niacin in the diet, two servings providing about 50% of the recommended allowance; veal and poultry are the richest sources.

The vitamin A, calcium, and ascorbic acid contents of meat are low. Liver is a rich source of vitamin A and riboflavin and a good source of ascorbic acid, but since it is not a consistent item in the diet, the meat group makes a limited contribution of these nutrients in the diet.

Table 14-8. Amount of meat or meat substitutes needed to provide 20 g of protein

Food	g
Chicken	67
Cod	70
Veal	74
Beef liver	77
Peanut butter	80
Lamb	90
Dried peas	90
Pork	90
Salmon (pink)	100
Luncheon meat	105
Frankfurters	160
Eggs	160

One of the most important contributions of the meat group is vitamin B_{12}, or cobalamin, which is derived only from foods of animal origin.

Meat is often the most expensive single item on the menu, often accounting for over a third of every food dollar. Thus consumers have come to plan meals around the meat or protein dish. The cost of a serving of meat may range from a low of 12 cents for pork liver to a high of $1.60 for filet mignon for a 3- to 4-ounce serving in 1978.

The utilization of the meat supply in the United States has been increased by a process of mechanically removing the flesh from the bone of both poultry and beef. This product contains the same high-quality protein, vitamins, and minerals of meat and some calcium extracted from the bone. It is a nutritious, palatable, and economical product to be used in processed meats.

In general, American dietary patterns provide adequate intakes of protein; thus there is little reason to promote the use of additional servings of foods from this group. The exclusion of meat from the diet, however,

Table 14-9. Content of B complex vitamins in 100 g of meat and eggs*

Food	Thiamin (mg)	Riboflavin (mg)	Nicotinic acid (mg)	Vitamin B_6 (mg)	Pantothenic acid (mg)	Folic acid (μg)	Vitamin B_{12} (μg)
Beef	0.08	0.15	4.5	0.35	0.7	14	2.5
Veal	0.17	0.35	7.0	0.35	0.7	20	1.2
Pork	0.80	0.18	4.1	0.45	0.7	7	1.0
Lamb	0.15	0.20	4.6	0.35	0.7	7	2.8
Poultry	0.08	0.16	7.0	0.50	0.8	3	3.2
Eggs	0.10	0.35	0.1	0.25	1.3	8	0.7

*From Siedler, A. J.: Nutritional contributions of the meat group to an adequate diet, Borden Rev. Nutr. Res. **24**:29, 1963.

makes it increasingly difficult to obtain adequate vitamin B_{12} and has implications for the effectiveness of iron absorption.

Cereal and cereal products

Four servings of enriched or whole-grain cereal products are recommended primarily for their contribution of the day's intake of thiamin, riboflavin, niacin, and iron (Fig. 14-6). Current standards of identity for cereal products are provided in Table 14-10. The contribution of this group to the protein intake may be significant. Although most cereal products, with 7% to 14% protein, contain incomplete or low-quality protein, they are so frequently served in conjunction with a complete protein that will provide the essential amino acid lacking that the quality of the cereal protein is improved. Examples are macaroni and cheese, rice with chicken, poached egg on toast, or cereal and milk. In addition, two or more vegetables, cereals, or legumes served at the same time can supplement each other. The current practice of

Table 14-10. Standards of identity for enriched flour, bread, rolls, and buns

	Thiamin (mg/lb)	Riboflavin (mg/lb)	Niacin (mg/lb)	Iron (mg/lb)
Enriched flour	2.9	1.8	24	25
Enriched self-rising flour	2.9	1.8	24	25
Enriched bread, rolls, or buns	1.8	1.1	15	25

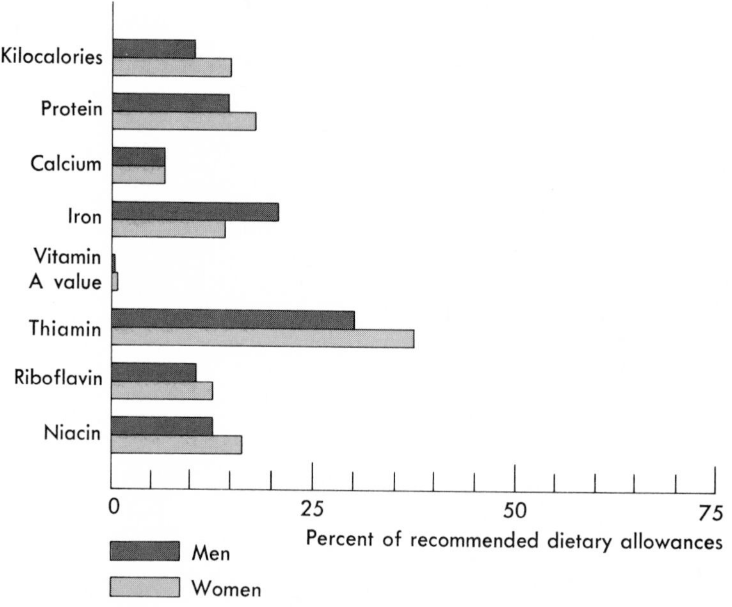

Fig. 14-6. Nutritive contribution of four servings of whole-grain or enriched cereal to diet of an adult.

using dried milk solids in commercially prepared bakery products enhances their protein quality.

The enrichment of both wheat and rice with the amino acid lysine is being used as a means of improving the quality of these two relatively inexpensive cereal proteins. It has, however, limited merit in countries where most persons consume some animal protein. The addition of methionine and tryptophan may further enhance the quality of some cereal proteins. This technique has the greatest potential for developing countries in which staple cereals may provide as much as 80% of the calories and for those on limited incomes who consume a relatively high proportion of cereals and relatively less animal protein. Here, also, the potential of using one vegetable protein to supplement another should be exploited.

The concept that only such products as bread, rice, macaroni, and dry or cooked cereal would satisfy the recommendation for four servings of cereal has been modified so that any product made primarily of flour is considered in the group. Although only thirty states have compulsory enrichment of bread and flour, over 90% of the flour now sold in the United States is enriched, and it is believed that most products made from flour contain appreciable amounts of the B vitamins and iron. Thus waffles, muffins, pancakes, pastry, cakes, and cookies can all be considered part of the cereal group. Commercially prepared mixes, fortunately, are now made with enriched flour, as the result of the food industry's decision to make more universal use of enriched flour. The use of milk or nonfat milk solids in many of these products increases the calcium to significant levels and supplements the cereal protein.

The value of iron in enriched cereals depends on the form in which it is added, the specific cereal, and the method by which the cereal is prepared. Legislation proposed in 1974 to raise the level of enrichment of iron in cereals is still under consideration but is unlikely to be passed.

One of the major justifications for the inclusion of cereal products in the diet is the contribution of relatively significant amounts of many nutrients at minimum cost. It should be pointed out, however, that the current enrichment program calls for the addition of only four of the many nutrients that are removed with the germ and outer husk of the grain. Therefore while enriched cereals are comparable to whole-grain cereal in nutritive content of iron, thiamin, riboflavin, and niacin, they provide smaller amounts of other nutrients including magnesium, vitamin E, pyridoxine, and some trace elements.

Currently about 85% of the ready-to-eat cereals are fortified, which means they have nutrients restored to the level originally in the unmilled cereal or higher. There has been a trend in the highly competitive breakfast cereal business to promote a cereal product enriched with any number of nutrients in addition to thiamin, riboflavin, niacin, and iron (which must be added to enriched cereals) and calcium, an optional nutrient. Little justification can be found for adding ascorbic acid or vitamins A, D, and B_{12} to cereal products. None of these are nutrients normally present in whole-grain cereal. Current legislation places a limit of 150% of the recommended dietary allowance for a nutrient on the amount that can be added to a food product for trade advantage. A more rational approach to fortification would be the addition of nutrients to assure an INQ of 2 for each nutrient added. The charge that most breakfast cereals are devoid of nutritional value is not justified.

The addition of sugar to ready-to-eat cereals has become a highly controversial issue. Opponents question the value of having sugar as an integral part of the product at what they believe to be excessive levels. Those in favor point out that the amount present may be less than the individual might add himself. Cereal with 1 tablespoon of sugar added per 1-ounce serving is 50% sugar by weight. That with 1 teaspoon is 16% sugar. Both are generally available.

One ounce of cereal, dry weight, is considered as one serving. Thus 1 ounce of a prepared cereal such as bran flakes or 1 ounce of dry oatmeal, when cooked, constitutes an average serving. The volume of 1 ounce of puffed cereal is usually so large that only ½ ounce will be used as a serving. Fig. 14-7 shows the pattern of consumption of grain products in the United States.

Converted rice is prepared by parboiling the rice kernels prior to polishing. During this process the nutrients normally concentrated in the outer husk are driven into the kernel, where they remain when the husk is removed. Thus a refined cereal that has been enriched with its own nutrients is produced. This process has been used in India for many years, and should be distinguished from the method of preparing quick-cooking rice.

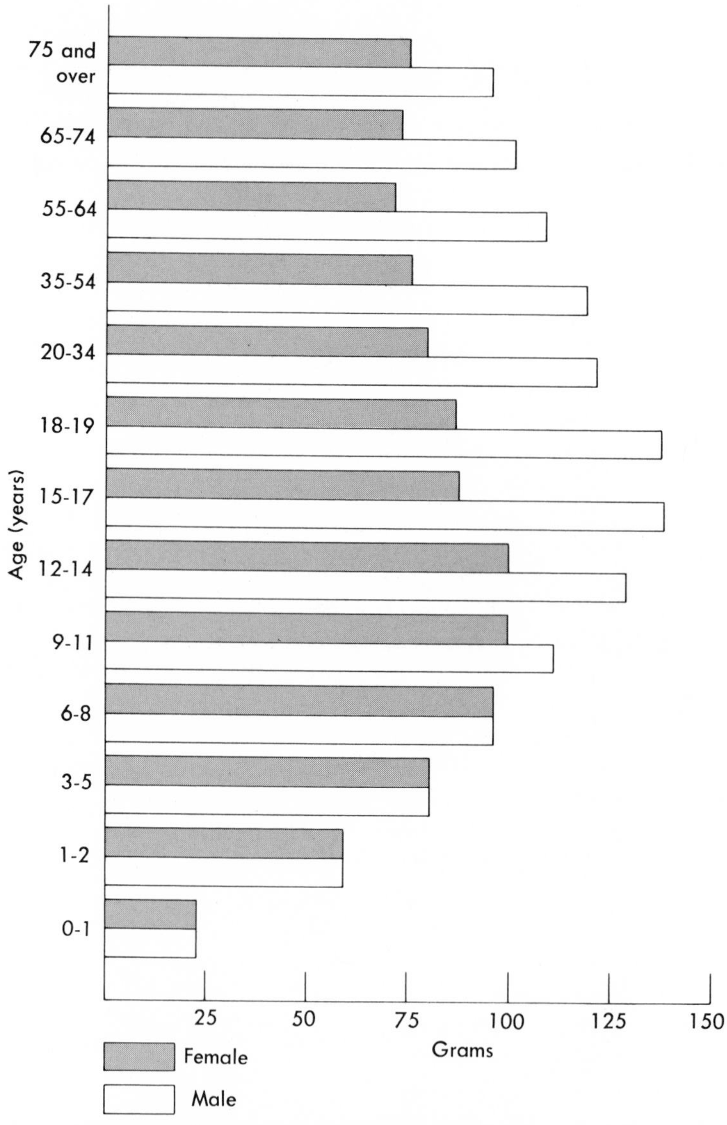

Fig. 14-7. Consumption of grain products (flour equivalent, quantity per person per day) as related to age in the United States—spring, 1965; 28 g = 1 oz. (From Agricultural Research Service, U.S. Department of Agriculture, 1969.)

FOUNDATION OF AN ADEQUATE DIET

As can be seen from Fig. 14-8, the inclusion of 2 cups of milk or its equivalent, two servings of meat or meat substitutes, four servings of fruit and vegetables, and four servings of enriched or whole-grain cereals will assure an intake of over 75% of the NRC recommended dietary allowances of all nutrients except calories for the adult man and iron for the adult woman. With this foundation there is little need for guidance in the selection of additional foods to provide the calories needed to meet individual requirements, but the greater the variety of foods used, the greater the chance of providing adequate amounts of trace elements.

In many cases the calorie requirement will be met at least partially through additional servings of the four food groups. The use of the visible fats and oils, which are natural accompaniments to the cereals and vegetables and which constitute about a third of the total fat intake, will provide about 15% of the total calories. The use of carbohydrate-rich foods, which is sometimes advocated as the least expensive way of obtaining the additional calories, does not receive the wholehearted endorsement of nutritionists because simple sugars with possible detrimental effects on dental health rather than complex carbohydrates are often used. The use of whole-grain and enriched cereals and additional servings of fruits and vegetables has the advantage of providing both fiber and trace elements along with the additional calories. Once the basic nutritional needs are met, there is no reason to condemn the use of foods of low nutrient density. In fact, the psychological and palatability advantages of their limited use should not be overlooked. It

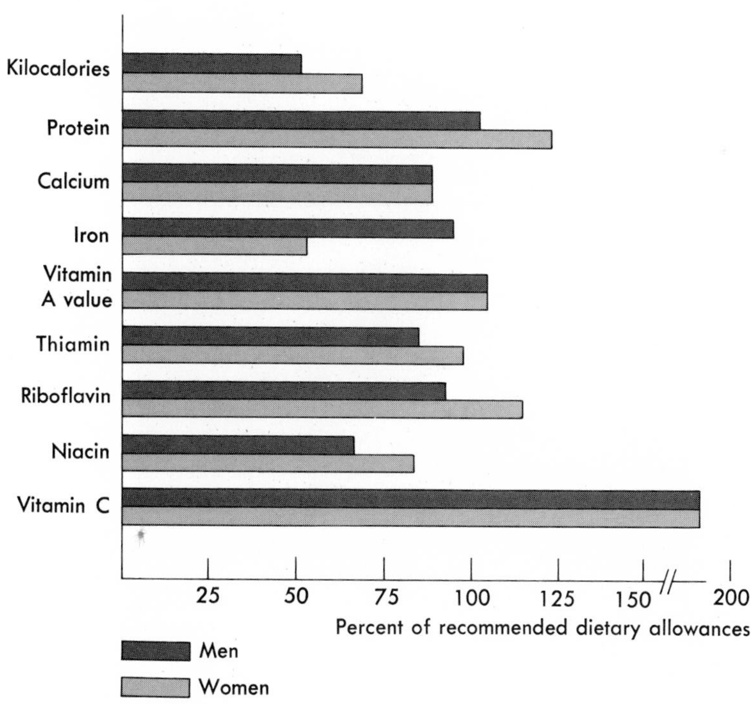

Fig. 14-8. Contribution of all four food groups of essentials of an adequate diet to nutritive intake of an adult.

is only when they replace foods that provide the nutritional foundation of the diet that their use is of concern.

For women, need exists to stress the use of foods high in iron as sources of the additional calories, since women are most likely to have an intake inadequate in iron. In fact, it is virtually impossible to obtain the recommended 18 mg of iron on a diet of less than 3000 kcal, which is considerably more energy than is required by this group. A supplemental source of dietary iron is indicated if there is any evidence of a depletion of iron stores.

The number of calories provided by the four basic food groups will depend on the selection of foods made within each category. To illustrate the range possible within the specifications of the four-group plan, the caloric value of two extremes is calculated in Table 14-11. Admittedly, differences will exist in the level of other nutrients also, but the selection was made within the framework of the plan.

As the Food and Nutrition Board of the National Research Council emphasized with the publication of its first dietary standards, the level of nutrition it advocated as a goal in planning the food supplies of the nations could be met in innumerable ways by an unlimited combination of foods. The suggestions made in the basic four groups represent but one pattern that reflects dietary practices acceptable to a large number of persons living in the United States. Although adherence to such a plan will usually ensure at least a minimal level of nutritional adequacy, failure to follow such a plan must never be construed as evidence of dietary inadequacy. Other cultures have developed eating patterns entirely different from these but which result in quite adequate nutrient intake. However, such a guide provides a quick and easy basis for evaluating the adequacy of a

Table 14-11. Caloric value of two diet patterns meeting requirements of essentials of an adequate diet*

Food group	Diet I foods	kcal	Diet II foods	kcal
Milk	Nonfat milk (2 cups)	160	Whole milk (1½ cups)	290
			Ice cream (1 cup)	145
Meat	Chicken, broiled (3 ounces)	185	Chicken, fried (3 ounces)	245
	Salmon, canned (3 ounces)	120	Ham (3 ounces)	340
Fruits and vegetables	Tomato juice (½ cup)	25	Sweet potatoes, baked	155
	Carrots (½)	22	Lima beans (½ cup)	75
	Apple (1 medium)	70	Grape juice (½ cup)	82
	Green beans (½ cup)	12	Figs (4)	120
Cereal	Puffed wheat (1 cup)	50	1 waffle	240
	Bread, thin-sliced (3 slices)	135	2 cookies (3-inch diameter)	220
			Oatmeal (1 ounce)	115
			Muffin	135
TOTAL		879		2162

*Calculations are based on energy value of the food prepared and served without any flavor adjunct, such as butter, sugar, syrup, sauces, etc. Based on Nutritive value of foods, Home and Garden Bulletin, No. 72, Washington, D.C., 1976, U.S. Department of Agriculture.

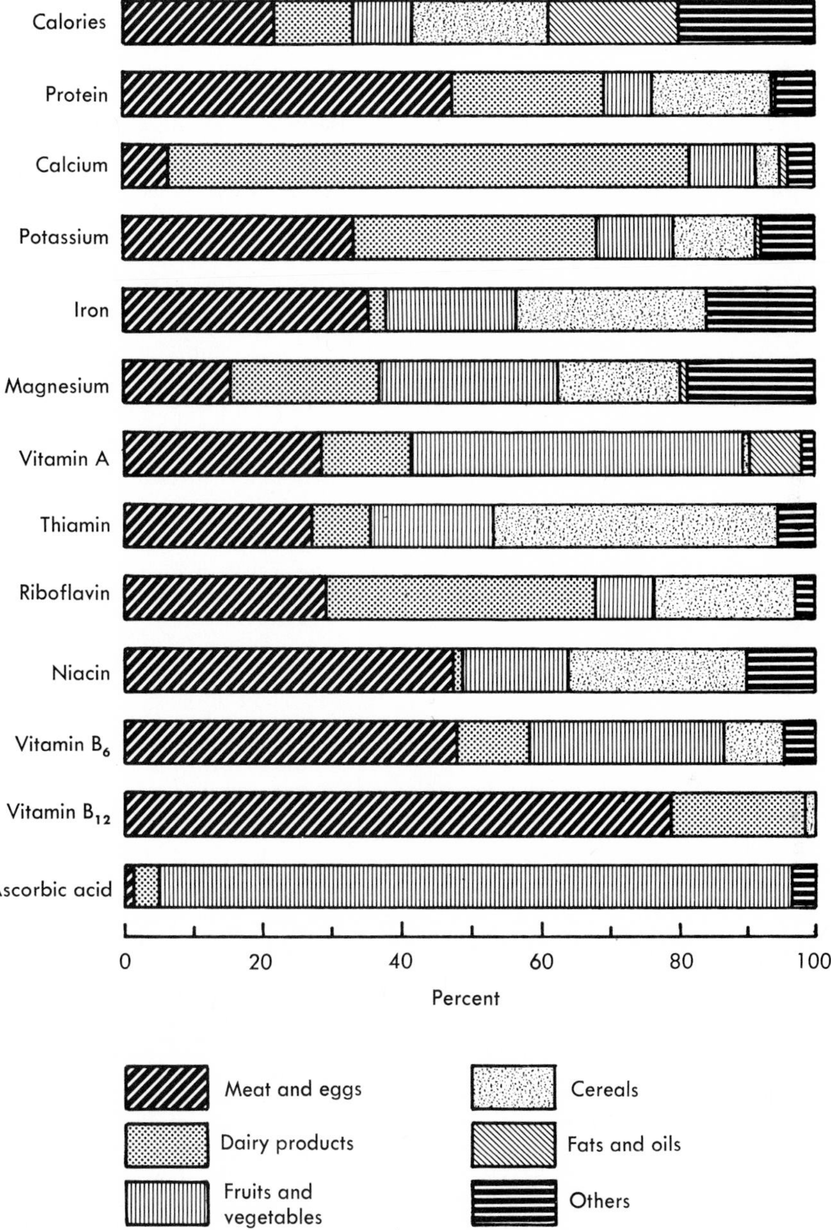

Fig. 14-9. Contribution of the various food groups to the nutrients available in the food supply, 1976. (Based on data from National Food Situation, NSF-159, Washington, D.C., 1977, Economic Research Service.)

prescribed or popular diet. If the minimum recommendations are met, one can be reasonably confident that the diet has a sound nutritional basis.

There is some concern that the food guide does not assure an adequare intake of some critical nutrients such as magnesium, pyridoxine, and folic acid. Attempts to formulate food guides that would overcome the limitations of the present plans have results in recommendations so much more cumbersome and complex that they may be no more effective. Clearly there is a need for alternative plans that compliment and supplement one another.

That the food supply available to the American public has the potential for meeting the nutritional needs of all citizens is evident in Table 14-12, in which estimates of the amount of each nutrient available per person at the retail level are tabulated. The contribution of the major food groups to the available nutrients is illustrated in Fig. 14-9.

Table 14-12. Estimate of nutrients available per person per day on the retail markets in the United States compared to NRC recommended allowances for the adult male*

Nutrients	Amount available	Recommended allowances
Energy (kcal)	3380	2700
Protein (g)	103	56
Fat (g)	159	—
Carbohydrate (g)	391	—
Calcium (g)	0.94	0.8
Magnesium (mg)	347	300
Phosphorus (g)	1.57	0.8
Iron (mg)	18.6	10
Vitamin A (IU)	8200	5000
Thiamin (mg)	2.09	1.4
Riboflavin (mg)	2.50	1.6
Niacin (mg)	25.6	16
Ascorbic acid (mg)	116	75
Vitamin B_6 (mg)	2.29	2.0
Vitamin B_{12} (mg)	9.7	3.0

*From Nutritive value of food available for consumption, United States, 1909-1976, National Food Review, No. FR-1, 1978, U.S. Department of Agriculture.

DIETARY STANDARDS

Although the concept that food contained more than the energy-yielding nutrients was well established by 1920 and a knowledge of the role and need for many other nutrients had been ascertained by 1935, it was not until 1940 that any formal effort was made in the United States to evaluate existing knowledge and to establish dietary standards. Previous efforts on the part of individuals and groups had attracted little attention. The economic depression of the 1930s focused attention on some nutritional deficiencies, and effort was made to incorporate the then-current knowledge of nutrition in programs of food subsidization. Only in the face of threat of war in 1940, however, did any strong feeling develop that nutritional science could make a contribution to the national security. The country had been appalled at the high rejection rate among young service recruits for reasons that could be attributed to suboptimal nutrition. Against this background twenty-five scientists met in 1940 as the first Food and Nutrition Board of the National Research Council, charged with the responsibility of establishing dietary standards that could be used to evaluate the dietary intake of large population groups and to provide a rational guide for practical nutrition and for the planning of agricultural production schedules. It was recognized that although insufficient evidence of the nutritional needs of humans had been compiled to propose exact requirements, a need did exist for a standard that reflected more than minimum needs. It was believed that even if the quantitative standards based on the available information should later prove to be inaccurate, they were very necessary. Indeed, it was with the belief and hope that they would soon be revised that the first standards were proposed.

National Research Council recommended allowances

The task of determining dietary standards was not an easy one. In the case of some nutrients very little information was available, for others little agreement was found among the fifty or more scientists consulted, and for still others it was recognized that such a wide range of requirements for the individual made it difficult to arrive at an acceptable figure. The data on which judgments were made were obtained from (1) surveys of large groups of individuals to determine presence or absence of disease in relation to nutritive intake, (2) controlled feeding experiments with limited numbers of individuals, and (3) critical metabolic studies on several species of animals.

The first National Research Council Recommended Dietary Allowances (RDA) were published in 1943. These allowances were numerical expressions of the quantities of certain nutrients believed to be adequate to meet the known nutritional needs of practically all healthy persons in the United States. Individuals were classified into several age and sex categories. The allowances did not represent average requirements, which would be adequate for only half the population, but were set sufficiently high to include the whole range of requirements that would maintain good nutrition in practically all healthy persons in the United States. As such, they became goals to be used in planning national food supplies and meals for large groups.

The term *allowance* was purposely chosen to avoid any implication of finality and to encourage a reevaluation of the figures as more information on which to base judgments became available. To allow for nutrient losses that might occur in cooking and storage of food, to cover the wide range of requirements in the population, and to provide a buffer under stress conditions a margin of safety at least 2 standard deviations above the mean was used in setting the recommended allowances. Some other factors that were considered were the stability of the nutrients, the body's ability to store the nu-

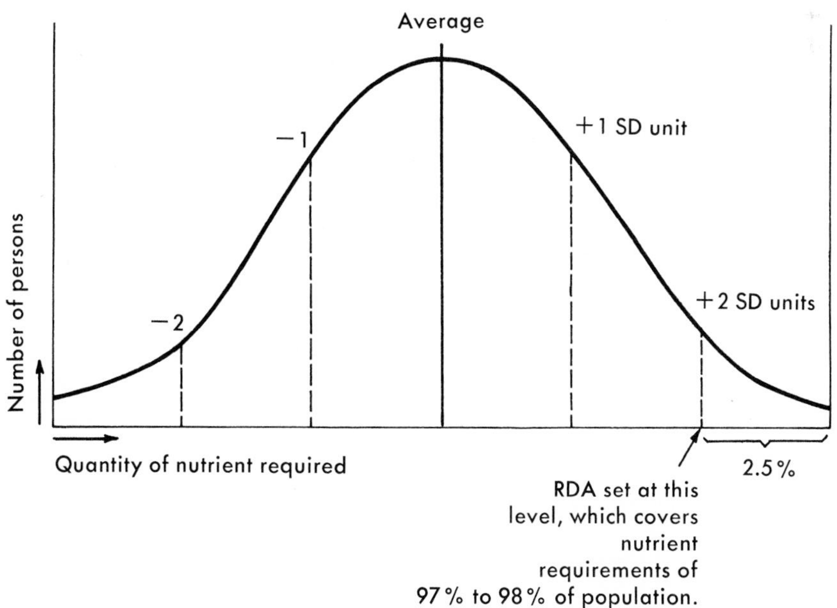

Fig. 14-10. Basis for establishing Recommended Dietary Allowances.

trient, the range of observed requirements, the availability of the nutrient in the American diet, the possible hazards from an excessive intake, and the difficulties involved in establishing precise requirements. The philosophy of setting requirements is depicted in Fig. 14-10.

It was emphasized that the allowances did not provide a criterion for judging the nutritional status of an individual but were a valuable guide for persons involved in feeding a population group. For individuals they served as a point of reference for judging nutritional adequacy, but only when an individual showed clinical, physical, or biochemical evidence of a dietary lack in addition to the suboptimal intake could he be considered deficient in the nutrient.

The original recommended dietary allowances have undergone eight revisions; the latest is to be published in 1979. (See Appendix C for 1974 revision.) The philosophy on which the allowances are based has remained essentially the same, but improved analytical techniques and increased knowledge of the biological importance of most nutrients have led to some change and to an increasing level of confidence in the recommended allowances. Complete agreement among nutritionists has not been reached, however. It is believed that the allowances provide sufficient buffer in cases of nutritional stress but will not meet the additional requirements of persons depleted by disease.

The major goal of the allowances is to permit and to encourage the development of food practices by the population of the United States that will provide the greatest dividends in health and resistance to disease.

The 1974 allowances differed from previous ones in that recommendations were made for an additional nutrient, zinc. In 1979, for the first time, scientists believe they should have enough information to propose provisional dietary allowances expressed as a range of values for several trace elements for a restricted number of age and sex categories. These recommendations will be included in the next RDA. Since revisions appear approximately every five years as research provides more information on which to base recommendations, the reader should be alerted to look for the next revision in about 1984.

Although the RDA have never been assumed to represent either a minimal or optimal level of intake, they have served several useful purposes. They provided a yardstick in planning diets for groups, and they have been widely accepted as a basis for evaluating diets. They have been used as an official guide for many nutrition intervention programs, such as the school lunch, congregate feeding, and WIC, and as a basis for formulating regulations governing the composition of foods, dietary supplements, and nutrient labelling. They are admittedly high for use under conditions of economic stringency or national emergencies, but under normal conditions they are a worthwhile goal.

Many nutritionists become concerned when the RDA is used as a basis for evaluating the nutrient intake of an individual. However, since there is no more precise yardstick against which to measure dietary adequacy, they remain the only criteria and must be used with the full recognition of their limitations. They must be interpreted with caution, but certainly the alternative—no standard against which to compare an individual's intake—is even less acceptable. For a few of the nutrients the Recommended Dietary Allowances published by the Food and Nutrition Board each time the allowances are revised provides the rationale for the allowances and offers formulas for calculating more individual allowances.

In addition to the nutrients and energy for which discrete recommendations are made by the Food and Nutrition Board, many other nutrients are discussed in the light of our current knowledge of their requirements and major biological roles. Among those discussed are carbohydrate, fat, alcohol, water, several micronutrient elements, choline, pantothenic acid, biotin, and vitamin K. It is hoped that the lack of information on requirements for these nutrients will stimulate research to more clearly define human needs.

Other dietary standards

Many other countries have established dietary standards for their populations. However, comparison or evaluation of these is not valid until one recognizes the philosophy behind each of them. Care must be taken to distinguish among terms such as standards, requirements, and allowances, which must be defined before an interpretation of proposed nutrient intake can be made.

The different recommendations reflect differences in judgment of the implications of the available data or differing opinions on the purpose and function of dietary standards. Although most standards make adjustments for age, sex, size, and activity, they are made on the basis of little precise data.

The British Medical Association, in establishing the British dietary standards, chose levels they believed represented the needs of the average healthy individual; these levels were never intended, as were the American standards, to cover the needs of all persons. British standards tend to be lower for some nutrients than American standards, although in a few instances they are the same in spite of the differences in philosophy behind them. The Canadian standard is based on a sufficient excess above minimum requirements for the maintenance of health among the majority of Canadians. Variations are made for age, sex, body weight, and degree of activity. The Canadian Recommended Daily Nutrient intakes are shown in Appendix E. Before 1964 they had considered their standards a nutritional floor below which adequate nutrition cannot be assumed but one well above the level required to prevent clinical deficiency symptoms.

Table 14-13. Comparison of United States, British, Canadian, and FAO dietary standards for the adult male and adult female

Classification	kcal	Protein (g)	Calcium (g)	Iron (mg)	Vitamin A (IU)	Thiamin (mg)	Riboflavin (mg)	Ascorbic acid (mg)
United States								
Female (57.6 kg, 1.62 m)	2100	46	0.8	18	4000	1.0	1.2	75
Male (69.3 kg, 1.72 m)	2700	56	0.8	10	5000	1.4	1.6	75
Britain*								
Female	2200	55	0.5	12	750*	1.0	1.3	30
Male	2750	75	0.8	12	750*	1.0	1.7	30
Canada								
Female (55.8 kg)	2100	41	0.7	14	800*	1.10	1.3	30
Male (71.1 kg)	3000	56	0.8	10	1000*	1.50	1.8	30
FAO								
Female	2300	39	0.4-0.5	18	750*	0.90	1.3	—
Male	3200	46	0.4-0.5	10	750*	1.30	1.8	—

*μg retinol equivalents (1 μg retinol equivalent = 1 μg retinol = 3.3 IU).

The Food and Agricultural Organization (FAO) of the United Nations, charged with devising a standard to meet the needs of fully active, healthy individuals that is equally applicable in all cultures, has thus far proposed practical allowances for kilocalories, calcium, protein, thiamin, riboflavin, niacin, vitamin A, iron, ascorbic acid, folacin, vitamin D, and Vitamin B_{12}. A comparison of the American, Canadian, British and FAO standards for adults is given in Table 14-13.

U.S. Recommended Daily Allowances

In March 1973 with the introduction of legislation requiring that a processor of food who chooses to reveal any nutritional information regarding his product or who adds any nutrient to the food must make a full nutritional declaration, the Food and Drug Administration proposed that a new dietary standard, the U.S. Recommended Daily Allowance replace the Minimun Daily Requirements which had previously been used as a standard for labelling purposes. The new standard represents the highest recommended level of intake for any age group (except for pregnant and lactating women) proposed in the 1968 Recommended Dietary Allowances. In most cases this is the U.S. RDA for 18-year-old males. Nutrient infor-

Nutrition information
(Per serving)
Serving size = 8 oz
Servings per container = 2

Calories	**560**
Protein	**23 g**
Carbohydrate	**43 g**
Fat	**33 g**

(Percent of calories from fat = 53%)

Polyunsaturated*	22 g
Saturated	9 g
Cholesterol* (18 mg/100 g)	40 mg
Sodium (365 mg/100 g)	810 mg

Percentage of U.S. Recommended Daily Allowance (U.S. RDA)

Protein	**35**	**Niacin**	**25**
Vitamin A	**35**	**Calcium**	**2**
Vitamin C	**10**	**Iron**	**25**
Thiamin	**15**	**Vitamin B_6**	**20**
Riboflavin	**15**	**Vitamin B_{12}**	**15**

*Information on fat and cholesterol content is provided for individuals who, on the advice of a physician, are modifying their total dietary intake of fat and cholesterol.

Fig. 14-11. Label format providing optional (light type) as well as mandatory (boldface type) information.

Nutrition information per serving

Serving size: One ounce (1⅓ cup) corn flakes alone and in combination with ½ cup vitamin D fortified whole milk.
Servings per container: 12

	Corn flakes	
	1 oz	*with ½ cup whole milk*
Calories	110	190
Protein	2 g	6 g
Carbohydrates	24 g	30 g
Fat	0 g	4 g

Percentage of U.S. Recommended Daily Allowance (U.S. RDA)

	Corn flakes	
	1 oz	*with ½ cup whole milk*
Protein	2	10
Vitamin A	25	25
Vitamin C	25	25
Thiamin	25	25
Riboflavin	25	35
Niacin	25	25
Calcium	*	15
Iron	10	10

*Contains less than 2% of the U.S. RDA of these nutrients.

Fig. 14-12. Nutrient label showing only mandatory information.

mation is expressed as a percentage of the U.S. RDA with amounts up to 10% being indicated in increments of 2% and amounts above 10% in increments of 5%. If any information is provided on the label, it must be given for carbohydrate, fat, and protein in weights and for protein, vitamin A, ascorbic acid, thiamin, riboflavin, niacin, calcium, and iron in terms of the newly proposed standard. Data on twelve other nutrients—zinc, pyridoxine, magnesium, folic acid, vitamin D, vitamin E, vitamin B_{12}, phosphorus, iodine, biotin, copper, and pantothenic acid—can also be provided. Beginning July 1975, any label information on nutritive value had to conform to this format. Nutrients for which the amount is less than 2% of the U.S. RDA can be identified by an asterisk and a footnote indicating that they were present in this insignificant amount.

Since this new labelling standard includes the highest amount recommended for any nutrient for any age group, it is comprised of very generous allowances. The new labelling standards are shown in Appendix D.

Examples of labels providing nutrient information according to the current standards are shown in Figs. 14-11 and 14-12. Table 14-14 presents data on the nutrient values of representative foods according to labelling standards. Similar information on 889 foods is available in the government publication *Nutrient Labelling—Tools for Its Use.*

Since this type of information is applicable only for labelling foods of known compositions or whose composition can be carefully controlled, it is given only on processed foods, bread, and milk. Information on fresh fruits and vegetables, meat, fish, poultry, and eggs is not available at time of purchase. Thus a consumer can use nutrient labelling information to compare different brands or to choose among comparable products but does not have enough information to assess the total nutrient content of each meal served. Nutrient information does, however, satisfy the consumer's right to know the content of available food. There is considerable question about how much of the mandatory information is understood by the consumer.

Once given nutrient information the consumer is faced with the problem of determining whether a food is nutritious. To provide some guidance, nutritionists have developed the concept of an *index of nutrient quality* (INQ). This is an expression of the nutrient density of a food—the relationship between the extent to which it meets the requirement for a specific nutrient compared to the extent to which it meets the needs for energy. Thus the definition of an INQ becomes:

$$\frac{\text{Percent U.S. RDA for a nutrient}}{\text{Percent energy requirement*}}$$

A food that has an INQ of 1 or more for a nutrient is making as great a contribution to the needs for that nutrient as for energy. If that particular food were the sole source of energy in the diet, the food would provide the full day's requirement for all nutrients for which it has an INQ of 1 or more.

It has been proposed that if a food has an INQ of 1 or more for four nutrients or an INQ of 2 for two nutrients that it makes a significant contribution to the nutrient intake and may be identified as nutritious. Most foods that have traditionally been considered wise choices nutritionally meet these criteria. Those that don't are foods with a high caloric density, usually due to the addition of sugar, starch, or fat in preparation. In Fig. 14-13, representing nutrient profiles for three foods, food A qualifies as nutritious because of the four nutrients with an INQ greater than 1 and food B on the basis of 2 nutrients with a INQ greater than 2. Food C does not qualify, since it provides no nutrients in greater amounts than it does energy.

A food is considered a source of a nutrient if it has an INQ of 1 and if one serving provides at least 2% of the U.S. RDA for the nutrient. To qualify as a good or excellent

*Energy requirement will vary from one individual to another, but for the sake of consistency it is usually based on 2000 or 2500 kcal.

Table 14-14. Food energy and percentage of U.S. RDA for eight nutrients provided by a serving of selected foods*†

Food‡	Size of serving (ready-to-eat)	Food energy (kcal)	Protein (%)	Vitamin A (%)	Vitamin C (ascorbic acid) (%)	B Vitamins			Calcium (%)	Iron (%)
						Thiamin (%)	Riboflavin (%)	Niacin§ (%)		
Milk, whole fluid	1 cup	160	20	6	4	4	25	—	30	—
Cheese, process Cheddar	1 ounce	110	15	6	0	—	8	—	20	—
Meat, poultry, fish (lean)	3 ounces	220	50	15	—	10	15	25	—	15
Eggs	1 large	80	15	10	0	4	8	—	2	6
Dry beans	¾ cup	230	20	2	6	10	4	6	15	20
Peanut butter	2 tbs	190	10	—	0	2	2	25	—	4
Bread, enriched	2 slices	140	6	—	—	8	6	6	4	6
Cereal, ready-to-eat‖	1 ounce	110	4	20	20	35	25	20	—	20
Citrus juice	½ cup	60	—	6	100	8	—	2	—	—
Other fruit, fruit juice	½ cup	60	—	6	15	2	2	2	—	4
Tomatoes, tomato juice	½ cup	25	—	20	35	4	2	4	—	4
Dark-green and deep-yellow vegetables	½ cup	45	4	140	40	6	6	4	6	6
Potatoes	Medium	80	4	—	35	8	2	6	—	4
Other vegetables	½ cup	45	4	8	20	4	4	2	2	4
Butter, margarine	1 tbs	100	—	10	0	—	—	—	—	0
Sugar	2 tbs	25	—	0	0	0	0	0	0	—
Molasses	2 tbs	100	—	—	—	2	2	2	15	25

*From Family Economics Review, ARS 62-5, USDA, Summer 1973.

†Percentages expressed in increments as required by regulation for nutrition labeling ("Food labeling," Federal Register, vol. 38, No. 49, part II, March 14, 1973): 2% increments up to and including 10% level: 5% increments above 10% and up to and including the 50% level, and 10% increments above the 50% level.

‡"Nutritive Value of Foods," USDA, HG-72, was used as a basis for percentages for specific foods. Values for food groups are based on average selections of foods in the group by United States families.

§In addition, niacin equivalent from the amino acid, tryptophan, found principally in animal products, would contribute substantially toward meeting the body's need for this nutrient.

‖Based on average of values on labels of 59 varieties of ready-to-eat cereals, February 1973.

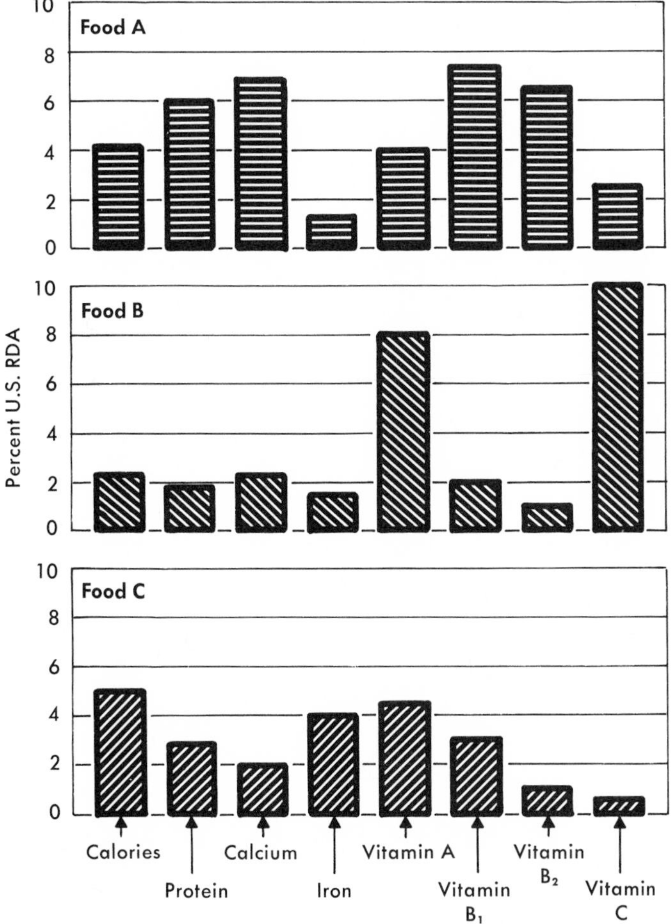

Fig. 14-13. Nutrient profiles. Food A has an INQ > 1 for four nutrients; food B has an INQ > 2 for two nutrients; food C has no nutrients with INQ > 1.

source, it must have an INQ of 1.5 and provide 10% of the U.S. RDA in each serving.

TABLES OF FOOD COMPOSITION

Although data from food composition tables as applied to food intake records provide the least expensive and most widely used tool in estimating the nutrient intake of an individual or group, it is only with an understanding of the method by which the tables were developed that one can recognize their limitations and make an intelligent interpretation of the results. The food composition tables in Appendix G are based on values in the standard publication for food composition in the United States, U.S. Department of Agriculture Handbook, No. 456, *Nutritive Value of American Foods.* These values in turn are based on data from the U.S. Department of Agriculture Handbook No. 8, *Composition of Foods—Raw, Processed, and Prepared.* Originally published in 1950 and revised in 1963, this publication presents food values in terms of 100 g edible portion (EP) and 1 pound as purchased (AP) of the foods. In the 1963 edition information is given for the energy value and contribution of sixteen different nutrients for 2483 food items. This represents an expansion from values on energy and eleven nutrients for 751 foods in 1950. In

Appendix G, as in the U.S. Department of Agriculture Home and Garden Bulletin No. 72 (1977), food values for over 730 foods are expressed in terms of average servings or common household units. Differences in values for the same foods in these two editions may reflect changes in marketing and processing techniques as well as improved analytical techniques. For instance, selective breeding of poultry has produced a product with a reduced fat content; the use of dried milk solids in bread has led to an increase in its calcium content; and the use of cooking oils with higher percentages of unsaturated fatty acids has changed the character of fat in many food products.

In 1977 and 1978 segments of a revision of Handbook No. 8 appeared, providing data on over sixty different nutrients. Each section of the 21 planned is devoted to a particular food grouping. Altogether data on 4000 foods will be included. In addition to providing information on the nutrient content of 1 pound as purchased, 100 g, and an average serving of a food, it indicates the number of analyses on which each piece of information was based and the range of values obtained. The Department of Agriculture has now set up a computerized nutrient data bank that can be constantly updated to provide the kinds of nutrient information needed by those concerned with nutritional evaluation and counselling. The requirement that industries using nutrient labelling provide analytical data to support their label claims has increased manyfold the nutrient information data that are available.

Although the details of the biological and chemical techniques by which the values are derived are beyond the scope of this discussion, some mention of the methods by which the data are compiled should provide a rational basis on which to evaluate the values obtained in dietary calculations.

Great variation exists in the amount and specificity of data available for different foods and different nutrients. Much data that are potentially useful cannot be used because of lack of an adequate description of the product, the source of the product, the method of processing, or the basis on which data were presented. Most of the data were obtained from published and unpublished analyses made by laboratories of government agencies, colleges, universities, and private industry. Only data on food samples adequately identified were usable. In some cases few or only a single analytical report was available. In other cases data were available on several varieties of the same food at several seasons of the year and from various geographical areas. An example is the ascorbic acid in oranges. The single value appearing in the table represents a weighted average obtained by making use of marketing information on the extent to which each variety was consumed, the percentage of the domestic production coming from each geographical area, and the size of the crop in each season. Thus, although the value may not be accurate for any one specific orange, it does provide a value representative of all oranges consumed in the United States.

Similarly, values for other foods and nutrients take into account varietal, seasonal, and geographical differences in the nutrient content of foods and loss or gain of nutrients through harvesting, handling, commercial processing, packaging, storage, home practices of preparation, cooking, and serving, and consumption statistics. The factors that result in changes in the content of important nutrients vary with both the food and the nutrient. As examples, the vitamin A value of sweet potatoes varies with the variety; the ascorbic acid in potatoes varies with the maturity and conditions of storage; vitamin A in butter varies with the season; ascorbic acid in oranges varies with the site of production and the time of harvesting; and vitamin A in plants varies with the part used.

In addition to Handbook No. 8, many other food composition tables in wide use today are based on sound analytical data. The beginning student is cautioned not to be concerned over differences between values from different tables, since they often merely represent slightly different interpretations of the same analytical data. Usually the differences are small when one considers the errors in the methods of collecting data. To be concerned over minor differences is to attribute an unwarranted degree of accuracy to the tables.

The nutrients for which values are presented in the table are those for which data were available for a sufficient number of foods to justify their inclusion. For nutrients such as pantothenic acid, folic acid, pyridoxine, amino acids, vitamin B_{12}, and magnesium tables have been published separately. A compilation of available data on these nutrients for some representative foods is given in Appendix H. As more precise analytical methods become available, tables for other nutrients will undoubtedly be published.

Derivation of values. Energy value expressed as kilocalories is calculated by a modification of a method used by Atwater in 1899 when the first table of chemical composition of food was published. An energy equivalent is determined for each gram of carbohydrate, fat, and protein in a range of separate food groups such as eggs, milk, meat, fruits and vegetables, and cereals. These are based on the heat of combustion (as measured in the bomb calorimeter) for each of these energy-yielding nutrients and the coefficients of digestibility for each of these in each general class of food. From data on the carbohydrate, fat, and protein in a food, it is then possible to calculate its energy value.

The values of 4, 9, and 4 kcal/g of carbohydrate, fat, and protein, respectively, are widely used to represent their physiological fuel values. Their use is justified when applied to whole diets, but because these values vary from one food to another, they must be used with reservation for individual foods. For instance, the physiological fuel value of protein is 4.35, 4.25, 3.70, 3.20, 3.15, and 2.90 kcal from eggs, meat, cereals, legumes, fruits, and vegetables, respectively. The calculations shown in Table 14-15 illustrate variations in heat of combustion, coefficients of digestibility, and hence physiological fuel values observed with different foods.

Protein is determined by measuring the nitrogen in a food; from knowledge of the percentage of nitrogen in a specific protein, it is possible to calculate the amount of protein. Many proteins, such as eggs, meat, corn, and beans, contain 16% nitrogen, but others such as milk contain less and nuts and many cereals slightly more. Assuming an average of 16% nitrogen in protein, a factor of 6.25 has been widely used to convert nitrogen values

Table 14-15. Calculations of physiological fuel value of energy-yielding nutrients in two classes of foods

Food	Heat of combustion	Coefficient of digestibility	Physiological food value
Eggs			
Carbohydrate	3.75	98	3.68
Fat	9.50	95	9.02
Protein	4.50	97	4.36
Potatoes			
Carbohydrate	4.20	96	4.03
Fat	9.30	90	8.37
Protein	3.75	74	2.78

to protein values, especially in mixed diets, but if a more precise figure is needed, factors of 6.38 for milk, 5.7 for refined flour, 5.8 for whole wheat flour, and 5.3 for nuts give more accurate estimates. The fact that all foods especially vegetables, contain some nonprotein nitrogen is a source of error in protein calculations.

Fat values are admittedly difficult to determine and have been obtained largely by simple solvent extraction methods. These methods may overestimate by including nonfat material and may underestimate by failing to separate the fat from a protein-fat or carbohydrate-fat complex in which it frequently occurs in food.

Carbohydrate values are obtained by subtracting the total percentage of water, mineral, protein, and fat from 100. This is known as *carbohydrate by difference* and is used because no satisfactory method exists for determining carbohydrate by direct analysis. The values for carbohydrate include sugars, starches, fiber, organic acids, and other complex forms of carbohydrate, some of which are not available to the human as a source of energy. The values reported for indigestible fiber, or cellulose, are based on methods that now appear to yield low values as new procedures suggest values three to four times as high. The values now appearing in tables represent only the cellulose or fiber that is not digested by strong acid or alkali. From a physiological standpoint many other substances such as hemicellulose and lignin, which are not digested, contribute to the dietary fiber content, or plantix, in food.

Newer approaches using data on starch, sugar, and dextrin analyzed separately yield low-energy values, since they ignore the contribution of organic acids, which in foods such as lemon juice account for 62% of the energy.

The food composition tables record values for vitamin A in food and the potential vitamin A from the precursor carotenoids. In foods such as oranges and corn, in which cryptoxanthine, a biologically active precursor of vitamin A, is present in large amounts, the vitamin A may be underestimated, since methods for determining carotenes do not include cryptoxanthine. On the other hand, some yellow- and red-pigmented foods have carotenoids that are not physiologically available but that will be measured. Even when it is accurately measured, the extent to which carotene is utilized varies from 33% to 100%. Some vitamin A values are obtained by biological assay and others by physiochemical means. Since recommended dietary allowances are now expressed as retinol equivalents, dietary data must be converted into retinol equivalents before a comparison of intake and requirement can be made. It will undoubtedly be some time before this is done easily.

Thiamin values are determined by chemical or microbiological methods but make no allowances for the losses that may occur through solution or destruction by heat or alkali during home preparation and storage.

Riboflavin is generally determined by fluorometric and microbiological methods, but no method has been developed to assess the increase in riboflavin that occurs with cooking, which may reflect the liberation of bound riboflavin not measured by current methods.

Methods of determining niacin involve the conversion of the amide form that occurs in many foods to the acid form. Although it has been well established that tryptophan in excess of the body's needs for protein synthesis can be converted into niacin (60 mg of tryptophan yielding 1 mg of niacin), the values in the tables report only niacin content and not niacin equivalents (niacin content plus niacin that could be formed from tryptophan). It is suggested that equivalents will be about 50% higher than the niacin values recorded in the tables even after subtracting about 500 mg of tryptophan to meet the needs for protein synthesis.

The National Research Council, on the other hand, has recognized that the body does not discriminate between niacin that is preformed in food and niacin obtained from tryptophan and has established its allowance in terms of niacin equivalents. It is possible, then, that the calculated niacin values for a diet may be considerably lower than the actual niacin available; therefore, failure of a calculated diet to meet an established standard cannot be considered evidence of an inadequate intake of the nutrient.

One interesting aspect of the niacin content of foods is the presence of a biologically inactive form of the vitamin, trigonelline, in many seeds and nuts. The roasting process for coffee beans tends to convert it into an active form so that coffee beverage provides some niacin in the diet.

A similar situation exists in regard to the data for ascorbic acid in food composition tables. It is known that the body uses both reduced ascorbic acid and dehydroascorbic acid. However, the limited data available on dehydroascorbic acid and total ascorbic acid values had led to the inclusion of only reduced ascorbic acid values in the current food composition tables for raw, canned, and dehydrated fruit and vegetables. For some foods this may lead to markedly low values, whereas for others the differences may be insignificant. It is highly possible that for such a labile nutrient any underestimate caused by failure to include the variable dehydroascorbic acid values will merely compensate for losses during storage and preparation or for the measurement of other reducing substances as ascorbic acid. It is also possible that some dehydroascorbic acid undergoes further oxidation to an inactive form. The data for frozen foods include the total for dehydroascorbic acid and reduced ascorbic acid and were obtained on foods under rather ideal conditions, permitting almost complete retention of the vitamin. These values may be high, since much storage of frozen foods is under less than ideal conditions and treatment of food during thawing and serving may cause considerable loss.

In spite of their recognized limitations, the food composition tables allow estimates of the nutritive content of diets that approximate those determined by direct chemical analysis but at a much lower cost in time, equipment, and money. These tables represent an indispensable tool for persons concerned with evaluating national food supplies, developing programs of food distribution, planning and evaluating food consumption surveys, and estimating the nutritive intake of individuals. The availability of the information from food composition tables on cards and magnetic tapes for storage in computers has greatly facilitated the use of this information in menu planning, in the analysis of dietary intake, and as a basis for nutrition counselling and has increased tremendously the scope of calculations that can be reasonably made with this information.

Recently, the appearance of engineered foods and food analogues on the market has compounded the problem of keeping tables of food composition up to date. As the character of the food supply changes, the Department of Agriculture attempts to make available information that will help the public assess the nutritive quality of the diet.

BIBLIOGRAPHY

Food selection guides

American Medical Association, Council on Food and Nutrition: General policies on the improvement of nutritional quality of foods, J.A.M.A. **225**:1116, 1973.

Bronner, F.: An aid to teaching nutrient requirements and allowances, Am. J. Clin. Nutr. **30**:726, 1977.

Guthrie, H. A.: Concept of a nutritious food, J. Am. Diet. Assoc. **71**:14, 1977.

Hertzler, A. A., and Anderson, H. L.: Food guides in the United States, J. Am. Diet. Assoc. **64**:19, 1974.

King, J., Cohenour, S. H., Coruccini, C. G., and Sheenan, P.: Evaluation and modification of the Basic Four Food Guides, J. Nutr. Ed. **10**:27, 1978.

Marston, R., and Friend, B.: Nutrient content of the national food supply, National Food Review, Washington, D.C., 1978, U.S. Department of Agriculture.

Peterkin, B., Nichols, J., and Cromwell, C.: Nutrition labeling—tools for its use, Publication AIB-382, 1975, Washington, D.C., U.S. Department of Agriculture.

Phipard, E. F., and Page, L.: Meeting nutritional needs through foods, Borden Rev. Nutr. Res. **23**:31, 1962.

Sorenson, A. W., and Hansen, R. G.: Index of food quality, J. Nutr. Ed. **7**:53, 1975.

Sorenson, A. W., Wyse, B. W., Wittwer, A. J., and Hansen, R. G.: An index of nutritional quality for a balanced diet, J. Am. Diet. Assoc. **68**:236, 1976.

Wittwer, A. J., Sorenson, A. W., Wyse, B. W., and Hansen, R. G.: Nutrient density—evaluation of nutritional attributes of foods, J. Nutr. Ed. **9**:26, 1977.

Dietary standards

Campbell, J. A.: Canadian, U.S., and international standards compared: approaches in revising dietary standards, J. Am. Diet. Assoc. **64**:175, 1974.

Dietary standards for Canada, Can. Bull. Nutr. **6**:1, 1964, rev. 1974.

Feeley, R. M., Criner, P. E., Murphy, E. W., and Toepfer, E. W.: Major mineral elements in dairy products, J. Am. Diet. Assoc. **61**:505, 1972.

Food and Agricultural Organization: Calorie requirements, FAO Nutr. Stud., No. 15, 1957.

Food and Agricultural Organization: Protein requirements, FAO Nutr. Stud., No. 16, 1957.

Food and Agricultural Organization: Calcium requirements, FAO Nutrition Report Series No. 30, 1962.

Food and Agricultural Organization: Requirements of ascorbic acid, vitamin D, vitamin B_{12}, folate and iron, WHO Techn. Rep. Ser., No. 452, 1970.

Food and Agricultural Organization: Requirements of vitamin A, thiamine, riboflavin and niacin, FAO Nutrition Report Series, No. 41, 1967.

Food and Nutrition Board: Recommended dietary allowances, ed. 9, Washington, D.C., 1979, National Academy of Sciences–National Research Council.

Harper, A. E.: Recommended dietary allowances: Are they what we think they are? J. Am. Diet. Assoc. **64**:151, 1974.

Hegsted, D. M.: On dietary standards, Nutr. Rev. **36**:33, 1978.

Munro, H. N.: How well recommended are the Recommended Dietary Allowances? J. Am. Diet. Assoc. **71**:490, 1977.

Peterkin, B.: The RDA or the USRDA? J. Nutr. Ed. **9**:10, 1977.

Schrimshaw, N., and Young, V. R.: The requirements of human nutrition, Sci. Am. **235**(3):50, 1976.

Tables of food composition

Adams, C. F.: Nutritive value of American foods in common units, Agric. Handbook No. 456, Washington, D.C., 1975, U.S. Department of Agriculture.

Agricultural Research Service. Comprehensive Evaluation of Fatty Acids in Foods:

I. Dairy products, J. Am. Diet. Assoc. **67**:482, 1975.

II. Beef products, J. Am. Diet. Assoc. **67**:35, 1975.

III. Eggs and egg products, J. Am. Diet. Assoc. **67**:111, 1975.

IV. Nuts, peanuts, and soups, J. Am. Diet. Assoc. **67**:351, 1975.

V. Unhydrogenated fats and oils, J. Am. Diet. Assoc. **68**:224, 1976.

VI. Cereal products, J. Am. Diet. Assoc. **68**:335, 1976.

VII. Pork products, J. Am. Diet. Assoc. **69**:44, 1976.

VIII. Finfish, J. Am. Diet. Assoc. **69**:243, 1976.

IX. Fowl, J. Am. Diet. Assoc. **69**:517, 1976.

X. Lamb and veal, J. Am. Diet. Assoc. **70**:53, 1977.

XI. Leguminous seeds, J. Am. Diet. Assoc. **71**:412, 1977.

XII. Shellfish, J. Am. Diet. Assoc. **71**:518, 1977.

Folic acid content of foods, Handbook No. 29, Washington, D.C., 1951, U.S. Department of Agriculture.

Food and Agricultural Organization: Amino acid content of foods, Nutr. Stud., No. 24, 1967.

Freeland, J. H., and Cousins, R. J.: Zinc content of selected foods, J. Am. Diet. Assoc. **68**:526, 1976.

Friend, B.: Nutritive value of the United States per capita food supply, Am. J. Clin. Nutr. **27**:1, 1974.

Goldblith, S.: Thermal processing of foods: A review, World Rev. Nutr. Diet. **13**:167, 1971.

Hardinge, M. G., and Crooks, H.: Lesser known vitamins in foods, J. Am. Diet. Assoc. **38**:240, 1961.

Harris, R. S.: Reliability of nutrient analyses and food tables, Am. J. Clin. Nutr. **11**:377, 1962.

Hertzler, A. A., and Hoover, I. W.: Development of food tables and use with computers, J. Am. Diet. Assoc. **70**:20, 1977.

Institute of Food Technologists: The effects of food processing on nutritional values, Nutr. Rev. **33**:123, 1975.

Lang, K.: Influence of cooking on foodstuffs, World Rev. Nutr. Diet. **12**:267, 1970.

Leung, W. T. W.: Problems in compiling food composition data, J. Am. Diet. Assoc. **40**:19, 1962.

Mayer, J.: Food composition tables: basis, uses, and limitations, Postgrad. Med. **28**:295, 1960.

Murphy, E. W., Willis, B. W., and Watt, B. K.: Provisional tables on the zinc content of foods, J. Am. Diet. Assoc. **66**:345, 1975.

Nazir, D. J., Moorecroft, B. J., and Mishkel, M. A.: Fatty acid composition of margarines, Am. J. Clin. Nutr. **29**:331, 1976.

Pantothenic acid, vitamin B_6 and vitamin B_{12} in foods, Home Economics Research Report No. 36, Washington, D.C., 1969.

Schroeder, H. A.: Losses of vitamins and trace minerals resulting from processing and preservation of foods, Am. J. Clin. Nutr. **24**:562, 1971.

Watt, B. K.: Concepts in developing a food composition table, J. Am. Diet. Assoc. **40**:297, 1962.

Watt, B. K., Gebhardt, S. E., Murphy, E. W., and Butrum, R. R.: Food composition tables for the 70's, J. Am. Diet. Assoc. **64**:257, 1974.

Watt, B. K., and Merrill, A. L.: Composition of foods—raw, processed and prepared, Handbook No. 8, Washington, D.C., 1963, U.S. Department of Agriculture.

15

Evaluation of nutritional status

The effect of diet on health is measured by an assessment of nutritional status. Although some indices of nutritional status reflect relatively recent nutrient intake, others reflect long-standing dietary habits. Current research is directed toward determining the key factors that can be easily assessed to identify individuals at nutritional risk. Such measures are also needed to monitor the nutritional status of a population over a period of time as a basis for establishing both agricultural and health policies.

Just as it is relatively easy to identify individuals who are markedly obese or markedly undernourished from casual observations, it is a simple matter to diagnose severe nutritional deficiency states, such as beriberi, pellagra, or scurvy, without the aid of any sensitive biochemical assessment technique. However, these deficiency diseases are encountered relatively infrequently, especially in developed countries, and they represent only the severest manifestation of the deficiency. As a result, nutritionists are concerned with developing techniques of evaluating nutritional status sufficiently sensitive to identify individuals who have a marginal nutritive intake, which fosters a low level of vitality and health and possible behavioral changes, and which may eventually result in subclinical nutritional deficiency symptoms. It is important to identify these persons in the early stages of undernutrition so that preventive measures can be taken before the deficiencies result in overt functional or anatomical changes.

The severe deficiency state will often become evident only when the deficiency has persisted for a long period of time or when it is precipitated by a severe stress, such as surgery, prolonged fever, or infection.

In the case of nutrients such as thiamin or ascorbic acid, for which there are limited body stores, symptoms will develop quickly on a deficient diet. For others such as vitamin A and calcium, for which body stores are adequate for years, symptoms develop much more slowly.

Although primary and secondary causes of nutritional deficiencies lead to the same results, it is important to identify the cause. For instance, the symptoms developing on a strict vegetarian diet devoid of vitamin B_{12} and those resulting when a genetic defect in the gastric mucosa prevents vitamin B_{12} absorption will be the same, but the conditions will be treated differently because the causes differ.

Because of the multiple causes of nutritional deficiencies and the diverse ways in which deficiencies of various nutrients manifest themselves, no one method of assessing nutritional status has proved completely satisfactory. As a result, several techniques are used to identify individuals whose limited nutritive intake or inability to absorb or utilize a nutrient have resulted in biochemical changes in tissues. If continued sufficiently long, these changes will lead to clinically observable symptoms. The techniques by which attempts are made to assess the nutritional status of an individual include clinical obser-

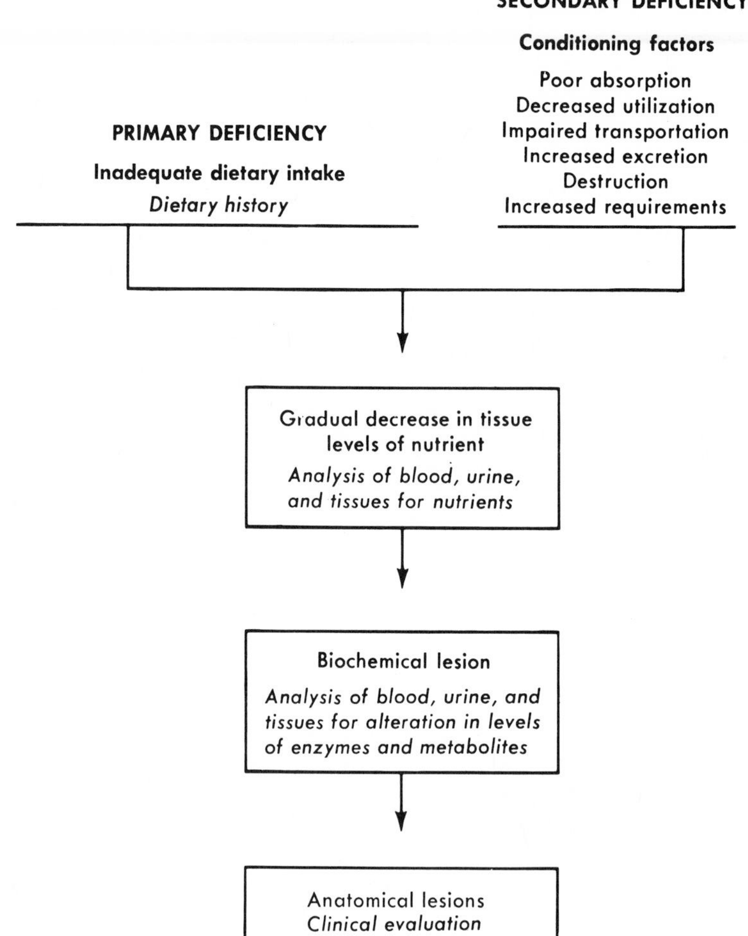

Fig. 15-1. Development and evaluation of nutritional deficiencies. (Modified from Krehl, W. A.: Med. Clin. N. Am. **48:**1129, 1964.)

vations, biochemical analyses, physical or anthropometric measurements, and dietary evaluations. In addition, some information on nutritional adequacy of population groups can be elucidated from the vital statistics of a country. The general features and unique advantages and limitations of each of these approaches to evaluating nutritional status will be discussed.

The ways in which nutritional deficiencies develop are outlined in Fig. 15-1. The techniques for detecting the changes at each stage are shown in italics.

CLINICAL OBSERVATIONS

Clinical observations, the least sensitive approach, lend themselves to use in nutritional surveys of population groups because they involve an assessment of the health of those parts of the body that can be readily observed in a routine physical examination and do not involve obtaining blood, urine, or tissue samples. The most commonly observed tissues are the eyes, mucous membranes, skin, hair, mouth, teeth, tongue, thyroid gland, and lower extremities. Although many of the changes in these tissues are often specific for a single nutrient, others are nonspecific and should not be considered as diagnostic of a specific nutrient deficiency. In some cases the same changes may be caused by the lack of several nutrients. Even though some symptoms do not occur until the deficiency is well advanced, the presence of clinical deficiencies in some persons suggests the presence of subclinical symptoms in others in the same population.

Although clinical observations are of limited value in the early diagnosis of a deficiency state or in identifying marginal intakes that prevail for short periods, they are widely used to confirm biochemical and dietary data. Because of the subjective nature of the judgement in a clinical evaluation, this method is extremely unreliable even when used by highly skilled observers.

The most useful findings in each tissue will be discussed.

Eyes. The most commonly observed symptom is a dryness of the cornea and conjunctiva (xerosis conjunctiva) usually associated with a lack of vitamin A. An increase in severity of vitamin A and possibly other deficiencies show up as Bitot's spots (Fig. 11-10) (foamy spots in the cornea) followed by a complete opacity in the cornea in a condition known as xerophthalmia. Infiltration of the cornea by blood vessels (corneal vascularization) is associated with a low intake of riboflavin.

Membranes. The color of the mucous membranes, such as those on the underside of the eyelid, in which the blood supply is close to the surface, provides an opportunity to observe the pigmentation of the blood. A pale mucous membrane is suggestive of anemia, whereas a more highly colored membrane usually occurs in persons with adequate hemoglobin levels.

Skin. The condition of the skin is often a reflection of the nutritional state of the individual, although all skin changes are by no means of nutritional origin. Deficiencies of some of the vitamins manifest themselves in varying forms and degrees of dermatitis. Skin lesions on areas of the skin exposed to sunlight occur in niacin deficiency, and a roughness and hardness of the papillae at the base of the hair follicle previously associated only with a lack of vitamin A is now thought to be due also to fatty acid and B-complex deficiencies. The dermatitis occurs primarily on the arm, chest, back, and thighs. Pyridoxine and/or riboflavin deficiency sometimes causes a dermatitis in the area surrounding the nose (nasolabial area). In infants eczema may indicate an essential fatty acid deficiency. A dry inelastic skin is most frequently observed after dehydration. The presence of small pinpoint hemorrhages under the skin after the application of either positive or negative pressure is indicative of fragility in the capillary wall, often a manifestation of ascorbic acid deficiency.

Mouth and teeth. Cracks at the corners of the mouth, referred to as angular stomatitis, and vertical cracks followed by redness, swelling, and ulceration in areas other than the corners of the lips reflect a lack of riboflavin. Loss of the papillae on the tongue and a scarlet and raw appearance of the tongue are associated with a niacin deficiency. A magenta color reflects a riboflavin deficiency. Similar changes have been observed in folacin and vitamin B_{12} deficiencies. Soft, spongy, and bleeding gums observed in dentulous persons are indicative of a lack of ascorbic acid. The presence of mottling on the tooth enamel results from a high intake of fluorine. The incidence of dental caries reported as a DMF index may be an indication of nutritional status but usually reflects diet during the early years of life when the teeth were forming. Loss of teeth and poor periodontal tissue are indicative of bone changes associated with osteoporosis and a high phosphorus/calcium ratio.

Other tissues. One of the first clinical observations to be correlated with a nutritional factor was the enlargement of the thyroid gland traditionally associated with a deficiency of iodine or an intake of food goitrogens but now suggestive of an iodine excess. Other clinical observations that may be significant are edema, especially of the lower extremities, which accompanies thiamin deficiency and protein inadequacies; depigmentation, lack of luster, and decreased hair diameter in protein deficiency; the cupping of the nails when iron is inadequate; bowed legs and the beading of the ribs, especially at the junction with the breastbone associated with a lack of vitamin D. Neurological abnormalities associated with thiamin and vitamin B_{12} deficiencies are identified by testing reflexes in the lower extremities.

BIOCHEMICAL ANALYSES

The biochemical evaluation of nutritional status involves quantitative determinations of nutrients or related metabolites in such tissues as the blood and urine. Low blood levels of a nutrient may reflect a low dietary intake, defective absorption, or increased utilization, destruction, or excretion. Occasionally, analysis will be made of a biopsy sample of liver or bone, but the use of this rather hazardous and involved technique is not justified in routine nutritional evaluations. The potential of the analysis of carefully sampled hair as an indicator of nutritional status, especially for micronutrient elements, is now being investigated. Saliva, another readily available tissue, is being investigated to determine its usefulness in assessing nutritional status.

Since variations in composition of the blood and other tissues often reflect recent changes in quantity and composition of the diet, an understanding of the metabolism of the nutrient is necessary to interpret the findings. In many instances the homeostatic mechanisms of the body will mask changes that would otherwise reflect nutritional status. Biochemical data serve either to confirm findings from clinical observations and dietary studies or to identify subclinical deficiencies before clinical symptoms are evident. They can be used for some nutrients to assess the range from frank deficiency levels through adequate, optimal, and excessive levels of nutritive intake.

The interpretation of findings from biochemical data is complicated by the fact that the levels of many nutrients and metabolites in the blood and urine vary sufficiently throughout the day that the use of values from a single determination may be misleading. In addition, only when the body's ability to compensate for deficiencies is overwhelmed will diagnostic changes occur in the nutrient or metabolite levels in the blood and urine. The causes of the observed deviations—whether dietary, genetic, environmental, or physiological—cannot always be identified on the basis of biochemical data.

Many of the analytical techniques for evaluating the constituents of the blood and urine have been adapted for use on very small samples. These microtechniques enable biochemists to make determinations for as many as fifteen or twenty nutritional factors or metabolites with a single 1 ml sample of blood.

A discussion of some of the information that can be obtained biochemically follows. The selection of measures to be used depends on the purpose of the study and the facilities, money, and technical help available.

Blood levels of nutrients

The determination of either blood serum or blood plasma nutrient level may reflect the most recent intake of a nutrient or may be indicative of the body's reserves. For instance, levels of ascorbic acid in the blood reflect recent intake. After about six weeks of a deficient diet, however, normal vitamin C serum levels of 0.5 mg will drop to zero when reserves are only 50% depleted. The level of the vitamin in the white blood cells, however, will drop only when tissue saturation is down to 20% of normal, which will occur only at the time other symptoms of scurvy are about to appear.

On the other hand, blood levels of calcium are of little value in assessing nutritional status; the body has so many mechanisms that operate to maintain normal blood levels that only when these mechanisms fail or body reserves are depleted will any change occur in blood calcium levels. However, when the product of calcium and phosphorus values falls below 30, the possibility of rickets is suggested.

Amino acid analysis of blood is expensive and of little value, since values are readily altered by recent intake and mobilization of body reserves.

The large reserves of vitamin A maintained in the liver make blood levels of vitamin A rather meaningless as an indicator of current intakes. Failure to release vitamin A may keep blood levels low in spite of adequate stores in the liver.

Recently use has been made of serum lipid values, especially cholesterol, triglycerides, and lipoproteins, to screen persons who may be at high risk of coronary heart disease.

Since both activity and recent food intake may influence biochemical data, an early morning fasting blood sample is preferred.

Blood levels of metabolites

In many cases the absence of a vitamin leads to a block in the normal series of reactions in the metabolism of carbohydrate, fat, or protein. An accumulation of one of the intermediary products in the blood often indicates a lack of the nutrient required for metabolism to proceed beyond that point. For instance, an increase in the pyruvic acid in the blood occurs when insufficient thiamin is available to form the enzyme necessary to decarboxylate the pyruvic acid formed in carbohydrate metabolism.

Other blood components such as albumin and total protein are insensitive indices except in severe deficiencies.

Blood enzyme levels

Since many nutrients act as parts of enzymes or as coenzymes, it is frequently possible to determine the level of enzyme as a measure of the amount of the nutrient available. For instance, the level of the enzyme transketolase in the red blood cells is a sensitive indicator of the available thiamin, which is part of a coenzyme that works in conjunction with transketolase in the metabolism of glucose. Transketolase values are easily determined, and a drop in the level precedes any other signs of a deficiency. As such, they are a valuable diagnostic tool in detecting subclinical thiamin deficiency. Similarly, the level of the enzyme glutathione reductase is indicative of riboflavin status.

An increase in the amount of another enzyme, alkaline phosphatase, occurs in a vitamin D deficiency. On the other hand, a drop in the level of this enzyme has also been reported in protein deficiency; therefore these two forces in some instances may counteract one another. Since all enzymes are protein in nature, a drop in all enzyme levels could be expected when labile protein reserves are depleted.

Carrier proteins

The determination of specific proteins that serve to transport nutrients in the blood provides some information on nutritional status. For instance, the amount of transferrin or retinol-binding proteins reflect nutritional status in regard to iron and vitamin A.

Urine analysis

Biochemical determinations of the nutrients or metabolites in the urine often give valuable information about the nutritional status of an individual. Not only is the amount of a nutrient found in the urine significant, but the presence of substances not normally found in the urine is also informative.

In a saturation test, the urine is analyzed to determine the proportion of a large test dose of a water-soluble vitamin that is excreted. It is assumed than an individual whose tissues are saturated with the nutrient will retain little and excrete most of the dose, whereas a person who has had low intakes will retain more in an effort to raise tissue levels to normal. This test has been widely used in efforts to assess the ascorbic acid status. Test doses of 200 to 1000 mg are used.

A variation of this is the load test. For example, the amino acid tryptophan requires the vitamin pyridoxine if it is to be metabolized and excreted in a normal manner as

N-methyl nicotinamide. If insufficient pyridoxine is available, an abnormal urinary constituent, xanthurenic acid, appears. The level of xanthurenic acid in the urine is low when pyridoxine reserves are high and high when little pyridoxine is available for tryptophan metabolism. Similarly, histidine load tests are used to evaluate folic acid nutriture. In the absence of folic acid, formiminoglutamic acid (FIGLU), an intermediary product of histidine metabolism, accumulates and appears in increased amounts in the urine.

Hydroxyproline appears in the urine only as the result of the breakdown of the protein collagen. Determination of hydroxyproline in the urine is a useful indicator of the extent of collagen metabolism. High levels occur during active growth and are considered desirable while low levels are undesirable.

The amount of creatinine in the urine is a direct reflection of the muscle mass of an individual and has been assumed to be constant. Such information is helpful in determination of body composition, in which it is desirable to know the percentage of body weight represented by fat or muscle tissue. Some other urinary data may be more meaningful when expressed in terms of the amount of creatinine excreted at the same time. This is especially true when data are obtained from a casual urinary sample rather than from a complete 24-hour specimen. For instance, urinary nitrogen in relation to creatinine excretion in a 4-hour specimen has been used as one of the best indicators of protein nutrition, although its value is now being questioned. The excretion of several vitamins such as thiamin and riboflavin is recorded in relation to creatinine excretion. However, interpretation of such data is often difficult because of observed diurnal and day-to-day variations in both creatinine and vitamin excretion, which often do not vary in the same pattern.

The excretion of riboflavin for which no other metabolites appear in the urine reflects fairly accurately the daily intake of the vitamin. An excretion of 50 μg or less per day is usually associated with other riboflavin deficiency symptoms. Since about 10% of the intake under 1 mg is excreted, an excretion as low as 50 μg would result from an intake of less than 0.5 mg, generally regarded as a suboptimal intake.

Other biochemical tests

The rate of hemolysis, or breakdown, of the red blood cell membrane is sufficiently influenced by the amount of vitamin E available to be an adequate test for vitamin E status. The prothrombin time (the length of time required for clotting) is related to vitamin K nutriture.

Hemoglobin and hematocrit (blood solids or packed cell level) values reflect the amount of available iron but fall only when stores are depleted. Plasma albumin levels are maintained by synthesis of protein within the body and will be normal when adequate amounts of amino acids are available. However, the serum levels usually fall only after other signs of protein deficiency are evident. The free amino acid pool in the blood drops in a protein deficiency.

The types of biochemical tests used in the evaluation of nutritional status in the National Nutrition Survey are listed in the following outline. Those also used in the Health and Nutrition Evaluation Survey, which is an ongoing surveillance program are indicated with an asterisk. Those used in HANES but not in the Ten-State Survey are indicated by a dagger.

Blood analysis

Hemoglobin
Hematocrit
*Total serum protein
*Serum albumin
*Plasma vitamin A and carotene
*Serum vitamin C
†Magnesium
*Total serum iron and iron-binding capacity
*Serum and whole blood folic acid
*Serum globulin } Optional
*Serum cholesterol } Optional
Transketolase } Optional
*Plasma amino acid ratio } Optional

Urine analysis

- *Creatinine
- *Thiamin
- *Riboflavin
- *Iodine
- *Albumin
- *Glucose
- Urea nitrogen
- *N*-Methyl nicotinamide (Optional)
- Hydroxyproline (Optional)
- Creatine (Optional)

Other studies have used additional data.

Although a set of standards for evaluating these biochemical data has been proposed (Table 15-1), interpretation of much of the data is difficult. The need for improved methodology and for more sensitive measures for the biochemical evaluation of nutritional status is being increasingly recognized. Efforts are also being directed at identifying a smaller number of measures to be used in screening population groups. Statistical analysis now shows that the thirty to forty biochemical measurements routinely made could be reduced to ten tests with no loss of screening potential.

ANTHROPOMETRIC DATA

Scientists have attempted for years to establish a criterion of nutritional adequacy that involves the use of simple body measurements, such as height, weight, chest circumference, ankle circumference, and skinfold thickness (Fig. 15-2). So far their efforts have met with only limited success. This is partly caused by the difficulties of standardizing the techniques by which the measurements are obtained. Height and weight measurements

Table 15-1. Criteria for evaluating some frequently used biochemical measures of nutritional status (levels indicative of a deficiency state)*

	Adult males	Children	
		2-5 years	6-12 years
Blood data			
Hemoglobin (g/dl)	<12	<10	<10
Hematocrit (% packed cell volume)	<37	<30	<30
Serum albumin (g/dl)	<2.8	†	†
Serum ascorbic acid (mg/dl)	<0.1	<0.1	<0.1
Plasma vitamin A (μg/dl)	<10	<10	<10
Serum iron (μg/dl)	<60	<40	<50
Transferrin saturation (%)	<20	<20	<20
Serum folacin (mg/ml)	<2	<2	<2
Serum vitamin B_{12}	<100	<100	<100
Plasma vitamin E (mg/dl)	<0.2	<0.2	<0.2
Urinary data			
Thiamin (μg/g creatinine)	<27	<85	<70
Riboflavin (μg/g creatinine)	<27	<100	<85
Tryptophan load (100 mg/kg) (mg xanthurenic acid/24 hr)	>75	>75	>75

*Modified from Christakis, G., editor: Nutritional assessment in health programs, Am. J. Public Health **63**(suppl.), Nov. 1973.

†No values available.

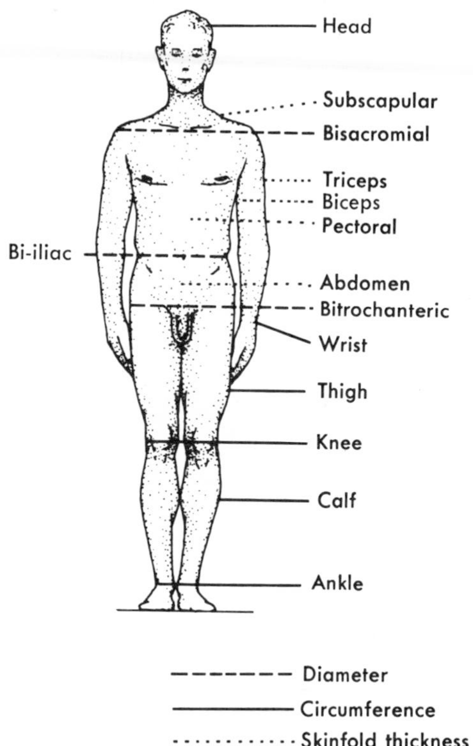

Fig. 15-2. Anthropometric measurements used in various formulas for evaluating nutritional status.

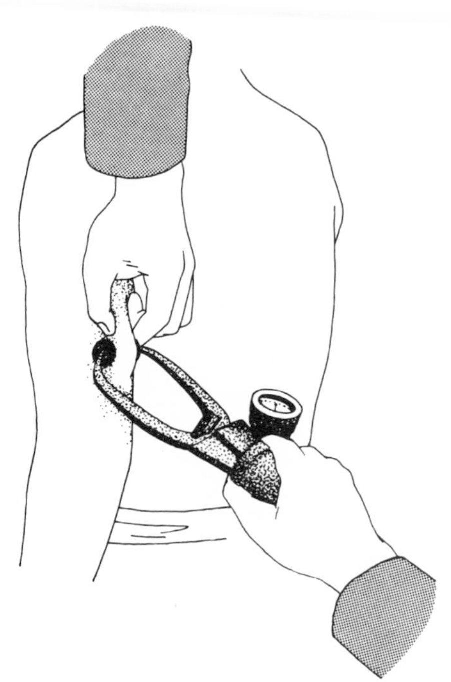

Fig. 15-3. Measuring triceps skinfold with calipers.

can be obtained fairly readily, but the others involve a high degree of skill if they are to be useful. Techniques for employing calipers, which can be used to measure bone structure or skinfold thickness (Fig. 15-3) are difficult to master. A second problem is whether or not standards such as the widely used Iowa Growth Standards developed twenty to thirty years ago are still valid criteria.

Although height and weight tables, long used as a growth standard, have many limitations, they still remain useful. If they fail to recognize differences in body build for persons of the same age and sex they are assuming too high a degree of hereditary homogeneity in the population. On the other hand, the use of tables based on different body builds with no basis on which to choose the proper category—small, medium, or large frame—requires a subjective evaluation, which reduces the usefulness of this refinement.

Two general types of tables have been used for adults. The first type merely records the average weight for height and age based on insurance statistics. The most recent table of this type was released in 1959 by the Society of Actuaries in a publication entitled *Build and Blood Pressure Study* and was based on measurements of nearly 5 million insured persons from ages 15 to 69 in ordinary indoor clothing and shoes. Values in this table tended to be lower for women and higher for men than earlier tables published in 1912 and 1952.

The second type of table, which is more useful in evaluating nutritional status, is one giving "ideal" or desirable weights for height. These tables ignore age and use three classifications of body build—small, medium, and large frame—for each increment in height. In each of these is presented the range of weights that is associated with the lowest mortality. These weights are essentially the average weights at age 27 for men and age 23 for women. Unfortunately, no criterion is given on which to base a judgment of body size.

Currently used tables designating desirable weights based on the 1959 *Build and Blood Pressure Study* show weights believed compatible with lowest mortality to be about 2 kg lower for men and 0.5 to 1 kg lower for women than those in earlier tables. These tables are presented in Appendix F. Desirable weights are generally 7 to 11 kg below average weights for both sexes. All these standards have been criticized because they represent measures only of persons that buy insurance, who may not be a representative population group. In addition, the standards imply that overweight is a cause of early mortality, whereas their data show only the relationship.

Until 1975 the most commonly used growth standards for children were the Stuart-Meredith growth curves, based on measurements of a limited number of white children in Iowa and Boston forty to fifty years ago. With the availability of current data based on a larger number of children from birth to 18 years of age which are more representative of the population, it is now recommended that curves based on these data be used as standards. In these standards height for age, indicative of shortness or tallness, and weight for height, indicative of thinness or fatness, are considered the most useful relationships. Consideration of weight for age is of limited usefulness. Curves (Figs. 15-4 to 15-7) showing the 5th, 10th, 25th, 50th, 75th, 90th, and 100th percentile values of weight for height for prepubertal boys from 2 to 11½ years of age and girls from 2 to 10 years and of weight and height for age for boys and girls 2 to 18 years of age. Charts from birth to 3 years are shown in Chapter 17. By plotting actual measurements on the appropriate chart, one can determine how a child is developing relative to others of the same age or stature. Those who fall below the 5th percentile (meaning that only 5% of the population are lighter for age or height) should be screened further to determine if there is a nutritional or other environmental cause of the retarded growth or whether the child is merely genetically smaller than others. Any deviation in the percentile ranking from one measurement to another should be assessed to determine if it represents an improvement or a deterioration in nutritional status. In general, weight for height is an excellent indicator of recent nutritional status (undernutrition or overnutrition) whereas height for age is more indicative of long-term nutrition, which will have had an effect on stature.

For more individual assessments the Wetzel Grid (Fig. 15-8), on which successive measurements of weight in relation to height are plotted, has been widely used. In this the child serves as his own control and falls into one of the nine developmental channels ranging from channel B4 for a tall, thin person to channel A4 for an obese individual. On the basis of subsequent measurements the growth progress is assessed by advancement within a developmental channel. Deviations into channels away from the median channel are often diagnostic of some medical or nutritional abnormality. A trend in the direction of channel A4, which is indicative of excess weight for height, may serve as a warning to initiate caloric restriction and to try to determine the underlying cause of the developing obesity. Trends in the other direction, toward channel B4, may signal infection or other conditions that have resulted in loss of appetite and weight. Again, the value of the grid is in presenting a visual record of a growth trend. Such records have proved useful in medical evaluations in developing countries.

Kram and Owen propose to evaluate weight gain in relation to expected rate of gain. They consider rate of gain unacceptable if it is less than half that expected. Since factors accelerating or retarding growth will

Text continued on p. 398.

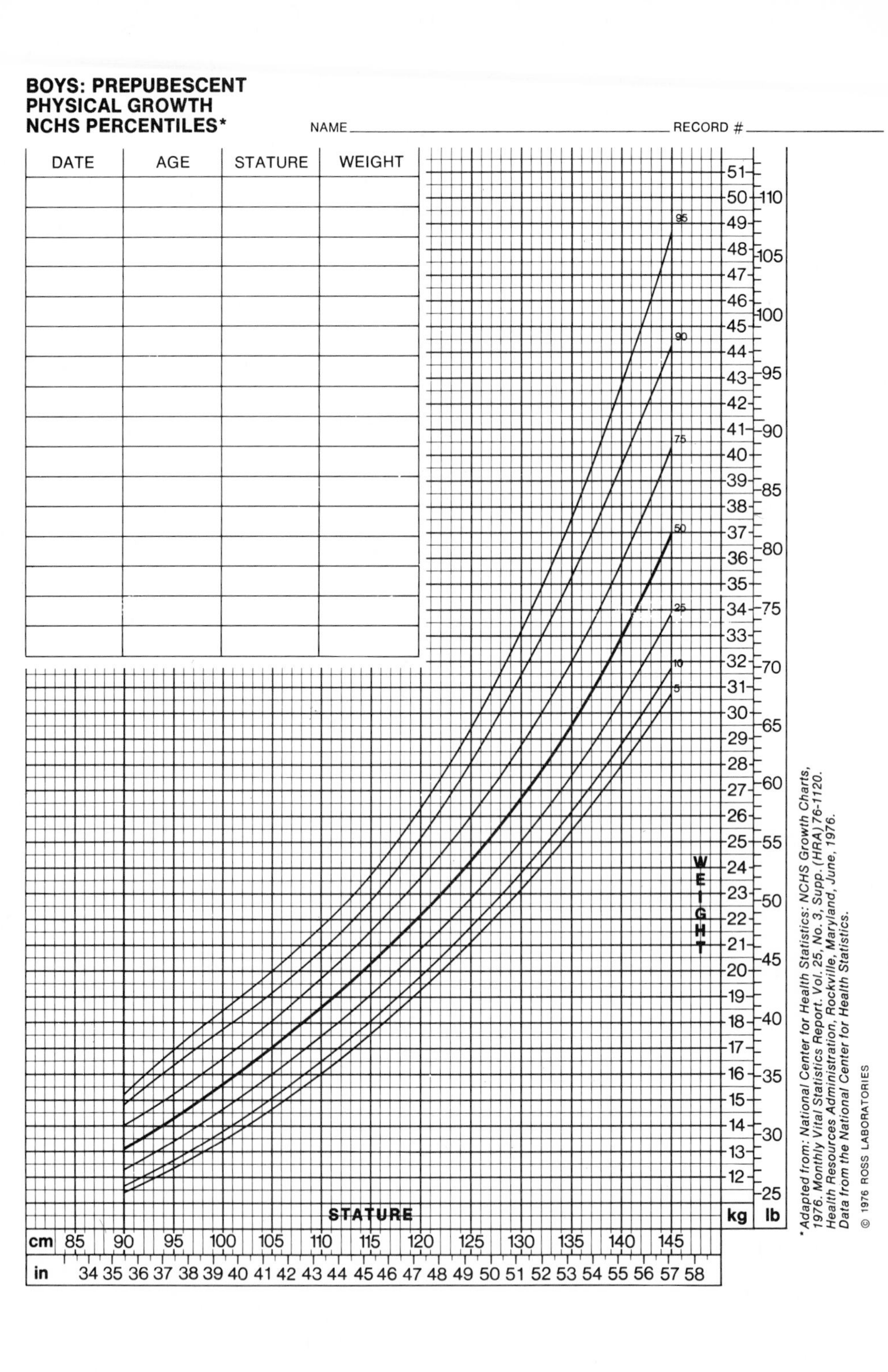

Fig. 15-4. Weight for height for prepubertal boys, age 2 to 11½ years. (Courtesy Ross Laboratories.)

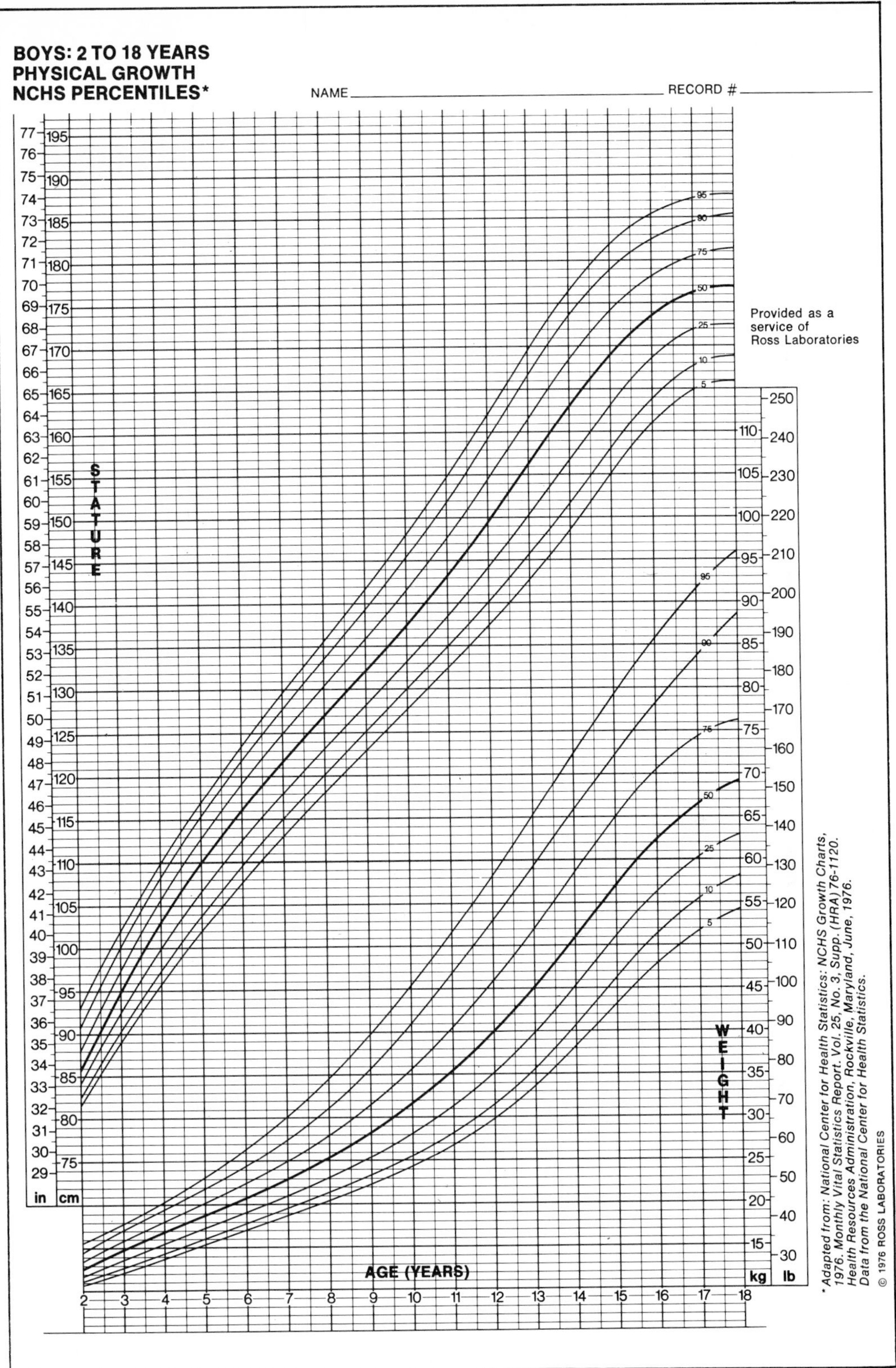

Fig. 15-5. Height and weight for age for boys from 2 to 18 years of age. (Courtesy Ross Laboratories.)

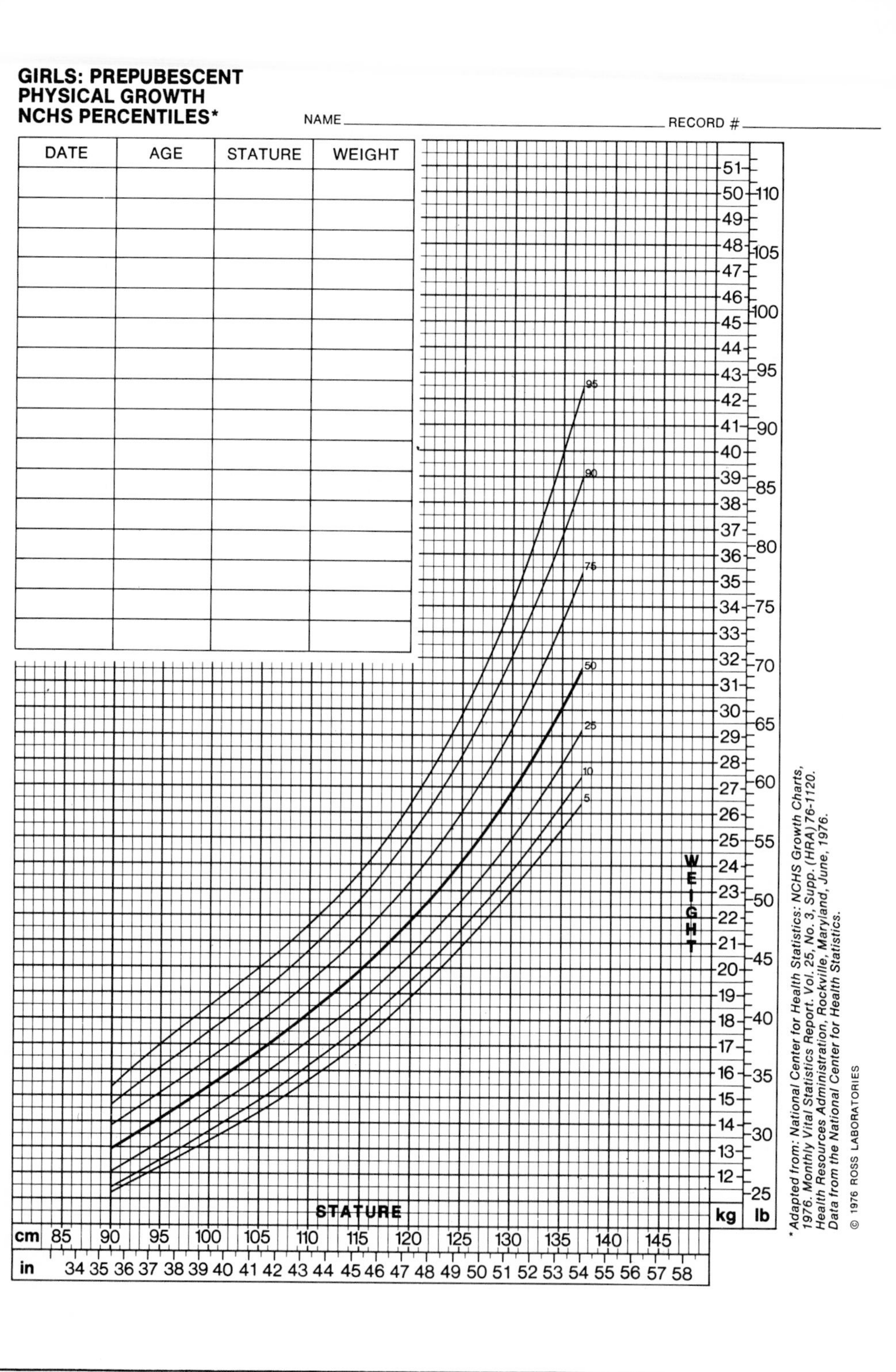

Fig. 15-6. Weight for height for prepubertal girls, age 2 to 10 years. (Courtesy Ross Laboratories.)

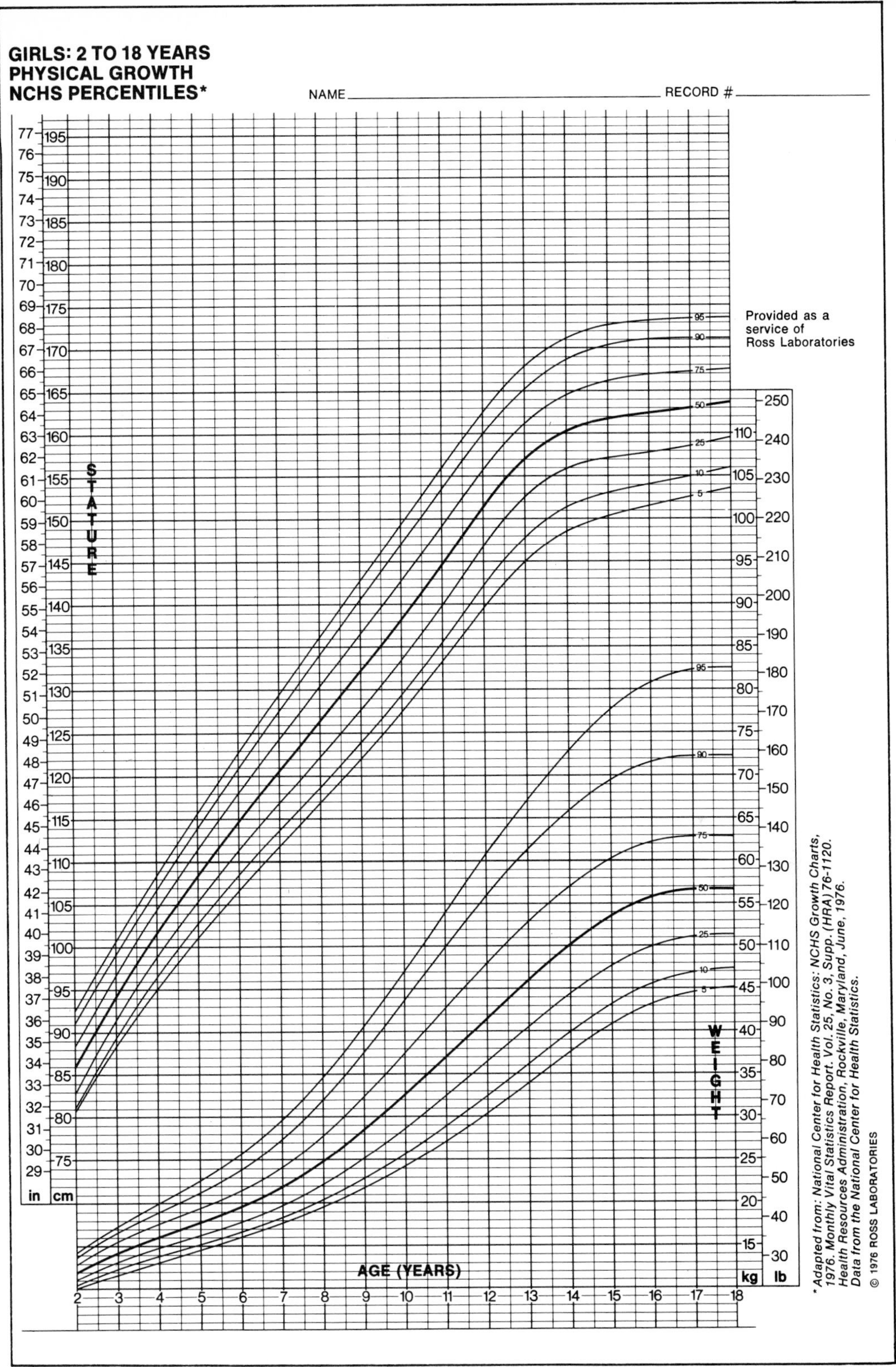

Fig. 15-7. Height and weight for age for girls from 2 to 18 years of age. (Courtesy Ross Laboratories.)

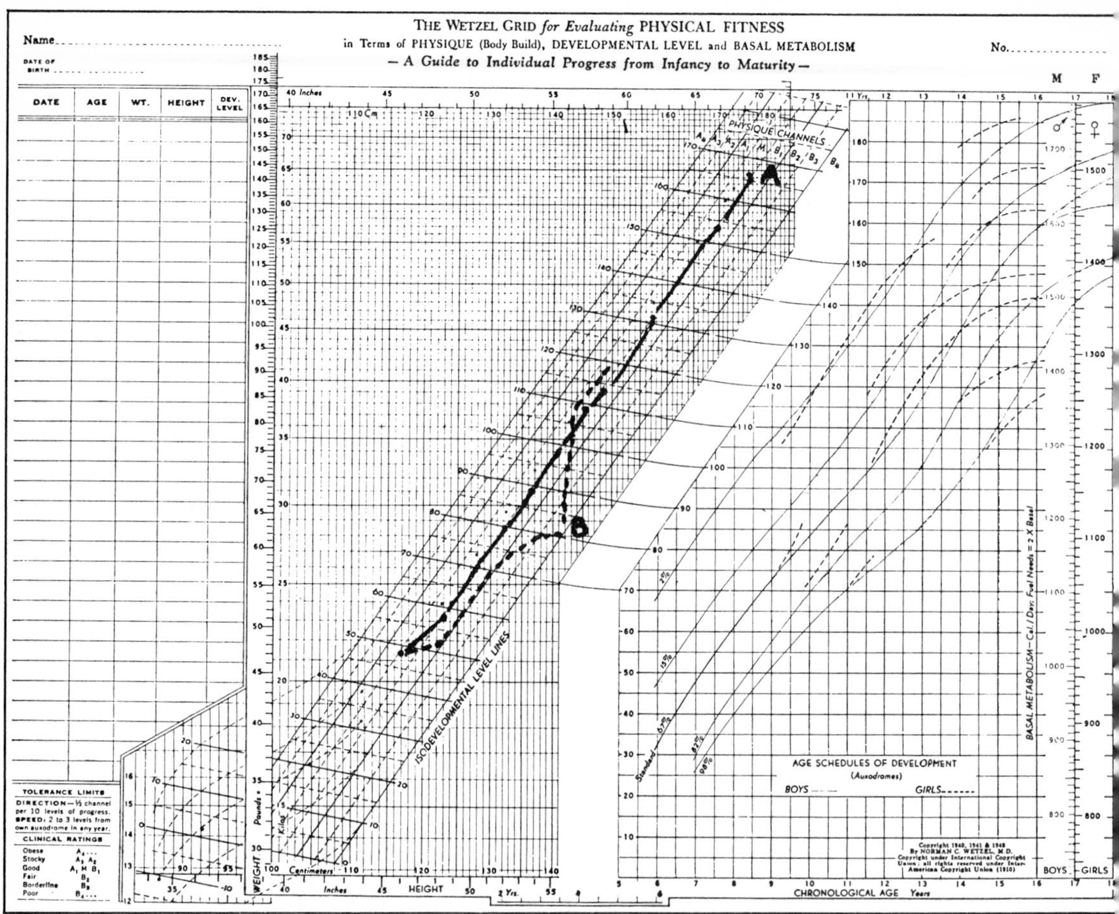

Fig. 15-8. Wetzel grid. Grid is used to assess growth and physical fitness on the basis of successive weight measurements. Growth curve *A* represents a normal growth pattern. Growth curve *B* represents simple growth failure with subsequent recovery. (Courtesy Dr. Norman Wetzel and the National Education Association, Cleveland Heights, Ohio.)

affect weight sooner than stature, gain in weight substantially greater or less than expected from gain in stature is considered undesirable.

Body fatness

With the continuing high incidence of obesity in the population and the need to recognize those individuals with excess body fat as distinct from those with above-average body weights, attempts have been made to find a method of assessing body fatness. Determination of body density, which involves a comparison of the weight of the body under water with that in air and correcting for the air in the lungs, is the most precise way of estimating body fat but is impractical for use on large groups. Special skinfold calipers that exert a specific pressure on a specific area of skinfold have been developed to measure the thickness of a skinfold in various parts of the body as an indication of the amount of subcutaneous fat (Fig. 15-3). Although skinfold measurements in the lower thoracic region give the best indication of body fat, measurement of triceps skinfold is the single most useful measurement in diagnosing obesity. A thickness of 16.5 mm for females and 12.5 mm for males is considered standard.

A simple index known as body mass index (BMI) makes use of measurements of height and weight and proposes that weight (kg)/height (cm^2) provides an indication of body fat. An index value over 30 is indicative of excess body fat and under 15 of undernutrition.

A formula using four of the anthropometric measurements shown in Fig. 15-2 has been devised for estimating body fat, which reportedly correlates well with the other methods. It involves measurement of arm and thigh circumference, abdominal skinfold, and weight. The formula for calculating body fat in white females between 25 and 34 years of age, for example, has been established as follows:

$$\text{kg of body fat} = \text{arm circumference (cm)} \times 0.354 + \text{thigh circumference (cm)} \times 0.403 + \text{abdomen skinfold (mm)} \times 0.159 + \text{weight (pounds)} \times 0.083 - 26.189$$

The difficulties of making accurate anthropometric measurements of body structure in extremely obese individuals impose limitations on the usefulness of some of these indices. As a result several alternative methods have been proposed.

X-ray films have made it possible to measure body fat in such areas as the hips, where caliper measurements of skinfold thickness are of little value. This technique has been validated to establish that each millimeter of outer fat represents 1 to 2 kg of total body fat.

Body fat may also be estimated from the relationship between body weight and lean body mass based on the whole body counter assessment of potassium 40, as discussed in Chapter 7.

In addition to wishing to know something of body composition for purposes of identifying obese persons, physicians use fat-free weight estimates to determine drug-dosages.

In field studies in developing countries the measurement of arm circumference or arm circumference in relation to height, the Quaker Arm Circumference (QUAC) stick, has been useful in identifying undernourished children with low fat reserves. In 1- to 4-year-old children in whom there is normally little change with age, arm circumference measurements below 14.6 cm are considered indicative of undernutrition.

A combination of arm circumference and triceps skinfold measurements has been used to calculate muscle circumference, believed to be a sensitive indicator of caloric adequacy and muscle mass. Muscle circumference is represented by the formula:

$$\text{Muscle circumference} = \text{Midarm upper circumference (cm)} - (\pi\ [3.14] \times \text{triceps skinfold thickness})$$

For women 23.2 cm is considered standard muscle circumference and for men, 25.3 cm.

In the National Nutrition Survey, the following anthropometric measurements were obtained to provide a basis for the evaluation of nutritional status: height, weight, knee height, knee, wrist, and shoulder diameter, calf, arm, shoulder, and head circumferences, and triceps and subscapular skinfolds. In addition, a wristbone x-ray film is routinely taken. The relative usefulness of these data will become known only after it has been possible to correlate them with other measures of nutritional status.

DIETARY EVALUATION

The analysis of food intake as part of an assessment of nutritional status is useful in providing evidence of nutritive intakes that may be suggestive of inadequacies. It can help to identify individuals or groups in need of further study. However, unless low intakes are accompanied by some biochemical or physical evidence of a deficiency state, they can be used only to infer nutritional deficiencies as a basis for nutritional education programs or for agricultural and health policies.

On the other hand, when a low dietary intake of a specific nutrient is found in conjunction with biochemical and clinical signs of a deficiency, the dietary data serve to confirm a diagnosis and provide a basis on which to build a dietary treatment. An apparently adequate diet may be taken by a person exhibiting deficiency symptoms, and, conversely, persons with apparently suboptimal intakes may show no evidence of deficiency symptoms. In these cases the discrepancy can often be explained on the basis of wide individual variability in nutritive needs resulting from differences in ability to absorb a nutrient, in efficiency or utilization, or in the actual nutrient content of a food compared to the values used in calculating the diet. In addition, a dietary evaluation reflects only the immediate intake, whereas much of the biochemical and clinical evidence reflects long-term nutritive intake. A recently improved diet would not immediately result in relief of the symptoms; thus a discrepancy between dietary and clinical findings can be explained on the basis of the continuation of deficiency symptoms after the initiation of a better diet. Conversely, failure to find biochemical or clinical evidence of a deficiency in conjunction with low intakes may be a reflection of the time required to deplete nutrient reserves when the quality of the diet declines.

Evaluations of nutrient intake are carried out in a number of ways, each with its own merits and limitations. In a general way they can be categorized as *indirect* and *direct.*

Indirect methods

Food balance sheet or food disappearance data. The most common of the indirect methods is the national food balance sheet. In this the records of agricultural productivity and of the export and import of food products of a country and estimates of food wastage are used to obtain a measure of the kinds and amounts of food and hence of nutrients available to a country. Adjustment must be made for food directed to animal feeding and nonfood uses. Since no information is provided on the distribution of food within a country, this is in no way an assessment of the nutritive intake of individuals, nor does it provide information of the variation of intake that occurs with socioeconomic status, cultural background, age, occupation, or sex. It is, however, useful in detecting year-to-year trends in the availability of nutrients, in providing a basis for planning the emphasis that should prevail in agricultural production and processing, and in pinpointing possible nutritional shortages.

Vital statistics. The vital statistics of a country provide a second indirect method of assessing nutrition adequacy. Records of the ages and causes of illness and deaths provide a measure of the extent and nature of morbidity and mortality of a population. Where the incidence of nutritionally related conditions such as beriberi or kwashiorkor is high, malnutrition is undoubtedly present. Where the recorded incidence is low, it may reflect adequate nutrition in regard to these nutrients, but it is equally possible that the recording of mortality and morbidity statistics has not been sufficiently accurate to reflect these less well known causes of death and sickness. Instead, they may only reflect the ultimate cause of death, such as heart failure or tuberculosis. The incidence and death rate from infectious diseases, such as measles or tuberculosis, is often higher in a malnourished population that lacks the ability to combat the infection. In these cases, however, it is difficult to distinguish the role played by nutrition from that of environmental hygiene and medical practices. When used with a recognition of their limitations, vital statistics or public health indices provide a useful tool in evaluating trends in the nutritional status of a population.

Not until 1970 was malnutrition considered a reportable disease in the United States and then only in a few states.

Direct methods

Direct methods involve an evaluation of the dietary intake of a much smaller unit, such as an institution, a family, or an individual. These methods will be discussed in increasing order of specificity of data obtained.

Food inventory. The food inventory method is used with either a socially homogeneous group such as residents in an institution or members of a family who are fed from a common kitchen. A record is made of all the foods available at the beginning of the study, all food purchased, contributed, or grown for consumption during the period of the study (usually two weeks to a month), the food remaining in the inventory at the end, and an estimate of the waste of food occurring during the course of the study and the food used in feeding animals. From this information an approximation of the nutritive value of the food available to those eating in the group during this period is calculated. Adjustments are usually made for food eaten away from home.

Another method of obtaining this information is a list-recall procedure in which the homemaker is given a list of food items to assist in recalling the kinds and amounts of foods purchased or acquired during the study period.

These methods have several limitations. First, with no indication of who consumes the food, it is quite possible that some members of the group are adequately nourished or even overnourished, whereas other may lack one or more nutrients even though the amount consumed by the group would have been adequate for all had it been properly distributed. Second, studies on small family units have shown that homemakers modify their habits of purchasing food during a time when they are made more conscious of their buying habits. The mere presence of a person recording the food inventory creates a situation in which food habits may vary from normal. It may also increase the reluctance of families, especially in higher income groups, to participate. Weighed records of the family food consumption have also been obtained, but these require a high level of cooperation from the participating families and yield no data on the distribution of food among family members.

Individual food intake. No matter what standard of evaluating an individual's dietary habits is used, whether it be a dietary score or nutritive value calculated from tables of food composition, it is necessary to have as complete a record as possible of the food intake for a specified period of time or to have typical food patterns. These are obtained in several ways. The choice of method depends on several factors—the purpose of the study, the funds and personnel available to carry it out, the target population (children, elderly, pregnant women), and the literacy level of the group.

Twenty-four–hour recall. The subject is interviewed by a trained interviewer who asks him to describe the kinds and amounts of food consumed in the previous 24 hours. The subject is often given food models, measuring cups, or a ruler to help him describe the amounts of food consumed. This method has two major advantages. Since it is a retrospective account taken at an unannounced time, it reduces the possibility of the subject modifying his food habits during a time when he knows they are being assessed. The use of the immediately past 24 hours does not involve an appreciable memory span, thus increasing the likelihood of obtaining a complete record. It is suitable for use in illiterate populations. By asking appropriate questions, the trained interviewer is able to probe further and elicit information on the use of condiments, beverages, snacks, and food adjuncts such as catsup, mayonnaise, butter, cream, and relishes that might otherwise be overlooked.

Validation studies have confirmed that larger intakes are often underestimated and small intakes overestimated. In the usual ranges of intake these discrepancies have limited significance, but at either very high or very low intakes, these variations assume greater importance.

Individual interviews are a rather costly method of obtaining dietary information. If data are desired on a group such as schoolchildren, 24-hour diet records are sometimes obtained as written records.

Comparison between diet records from 24-hour recall and seven-day written records shows that intakes from the 24-hour recall tend to be higher. This has been interpreted as reflecting the desire of the subject to make a good impression on the interviewer.

The 24-hour recall is considered a feasible method of obtaining data that can be used to compare the nutritive intake of groups of individuals, but the high variability in diet from day to day in many segments of society precludes its use in evaluating intake for individuals or in relating daily intake to biochemical data.

The use of the 24-hour recall requires that the subject have a fairly acute memory. Research has shown that data from women is better than from men and that data from younger persons is more valid than that from older individuals. Probing by the interviewer has been shown to increase the extent to which actual food intake is recalled by as much as 25%.

The use of data from a one-day period fails to provide information on variations in intake associated with season, day of week, or emotional state, all of which may account for variability in intake for one individual. Attempts to use longer recall periods ranging up to twenty-eight days have shown that, although four days is a maximum for many, if the respondent can tie food intake to activities, memory is greatly enhanced. In many cases a seven-day recall is possible.

Dietary history. A dietary history is an effort to obtain qualitative rather than quantitative information on long-standing food habits that influence the appearance of clinical signs and symptoms. Used in conjunction with the 24-hour recall of food intake and a three-day food record, it is considered by many as a very effective method of assessing nutritive adequacy. The subject is asked for information on his past dietary habits—the number and type of meals he normally eats, the frequency and extent to which he uses the various food groups (green and yellow vegetables, milk or milk substitutes, meat, eggs, cereals, etc.), his food likes and dislikes, food allergies, and seasonal variations in intake. From this data it is possible to establish whether the pattern observed in the 24-hour record represents a typical or an atypical food intake. Much of the success of this method depends on the cooperation of the subject and the effectiveness of the interviewer. It is relatively costly in time and money, a typical interview requiring at least 45 minutes. Estimates of dietary intake from a dietary history tend to be higher compared to those from weighed records.

With the widespread availability of computers, several groups are marketing nutrient intake analyses based on information provided by the subject, who fills out a form that asks for dietary history and food frequency information. These analyses have not yet been evaluated and the hazards of having an unqualified individual interpret such data suggest that they be used with great caution.

Food intake records. When evaluating the diets of large groups of literate subjects, the use of written food intake records has proved an inexpensive and relatively satisfactory method of obtaining data. The question not yet answered satisfactorily is how many and which days should be used. In a country such as the United States, with a varied food supply and a tradition for consuming a varied diet, a one-day food record is considerably less representative of usual dietary patterns than in a country where the diet seldom varies. It is recognized that for many persons dietary patterns on weekends differ from those on weekdays. Yet experience has shown that persons asked to keep a seven-day food record lose interest in the task as the period progresses and keep increasingly less satisfactory records or stop entirely. Some investigators have found that three weekdays and one weekend day provide an accurate picture. If no provision is made to see that records are kept daily, there is always the possibility that the task will be put off until the end of the period, leading to errors from incomplete or inaccurate recall.

Many investigators have chosen to use the

three-day written food record as the one giving sufficiently useful information within a period of time in which one could expect to maintain the cooperation of subjects. Some studies in a highly selected group have made use of twenty-eight–day records at four seasons of the year, but this involves a strong commitment and a high degree of cooperation on the part of the subjects.

Whether food intake is assessed on the basis of a food inventory, a 24-hour recall, or a written food record the problems of the subject's estimate of serving size and the investigator's interpretation of the resulting records must be considered.

The concern that after a person is asked for information on his food intake, he will modify his intake or provide an inaccurate record has led nutritionists to seek an unobtrusive measurement of food intake in which the subject is more likely to retain typical eating patterns. So far such methods have proved costly and in some cases a violation of the individual's right to privacy.

Weighed food records. When a precise individual dietary analysis is required, the weighed food record provides the most accurate means of obtaining it. All food taken by the subject must be accurately weighed and then adjusted for any plate waste. This involves training the subject to keep accurate records or assigning an investigator to be present at all times to help. In either case the problem exists that the work involved in record keeping and/or the presence of a stranger may lead to a modified eating pattern. In addition to the high cost, the fact that it can be used only with highly motivated persons or those that can be paid to participate, and cannot be used with persons who eat away from home all present limitations in the use of the method.

Dietary score. The need for a simple scoring system for the rapid evaluation of dietary adequacy for use by nonprofessionals has been recognized for some time. Two such approaches that do not require the extensive computations involved in using food composition tables and dietary standards have been developed. The one shown in Table 15-2, which permits a maximum score of 100, places slightly more emphasis on the milk and fruit and vegetable groups than on the cereal and protein groups. The application of this approach requires a judgment of the serving size of the food with 8 ounces of milk or its equivalent, one half cup or 4 ounces of fruits or vegetables, 1 ounce of cereal, one slice of bread, or their equivalent, and 3 ounces of meat, fish, or poultry or its equivalent generally considered the average serving sizes required to earn points. To keep the scoring simple, no points are given for partial servings. The scoring system shown here is typical of several with the same intent developed by groups ranging from the U.S. Department of Agriculture to commodity-oriented associations such as the National Dairy Council and the National Livestock Board. A score of 100 is earned when all food groups are represented.

An even simpler system, placing equal emphasis (4 points) on each of the major food groups, assigns points whenever a food item appears in the diet, regardless of the amount. This system, which assigns 2 points for each of two servings of milk, 2 points for each of two servings of protein foods, 1 point for each of four fruits or vegetables, and 1 for each of four cereal or bread items, has been used in evaluating the effectiveness of nutritional intervention programs. It is shown in Table 15-3.

Each of these evaluation systems is based on the assumption that diets providing foods from each of the four major food groups will likely, but not necessarily, provide the foundation for an adequate dietary intake. Adopting these systems to evaluate a diet that may be nutritionally adequate but which follows a less conventional pattern requires considerable knowledge of nutritional equivalents of different foods. Research has shown a sufficient degree of agreement between the results from the use of these simple scoring tools and more involved dietary analyses that they can be used with confidence as a basis for counselling.

Table 15-2. Food selection check sheet

Food		Maximum score	Daily score						
Milk		30							
One cup of milk or equivalent	10								
Second cup of milk	10								
Third cup of milk or more	10								
Fruits and vegetables		30							
One serving of green or yellow vegetables	10								
One serving of citrus fruit, tomato, or cabbage	10								
Two or more servings of other fruits and vegetables, including potato	5 each								
Breads and cereals		15							
Three servings of whole-grain or enriched cereals or breads	5 each								
Protein-rich foods		25							
One serving of egg, meat, fish, poultry or cheese (or dried beans or peas)	15								
One or more additional servings of egg, meat, fish, poultry or cheese	10								
TOTAL		100							

Table 15-3. Dietary score

	Score each time food is mentioned	Maximum score
Milk and milk products	2	4
Protein foods—meat, fish, poultry, eggs	2	4
Fruits and vegetables	1	4
Cereals	1	4
TOTAL		16

Calculations from tables of food composition. Many tables based on chemical analyses of food composition are available. The standard reference is the U.S. Department of Agriculture Handbook No. 8, first published in 1908, which has been compiled after a careful analysis of data available from many research laboratories. It is currently being revised and will be published in twenty-one different sections, each dealing with a specific class of foods such as milk products, spices, or baby foods. Data on these classes will be given for 61 nutrients, on the basis of 100 g, 1 pound, and 100 kcal portions. In addition, it will give information on the number of analyses on which the data were based and the range of values reported. Consideration is given to variety, method of preparation, sources in terms of climates and soil environment, degree of maturity, and many other factors that influence the nutritive value of foods as consumed by the American public.

The rapid rate at which the food industry is marketing new food products and fabricated foods has complicated the task of providing an accurate, up-to-date compilation of the nutritive contribution of available foods. Much of this information is included in the most recent revision of Home and Garden Bulletin No. 72, *Nutritive Value of Foods,* reproduced in Appendix G. However, if exact information on the composition of new foods is essential, as for therapeutic diets, it is wise to obtain the information from the manufacturer or processor. The U.S. Department of Agriculture is planning to establish a nutritive data bank in which all such data would be stored in a computer.

With an accurate description of the kind and amount of food eaten, it is possible to use tables to calculate the amount of various nutrients present in a diet. This method assumes that the food consumed can be represented by the food described in the table. Among the major limitations to the analysis of diets from food records are the variations and limitations in an individual's estimate of the amount of food eaten and his failure to describe the food in sufficient detail. Tables for a short method of dietary calculation have been developed in which similar foods are grouped in broad categories, and one figure is given for the nutritive value of the whole group. Estimates of nutritive content using the short method agree rather closely with those obtained from the long method and may be satisfactory for analysis of diets in which the amount of food has been estimated in the first place. Persons using data derived from calculations from diet records should be cautioned against reporting the values as precise figures (that is, protein to 0.1 g or thiamin to 0.01 mg), since this represents a degree of accuracy not justified within the limitations of the method of collecting the data.

Chemical analysis. In research situations, when it is essential to know as exactly as possible the intake of a nutrient, the food intake is weighed accurately and a representative or aliquot sample is saved for chemical analysis in the laboratory. The cost of such means of determining nutritive value of a diet precludes its use in routine dietary studies. It is useful when a carefully prescribed diet is being consumed but has many limitations on a freely selected diet.

Standards for evaluating dietary intake. Knowledge of the nutritive content of a diet is meaningless unless it can be compared to some standard. In the United States the most commonly used standard is the Recommended Dietary Allowances (RDA) prepared by the Food and Nutrition Board of the National Research Council. These standards, shown in Appendix C, were established as the result of careful evaluation of evidence of nutritional needs for various nutrients by various population groups and of an evaluation of figures on agricultural productivity, imports, and exports to determine the availability of nutrients in the food supply. These standards do not represent minimum requirements, and any failure to consume the recommended amounts must *not* necessarily be interpreted as evidence of dietary deficiencies. In fact, a large segment of the population can maintain a high level of health on intakes well below the recommended amounts, although a small group may require the full amounts. It most studies of dietary adequacy, intakes of two thirds the recommended allowances have been considered adequate and those below this level as indicative of a possible suboptimal state of nutrition. Because of the wide individual variation in need for a specific nutrient, a great deal of caution must be observed in comparing the intake of an individual to that of the recommended allowances.

To interpret dietary data from the National Nutritional Survey, The U.S. Public Health Service developed a standard of acceptable intakes, which is outlined in Table 15-4. A further modification was made to interpret data from the Health and Nutrition Examination Study (HANES) (Table 15-5). In

Table 15-4. Dietary standards used by the U.S. Public Health Service in evaluating dietary intake in the National Nutritional Survey, 1970

Age	Energy (kcal/kg)	Protein (g/kg)	Calcium (mg)	Iron (mg)	Thiamin (per 1000 kcal)	Riboflavin (per 1000 kcal)	Vitamin A (IU)	Ascorbic acid (mg)
6-7 yr	82	1.3	450	10	0.4 mg	0.55 mg	2500	30
10-12 yr								
Male	68	1.2	650	10	0.4 mg	0.55 mg	2500	30
Female	64	1.2	650	18	0.4 mg	0.55 mg	2500	30
17-19 yr								
Male	44	1.1	550	18	0.4 mg	0.55 mg	3500	30
Female	35	1.1	550	18	0.4 mg	0.55 mg	3500	30
Adults								
Male	38	1.0	400	10	0.4 mg	0.55 mg	3500	30
Female	38	1.0		18	0.4 mg	0.55 mg		
Pregnant	+200	+20	800	18	0.4 mg	0.55 mg	3500	30
Lactating	+1000	+25	900	18	0.4 mg	0.55 mg	4500	30

Table 15-5. Standards for HANES dietary intake data*

Evaluation of daily dietary intake used in the Health and Nutrition Examination Survey, United States, 1971-1974

Age, sex, and physiological state	Calories (per kg)	Protein (g/kg)	Calcium (mg)	Iron (mg)	Vitamin A† (IU)	Vitamin C (mg)	B vitamins (all ages)
Age and sex							
1-5 yr							Thiamin
12-23 mo, male and female	90	1.9	450	15	2000	40	0.4 mg per 1000 calories
24-47 mo, male and female	86	1.7	450	15	2000	40	Riboflavin
48-71 mo, male and female	82	1.5	450	10	2000	40	0.55 mg per 1000 calories

*U. S. Department of Health, Education, and Welfare: First Health and Nutrition Examination Survey (1971-1972). Dietary intakes and biochemical findings, Publication No. (HRA) 74-1291-1, p. 181, Rockville, Md., 1974, National Center for Health Statistics.

†Assume 70% carotene, 30% retinol.

‡For all pregnancies.

Table 15-5. Standards for HANES dietary intake data—cont'd

Evaluation of daily dietary intake used in the Health and Nutrition Examination Survey, United States, 1971-1974

Age, sex, and physiological state	Calories (per kg)	Protein (g/kg)	Calcium (mg)	Iron (mg)	Vitamin A† (IU)	Vitamin C (mg)	B vitamins (all ages)
6-7 yr, male and female	82	1.3	450	10	2500	40	Niacin 6.6 mg per 1000 calories
8-9 yr, male and female	82	1.3	450	10	2500	40	
10-12 yr							
Male	68	1.2	650	10	2500	40	
Female	64	1.2	650	18	2500	40	
13-16 yr							
Male	60	1.2	650	18	3500	50	
Female	48	1.2	650	18	3500	50	
17-19 yr							
Male	44	1.1	550	18	3500	55	
Female	35	1.1	550	18	3500	50	
20-29 yr							
Male	40	1.0	400	10	3500	60	
Female	35	1.0	600	18	3500	55	
30-39 yr							
Male	38	1.0	400	10	3500	60	
Female	33	1.0	600	18	3500	55	
40-49 yr							
Male	37	1.0	400	10	3500	60	
Female	31	1.0	600	18	3500	55	
50-54 yr							
Male	36	1.0	400	10	3500	60	
Female	30	1.0	600	18	3500	55	
55-59 yr							
Male	36	1.0	400	10	3500	60	
Female	30	1.0	600	10	3500	55	
60-69 yr							
Male	34	1.0	400	10	3500	60	
Female	29	1.0	600	10	3500	55	
70 yr and over							
Male	34	1.0	400	10	3500	60	
Female	29	1.0	600	10	3500	55	
Physiological state							
Pregnancy (fifth month and beyond), add to basic standard	200	20	200		1000	5	‡
Lactating, add to basic standard	1000	25	500		1000	5	

comparing results of various surveys, it is important to know which standard was used.

Unless low dietary intakes are accompanied by some clinical or biochemical abnormalities associated with a lack of the nutrient, it is dangerous to assume that the intake is below the need of that individual. However, low intakes should prompt an evaluation of nutritional status and nutrition counselling, since an intake increased to recommended levels should be associated with a higher degree of health.

In summary, in the evaluation of nutritional status, dietary data provide evidence that is suggestive but not diagnostic of nutritional deficiency. Nutrient levels in the blood are indicative of either recent intake or available stores. Amount of nutrient-related enzymes and metabolites in the blood and urine reflect early changes associated with nutrient inadequacies, while clinical changes occur only as manifestations of advanced symptoms. Only when evidence associated with a nutrient deficiency is provided by more than one approach to assessment is it likely that a nutrient inadequacy does exist.

BIBLIOGRAPHY

Anthropometry in nutritional surveillance: an overview, PAG Bull. **6:**12, 1976.

Bowering, J., Morrison, M. A., Lowenberg, R., and Tirado, N.: Evaluating 24-hour dietary recalls, J. Nutr. Educ. **9:**22, 1977.

Brin, M.: Erythrocyte as a biopsy tissue for functional evaluation of thiamin adequacy, J.A.M.A. **187:**762, 1964.

Byron, A. H., and Anderson, E.: Retrospective dietary interviewing, J. Am. Diet. Assoc. **37:**558, 1960.

Christakis, G. M., editor: Nutritional assessment in health programs, Am. J. Public Health **63**(suppl.):1 Nov. 1973.

Cinnamon, A. D., and Beaton, J. R.: Biochemical assessment of vitamin B_6 status in man, Am. J. Clin. Nutr. **23:**696, 1970.

Clark, F.: Recent food consumption surveys and their uses, Fed. Proc. **33:**2270, 1974.

Committee on Procedures for Appraisal of Protein-Calorie Malnutrition, International Union oif Nutritional Science: Assessment of protein nutritional status, Am. J. Clin. Nutr. **23:**807, 1970.

Demming, S. B., and Weber, C. W.: Evaluation of hair analysis for determination of zinc status using rats, Am. J. Clin. Nutr. **30:**2047, 1977.

Ferro-Luzzi, G.: Rapid evaluation of nutritional level, Am. J. Nutr. **19:**247, 1966.

Frank, G. C., Berenson, G. S., Schilling, P. E., and Moore, M. C.: Adapting the 24-hour recall for epidemiologic studies of school children, J. Am. Diet. Assoc. **71:**26, 1977.

Gersovitz, M., Madden, J. P., and Smiciklas-Wright, H.: Validity of 24-hour recall and seven-day record for group comparisons, J. Am. Diet. Assoc. **73:**48, 1978.

Gueney, M. J., and Jelliffe, D.: Arm anthropometry in nutritional assessment: monogram for rapid calculation of muscle circumference and cross-section muscle and fat areas, Am. J. Clin. Nutr. **26:**912, 1973.

Guthrie, H. A., and Gurthrie, G. M.: Factor analysis of nutritional status data from Ten State Nutrition Survey, Am. J. Clin. Nutr. **29:**1238, 1976.

Hollingsworth, D.: Dietary determination of nutritional status, Fed. Proc. **20:**50, 1960.

How to control your weight, supplement (based on 1959 Body build and blood pressure study), New York, 1960, Metropolitan Insurance Co.

Huenemann, R. L.: Interpretation of nutritional status, J. Am. Diet. Assoc. **63:**123, 1973.

Kelsay, J. L.: A compendium of nutritional status studies and dietary evaluation studies conducted in the United States, 1957-1967, J. Nutr. **99**(suppl. 1, part II):123, 1969.

Klevay, L. M.: Hair as a biopsy material. Assessment of zinc nutriture, Am. J. Clin. Nutr. **23:**284, 1970.

Kram, K. M., and Owen, G.: Evaluation of nutritional status in preschool children in the United States, U.S. Government Printing Office, 1972.

Krehl, W. A., and Hodges, R. E.: The interpretation of nutrition survey data, Am. J. Clin. Nutr. **17:**191, 1965.

Madden, J. P., Goodman, S. J., Guthrie, H. A.: Validity of the 24-hour recall. Analysis of data obtained from elderly subjects, J. Am. Diet. Assoc. **68:**143, 1976.

Marr, J. W.: Individual dietary surveys—purposes and methods, World Rev. Nutr. Diet. **13:**106, 1971.

Medical assessment of nutritional status, Report of the Joint FAO/WHO Expert Committee, WHO Techn. Rep. Ser. No. 258, 1963.

Nutritive value of foods, Home and Garden Bulletin No. 72, Agriculture Research Service, Washington, D.C., 1977, U.S. Department of Agriculture.

O'Neal, R. M., Johnson, O. C., and Schaeffer, A. E.: Guidelines for classification and interpretation of group blood and urine data collected as part of the National Nutritional Survey, Pediatr. Res. **4:**103, 1970.

Pekkarinen, M.: Methodology in the collection of food consumption data, World Rev. Nutr. Diet. **12:**145, 1970.

Pollack, H.: Creatinine excretion as an index for estimating urinary excretion of micronutrients or their metabolic end products, Am. J. Clin. Nutr. **23:**865, 1970.

Population screening for iron deficiency, Nutr. Rev. **35:**271, 1977.

Roche, A. F., and McKigney, J. I.: Physical growth of ethnic groups comprising the United States population, Am. J. Clin. Nutr. **28:**1071, 1975.

Sabry, A. I., Campbell, E., Campbell, J. A., and Forbes, A. L.: Nutrition Canada—a national nutrition survey, Nutr. Rev. **32:**105, 1974.

Selzer, C. C., Goldman, R. F., and Mayer, J.: The triceps skinfold as a predictive measure of body density and body fat in obese adolescent girls, Pediatrics **36:**212, 1965.

Shemesh, A.: Threshold weight and ponderal index (letter to the editor), J.A.M.A. **236:**2173, 1976.

Simmes, M. A., Addiego, J. E., Dallman, P. R.: Ferritin in serum: Diagnosis of iron deficiency and iron overload in infants and children, Blood **43:**581, 1974.

Smith, D. P., and Boyce, R. W.: Prediction of body density and lean body weight in females 25 to 37 years old, Am. J. Clin. Nutr. **30:**560, 1977.

Wadsworth, G. R.: Nutritional surveys—clinical signs and biochemical measurements, Proc. Nutr. Soc. **22:**72, 1963.

Walker, A. R. P.: Interpretation of biological data on one ethnic or regional group may not be equally applicable to other groups, Am. J. Clin. Nutr. **20:**1025, 1967.

Wilson, C. S., Schaeffer, A. E., Darby, W. J., and others: A review of methods used in nutrition surveys conducted by the Interdepartmental Committee on Nutrition for National Defense (ICNND), Am. J. Clin. Nutr. **15:**29, 1964.

Youland, D. M., and Engle, A.: Practices and problems in HANES: dietary data methodology, J. Am. Diet. Assoc. **68:**22, 1976.

16

Nutrition in pregnancy and lactation

The relationship between the quality of health of the offspring and the nutritional status of the mother at the time of conception and during pregnancy has been recognized since the 1940s. More recently, the realization that the United States has a relatively unfavorable record in regard to perinatal morbidity and mortality has directed attention to sound nutritional practices as a possible form of preventive health care.

PREGNANCY

From a nutritional point of view the nine months of pregnancy, although physiologically normal, must be considered a period of stress during which the nutrient demands of the developing fetus are superimposed on those for normal maintenance of the adult woman.

The importance of adequate nutrition for the fetus cannot be overemphasized, since the future health of the individual depends to a large extent on the nutritional foundation established in prenatal life. Fortunately, the needs of the growing fetus are not added totally to those of the adult woman. The pregnant woman experiences a series of physiological adaptations, which result in improved utilization of nutrients either through increased absorption, decreased excretion, or alterations in metabolism. In addition, the mother who has been well nourished prior to conception enters pregnancy with a reserve of several nutrients that can meet the needs of the growing fetus without jeopardizing her health. The capacity of the maternal organism to adapt to meet the needs of the infant is generally sufficient; thus the mother whose diet has been reasonably adequate prior to pregnancy is usually able to bear a full-term, viable infant without extensive modification of her diet. It is recommended, however, that the mother consume a diet sufficiently adequate so that (1) maternal stores will not be depleted and (2) the mother will be able to produce enough milk to adequately nourish her child after birth.

Concern over the quality of the diet during pregnancy is prompted by evidence that up to 15% of all infants, or over a quarter of a million, are **low–birth weight (LBW)** babies weighing less than 2500 g. More than two thirds of these babies are premature (less than 37 weeks of gestation) and the rest suffer from **intrauterine growth retardation (IUGR),** being born after 40 weeks of gestation but small because of malnutrition during uterine growth. In either case they enter life with a risk of neonatal death thirty times that of normal weight infants. They also have an increased susceptibility to infection, immature kidneys, difficulty regulating body temperature, and problems in both carbohydrate and protein metabolism.

These risks are high among babies born to adolescent mothers who themselves have high nutritional requirements for their own growth needs. In addition, many teenage pregnancies involve girls of low socioeconomic status who have been identified as a generally undernourished group themselves and are often incapable of providing adequate nutrients to promote intrauterine growth. As a result children born to mothers under 18 years of age are more likely to suffer from defects in physical, social, and psychological development. This assumes increased importance in light of the fact that at present over half the girls in the United States are married by age 19 and that a fifth of the 3 million babies born each year are born to teenagers, a third of whom are under 16.

Intrauterine growth retardation, which results in babies who are "small for date" (SFD) is most likely to occur in offspring of mothers who are of low socioeconomic status, women with poor nutritional status who are shorter and lighter than their better nourished counterparts at the time of conception, mothers who experience hypertension, viral infections, or other diseases, and women who use drugs extensively during pregnancy. These infants may be undernourished because of poor circulation to the fetus resulting in lack of oxygen, inhibition of the transfer of nutrients to the fetus because of reduced size of placenta, or hormonal changes.

Prematurity as a cause of low–birth weight infants is most likely to occur with multiple births or when mothers gain too little (<7 kg) or too much (>13 kg) weight during pregnancy or smoke excessively (over eleven cigarettes a day). Since much of the neurological development and maturation of the kidneys and lungs occur in the latter part of pregnancy, the chances of defects in these aspects of development increase markedly among premature babies.

There are many ways by which the malnourished mother is protec[illegible]against carrying a potentially undernou[illegible]hed child to term. It is estimated that only 60% of conceptions survive the critical first four weeks of gestation. Of these another 10% fail to survive to twenty weeks. Intrauterine deaths from twenty weeks to term reduce to 50% the proportion of conceptions that result in the birth of viable infants. Approximately 1% of these suffer from perinatal handicaps necessitating special care. The death rate in the first two years is approximately 25 per 1000 live births. There is general agreement that much of this pregnancy wastage is due to undernutrition and malnutrition prior to and during pregnancy and thus is preventable.

The developing fetus is parasitic on the mother for all nourishment. This nourishment is obtained primarily from the mother's blood, which comes in sufficiently close contact with the fetal circulation system in the **placenta** that required nutrients can be transferred. During the latter part of gestation, some nutrients are available to the fetus through the **amniotic fluid.** Nutrients may be provided from the mother's immediate diet, from her stores of nutrients (primarily in the bones and liver), or from synthesis in the placenta. Because the placenta controls the transfer of nutrients, hormones, and other substances such as drugs to the fetus, the development of the placenta itself is crucial to the health of the fetus. There is now considerable evidence to show that placentas of poorly nourished mothers contain fewer and smaller cells than those of well-nourished mothers. This reduction in the number of cells reduces the ability of the placenta to synthesize substances needed by the fetus, to facilitate the flow of needed nutrients, and to inhibit the passage of potentially harmful substances. Intrauterine nutrition is especially important in terms of the development of the central nervous system and the kidneys, whose growth occurs to a large extent in the latter part of pregnancy. Nutritional deficits encountered prenatally cannot be wholly reversed by adequate postnatal nutrition.

Further evidence that attention should be focused on the adequacy of the diet during pregnancy comes from data on the dietary intake of pregnant women participating in the Ten-State Nutritional Survey. Analysis of their nutrient intake showed that it fell below standards for calories, iron, calcium, vitamin A, and protein. These same nutrients were the ones identified by McGanity and co-workers as lacking in the diets of 800 low-income pregnant women in Texas. These findings are not surprising since 63%

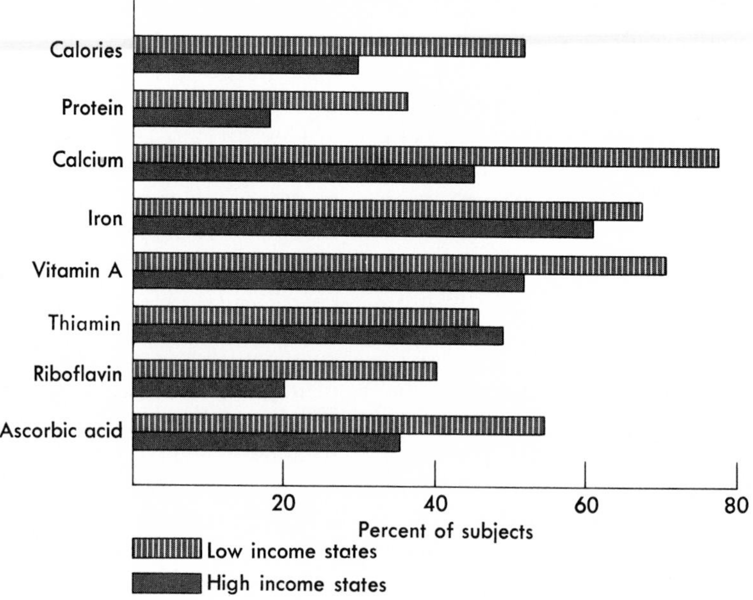

Fig. 16-1. Percentage of pregnant women in the United States with dietary intakes below two-thirds RDA by income. Data from Ten-State Nutrition Survey (1968-1970).

of the women consumed diets providing fewer than 1750 kcal, which is known to be inadequate to assure the recommended intake of the other nutrients. Results of the nutrient intake of pregnant women in the Ten-State Nutrition Survey are shown graphically in Fig. 16-1.

Physiological adjustments

During pregnancy many physiological, biochemical, and hormonal changes occur that influence the need for nutrients and the efficiency with which the body uses them. Total blood volume is known to increase about 33% above normal levels, and plasma volume 50% in **primiparas** and higher in multiparas. This is—partially, at least—a response to the need for an increased amount of blood to carry nutrients to the fetus and metabolic waste (such as carbon dioxide and nitrogenous end products) away from the fetus. With the increase in blood volume, more fluid carrying nutrients is available to the placenta. At the same time the 50% increase in the rate at which the blood filters through the kidneys increases the ability of the mother to excrete the waste products from fetal development. Any loss of needed nutrients is prevented by an increase in the ability of the kidneys to reabsorb nutrients from the filtered blood. To facilitate the circulation of the larger amount of blood the capacity of the heart to pump fluid is increased by a third (from 45 to 60 L/min). In addition to the increase in fluid within the circulatory system there is an increase of another 5 to 6 liters in intercellular water.

This hemodilution, occurring as blood volume increases, results in decreased hemoglobin and plasma protein values as well as a lowered per unit volume concentration of red blood cells and many nutrients. These observations are often erroneously interpreted as evidence of a deficiency. Frequently the total amount may have increased, although the per unit measurement will have dropped.

The decrease in gastric motility and intestinal tonus common in pregnancy has the advantage of slowing the passage of food through the gastrointestinal tract and enhancing the possibility of absorption of nutrients. On the other hand, it may be a factor in nausea of pregnancy and may lead to considerable discomfort when it results in constipation because of an inability to empty the gastrointestinal tract in the latter part of pregnancy.

The observed decrease in the secretion of hydrochloric acid reduces gastric acidity, which could have a depressing effect on calcium and iron absorption, in which the ionization of the element from its complex depends on acid. However, any such effect is counterbalanced by other factors that lead to an increased absorption of these two elements in the last trimester of pregnancy.

Among the hormonal changes associated with pregnancy that have nutritional implications are increased secretion of (1) aldosterone (the salt-conserving hormone) by the adrenal gland, (2) growth hormone by the pituitary, (3) thyroxin, which regulates metabolism, by the thyroid, (4) parathyroid hormone, which controls calcium and magnesium metabolism, by the parathyroid, and (5) the increased uptake of iodine by the thyroid gland.

Physiological stages of pregnancy

Implantation. Pregnancy can be divided into three main phases, each with specific nutrient needs, from a physiological point of view. The first two weeks of gestation is a period of **implantation,** during which the fertilized ovum becomes embedded in the wall of the uterus. At this time the fetus is nourished from the outer layers of the germ plasm and from the secretions of the uterine glands, known as *uterine milk.*

Organogenesis. The next six weeks are known as the period of **organogenesis,** during which the developing fetal tissue, known as the embryo, undergoes differentiation into functional units. During this period, nourishment is obtained from the blood and degenerating cells in the space between the embryo and the maternal tissue. The beginnings of the individual organs and the various aspects of skeletal formation are established during this period, and the presence or absence of many nutrients may be crucial for the continued growth of a normal fetus.

Considerable evidence exists in animal studies linking the absence of certain nutrients during specific periods of organogenesis with specific congenital abnormalities in the newborn. For instance, riboflavin deficiency has been associated with poor skeletal formation, pyridoxine deficiency with neuromotor problems, vitamin B_{12} deficiency with hydrocephalus, and niacin and folic acid deficiency with cleft palate.

From studies on animals it is evident that the stage in pregnancy at which the deficiency occurs determines susceptibility to the deficiency and the way in which it is manifest. If the inadequacy occurs in the very early stages, the result may be a failure in pregnancy, reflected in a spontaneous abortion; at certain stages during differentiation it may show up in a variety of forms of congenital abnormalities; and again, there are stages, especially after differentiation is complete, at which a deficiency will have virtually no effect on the developing fetus.

It has been difficult to demonstrate a relationship in human nutrition because any dietary information must come from retrospective accounts and not from experimental manipulation of the diet. Once the abnormality is observed, however, it is sometimes possible to implicate nutritional factors. The possibility of a nutritional inadequacy with its potential hazards to the fetus during organogenesis is increased since this rather critical period occurs at an early stage in pregnancy before it is customary for a pregnant woman to seek medical advice. In addition, many women experience nausea during pregnancy that depresses appetite and food intake and in many cases reduces the nutrients available for absorption to a critically low level. It is under such conditions that the mother who has had good dietary habits prior to conception has an advantage over her less well-fed counterpart who may not have entered pregnancy with such good reserves. By the end of the period of organogenesis the immune system, which allows the infant to combat infection, is beginning to develop.

Growth. The remaining seven months of pregnancy are known as the growth period. During this time the differentiated tissues continue to grow until they reach a functional size capable of supporting extrauterine life. The needs for nutrients at this time are high both quantitatively and qualitatively, although a deficiency will usually result only in a premature or smaller infant, rather than the serious deficiency symptoms observed as a result of a dietary lack during organogenesis.

Growth occurs in three phases. During the first, known as **hyperplasia,** increase in size is almost totally due to rapid increase in the number of cells. In the next phase, cell proliferation continues but there is also **hypertrophy,** an increase in cell size. In the final phase there is practically no further cell division, and growth is entirely due to an increase in cell size. The age that a particular tissue reaches the final stage at which cell number no longer increases varies from the first year of life for the brain to several years for the liver. A depressed increase in cell number due to an inadequate diet during a critical period of cell division cannot be reversed by an adequate diet at a later time. Conversely, if cell growth is depressed during a period of undernutrition, growth can be stimulated again when an adequate diet is available. Thus nutritional effects on cell number are permanent, whereas those on cell size are reversible.

Early in this growth stage, the placenta develops and takes over its role in providing nourishment for the fetus. The placenta, which weighs from 325 to 1000 g at birth, is the tissue through which the nutrients and oxygen needed for fetal growth are transferred from the maternal tissue to the fetus and through which fetal waste is excreted. No direct circulatory connection between the fetus and the mother exists, but in the placenta the two independent circulatory systems come in sufficiently close contact with one another that nutrients are able to pass from one to the other. In the placenta approximately 13 square meters of contact exist between the two circulations. For some nutrients, such as iron and vitamin C, the placenta allows the passage of sufficient amounts to meet the demands of the growing fetus even at the expense of maternal reserves. For others, such as thiamin, riboflavin, vitamin B_{12}, folacin, pyridoxine, and vitamin D, it allows the maternal and fetal tissue to compete. Vitamins A and E are present in lower amounts in fetal than in maternal blood. Thus the placenta becomes the regulator of fetal nutrition, the success of which depends not only on the nutrients available in the bloodstream of the mother but also on the way in which the placenta governs their transfer. In addition to promoting the active transfer of nutrients, the placenta is capable of synthesizing some body compounds. It is postulated that nutritional failure is as often the result of an inadequate supply of blood to the placenta as of a low level of nutrients in the maternal blood.

Table 16-1. Fetal weight and maternal weight gains at different ages in gestation

Age (weeks)	Total fetal weight (g)	Maternal gain (g)
10	5	650
12	30	
20	300	4000
24	900	
28	1240	
30	1484	8500
32	1750	
34	2278	
36	2750	
38	3052	
40	3230	12,500
42	3310	

Rate of growth

The rate of fetal growth is very slow in the first half of pregnancy. At a gestational age of 25 weeks the growth increment is only 6 g/day. By 34 weeks it is estimated at 40 g/day and by term has dropped again to 13 g. The fetal weights at various ages of gestation and comparable increases in maternal weight are shown in Table 16-1. During the first trimester growth is almost entirely in maternal tissue; during the second trimester gain is primarily in maternal tissue and in the third trimester in fetal tissue. Gain during the latter two periods is 350 to 450 g each week.

The relatively slow development of the human fetus means that nutritional deficiencies must prevail over a long period of time if they are to have a marked effect on fetal development. In contrast, many animals used in nutrition investigations develop at a very rapid rate, produce litters of larger size relative to maternal size, and thus are much more susceptible to short-term dietary deviations. A comparison of the rate of development and the relationship of litter size to maternal weight is shown in Fig. 16-2. It will be observed that mice produce a litter weighing 30% of maternal weight in three weeks, whereas the human mother takes nine months to develop a fetus representing 5% of her weight.

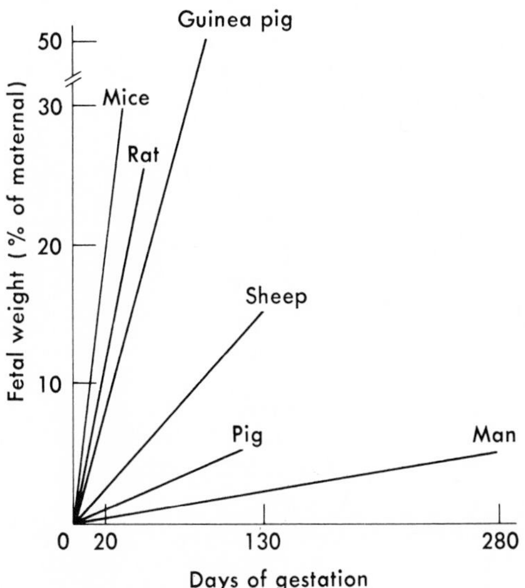

Fig. 16-2. Products of conception of six mammalian species in percentage of maternal weight.

Nutritive needs

The recommended increase over the normal nutrient needs of the mother to meet the demands of pregnancy varies from one nutrient to another, as shown in Table 16-2. For some nutrients, such as iron and vitamin A, the recommended intake allows the infant to accumulate sufficient amounts to establish a storage supply to last through the early stages of infancy. For others, such as vitamin D,

Table 16-2. Increase in nutritional requirements during pregnancy and lactation

Nutrient	Percentage increase over normal	
	Pregnancy	Lactation
Energy	15	25
Protein	65	43
Vitamin A	25	50
Vitamin D	+ +	+ +
Vitamin E	25	25
Ascorbic acid	33	33
Folacin	100	50
Niacin	15	31
Riboflavin	24	38
Thiamin	30	30
Pyridoxine	25	25
Cobalamin	33	33
Calcium	50	50
Phosphorus	50	62
Iodine	25	50
Iron	0 (+ suppl.)*	0
Magnesium	50	50
Zinc	33	53

+ + = No requirement for adult woman except during pregnancy and lactation.
*Supplement of 30 to 60 mg of elemental iron recommended.

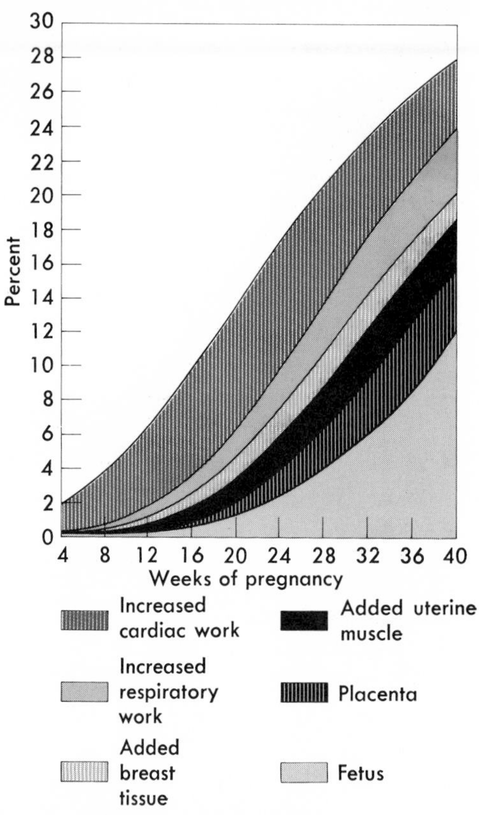

Fig. 16-3. Components of increased oxygen consumption in pregnancy. (From Hytten, F. E., and Leitch, I.: The physiology of human pregnancy, Philadelphia, 1963, F. A. Davis Co.)

ascorbic acid, and calcium, virtually no storage occurs in the infant's body prior to birth; thus the mother need provide only enough for fetal growth. The recommended increase to meet the nutritional stresses of pregnancy depends on many factors, such as the mechanism for adjusting to increased demands, the nature of the metabolic changes of pregnancy, and the nutrient reserves of the mother. The National Research Council recommended dietary allowances, which vary from 15% above normal for energy and niacin to 100% for folacin, are based on rather scanty information regarding quantitative needs. For a better understanding of the kind of dietary adjustment that may be necessary during pregnancy, the needs for each nutrient will be discussed separately.

Energy. During pregnancy caloric needs are influenced by several factors. The growth of the fetus, although very slow at first, calls for additional energy (40,000 kcal stored as fat and protein at birth), as does the growth of the placenta, the normal increase in maternal body size (including fat reserves of 35,000 kcal), the additional work of carrying the growing fetus, and the steady but slow rise in basal metabolism. On the other hand, the decreased activity of the mother depresses the caloric requirement.

Table 16-3. Components of maternal weight gain in pregnancy

Tissue	Weight (g)		Weight (lb)		
Fetus	3,150		7		Range, 5-10
Placenta	675		1.5		Relatively constant
Amniotic fluid	900		2		
Subtotal		3,725		10.5	
Mother					
Uterus	900		2		
Breasts	450		1		
Increase in blood volume	1,350		3		
Tissue fluids	1,350		3		
Fat	4,050		9		
Subtotal		8,100		18.0	
TOTAL		11,825		28.5	

It is estimated that the growth of the fetus and maternal tissue and their maintenance (the cost of increased cardiac output and respiration rate) calls for approximately 80,000 kcal. Normal energy requirements are reduced through deceased activity resulting in a net increased requirement of 24,000 to 30,000 kcal. Fig. 16-3 shows the components of the increased energy need of pregnancy. For some mothers who greatly reduce their activity a demand for an increase in energy may never occur in spite of the increased basal energy requirement and fetal growth needs of the last trimester.

Along with the growth of the developing fetus itself, a concurrent increase in the size of supporting maternal tissues occurs. The components of maternal weight gain shown on Table 16-3 indicate that a normal pregnancy calls for considerable weight gain over and above that represented by the size of the fetus. Thus, if the net gain in maternal weight is less than 9 to 11 kg, one must assume that the growth of the child as a parasite on the mother has caused a depletion of the mother's tissue reserves. A failure in the development of mammary structures and fat reserves during pregnancy may preclude a normal and successful lactation period. The pattern and components of weight gain during pregnancy are shown in Fig. 16-4.

Energy stored as fat in the maternal tissue is concentrated almost exclusively in fat depots, with virtually none occurring in the reproductive tissues other than the mammary gland. Fat that is deposited throughout the whole period of pregnancy acts as a buffer against food deprivation and prevents the catabolism of the mother's tissue. The increase in ketones that appear in the urine in late pregnancy suggests that fat reserves are being utilized to provide for the high energy needs of the rapidly growing fetus and to spare protein for tissue growth. The increase in body fat during pregnancy represents storage of sufficient energy to subsidize lactation at 300 kcal/day for four months.

In the first trimester the fetus accumulates no fat other than that which is part of the essential lipids in the cell wall and the nervous system. At 20 weeks the fetus contains only 0.5% fat, but this rises steadily to 3.5% at 28 weeks, 7.5% at 34 weeks; and 16% of body weight at term. Fat is synthesized by the fetus from glucose, which crosses the placental barrier readily. The only fatty acids to be

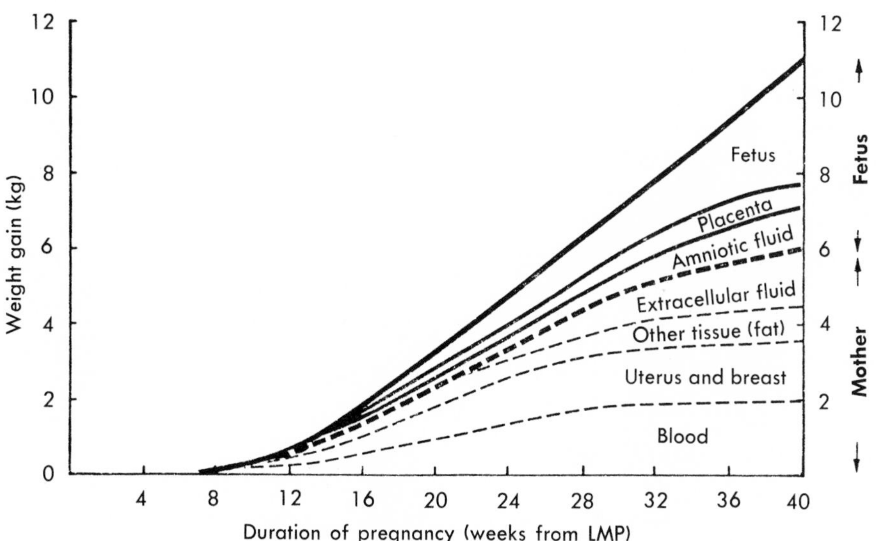

Fig. 16-4. Pattern and components of weight gain throughout the course of pregnancy. (From Pitkin, R. M.: Clin. Obstet. Gynecol. **19**:489, 1975.)

transferred from the mother to the child are the essential fatty acids. The rest are synthesized from glucose.

There has been much conflict in the literature regarding what constitutes a desirable gain in weight for a pregnant woman. The practice of allowing the mother unrestricted weight gain on the theory that she was "eating for two" was widely accepted in the early part of the century. The undesirable consequences of this regimen, such as toxemia, difficulties of labor with increased risk to the mother, and the birth of large babies who suffered many complications in early life, soon became evident. The proponents of unlimited weight gain were replaced by a group recommending caloric restriction sufficiently severe to limit weight gain to 4.5 to 5.5 kg, a regimen that resulted in equally undesirable consequences. Mothers who fail to gain weight in the second trimester are very likely to have premature deliveries, with increased risk to the health of the baby, and to experience toxemia or preeclampsia, with its symptoms of proteinuria, elevated blood pressure, headache, blurred vision, edema, and abnormalities in blood coagulation. Some edema, especially in the ankle region, is normal and in the absence of other symptoms is not considered suggestive of toxemia. Eclampsia with convulsive seizures is more common among women who are overweight at conception and those who gain excessively in the latter half of pregnancy. It is most severe, however, in women who are underweight at conception and who fail to gain weight. Women at greatest risk are those who experience a sudden and excessive weight gain, especially after the twenty-fourth week. Mothers who become eclamptic are frequently the ones who gain less than 7 kg or over 13 kg during gestation, especially during a first pregnancy.

The pattern of weight gain is as important as the total weight gain. In general, practically no gain in the first trimester followed by a steady increase of approximately 400 g is the normal course of pregnancy.

The relationship between weight gain and

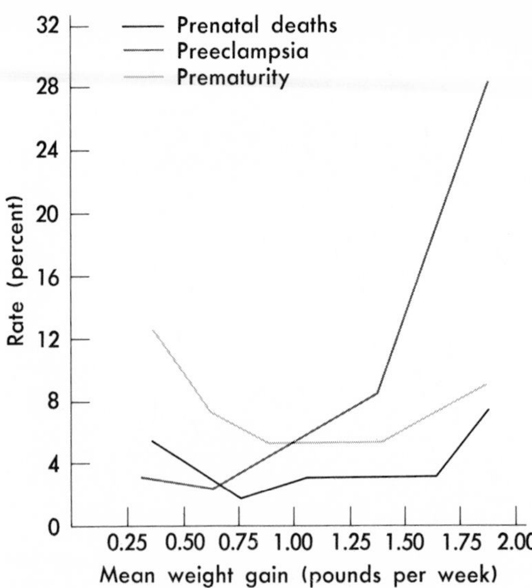

Fig. 16-5. Incidence of three major obstetrical complications by mean weight gain between 20 weeks and delivery. (From Hytten, F. E., and Leitch, I.: The physiology of human pregnancy, Philadelphia, 1963, F. A. Davis Co.)

complications of pregnancy is shown in Fig. 16-5. Research data showed that women consuming less than 1800 kcal a day were unable to maintain a positive nitrogen balance, which means that if the fetus continued to grow, it did so at the expense of maternal tissue that could not be replaced as fast as it was depleted.

For mothers on diets providing marginal energy, even a small daily increase in calories will result in an increase in fetal weight, which reduces the risk of morbidity and mortality in early life. The effect on a nutrient supplement of 20,000 kcal on the incidence of low–birth weight infants among Guatemalan women is shown in Fig. 16-6.

Many women restrict their weight gain in fear that a gain may remain a permanent weight increment. Studies show that about 4 kg of weight gained during pregnancy remains immediately after birth and only 2 kg at six weeks postpartum. All the gained weight is usually lost in six to eight months.

Although some workers maintain that the

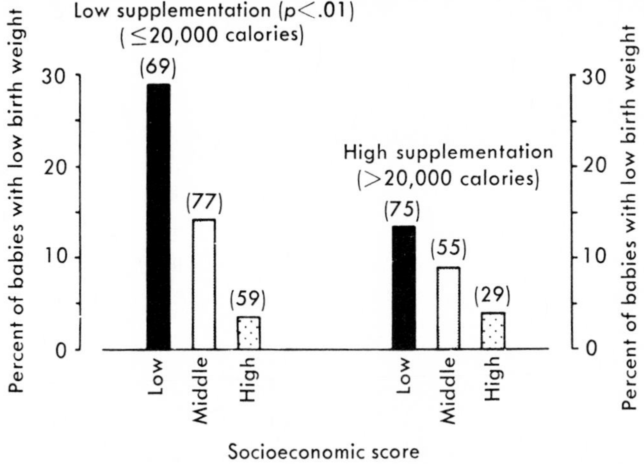

Fig. 16-6. Effect of caloric supplementation on relationship between socioeconomic score and proportion of babies with low birth weight. (From Lechtig, A., et al.: Am. J. Dis. Child. **129:**434, 1975; copyright 1975, American Medical Association.)

woman who is obese at the onset of pregnancy can successfully reduce her own body size without jeopardizing the health of the infant or herself if the qualitative aspects of the diet are guarded carefully, the preponderance of the evidence suggests that any major adjustments in the mother's weight should be undertaken under normal circumstances rather than during a period of nutritional stress such as pregnancy. Aside from the physiological stress produced by caloric restriction, the emotional tension accompanying it, especially in the face of a stimulated appetite, may have even more adverse effects. If weight gain is to be controlled, however, the only effective way to do it is through caloric restriction rather than by a restriction of salt or water intake.

The Food and Nutrition Board of the Committee on Maternal Nutrition of the National Research Council has concluded that a gain of 9 to 11 kg minimizes the risks of pregnancy and is most desirable in terms of the health of both the mother and baby.

After a careful evaluation of all relevant data the National Research Council has suggested that an additional 300 kcal daily in the last half of pregnancy will satisfy the energy demands of pregnancy and will lead to the desirable weight gain.

Protein. The National Research Council in establishing recommendations for protein intakes during pregnancy considered (1) estimates of the theoretical amounts of protein deposited in the fetus, placenta, and maternal tissues which amounts to 10 g/day; (2) data on nitrogen balance during pregnancy suggesting a retention twice estimates; (3) evidence that women with intakes throughout pregnancy higher than estimated needs have better reproductive histories; and (4) evidence that there is increased risk associated with low protein intakes. The NRC recommends that a pregnant woman have an additional 30 g of protein *throughout* pregnancy. FAO has suggested a much smaller increase of 9 g above normal needs.

Protein intake of the mother influences the birth length of the fetus within the limits determined by heredity. Taller babies are born to mothers with high-protein diets than to those with limited protein intake. The smaller babies born to mothers on diets inadequate in protein are more susceptible to the hazards of early life and have a decreased chance of survival. Recent research showed that a pregnant adolescent requires 1.25 g of protein per kilogram of body weight to maintain nitrogen balance.

Total weight gain during pregnancy includes 1 kg of protein, half of which is in fetal tissue. The greater part of this protein has been deposited at a rate of 4.5 to 5.7 g/day during the last half of pregnancy when the growth hormone produced during pregnancy stimulates the retention of nitrogen. Protein is transferred to the fetus in the form of amino acids. Since the fetus cannot oxidize amino acids, it appears that they are used exclusively for protein synthesis.

There is little storage of protein in maternal tissues other than reproductive tissues. When dietary protein is restricted, it is the amount in storage that is reduced, rather than the amount transferred to the fetus. The reserve of energy in the form of fat helps to spare protein during rapid fetal growth.

Protein restriction during fetal life is associated with a decrease in the number of cells in tissues at the time of birth. This is particularly serious in the case of the brain, which is relatively well developed in prenatal life and may be irreversibly stunted. This is in contrast to other tissues that achieve less of their mature size in the prenatal period and relatively more during postnatal development.

Studies on rats and humans suggested that a protein and caloric deficiency during gestation results in poor utilization of food by the offspring after birth and a failure to ever compensate for early food deprivation.

In addition to the amino acids that are transferred to the fetus, large protein molecules such as antibodies also cross the placental barrier and give the infant passive immunity to the antigens to which the mother has been exposed.

Calcium. Although the infant's bones are poorly calcified at the time of birth, a demand still exists for an appreciable amount of calcium for fetal development. The demand of approximately 7 mg a day for the first trimester increases to 110 mg a day in the second trimester and jumps to 350 mg in the last trimester. This leads to the deposition of approximately 30 g of calcium in the body of the newborn infant. About 80% of this occurs in the third trimester. Although the mother has more than 1000 g of calcium to draw on, she becomes more efficient in absorbing calcium. The decrease in absorption that occurs under conditions of emotional stress such as may prevail among unwilling mothers, may be counterbalanced by the twofold increase in absorption that is a normal response to the demands of pregnancy.

It is estimated that about 30% of fetal calcium has been obtained from maternal stores. The amount of dietary calcium needed is reduced if vitamin D is available and is increased if it is not. Ideally, there should be a storage rather than a depletion of calcium in the mother's tissues during pregnancy to help anticipate the demands for calcium, which are particularly high during lactation, but there is no evidence that this occurs. Although bones are poorly calcified at birth, the teeth begin to calcify at 5 months of gestation. To counteract any tendency toward osteomalacia, the maternal diet should contain reasonable calcium, no excess of phytic acid, and adequate vitamin D.

Iron. Since infants are born with high hemoglobin levels of 18 to 22 g/dl of blood and with a supply of iron stored in the liver to last from three to six months, the maternal organism transfers about 300 mg of iron to the fetus during gestation. In addition to this need for fetal growth, 70 mg are required for the placenta, 500 mg for the formation of hemoglobin, which is the result of the increase in maternal blood volume, and 280 mg to replace basal losses in skin, hair, and sweat. Of this total of over 1100 mg that represents almost twice the total iron reserves of the adult female, a saving of 100 to 200 mg is effected by the absence of menstrual losses. In addition, about 230 mg of the iron in the extra hemoglobin will be returned to the iron pools when the blood volume returns to normal after delivery. A need still exists however, for about 1 mg of iron a day over and above the needs of the nonpregnant woman if a 30% increase in red cells is to occur. If dietary iron is not available to meet this need, iron stores will be depleted, and there will be reduction in the expansion of red cell mass, rather than an impairment of fetal iron reserves. If the mother has no iron reserves, as appears to be the case in many young women, especially teenagers, maternal hemoglobin levels will drop and may reach the level of 10 g/dl, which is considered indicative of anemia in the pregnant woman.

In spite of the fact that the usual rate of iron absorption of 10% of dietary intake increases to 25% to 30% in the second half of pregnancy, the Food and Nutrition Board felt that the recommended dietary allowance of 18 mg suggested for the nonpregnant woman should be supplemented with 30 to 60 mg of elemental iron (150 to 300 mg of ferrous sulfate) to maintain maternal reserves and to meet fetal requirements during pregnancy. An increase in the amount of the protein transferrin, which influences the capacity for iron absorption, is observed during pregnancy. The absorption of dietary iron observed in the last trimester of pregnancy results in as much as 3.5 mg of iron being retained by the fetus each day. As under normal conditions, the amount of iron absorbed is influenced by the need for it and the food source. Iron from cereals is poorly absorbed and that from muscle is readily available. Such observations are of special significance in countries where cereals are the staple item in the diet.

It is believed that the best method of combating iron deficiency in pregnancy is to promote high intakes of available iron by the nonpregnant woman so that she enters pregnancy with at least 300 mg of iron stored. Some investigators have found that the injection of a single large dose of iron at the beginning of pregnancy builds iron stores and protects against iron depletion throughout pregnancy. Such a procedure may be justified in the light of the finding that lack of patient cooperation in taking iron is an important factor in the failure of iron supplementation in pregnancy. One study showed that women whose hemoglobin levels stayed below 12 g/dl had not been taking supplements despite claims to the contrary and the fact that the level given (130 mg) did not cause side effects.

Macrocytic (large cell) anemia, which frequently occurs in pregnancy, is believed to be caused by a relatively inadequate intake of dietary folate. There are indications that iron deficiency puts additional stress on folate metabolism and may convert a subclinical folate deficiency into a megaloblastic anemia.

Sodium. During pregnancy the increase in extracellular fluids calls for an increase in body sodium amounting to 500 to 900 mEq (or 11.5 to 20.7 g). As a result, rather than advising a restriction in sodium intake during pregnancy as has been a long-standing practice, obstetricians are recognizing the increased need. When salt is restricted, the maternal organism undergoes a series of hormonal and biochemical changes that help conserve sodium. When blood sodium levels drop, the kidneys produce more of the hormone renin. This in turn acts on a protein in the blood to convert it to angiotensin. The adrenal gland responds to the presence of angiotensin to produce more of the hormone aldosterone. Aldosterone acts on the kidneys to stimulate them to reabsorb and hence conserve more of the sodium in the blood being filtered through them. Thus the pregnant woman has a series of mechanisms to help her retain the sodium she obviously needs.

Because they lead to a loss of sodium, the use of diuretics during pregnancy should be discouraged. The use of lithium chloride as a salt substitute should likewise be discouraged because of evidence of hazards to pregnant women.

Iodine. Levels of iodine that will prevent goiter under normal circumstances frequently prove inadequate in pregnancy, leading to goiter in the mother, especially an adolescent mother. The relative deficiency may be due in part to the increased urinary losses of iodine observed in pregnancy.

When the mother has goiter, the chances that the child will develop goiter are increased ten times. In addition, the incidence of cretinism, the most severe form of iodine deficiency, among infants rises to 1% when the incidence of goiter among mothers reaches 55%.

In many parts of the country, diets are adequate in iodine only when iodized salt is used in cooking. Should salt intake be restricted in an attempt to control toxemia of pregnancy, the woman is deprived of her only reliable source of iodine and should be encouraged to use some other supplementary source as a protection against goiter. Iodine-containing drugs, however, should be avoided.

Other mineral elements. Little work has been done to determine quantitative needs for other mineral elements during pregnancy, but is seems reasonable to suggest that the body's ability to adapt to a state of stress by improved absorption and decreased excretion will take care of some but not necessary all of the additional needs for mineral elements. Evidence that infants develop teeth with increased resistance to dental caries when the mother's diet contains adequate fluorine is controversial. The fact that the tooth buds have little enamel suggest that the benefits may be minimal.

Low levels of zinc, magnesium, and manganese have all been associated with undesirable changes in the developing fetus. Excessively high levels also have adverse consequences. Although levels used in experimental studies far exceed those found in normal dietaries, these findings should be kept in mind when dietary supplementation or food enrichment is considered. Blood levels of copper and zinc are two and a half times higher in pregnant than in nonpregnant women.

Fat-soluble vitamins. Although it is fairly well established that the pregnant animal has a series of adaptive mechanisms to cope with increased demands for minerals during pregnancy, there is no evidence that such a system of adaptation exists for vitamins.

Vitamin A. Aside from the fact that animals on vitamin A-deficient diets have a poor reproductive performance, little is known about the need for vitamin A during pregnancy.

A child is born with a reserve of 24,000 IU, which can be provided by a small increase to 5000 IU (1000 RE) per day, especially if some is preformed vitamin A. Lack of vitamin A during the early stages of fetal development in animals has been implicated in cleft palate and skeletal and eye defects. Similar relationships in humans have not been established.

Vitamin D. The need for vitamin D is set at 400 IU/day to promote the absorption and utilization of calcium and phosphorus, which are so essential in bone formation. Unless milk fortified with vitamin D or a combination of other foods to which vitamin D has been added is used, a normal diet cannot be relied on to provide adequate amounts for women living in the temperate zone. Supplements providing 400 IU/day are recommended. However, evidence linking arteriosclerosis, mental retardation and renal acidosis in infants with excessive intakes by the mother during pregnancy suggests caution in the use of supplements along with fortified foods. If milk fortified with 400 IU of vitamin D per quart is used, there is no need for an additional source of the nutrient; in fact, it should be avoided.

Vitamin E. The observation of a role of vitamin E in promoting normal reproduction and reducing the number of spontaneous abortions and stillbirths in animals led to many studies to elucidate a similar role in humans. So far scientists have been unable to determine any unique role of the tocopherols in human reproduction, and, in spite of some evidence that tocopherol may be beneficial to women who have experienced repeated spontaneous abortions or failure to conceive, it has not been shown that vitamin E deficiency is responsible for reproductive failure. No evidence of any increased need for vitamin E in pregnancy has been found, and, as under normal conditions, the requirement appears to be adequately met by a balanced diet, with little likelihood of a deficiency unless the diet contains abnormally high amounts of polyunsaturated fatty acids. Little vitamin E crosses the placenta; therefore the human infant has low tissue concentrations. Although the effect of pregnancy on vitamin E requirements has not been established, the RDA are set at 15 IU/day, an increase of 3 IU above normal requirements.

Vitamin K. As the vitamin concerned with the synthesis of prothrombin necessary for normal coagulation of the blood, vitamin K has long been considered to play a role in preventing neonatal hemorrhaging, which was often fatal to either the mother or the fetus. It became routine practice to give menadione (synthetic vitamin K) orally to the mother in the last several weeks of pregnancy or even by injection during labor to prevent hemorrhage. However, evidence of some adverse effects (such as hyperbilirubinemia, especially in premature infants) from the use of large doses of the synthetic form has led to the recommendation that if a synthetic analogue is given it should be given in a controlled dose to the mother at a level sufficiently high to prevent hemorrhage but low enough to preclude adverse reactions. As a result, the inclusion of menadione in over-the-counter supplements for pregnancy is prohibited. Similar and safe protection is afforded by giving the natural form of the vitamin either by injection or orally to the infant or to the mother.

Water-soluble vitamins. Since water-soluble vitamins are not stored to any appreciable extent, the pregnant woman must rely on a daily intake sufficiently high to meet the added requirements of pregnancy.

Thiamin. The relationship between thiamin needs and caloric intake remains the same during pregnancy as under normal circumstances, thus calling for a 30% increase of 0.3 mg. The normal urinary excretion of thiamin drops, indicating that more is being retained and used by the tissues. Some investigations have shown that thiamin helps relieve the nausea of pregnancy.

Riboflavin. The increase in body size with the growth of the fetus and accessory tissues calls for an increase in riboflavin of 25%, which is present in higher amounts in fetal than in maternal blood.

Animal studies have shown that a lack of riboflavin in the thirteenth and fourteenth embryonic days interferes with cartilage formation, resulting in skeletal malformations such as shortening of the long bones and a fusion of the ribs.

Pyridoxine. Women under the normal stress of pregnancy exhibit an altered tryptophan metabolism with increased excretion of xanthurenic acid, decreased ability to handle sodium, and altered cell growth, all of which can be corrected by giving from 1.0 to 2.5 mg of additional pyridoxine daily.

There is an active transport of pyridoxine to the fetus to maintain a level in fetal blood five times that in maternal blood. Failure of pyridoxine to cross the placenta has been attributed to the lack of two enzymes—one needed to add phosphorus to transport it and one to convert it to pyridoxal, the form in which the placenta uses it. Levels of pyridoxine about a third of normal have been found in toxemia of pregnancy. Since it has been established that women taking contraceptive pills have an increased need for pyridoxine (vitamin B_6), it is possible that women who have been on the pill enter pregnancy with inadequate reserves and continue to have difficulty absorbing it. Although no experimental evidence exists to indicate the exact amount required to meet the needs of pregnancy, the RDA has been increased by 0.5 mg above that recommended for the nonpregnant woman. A study of 493 pregnant women showing that about 60% had suboptimal supplies of pyridoxine has led to the conclusion that pregnant women would benefit from supplementation to maintain enzyme saturation.

Pyridoxine has been used experimentally to help control the nausea of pregnancy, but the results, though encouraging for some individuals, have not been conclusive and no satisfactory theory explains this phenomenon.

Folic acid. Folate intake during pregnancy has been associated primarily with the promotion of normal fetal growth and the prevention of a macrocytic anemia of pregnancy. The need for folic acid in pregnancy is known to increase, and the recommended daily allowance is twice that of nonpregnant women. From 200 to 400 μg of supplementary folic acid is indicated for high-risk women such as those who have had many pregnancies and chronic hemolytic anemia. This amount is available only by prescription.

Although this level of intake may prevent the diagnosis of pernicious anemia, the incidence of undiagnosed cases is believed to be sufficiently low that the problem is minor. Evidence exists of a marked decrease in folate absorption and an increase in urinary excretion during pregnancy, which may contribute to the depletion of maternal reserves. Scientific opinion suggests that folic acid deficiency is a major cause for concern in pregnancy.

The importance of folic acid in promoting a normal pregnancy is emphasized by the fact that the use of a folic acid antagonist, aminopterin, induces the resorption of fetuses in animals. Its use in humans does not lead to resorption or abortion of a fetus but rather to the birth of a child with congenital malformations such as harelip, cleft palate, or hydrocephalus.

Current information suggests that complications such as abruptio placentae, hemorrhage, and fetal malformation previously identified as results of folic acid deficiency cannot be alleviated or prevented by folic acid supplementation.

Vitamin B_{12}. It has been confirmed that the infant is parasitic on the mother for vitamin B_{12}, as evidenced by the higher levels found in fetal blood than maternal blood even when maternal levels are depleted. Low maternal levels are associated with prematurity and occur more often in smokers than in nonsmokers.

The capacity to absorb vitamin B_{12} is increased in pregnancy, but a large amount is transferred to the fetus. The recommended daily intake of vitamin B_{12} to maintain constant serum levels is 4 μg. If these amounts are not supplied, the serum vitamin B_{12} levels drop but return to normal without supplementation after pregnancy.

Ascorbic acid. The NCR recommended allowances for ascorbic acid are increased by 15 mg during pregnancy, although there is little evidence on which to base this figure.

Table 16-4. Recommended dietary allowances during pregnancy

	FAO	RDA	British	Canadian
Energy (kcal)	2485	2300	2400	+500
Protein (g)	38	76	60	47.5
Calcium (g)	1.0-1.2	1.2	1.2	1.2
Iron (mg)	14-28	18	15	13
Vitamin A (IU)	2500	5000	2500	4200
Vitamin D (IU)	400	400	400	
Thiamin (mg)	1.0	1.3	1.0	0.3/100 kcal + 0.15
Riboflavin (mg)	1.4	1.5	1.6	0.5/100 kcal + 0.25
Pyridoxine (mg)	400	2.5		
Folate (μg)		800		
Vitamin B_{12} (μg)	403.0	4.0		
Ascorbic acid (mg)		60	60	40

Ascorbic acid does pass the placental barrier freely, and serum values of a fetus have been established at two to four times that of the mother. Some evidence has been established to indicate that the placenta is capable of synthesizing ascorbic acid, which could account for the higher levels in fetal tissues. Low maternal intakes of ascorbic acid are associated with premature rupture of fetal membranes and increased neonatal death rates. A comparison of the recommended dietary intakes during pregnancy from various groups is shown in Table 16-4.

Role of nutritional supplements during pregnancy

The reproductive period is one in which heavy demands are made on the mother to provide the nutrients needed for normal fetal development. It has been shown that the increase in need varies from one nutrient to another with a small increase for calories. To provide the amount of protein, minerals, and vitamins recommended without exceeding the caloric allowance, a woman must choose her food carefully and almost exclusively from protective foods (i.e., those that provide as high a percentage of the day's requirements of as least two nutrients as they do of calories).

The selection of a diet adequate for pregnancy is relatively easy if one is concerned with an isolated day or two, but the pregnant woman must maintain this high level of nutritive intake for the 280 days of the normal gestation period. To do this, she must constantly be conscious of her food choices. The woman who takes such a responsibility seriously is subjecting herself to a constant pressure during a period that is frequently characterized by at least some degree of emotional stress. To allow her a little more freedom in the selection of food and an occasional indulgence in a favorite low nutrient food, it may be reasonable to suggest that she use a supplement that provides a balanced formula at protective levels—possibly 25% of the day's recommended allowance.

Because of the competitive nature of the drug market, most manufacturers found it necessary to market supplements providing an excessive amount of the nutrients needed, to include many for which there is little likelihood of a deficiency occurring even in pregnancy, or to include ineffectual amounts of others. The use of such supplements was not only an economic waste and unnecessary from a nutritional point of view but also a practice that could produce nutritional imbalances, especially if the product contained mineral elements, and could adversely affect the fetus if the fat-soluble vitamins were too high. The FDA ruled in 1977 that nutritional supplements for pregnant women provide between 50% and 150% of the U.S. RDA for ten vitamins and five minerals for which evidence of need had been established.

Iron supplements, often not incorporated in the multivitamin-mineral preparations, are recommended for all women but especially those whose hemoglobin drops below 10.5 g/dl, a level indicative of depletion of iron reserves as well as hemodilution. Therapeutic iron in doses of 30 to 60 mg as ferrous sulfate or ferrous gluconate is most frequently recommended. Calcium to meet the needs of the growing fetus can be provided in calcium supplements, but the amounts in routine vitamin-mineral preparations are seldom significant.

One additional basis for caution in the use of high-level nutritional supplementation during pregnancy has been brought to light with the observation that infants may become conditioned to a high intake during fetal life if the intake of the maternal organism is high. This may be reflected in an increased need in the postnatal period. This has been advanced as a possible explanation for the increase in infantile scurvy in technically advanced countries. The toxic effects of too much of the fat-soluble vitamins A and D have been well documented.

Some research workers believe that the mother can adapt to such a wide range of nutrient intake during the stress of pregnancy that there is no need for supplementation.

Pica or geophagia, the practice of eating nonnutritive substances such as clay or laundry starch, is relatively common in pregnant women. The hypothesis that these food cravings represented sources of a particular nutrient that was lacking in the diet has not been substantiated by research. One study reported consumption of up to 1 kg of laundry starch a day. Nutrients such as calcium and iron found in some of the substances craved are not in a form that can be utilized. On the other hand, it has not been possible to demonstrate any adverse effects from the practice.

Dietary modifications in pregnancy

In addition to a need to modify the normal diet pattern to provide for the quantitative needs for nutrients, other modifications may have value. From the fifth to fourteenth week of pregnancy when 75% of women experience nausea and when appetite may be disturbed, the consumption of smaller and more frequent meals has been helpful to many women. The same pattern is useful in the latter part of pregnancy when the problem is one of discomfort after large meals because of crowding of the abdominal cavity.

Between the fourth and seventh months particularly, many women experience an insatiable appetite. Eating a small meal slightly before the time when hunger sensations become most severe has been found a useful method of controlling the total intake. It is important to maintain food intake at a level that results in a steady gain of 400 g/week in the second and third trimesters.

The use of a diet relatively high in bulk may be helpful in maintaining normal gastric motility at a time when a tendency toward constipation occurs.

The way in which the nutritive needs of pregnancy are met will vary with the preferred food habits or likes and dislikes of the woman. Usually a diet containing three cups of milk or its equivalent, two servings of meat, fish, poultry, or eggs, a dark green or yellow vegetable, and a generous serving of a citrus fruit daily will provide a foundation for a nutritionally adequate diet.

EFFECT OF NUTRITION ON PREGNANCY

It has been fairly well established that the nutritional status of the mother at the time of conception is as important for the outcome of pregnancy as is the diet during the period of gestation. The nutritional status of the mother at conception is generally a reflection of long-standing food habits that change in relatively few women during pregnancy in spite of the motivation one would expect to prevail at this time. Because of the influence of many factors, such as the maternal age, birth rate, birth interval, and metabolic interrelationships, it is difficult to delineate specific dietary effects.

The impact of the nutrition of the mother on the course of pregnancy and the condition of the infant at birth has been the subject of many investigations, but not all have led to the same conclusions. The now classic study by Burke, which has been described in Chapter 1, points most conclusively to a relationship between maternal diet and well-being of the infant. The chances of a child with a high pediatric rating being born to a mother with a good or excellent diet are much better than when the maternal diet is rated as poor or very poor. Studying Canadian women, Ebbs and co-workers found a similar relationship, with mothers on good diets experiencing few complications during pregnancy and giving birth to infants with a greater chance of surviving the neonatal period. More recently, however, a group of investigators at Vanderbilt University failed to demonstrate a relationship between quality of maternal diet and the course and outcome of pregnancy. They believed that complications of pregnancy led to suboptimal intakes rather than the converse. Although they found a relationship between diet and the course of pregnancy only at dietary intakes of less than 1500 kcal and 50 g of protein, they emphasized that these findings should not be interpreted to mean that good nutritional practices should not be encouraged. None of the subjects in their study had markedly suboptimal diets; therefore they may have entered pregnancy in sufficiently good nutritional status to provide a buffer against the stress of pregnancy.

Thomson in England in 1959 was unable to demonstrate any difference in the diet of mothers who had a normal clinical history during pregnancy and those who experienced some clinical abnormality. No relationship was found between diet and the duration of gestation, the birth weight of the infant, fetal malformation, perinatal deaths, or failure of lactation. From data in this study one can conclude that the abnormalities of reproduction were not caused by dietary deficiencies. However, this must not be interpreted to mean that dietary inadequacies could not cause abnormalities of pregnancy.

In 1963 after reviewing 4300 obstetrical cases, Thomson and Billewicz found that the incidence of prematurity, cesarean section, and perinatal deaths increased as the rating of the maternal health and physique fell. Their results are shown in Table 16-5.

Currently there are studies underway in the United States, Guatemala, and Taiwan to study the relationship of diet to the course of pregnancy. Results indicate that in lower socioeconomic groups the health of the mother and child is enhanced by the provision of adequate calories.

Other investigators have also indicated a relationship between specific dietary factors and specific complications of pregnancy. Toxemia of pregnancy is often associated with diets low in protein or pyridoxine, failure to gain enough weight, or too large a weight gain. The incidence of spontaneous abortion in early pregnancy among women with low-protein diets is almost twice as high as it is in women with high-protein diets.

The effect of diet prior to pregnancy can be illustrated from data on babies born during a period of wartime starvation in two different countries— Holland and Russia. In Holland the children born during a hunger period had been conceived prior to the period by mothers whose previous diet had been good. The babies were shorter and 10% lighter than babies born to mothers whose diets were adequate throughout pregnancy, but there was

Table 16-5. Incidence of obstetric abnormalities in Aberdeen primigravidas by maternal health and physique, as assessed at the first antenatal examination (twin pregnancies excluded)*

	Maternal health and physique			
	Very good	Good	Fair	Poor; very poor
Prematurity† (%)	5.1	6.4	10.4	12.1
Cesarean section (%)	2.7	3.5	4.2	5.4
Perinatal deaths per 1000 births	26.9	29.2	44.8	62.8
Number of subjects	707	2088	1294	223
Percentage tall (5 feet 4 inches or more)	42	29	18	13
Percentage short (under 5 feet 1 inch)	10	20	30	48

*From Thomson, A. M., and Billewicz, W. Z.: Nutritional status, maternal physique and reproductive efficiency, Proc. Nutr. Soc. **22**:55, 1963.
†Birth weight of baby 2500 g or less.

a decrease in stillbirths (20%), prematurity, and congenital malformation, all indications of the protective effect that a good diet prior to pregnancy may exert during the course of pregnancy. In contrast, mothers whose babies were born during the siege of Leningrad and whose diets had been poor prior to pregnancy experienced a stillbirth rate double the normal rate, a 41% incidence of prematurity among live births, and a 31% incidence of neonatal deaths among low–birth weight infants. A reduced rate of conception also occurred.

Additional evidence suggesting that the lifetime diet habits of the mother influence the outcome of pregnancy is advanced by Thomson, who found a prematurity rate of 32 per 1000 births and a neonatal death rate of 19 per 1000 births in children born to mothers over 1.6 m (64 inches) tall. These, he assumed, represented women who had been relatively well nourished throughout their lives. Similar statistics on women under 1.5 m (61 inches) tall who may have been less well nourished during their own growth period show a threefold increase in prematurity, with 91 per 1000 infants weighing less than 2500 g and a doubled incidence of neonatal deaths. Many other studies have suggested that the better the state of nutrition of the mother prior to or at the time of conception, the greater the chance of normal pregnancy leading to the birth of a healthy child.

LACTATION

In spite of the demonstrated advantages of human milk in infant feeding, in 1976 breast-feeding was practiced by less than half of all mothers in the United States, and the use of cow's milk formula is widespread.

The decision to breast- or bottle-feed an infant is one often surrounded with much emotion. The advantages of breast-feeding will be discussed in greater detail in Chapter 17, but some of the more cogent considerations are that it represents a very satisfying emotional experience for the mother, provides a source of nourishment uniquely suited to the growth demands and physiological capacity of the human infant, is a foolproof method that can be duplicated only by intelligent, carefully formulated, artificial feeding, and seldom, if ever, causes allergic reactions—an especially important consideration for parents with a family history of allergy. The decision to breast-feed is generally made before conception and certainly no later than the early part of pregnancy. For mothers who do not have a total commitment the attitudes of medical personnel at the time of delivery and opportunity to be in contact with the baby immediately following delivery become critical factors in the decision. Once the decision has been made the likelihood of success depends not only on the health and nutritional status of the mother but also on the mother's attitude toward breast-feeding, her understanding of the process of lactation, and the support and encouragement she receives from medical personnel and the family.

Nutritive needs

The nutritive demands on the mother during lactation far exceed those of pregnancy (Table 16-2), although she may cease to feel the responsibility of "eating for two." A normally developing infant doubles its birth weight accumulated in nine months of pregnancy in four months of life—evidence of the demands that the breast-fed infant makes on the mother. Milk secreted in one month represents more kilocalories than the net energy cost of pregnancy.

The health of the mother who is lactating successfully can be assured only if her own nutritive intake is satisfactory. In most cases a severe deficiency of a nutrient in the maternal diet will be reflected in a decreased secretion of milk, but in a few instances milk of inferior quality will be produced.

The NRC recommendations for dietary intakes during lactation are based on even less data on quantitative needs than are those for pregnancy. It is fairly well established that these levels will support the average production of 850 ml of milk, but it is entirely possible that satisfactory lactation can be maintained on somewhat lower levels of intake. Evidence also exists that many women produce much more than 850 ml of milk. For instance, one study among Budapest mothers of 19 to 23 years of age showed an average secretion of 1029 ml at three weeks, 1263 at seven weeks, and 1492 at fourteen weeks, with some mothers secreting over 2500 ml.

Recommended allowances

An adequate diet during pregnancy, which results in the accumulation of reserves of many nutrients, is one of the best bases for the initiation of breast-feeding, but the nutritional goals for successful continuation of lactation are less obvious. Lack of clear-cut information on the nutritive composition of milk, the volume of milk produced, and the efficiency of milk production has complicated the task of arriving at recommended levels of nutrients in the maternal diet to allow adequate milk production. There is lack of agreement about what constitutes normal composition of either colostrum, transitional, or mature milk, but just as cows of different genetic makeup secrete milks of different nutritive composition, human mothers with still greater biochemical, physiological, and psychological individuality can be expected to produce milks of varying composition. Analyses of human milk have shown considerable variation in composition not only among women but also in the same woman. The amount of some nutrients varies from day to day and from one time of the day to another. For other nutrients the composition remains constant. The fact that many mothers, especially in developing countries, are able to maintain a prolonged and satisfactory lactation period on diets well below currently accepted standards suggests a reappraisal of nutritional goals for lactating women. Since it is possible that in these cases lactation has been carried on at the expense of maternal reserves, which may be depleted to the point of endangering the maternal health, high standards for the maintenance of a satisfactory level of milk production are justified.

In general, the major constituents in human milk are maintained at the expense of the mother's stores while the content of vitamins and to a lesser extent minerals is more dependent on dietary intake. The basis for current standards will be discussed for individual nutrients. Table 16-2 shows the suggested increase in nutritive intake for lactation over that required under normal conditions. The increase suggested can be met by the equivalent of an additional meal of approximately 500 kcal of protective foods each day.

Energy. The energy required to provide for the needs of lactation is proportional to the amount of milk produced and will vary considerably from one woman to another. In general, 90 kcal are required for every 100 ml of milk produced. Thus, for the woman who secretes the typical 850 ml per day, energy needs are increased by 750 kcal. Of this, 150 kcal represent the energy required in the synthesis and secretion of the milk and the remaining 600 kcal the energy content of the milk itself. Since the 4 kg of fat stored during pregnancy represents a reserve of 200 to 400 kcal/day, recommended intake has been set at 500 kcal above normal. The long-standing belief that the mammary gland is only 60% efficient in transferring energy to milk has been challenged by data suggesting 80% efficiency.

Six months of lactation have an energy cost of 135,000 kcal, 100,000 above the amount stored in fat during pregnancy.

In addition to the energy needed to produce sufficient milk to meet the demands of a rapidly growing baby, the mother may have an increased energy requirement created by her return to a more active routine in caring for a small child.

Protein. Since human milk contains 1.0 to 1.5 g of protein per deciliter, the secretion of 850 ml of milk calls for about 10 g of protein and 1200 ml for 15 g. This assumes a protein of high biological value. To make allowances for consumption of less than ideal protein, the recommended dietary allowances have been set at 20 g above normal needs. The FAO in proposing practical allowances recommends that intake be increased by 17 g. Increasing the protein content of the mother's diet above a certain low level (approximately 35 g) does not result in an increased protein content of the milk secreted. Its effect on the quality of milk produced has not been ascertained.

Fat. No recommendations are made regarding the level of fat in the diet of a lactating woman. The amount of fat in the milk is not influenced by the amount in the mother's diet, but the character of the fat does reflect composition of her diet. The change in the American diet to one with an increasing proportion of polyunsaturated fatty acids has resulted in a similar increase in the P/S ratio of human milk. Medium-chain saturated fatty acids appear when the diet is high in carbohydrate and decrease when a large percentage of the calories comes from fat. Longer-chain and polyunsaturated fatty acids are derived from ingested fat. Human milk contains mostly medium-chain fatty acids and, in contrast to cow's milk, has virtually none with fewer than 10 carbon atoms. Human milk provides from 6% to 9% of its calories in the form of linoleic acid, most of which comes from the polyunsaturated fatty acids in the mother's diet.

Calcium. Although human milk contains only a fourth the level of calcium of cow's milk, normal milk production requires 250 mg. Even although calcium absorption improves when needs are greater, it is recommended that a lactating woman obtain an additional 400 mg from dietary sources to prevent depletion of her own calcium stores. The calcium content of milk will vary from one mother to another, but it is not influenced by the level of calcium in her diet.

Iron. Since relatively little iron is transferred to the infant through milk, the need for iron in the maternal diet does not increase above that for pregnancy.

The low level of iron in human milk may be the level that is best for assuring a good immune response in infants. Neither the Recommended Dietary Allowances nor the FAO/WHO standards call for any increase in dietary iron over the nonpregnant state.

The amount that does occur in human milk is independent of maternal intake. This iron is sufficiently well utilized that in spite of the fact that there is no increase in total body iron until age 4 months, the normal drop in hemoglobin levels may be delayed. This is especially true if adequate copper is present.

Thiamin. Thiamin is one nutrient for which a deficiency in the mother's diet is reflected in the production of a milk low in the nutrient rather than in a diminished output of milk. In addition, a mother whose diet is very low in thiamin may secrete a glyoxal, which accumulates in thiamin deficiency. The presence of this potentially toxic substance along with a low thiamin content in milk is associated with infantile beriberi. An intake of 0.5 mg/1000 kcal is recommended for the production of a milk with adequate thiamin levels. Although cow's milk may have a higher content than human milk, the fact that this heat-labile vitamin is destroyed during pasteurization and sterilization of the formula makes human milk a more dependable source.

Riboflavin. Milk is one of the most dependable sources of riboflavin in the adult diet, and human milk provides it for the infant. The mean content of 0.04 mg/dl of milk, which reflects dietary intake, would require that 0.34 mg be transferred to human milk each day. Since only 70% of additional riboflavin is utilized in milk production, it is recommended that the nursing mother increase her intake by 0.5 mg above normal.

Ascorbic acid. The amount of ascorbic acid in human milk is higher that that in cow's milk, which because of losses during heat processing, is incapable of meeting the needs of the infant after the first two weeks. The transfer of ascorbic acid to human milk calls for a maternal intake of 60 mg, which is easily obtained from a serving of citrus fruit or juice.

Vitamin B_6. The amount of pyridoxine in human milk is lower in women consuming less than 2.5 mg a day than in those consuming more. Intakes above this level, however, do not result in any further increase in the amount in milk.

Folic acid. The high incidence of folate deficient megaloblastic anemia in lactating women suggests that lactation imposes a drain on maternal reserves. This problem is complicated by the fact that folate deficiency is the most prevalent nutritional problem during pregnancy with the result that many women enter lactation with practically no reserves.

Vitamin B_{12}. The ingestion of Vitamin B_{12} is reflected in an increase in the vitamin in milk from one to six days later.

Vitamin A. Although most infants have a fair reserve of vitamin A stored in the liver at the time of birth, human milk provides both vitamin A and carotenoids. An intake of 6000 IU (1200 RE), easily achieved by the mother's regular use of green and yellow vegetables, allows production of milk with 170 IU (or RE)/dl which is sufficient to meet the needs of the infant. In one study of vitamin A supplementation of the diet of poor Indian women, no increase in the vitamin A in the milk was observed. The investigators hypothesized that once the mother's reserves have been restored, the levels in the milk would increase. The vitamin A in human milk continues to fall during the first thirty weeks of lactation. It can be increased within 12 hours by a single dose but falls again in 48 hours.

Vitamin D. The recent discovery of a water-soluble form of vitamin D in human milk explains its ability to protect the infant against rickets. It was previously believed that since little fat-soluble vitamin D was transferred to the milk, breast-fed infants received protection through exposure to sunlight. An intake of 400 IU is considered adequate for lactating women.

Vitamin K. Although the amount of vitamin K in breast milk is not sufficient to provide the needs of the infant, the amount can be increased by the addition of vitamin K to the mother's diet. However, vitamin K given to the mother is not transferred to the milk until the fourth day postpartum, which is too late to give the infant the resistance to postnatal hemorrhages during the critical first few days of life. As a result breast-fed infants are given a supplement of natural vitamin K either orally or by injection immediately following birth.

Other nutrients. The transfer of the micronutrient elements iodine and fluorine through the mother's milk to the infant is efficient and contributes appreciably to the intake of the infant when the mother's intake is adequate. These nutrients protect against goiter and increase resistance to tooth decay.

Ingested sodium is rapidly transferred to the milk, appearing within 20 minutes.

The effect of drugs, pesticides, herbicides, and other contaminants on the composition of mother's milk and on the infant is poorly understood. When DDT was more generally used there was some concern that it might reach questionably high levels in a mother's milk with her first lactation experience. There is also concern that the effect of oral contraceptives on milk composition may be detrimental to the infant. Infants of mothers who are taking sedatives suck less vigorously than normally.

The relatively high nutritional requirements of lactation require a significant increase in the quantity of food consumed and also dictate that the qualitative aspects of the food be carefully controlled. The use of an extra serving of meat, green and yellow fruits or vegetables, citrus fruit, and the equivalent of 2 cups of milk over and above a normal adequate diet will take care of the additional nutrients required. Obviously, this quantity of food cannot be incorporated into three regular meals without taxing the capacity of the stomach. Since most lactating women have very good appetites, it is feasible to suggest an eating pattern that includes five or six meals a day. If between-meal snacks are kept relatively low in satiety value, the appetite for regular meals shows little decrease.

Dietary supplements

In light of the very high level of nutritional intake prescribed for normal lactation, it is likely sound practice to recommend for the mother the use of a dietary supplement that provides protective levels of the nutrients for which the possibility of a dietary lack exists. This does not imply the endorsement of a supplement providing therapeutic levels of some nutrients and insignificant amounts of others and does not minimize the importance of a varied and balanced diet for the mother to provide trace elements not provided in most supplements.

Stimulation of lactation

Many techniques have been suggested to stimulate a satisfactory level of lactation. Lactation can be initiated only after the infant has begun to suck at the breast. Vigorous sucking stimulates both the anterior and posterior pituitary. The former produces prolactin, which leads to the production of milk in the mammary gland. The latter results in the secretion of a hormone oxytocin,

Table 16-6. Composition of colostrum, immature and mature human milk, and cow's milk per deciliter of milk*

Nutrient	Human			Mature cow's milk
	Colostrum (1-5 days)	Transitional (6-10 days)	Mature	
Energy (kcal)	58.0	74.0	71.0	69.0
Fat (g)	2.9	3.6	3.8	3.7
Lactose (g)	5.3	6.6	7.0	4.8
Protein (g)	2.7	1.6	1.2	3.3
Casein (g)	1.2	0.7	0.4	2.8
Lactalbumin (g)		0.8	0.3	0.4
Calcium (mg)	31.0	34.0	33.0	125.0
Phosphorus (mg)	14.0	17.0	15.0	96.0
Iron (mg)	0.09	0.04	0.15	0.10
Vitamins				
A (IU)	296	283	176	113
Carotene (IU)	186	63	45	63
D (IU)			0.42	2.36
E (mg)	1.28	1.32	0.56	0.06
Ascorbic acid (mg)	4.4	5.4	4.3	1.6
Folic acid (μg)	0.05	0.02	0.18	0.23
Niacin (mg)	0.075	0.175	0.172	0.085
Pantothenic acid (mg)	0.183	0.288	0.196	0.350
Pyridoxine (mg)			0.011	0.048
Riboflavin (mg)	0.029	0.033	0.042	0.157
Thiamin (mg)	0.015	0.006	0.016	0.042

*Based on Food and Nutrition Board: the composition of milks, Publication No. 254, Washington, D.C., 1953, National Academy of Sciences-National Research Council.

which stimulates the "let-down" reflex whereby the smooth muscles surrounding the alveoli of the nipple contract to allow the release of milk. The action of oxytocin counteracts the inhibition of the let-down reflex, which occurs as the result of pain, emotions, or embarrassment. Oxytocin also acts on the walls of the uterus causing strong contractions, which facilitate the return of the uterus to normal size.

Almost every culture has its own medicinal or food galactogogues, substances believed to stimulate lactation. These include garlic, cottonseed, candy, beer, ale, and large quantities of milk.

The relationship between fluid intake and volume of mammary secretion has not been established. Even when fluid intake is low, the volume secreted remains constant. A decreased intake of fluids will limit milk production only when total intake is less than the volume of milk produced. Drinking water beyond the level of natural thirst suppresses milk secretion through its action on the hormones of the pituitary that regulate milk production. Although high intakes do not stimulate milk production, liberal fluid intake is suggested to preclude the necessity of the formation of a highly concentrated urine to compensate for lack of fluid.

The first fluid secreted by the human breast, **colostrum**, is a thin, yellowish, watery fluid that bears little physical resemblance to milk and has its own unique nutritional composition, as shown in Table 16-6. The flow of colostrum may not begin for two to four days postpartum—a delay that is often erroneously interpreted as a failure of lactation. In the interval the child may be fed a glucose solution but only after he has been allowed to nurse to provide the stimulation necessary to initiate lactation.

Food avoidance

There are widespread beliefs, which are not based on any sound data, that lead many lactating women to avoid certain foods on the grounds that their infants can detect changes in their milk. One study reported that 59% of lactating women avoided cabbage, beans, garlic, and onions, 52% chocolate, 21% alcohol, and 18% carbonated beverages. However, there are no nutritional disadvantages and some advantages to limiting intakes of many of these foods.

Success and duration of lactation

Many attempts have been made to predict the success of lactation. Some evidence suggests that the output of milk is directly proportional to the metabolic size of the mother and that a strong positive correlation exists between rise in temperature of mammary skin due to nursing and milk supply. Other studies have shown that the course of lactation is established by the end of the first week, at which time the output should reach 500 ml. A positive attitude on the part of the mother is a determining factor in the success of breast-feeding. Although a great many undernourished women do succeed in breast-feeding satisfactorily, the woman who was severely malnourished in childhood may have impaired development of secondary sex characteristics, resulting in inadequate mammary tissue.

The period of time for which lactation is continued varies with a great many factors, both social and physiological. Mothers of higher socioeconomic and educational status are reported to be breast-feeding their infants more frequently and for longer periods but currently in the United States only one infant in five is breast-fed for six months.

Some mothers terminate lactation when the amount of milk produced declines to a point at which such extensive supplementary feeding is required that it is no longer feasible to continue breast-feeding.

In many cultures, breast-feeding is carried on for two to three years with milk being the sole source of food for a year or more. In other cultures, breast milk may be supplemented with other foods as early as three or four weeks. The latter case is believed to lead to less vigorous sucking, which in turn leads to a reduction in milk output and usually early weaning. Some evidence has been found that this same group experiences an earlier return to a regular pattern of ovulation with subsequent pregnancies occurring sooner.

Breast-feeding has merit as a contraceptive method, since when sucking is strong for a prolonged period both ovulation and the return of a regular menstrual cycle is delayed. At least half of the first postpartum menstrual cycles have not involved the production of an ovum. The risk of pregnancy during amenorrhea due to lactation is 5% but increases in each cycle. The use of artificial methods of contraception influences the course of lactation. The use of the IUD has a stimulating effect on lactation, whereas oral contraceptives tend to inhibit lactation.

Nutrition plays a role indirectly in human fertility in several ways. The undernourished woman has a delayed menarche, longer adolescent sterility, irregular menstrual cycles, longer amenorrhea during lactation, and an earlier menopause.

BIBLIOGRAPHY

Pregnancy

Adams, S. O., Barr, G. D., and R. L. Huenemann, Effect of nutritional supplementation on the outcome of pregnancy, J. Am. Diet. Assoc. **72:**144, 1978.

Agency for International Development: Malnutrition and infection during pregnancy. Determinants of growth and development of the child, Washington, D.C., 1975, National Academy of Science.

Albanese, A. A., editor: The effect of maternal nutrition on the development of the offspring, Proceedings of International Symposium, Nov., 1972, High Wycombe, Eng. Nutr. Rep. Intern. **7:**241, 1973.

Anderson, K. E., Bodansky, O., and Kappas, A.: Effects of oral contraceptives on vitamin metabolism, Adv. Clin. Chem. **18:**247, 1976.

Beaton, G. H.: Some physiological adjustments relating to nutrition in pregnancy, Can. Med. Assoc. J. **95:**622, 1966.

Behar, M., editor: Determinants of growth and development of child, Am. J. Dis. Child. **129:**549, 1975.

Behar, M., editor: Malnutrition and infection during pregnancy, J. Dis. Child. **129:**416, 1975.

Brenner, W. E., and Hendricks, C. H.: Interdependence of blood pressure, weight gain, and fetal weight during normal human pregnancy, Health Serv. Rep. **87:**236, 1972.

Burke, B. S., Stevenson, S. S., Worcester, J., and Stuart, H. C.: Nutrition studies during pregnancy. V. Relation of maternal nutrition to condition of infant at birth: study of siblings, J. Nutr. **38:**453, 1949.

Chase H. C.: Infant mortality and weight at birth: 1960 United States cohort, Am. J. Public Health **59:**1619, 1969.

Chopra, J. G., Forbes, A. L., and Habicht, J. P.: Protein in the U.S. diet, J. Am. Diet. Assoc. **72:**253, 1978.

Chow, B. F., Blackwell, R. Q., Blackwell, B. N., Hou, T. Y., Anilane, J. K., and Sherwin, R. W.: Maternal nutrition and metabolism of the offspring: studies in rats and man, Am. J. Public Health **58:**668, 1968.

Cohenour, S. H., and Calloway, D. H.: Blood, urine, and dietary pantothenic acid levels of pregnant teenagers, Am. J. Clin. Nutr. **25:**512, 1972.

Committee on Maternal and Child Health: Maternal nutrition and the course of pregnancy, Publication No. 1761, Washington, D.C., 1970, National Academy of Sciences—National Research Council.

Committee on Nutrition of the Mother and Preschool Child, Food and Nutrition Board, National Academy of Sciences: Oral contraceptives and nutrition, J. Am. Diet. Assoc. **68:**419, 1976.

Craft, I. L., Mathews, D. M., and Linnell, J. C.: Cobalamins in human pregnancy and lactation, J. Clin. Path. **24:**449, 1971.

Crosby, W. H.: Pica, J.A.M.A. **235:**2765, 1976.

Ebbs, J. F., Tisdall, F. F., and Scott, W. A.: Influence of prenatal diet on mother and child, J. Nutr. **22:**515, 1941.

The effect of oral contraceptive agents on plasma vitamin A in the human and the rat, Nutr. Rev. **35:**245, 1977.

Felig, P.: Maternal and fetal fuel homeostasis in human pregnancy, Am. J. Clin. Nutr. **26:**998, 1973.

Frisch, R. E.: Demographic implications of the biological determinants of femal fecundity, Soc. Biol. **22:**17, 1975.

Giroud, A.: Nutritional requirements of the embryo, World Rev. Nutr. Diet. **18:**195, 1973.

Gold, E. M.: Interconceptional nutrition, J. Am. Diet. Assoc. **55:**27, 1969.

Heaney, R. P., and Stillman, T. G.: Calcium metabolism and normal human pregnancy, J. Clin. Endocrin. Met. **33:**661, 1971.

Heller, S., Salkeld, R. M., and Korner, W. F.: Vitamin B_6 status in pregnancy, Am. J. Clin. Nutr. **26:**1339, 1973.

Influence of intrauterine nutritional status on the development of obesity in later life, Nutr. Rev. **35:**100, 1977.

Jackson, H. N., Burke, B. S., Smith, C. A., and Reed, D. E.: Effect of weight reduction in obese pregnant women on pregnancy, labor, and delivery and on the condition of the infant at birth, Am. J. Obstet. Gynecol. **83:**1609, 1962.

Jacobson, H.: Nutrition in pregnancy, N. Engl. J. Med. **297:**1051, 1977.

Jacobson, H. N.: Nutrition in pregnancy, J.A.M.A. **225**:634, 1973.

Jacobson, H. N.: Weight and weight gain during pregnancy, Clin. Perinatol. **2**:243, 1975.

King, J. C.: Nutrition during oral contraceptive use, J. Am. Pharm. Assoc. **17**:181, 1977.

Laboratory indices of nutritional status in pregnancy, summary report, Washington, D.C., 1977, National Academy of Sciences.

Larson, R. H.: Effect of prenatal nutrition on oral structures, J. Am. Diet. Assoc. **44**:368, 1964.

Lechtig, A., Yarbrough, C., Delgado, H., Habicht, J P, Martorell, R., and Klein, R. E.: Influence of maternal nutrition on birth weight, Am. J. Clin. Nutr. **28**:1223, 1975.

Lindheimer, H. D., and Katz, A. I.: Sodium and diuretics during pregnancy, N. Engl. J. Med. **288**:891, 1973.

Lowe, C. U.: Research in infant nutrition: the untapped well, Am. J. Clin. Nutr. **25**:245, 1972.

Macy, I. G.: Metabolic and biochemical changes in normal pregnancy, J.A.M.A. **168**:2265, 1958.

McCollum, E. B.: Symposium on prenatal nutrition, J. Am. Diet. Assoc. **36**:236, 1960.

McGanity, W. J., Bridgeforth, E. B., and Darby, W. J.: Vanderbilt cooperative study of maternal and infant nutrition; effect of reproductive cycle on nutritional status and requirements, J.A.M.A. **168**:2138, 1958.

McGanity, W. J., Little, H. M., Fogelman, A., Jennings, L., Calhoun, E., and Dawson, E. B.: Pregnancy in the adolescent, Am. J. Obstet. Gynecol. **101**:773, 1969.

Margen, S., and King, J. J.: Effect of oral contraceptive agents on the metabolism of some trace elements, Am. J. Clin. Nutr. **28**:392, 1975.

Martin, M. M., and Hurley, L. S.: Effect of large amounts of vitamin E during pregnancy and lactation, Am. J. Clin. Nutr. **30**:1629, 1977.

Naeye, R.L., Blanc, W., and Paul, C.: Effects of maternal nutrition on the human fetus, Pediatrics **52**:494, 1973.

Nutrition in pregnancy and lactation, Report of the Joint FAO/NRC Expert Committee, Techn. Rep. Ser. No. 302, 1965.

Pietarinen, G. J., Leichter, L., and Pratt, R. F.: Dietary folate intake and concentration of folate in serum and erythrocytes in women using oral contraceptives, Am. J. Clin. Nutr. **30**:375, 1977.

Pike, R. L.: Sodium intake during pregnancy, J. Am. Diet. Assoc. **44**:176, 1964.

Pike, R. L., and Smicklas, H. A.: A reappraisal of sodium restriction during pregnancy, Int. J. Gynecol. Obstet. **1**:1, 1972.

Pike, R. L.: Sodium requirement of the rat during pregnancy. In Invitational symposium on hypertension in pregnancy 1975, New York, 1976, John Wiley & Sons, Inc.

Pitkin, R. M.: Nutritional influences during pregnancy, Med. Clin. N. Am. **61**:3, 1977.

Pitkin, R. M.: Nutritional support in obstetrics and gynecology, Clin. Obstet. Gynecol. **19**:489, 1976.

Pitkin, R. M., Kaminetzky, H. A., Newton, M. and Pritchard, J. A.: Maternal nutrition—a selective review of clinic topics, Obstet. Gynecol. **40**:773, 1972.

Requirement of vitamin B_6 during pregnancy, Nutr. Rev. **34**:15, 1976.

Roeder, L. M.: Long-term effects of maternal and infant feeding, Am. J. Clin. Nutr. **26**:1120, 1973.

Rothman, D.: Folic acid in pregnancy, Am. J. Obstet. Gynecol. **108**:149, 1970.

Schwartz, N. E., and Barr, S. I.: Mothers—their attitudes and practices in perinatal nutrition, J. Nutr. Ed. **9**:169, Oct.-Dec., 1977.

Seifert, E.: Changes in beliefs and food practices in pregnancy, J. Am. Diet. Assoc. **39**:455, 1961.

Stearns, G.: Nutrition status of mother prior to conception, J.A.M.A. **168**:1655, 1958.

Teel, B. F.: Adaptations of digestive tract during reproduction in the mammal, World Rev. Nutr. Diet. **14**:181, 1972.

Thompson, A. M., and Hytten, F. Z.: Nutrition during pregnancy, World Rev. Nutr. Diet. **16**:23, 1973.

Thomson, A. M.: Diet in pregnancy. 3. Diet in relation to the course and outcome of pregnancy, Br. J. Nutr. **13**:509, 1959.

Thomson, A. M.: Nutrition in pregnancy, Br. J. Hosp. Med. **5**:600, 1971.

Thomson, A. M., and Billewicz, W. Z.: Nutritional status, maternal physique and reproductive efficiency, Proc. Nutr. Soc. **22**:55, 1963.

Thomson, A. M., Hytten, F. E., and Billewicz, W. Z.: The epidemiology of oedema during pregnancy, J. Obstet. Gynaec. Br. Comm. **74**(1):1, 1967.

Tsang, R. C.: Neonatal magnesium disturbances, Am. J. Dis. Child. **124**:282, 1972.

Weigley, E. S.: The pregnant adolescent. A review of nutritional research and programs, J. Am. Diet. Assoc. **66**:588, 1975.

Widdowson, E. M.: How the foetus is fed, Proc. Nutr. Soc. **28**:17, 1969.

Williams, M. L., Rose, C. S., Morrow G., Sloan, S. E., and Barness, L. A.: Calcium and fat absorption in neonatal period, Am. J. Clin. Nutr. **23**:1322, 1970.

Wong, N. P., La Croix, D. E., and Alford, J. E.: Mineral content of dairy products. 1. Milk and milk products, J. Am. Diet. Assoc. **72**:288, 1978.

Lactation

Aitchison, J. M., Dunkley, W. L., Canolty, N. L., and Smith, L. M.: Influence of diet on trans fatty acids in human milk, Am. J. Clin. Nutr. **30**:2006, 1977.

Bigwood, E. J.: Nitrogenous constituents and nutritive value of human and cow's milk, World Rev. Nutr. Diet. **4**:95, 1963.

Committee on Nutrition American Academy of Pediatrics: Commentary on breast-feeding and infant formulas, including proposed standards for formulas, Pediatrics **57:**278, 1976.

El-Minawi, M. F., and Foda, M. S.: Postpartum lactation amenorrhea, Am. J. Obstet. Gynecol. **111:**17, 1971.

Filer, L. J., Jr.: Maternal nutrition in lactation, Clin. Perinatol. **2:**353, 1975.

Gerrard, J. W.: Breast-feeding: second thoughts, Pediatrics **54:**757, 1974.

Goldman, A. S., and Smith, C. W.: Host resistance factors in human milk, Pediatrics **82:**1082, 1973.

Hadjimarkos, D. M., and Sheara, T. R.: Selenium in mature human milk, Am. J. Clin. Nutr. **26:**583, 1973.

Harrison, V. C., and Peat, G.: Significance of milk pH in newborn infants, Br. Med. J. **4:**515, 1972.

Herting, D. C., and Drury, E. E.: Vitamin E content of milk, milk products and simulated milks: relevance to infant nutrition, Am. J. Clin. Nutr. **22:**147, 1969.

Hook, E. B.: Dietary cravings and aversions during pregnancy, Am. J. Clin. Nutr. **31:**1355, 1978.

Jelliffe, D. B., and Jelliffe, E. F. P.: The uniqueness of human milk, Am. J. Clin. Nutr. **24:**968, 1971.

Jelliffe, D. B., and Jelliffe, E. F. P.: Pacifist factors in human milk, Pediatrics **83:**93, 1973.

Jelliffe, D. B., and Jelliffe, E. F. P.: Human milk, nutrition and the world resource crisis, Science **188:**557, 1975.

Jelliffe, D. B., and Jelliffe, E. F. P.: Breast-feeding *is* best for infants everywhere, Nutr. Today **13:**12, 1978.

Lakdawala, D. R., and Widdowson, E. M.: Vitamin D in human milk, Lancet **1:**167, 1977.

Macy, I. G., Kelly, H. J., and Sloan, R. E.: The composition of milks, Publication No. 254, Washington, D.C., 1953, National Research Council.

Metz, J.: Folate deficiency conditioned by lactation, Am. J. Clin. Nutr. **23:**843, 1970.

Meyer, H. F.: Current feeding practices in hospital maternity nurseries, Clin. Pediat. **8:**69, 1969.

Newton, M., and Newton, N.: The normal course and management of lactation, Clin. Obstet. Gynecol. **5:**44, 1962.

Newton, N., and Newton, M.: Psychologic aspects of lactation, N. Engl. J. Med. **277:**1179, 1967.

Perez, A., Vela, P., Potter, R., and Masnick, G. S.: Timing and sequence of resuming ovulation and menstruation after childbirth, Pop. Studies **25:**491, 1971.

Picciano, M. F., and Guthrie, H. A.: Copper, iron, and zinc contents of mature human milk, Am. J. Clin. Nutr. **29:**242, 1976.

Raphael, D.: The role of breast-feeding in a bottle oriented world. Eco. Food Nutr. **2:**121, 1973.

Sims, L.: Dietary status of lactating women, J. Am. Diet. Assoc. **73:**139, 1978.

Svanberg, U., Gebre-Medhin, M., Ljungqvist, B., and Olsson, M.: Breast milk composition in Ethiopian and Swedish mothers. III. Amino acids and other nitrogenous substances, Am. J. Clin. Nutr. **30:**499, 1977.

Thomas, E. B.: Neonate, mother interaction during breast feeding. Dev. Psych. **6:**110, 1972.

Thomson, A. M., Hytten, F. E., and Billewicz, W. Z.: The energy cost of human lactation, Br. J. Nutr. **24:**565, 1970.

Wades, N.: Bottle-feeding: adverse effects of a western technology, Science 184: 45, 1974.

Wichelow, M. J.: Success and failure of breast-feeding in relation to energy intake, Proc. Nutr. Soc. **35:**62A, 1976.

Williams, H. H.: Differences between cow's and human milk, J.A.M.A. **175:**104, 1961.

Woody, D. C., and Woody, H. B.: Management of breast feeding, J. Pediat. **68:**344, 1966.

17

Infant nutrition

With the emphasis in medical practice changing from curing to preventing disease and maintaining health there has been an increasing interest in the role of infant nutrition not only in early but later development. Infant feeding practices have changed rapidly in the past few decades in regard to the choice of early feeding method, the use of solid foods, and the frequency of feeding. Scientists are just now assessing the consequences of these changes and attempting to make recommendations for practices that are conducive to an optimal level of health in later life. Parents are concerned about the results of early feeding practices, and physicians and scientists are attempting to find the answers to their questions.

The state of nutrition of the mother prior to conception and throughout gestation is critical to the health of the infant at the time of birth. Similarly, the nutrition of the infant in the first year of life has long-term consequences for his survival and health throughout life.

The infant who is adequately nourished undergoes a normal rate of physical and mental development. On the other hand, one who is inadequately nourished in respect to one or more nutrients may experience a stunted growth and biochemical changes associated with undernutrition.

The impact of any nutritional deficiency is dependent on the timing and extent of the deficit. Many problems can be reversed if the inadequacy is corrected within a critical time period, but should the deficiency continue beyond the period when reversal is possible, the consequences will be permanent. The critical periods and critical nutrients vary from one tissue to another. Thus, in light of both mental and physical development the importance of an adequate nutritive intake throughout early infancy cannot be overemphasized.

The success of early nutrition will be dependent on the choice of early feeding methods, the correct use of nutrient supplementation, the pattern and timing of introduction of solid foods, and a careful monitoring of growth, morbidity, and nutritional status. For each of these factors the choice is determined to a certain extent by a complex of social, environmental, economic, and behavioral variables, as well as nutritional considerations.

BREAST-FEEDING

The incidence of breast-feeding in the United States underwent a decline from an almost universal practice at the turn of the century to 38% incidence in 1946, 21% in 1958, and 18% in 1966. By 1976, however, data showed 80% of mothers in the west and 45% of all other mothers were breast-feeding on discharge from the hospital. Further studies have indicated increased interest in breast-feeding among the more educated, higher socioeconomic groups. One report showed that 50% of mothers in a college town were breast-feeding successfully. Similarly, a study of 2233 mothers in the Boston area showed that, although only 22% of the total group were breast-feeding, 69.3% of those married to students breast-fed and that 39.8% of the upper social class and only 13.6% of the lower social class breast-fed. Current data show 37% of infants in the west and 20% in the rest of the country are breast-fed at 6 months. College-educated women tend to choose to breast-feed. Smokers breast-feed less often than nonsmokers.

Although other studies have shown that women report feeding their children in the way in which they themselves were fed, this study found no relationship between a daughter's decision and her mother's. The pattern of feeding used by the better-educated group is frequently followed several years later by less-educated mothers and those of lower socioeconomic status in a wavelike sequence, with the lower socioeconomic group emulating the higher. Whether such a trend prevails will not be ascertained for several years, but if it does, improved infant health might be expected. Any trend in this direction may be reinforced by the recommendation from many groups of pediatricians that breast milk or modified cow's milk formula, if breast-feeding is impossible, be the sole source of nutrition for the first six months of life and the major source for one year. It is doubtful that such a goal will be achieved, but any trend in that direction would be desirable.

Although many factors undoubtedly enter into the choice, the low incidence of breast-feeding has been attributed most often to the large number of women who are working, the availability of acceptable substitutes, and the lack of medical guidance and support. In a few cases, when the mother has tuberculosis or breast cancer, breast-feeding is precluded; in most cases, however, the decision will be made after a consideration of the relative merits of the two types, since for all intents and purposes either should be possible and successful in a Western culture. In developing countries, on the other hand, where suitable alternatives are too costly for most families, where the variable water supply is often a source of contamination, where refrigeration is unavailable, and where knowledge of aseptic techniques for handling the formula is limited, breast-feeding is almost essential if the child is to survive the neonatal period. Under these circumstances failure to breast-feed results in the loss of one of a country's best natural resources.

The following sections will be concerned with the relative advantages and disadvantages of breast-feeding.

Considerations favoring breast-feeding

Nutritional. In general, it is believed that the nutrient composition of the milk of each species is best suited to the growth needs of its offspring, and when possible it should be used. If this is not possible, the milk of another species should be modified to approximate the composition of the maternal milk.

The difference in nutritive composition of human and cow's milk is well documented, and some aspects are presented in Fig. 17-1. This graph show that breast milk contains more of some nutrients and less of others. The absolute amounts for some nutrients are given in Table 16-6, which includes a comparison of colostrum, the first secretion of the breast, and mature milk. The lower concentration of some nutrients such as calcium and protein in breast milk is believed to reflect the differing growth needs between the human infant and the calf. The latter doubles its birth weight in two months, compared to the human infant, which takes four months. Not only does the total amount of some nutrients differ but also the form in which they exist.

Energy. The caloric value of the two milks is similar, as is the total fat content. The lower protein is compensated for by a higher amount of lactose in human milk. Fat provides 51%, protein 7%, and carbohydrate 42% of the calories in human milk compared to 48%, 22%, and 30%, respectively, in cow's milk. Free fatty acids liberated by lipase present in human milk are an important source of energy for infants.

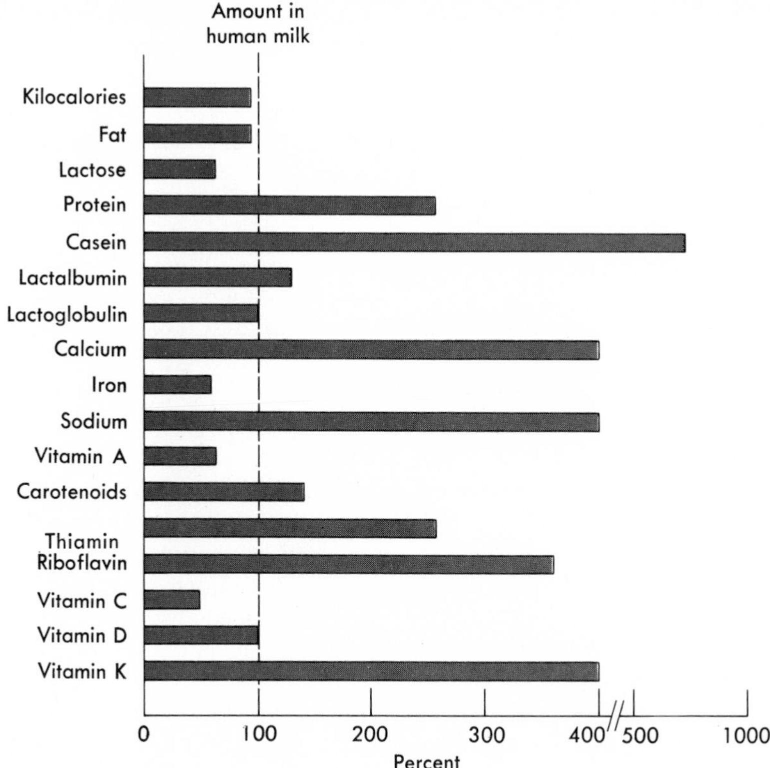

Fig. 17-1. Relative amounts of various nutrients in human and cow's milk, with amount in human milk represented as 100% and solid bars representing amount in cow's milk. (Based on data from Composition of human milk, Publication No. 254, Washington, D.C., 1953, National Academy of Sciences–National Research Council.)

Carbohydrate. The disaccharide lactose found in both human and cow's milk is present at a higher (42%) level in human milk. Lactose has several advantages in infant feeding over other carbohydrates in that it facilitates the absorption of calcium and magnesium and favors amino acid absorption and nitrogen retention. A source of lactose is also important to the infant, since it is the only source of the monosaccharide galactose, which is a structural part of the cerebrosides essential to the formation of myelin. Myelin surrounds nerve fibers and is essential to normal nerve function. Some evidence exists that lactose also favors riboflavin and pyridoxine synthesis, although this may be of little benefit to the infant if it occurs in the lower gastrointestinal tract and the nutrients cannot be absorbed.

Although the low solubility of lactose makes it impractical for use in formula prepared at home, it is the carbohydrate added to all milk-based commercially prepared formulas. In soy-based formulas, sucrose as the added carbohydrate may influence the growth of bacteria in the lower gastrointestinal tract.

Protein. Human milk, in which the protein is predominately (60%) lactalbumin, contains only half as much protein as cow's milk, in which most of the protein is in the form of casein. Lactalbumin not only has an amino acid pattern that more nearly approaches that of body proteins but also provides more of the essential amino acids than does casein. Casein forms a hard curd when subjected to the action of the enzyme rennin in the stomach, whereas lactalbumin forms a soft flocculent curd on which digestive enzymes act freely and which is more rapidly digested and absorbed.

Human milk protein has a higher cysteine to methionine ratio, which is important since the liver of the human infant lacks the enzyme necessary to allow it to use methionine as a sulfur-containing amino acid.

The presence of a protein-splitting enzyme in breast milk reduces proteins to the less complex peptone stage, on which digestive enzymes act more effectively. These enzymes in cow's milk are destroyed by the heat of pasteurization.

Lipid. The fat in human milk differs in several respects from that in cow's milk. Fatty acids in human milk are less saturated, have 10- to 14-carbon chains, and are utilized more effectively than are the short-chain, more saturated fatty acids in cow's milk. About 95% of human milk fat is retained after digestion compared to 61% of butterfat.

Palmitic acid, when present in human milk, is present in the number 2 (middle) carbon position, whereas in other milks it is attached in the number 1 or 3 position. Since human milk contains an enzyme that splits off the fatty acids in positions 1 and 3 before the monoglyceride with the fatty acid attached in position number 2 is absorbed intact, there is little free palmitic acid available in the intestine of the breast-fed infant. This is desirable, since free palmitic acid tends to interfere with calcium absorption.

Recent evidence has shown that the fatty acid pattern of human milk has been changing during the period in which the dietary fat intake of the population has shifted from saturated animal fats to more unsaturated vegetable oils. Current data suggest a higher proportion of the unsaturated fatty acids linoleic and linolenic acid contribute to an increasing P/S ratio in human milk.

The increase in the fat content of human milk from the beginning to the end of a feeding is believed to increase its satiety value and make it easier for the breast-fed infant to regulate his caloric intake and reduce the likelihood of excessive weight gain in early infancy.

Vitamins. The amount of the heat-labile vitamins thiamin and ascorbic acid found in human milk is almost completely absorbed by the infant, whereas the higher amount in cow's milk may be substantially less available because of its destruction as a result of the application of heat in the pasteurization of milk and sterilization of the formula.

Trace elements. With advances in knowledge of the role of trace elements in nutrition, there has been an increasing interest in determining the content of these in breast milk. This information is necessary to estimate the needs for infants and to provide a basis for formulating human milk substitutes. This is especially important since certain processes used to modify cow's milk so that it more closely resembles human milk may result in the removal of some of the trace elements. The use of distilled water by mothers concerned about environmental pollution may further reduce the amounts of these elements available to the bottle-fed child.

Of recent interest is the observation that the zinc to copper ratio (6:1) in breast milk compared to cow's milk is associated with decreased cholesterol synthesis.

For some elements such as selenium, for which both a deficiency and an excess may be harmful, the content in breast milk seems to be controlled within very narrow limits. Copper is present in human milk in amounts ranging from 22 to 144 ppm. Zinc is present in relatively large amounts of 130 to 1240 ppm. Data from the analysis of human milk suggest that for these and other elements such as chromium and vanadium there is a certain minimum amount that must be present in all breast milk. Until more complete information is available it will be impossible to judge whether formulas are indeed satisfactory substitutes for human milk in regard to trace elements. The extent to which the

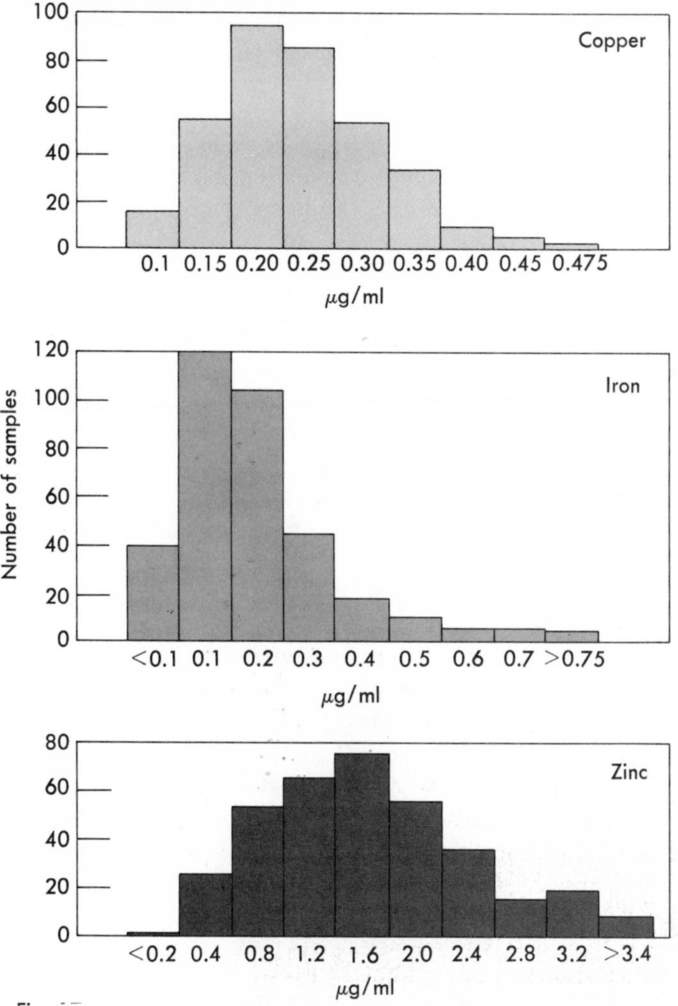

Fig. 17-2. Range of trace element content in human milk.

trace element content of human milk varies is illustrated in Fig. 17-2.

Infants fed human milk are afforded a high degree of protection against the accumulation of strontium in the body. Cow's milk, with a strontium content six times that of human milk, leads to doubling of body strontium by age 1 month.

The phosphorus content of human milk is appreciably lower than that of cow's milk, providing only a sixth as much per liter or per 100 kcal and a third as much per gram of protein. The high ratio of phosphorus to calcium in cow's milk may be a contributing factor in hypocalcemic tetany in infants who are fed whole cow's milk and whose parathyroid gland is not mature enough to respond to the low calcium levels.

Immunological properties. Colostrum, the secretion of the breast that precedes the secretion of mature milk, differs from milk in appearance and nutritional properties. This watery yellowish fluid is believed to contribute a high degree of **immunity** to the infant through its effect in the gastrointestinal tract rather than after absorption in the blood.

Between the fifth and tenth day after birth, colostrum undergoes changes in chemical and physical composition until by the tenth day it has usually assumed the characteristics of mature milk. Much effort has been directed toward identifying the substances responsible for the anti-infective properties of human milk. It is now believed that they are a group of substances called colostrum particles, or corpuscles, which are stable in the acid medium of the stomach and resistant to the digestive enzymes. Among these are lysozymes, which act by attacking and destroying the cell membrane after the bacteria have been inactivated by the peroxides and vitamin C present in colostrum. An enzyme, lactoperoxidase, acts by killing the *Streptococcus* organism. Another group contributing to the immune properties are macrophages (large eating cells). These molecules are not absorbed but contribute to the immunity of the infant by protecting against bacteria and viruses responsible for such diseases as poliomyelitis, influenza, and diphtheria. These cells also synthesize complement, a protein known to be involved in a series of reactions to establish immunity to infectious organisms. Another substance, lactoferrin, an iron-containing unsaturated fatty acid similar to linoleic acid, has been found in colostrum and mature milk. This substance inhibits the growth of *Staphylococcus* and *E. coli* by binding the iron needed for the growth of these organisms.

A nitrogen-containing carbohydrate in human milk has been designated as the **Lactobacillus bifidus factor**, since it creates a medium in the gastrointestinal tract conducive to the growth of the microorganism *Lactobacillus bifidus*. This microorganism, by producing acetic or lactic acid from lactose, depresses the growth of pathogenic organisms, thus decreasing the infant's susceptibility to infection. It also competes with undesirable *E. coli* to inhibit its growth. It is postulated that the factor in human milk is lactulose, a derivative of lactose known to occur in large amounts in breast milk and in higher amounts in heat-treated than in untreated cow's milk. The growth of *L. bifidus* is enhanced on a high-lactose, low-protein diet. The lactose-protein ratio is 7:1 in human milk compared to 4:1 in cow's milk.

Psychological. The psychological advantages of breast-feeding have been freely discussed but are poorly documented. Certainly many emotional and psychological considerations enter into the decision to breast- or bottle-feed. Once the decision has been made the psychological advantages or disadvantages are less well documented.

One study demonstrated that women who were allowed close physical contact with their infants in the delivery room immediately following birth were more likely to breast-feed and to do so successfully than were those who were separated from their infants for 8 hours or more.

The consensus of opinion is that the infant derives a sense of security and belonging in the early mother-child relationship from the warmth of the mother's body and from the comfort of being held rather than from the feeding process per se. It was shown in a classic study with monkeys that those fed by a surrogate mother (a bottle inserted in a wire screen covered with warm terry cloth) were as well adjusted as those fed by the real mother. Monkeys fed by a bottle alone showed more evidence of emotional instability. Research with dogs and ducks has identified a critical period during the first few days of life when imprinting, or learning, which is remarkably resistant to modification, occurs. It may be that the impact of the mother on the child in this critical period will have implications for later development. Although psychologists so far have been unable to elucidate consistent differences in personality between bottle-fed and breast-fed infants, it has been demonstrated that breast-feeding increases a mother's feeling of competence in dealing with her child. It is conceivable that more carefully controlled studies may show effects on personality that have so far largely evaded detection. There is some belief that the greatest psychological advantages accrue to the mother who feels that she is involved in a unique relationship with the child and is fulfilling her true maternal role.

Other factors. Various other advantages have been attributed to breast-feeding. Since the work of obtaining milk from the breast is much more difficult than from most bottles, it is believed that the use required of muscles of the mouth leads to the development of the jaw and reduces the incidence of crowded dentition in later years. Others maintain that the secretion of oxytocin in lactation favors the contraction of the uterus, thus speeding the return of the mother's abdomen to normal size. The reduced likelihood of contamination during preparation of the formula, the elimination of the possibility of mistakes in mixing the formula, or the necessity of finding a satisfactory formula are more salient factors favoring breast-feeding among the less well-educated segment of the population and in developing countries than they are for the intelligent middle-class mother. However, a mistake in the preparation of infant formula in a hospital when salt was used instead of sugar became a tragic example of the possibility of human error in preparing a formula. Contamination of milk with heavy metals such as lead occurs in human milk at 5%, the same level as in cow's milk.

Growth. The growth rate of breast-fed infants exceeds that of bottle-fed infants for the first four to five months of life. This may be due to the protein synthesizing properties of nucleotides in breast milk. After this period, bottle-fed infants experience a more rapid growth rate, but no differences between the two groups can be ascertained at 2 years of age.

Allergy. The use of breast milk virtually eliminates the possibility of a milk allergy, whereas reports on the incidence of cow's milk allergy range from 0.3% to 7% of artificially fed infants. One unsubstantiated explanation of "cot deaths," which account for 20% of mortality between 2 months and 2 years, is that it represents an allergic reaction after the aspiration of cow's milk protein regurgitated during sleep by a bottle fed infant sensitized to cow's milk protein in the first few months. Alternately, the lower incidence of this sudden unexpected death (SUD) in breast-fed infants has been attributed to the higher levels of vitamin E in breast milk, which serves as an antioxidant to prevent lipid oxidation in cell membranes in the lung and the subsequent respiratory distress, a yet unproven explanation of the syndrome.

Other considerations. Breast-fed infants, who absorb calcium very efficiently, seldom suffer from hypocalcemia and neonatal tetany that result when the calcium/phosphorus ratio decreases. It can occur when calcium absorption decreases in a vitamin D deficiency or when there is an excessive intake of phosphorus from the use of undiluted cow's milk or the early introduction of high-protein foods. This excess phosphorus cannot be excreted by the immature kidneys. High-fat diets, which cause the excretion of calcium, may also contribute to the imbalance.

At least one study has demonstrated that the chances of developing heart disease are almost twice as great in bottle-fed as in breast-fed infants, presumably due to altered lipid metabolism. The chances of developing ulcerative colitis are considerably greater.

There is considerable evidence that in nursing mothers, ovulation is delayed beyond the normal two-month period following delivery and that as long as the infant is fully breast-fed there is little likelihood of ovulation, and hence, subsequent pregnancies, occurring. The use of oral contraceptives inhibits lactation, whereas the use of the IUD enhances it.

Although the risk of breast cancer is lower among women who have had a child before 20 years of age or have breast-fed more children, there is also evidence that cancer-producing viruses may be transmitted to the milk by mothers who have a family history of breast cancer.

Disadvantages of breast-feeding

Since a majority of mothers choose not to breast-feed, there must be some objections or disadvantages to it or overriding advantages to bottle-feeding. Among these are the failure of the mother to secrete adequate milk, the constant fatigue reported by many mothers, the lack of freedom, the impossibility of turning the responsibility over to someone else, the possibility of breast infection, and a desire to quickly restore the mother's figure to normal.

From a physiological point of view the transmission of pregnanediol, a metabolite of the hormone progesterone, through the mother's milk can result in hyperbilirubinemia in some infants. Anticoagulants are also transmitted. Concern over high levels of DDT, PCBS, and other environmental contaminants in human milk has subsided as more rigid control over their use has been introduced.

For some mothers a failure to recognize that the onset of lactation may be delayed until three to five days after birth, that the physical appearance of colostrum is different from milk, and that their milk has not "turned to water" may explain their decision to abandon attempts at breast-feeding. The desire of mothers for either economic or psychological reasons to leave the hospital as soon as possible after delivery can mean that if lactation is not established shortly after birth, the mother will give up her plans in the interest of taking the infant home on a functioning bottle-feeding routine.

BOTTLE-FEEDING

Modified milk formula. The availability of safe and satisfactory preparations in which cow's milk has been modified to provide a suitable substitute for human milk leads many mothers to choose bottle-feeding. To be most satisfactory, cow's milk must be modified so that it resembles human milk as closely as possible in nutrient composition and in physiochemical properties. The dilution of cow's milk to provide a concentration of protein similar to that of human milk also causes a reduction in curd tension and leads to the formation of a softer, more flocculent curd that can be more readily digested by the proteolytic enzymes in the gastrointestinal tract of the infant. Other methods of modifying the character of the curd that are sometimes used in place of, or in addition to, dilution include the use of pancreatic enzymes, heat treatment, the addition of an acid such as citric acid or acid-producing microorganisms, or the addition of alkali. One method seems to have little advantage over another. The dilution of milk has the advantage of creating a calcium concentration more nearly approximating human milk and the disadvantage of reducing the caloric value from a normal level of 22 kcal/30 ml. The addition of a soluble and readily utilizable carbohydrate such as dextromaltose or sucrose can raise the caloric value to that of human milk but fails to provide the beneficial effects of lactose, which is suitable only for use in commercially prepared products.

The lower level of sodium (comparable to that in human milk) deemed desirable to reduce the burden on the kidneys through which sodium is excreted in the urine can be achieved by removing much of the electrolyte by dialysis, a method sometimes employed in commercial formula preparation. The possibility that essential trace elements may be removed at the same time must not be overlooked. Reduced sodium is especially important when fluid losses are high due to excessive heat or diarrhea.

Other products simulate the high linoleic content of human milk by replacing the butterfat (short-chain saturated fatty acid) with corn oil (long-chain unsaturated fatty acids). Fat in this form is tolerated better by the infant and provides more adequate levels of the essential fatty acid linoleic acid. Substitution of butterfat with coconut oil, which has saturated fatty acids, does not have any advantages. The use of too high a level of polyunsaturated fatty acids, however, increases the need for vitamin E. The use of medium chain triglycerides improves fat absorption but results in decreased absorption of vitamins A and E.

The safety of bottle-feeding has increased with greater awareness of the importance of aseptic techniques in the preparation of infant formula. Sterilization of feeding equipment and formula has reduced the transmission of pathogenic organisms and resulting disease. Prior to the recognition of microorganisms as the cause of disease, the hazards of bottle-feeding were so great that infant mortality and morbidity rates were considerably higher than those for breast-feeding. Some reports still indicate a markedly higher mortality and morbidity rate in bottle-fed infants than in breast-fed infants, but among infants born to middle-class parents in technologically developed countries there generally is no significant difference. The use of expensive but bacteriologically safe preprepared sterilized formulas in disposable bottles is increasing, offering advantages of convenience and safety to those who can afford them.

Since most commerical preparations are based on nonfat dried milk with vegetable oil added to provide the fat necessary to increase the caloric density, they contain practically no cholesterol. At this time it is unclear whether such a low cholesterol intake for infants is desirable. On the one hand, it is believed that with a low cholesterol intake the likelihood of the child developing cholesterol-containing arteriosclerotic deposits in the artery wall will be reduced. Those who believe that some dietary cholesterol should be available point to the fact that cholesterol is needed for the synthesis of myelin, which is essential for the normal functioning of the central nervous system. Additionally, evidence exists that if the child does not degrade dietary cholesterol early in life, he may not be able to regulate his degradation and synthesis to maintain normal blood cholesterol levels later in life. The fact that human milk does contain cholesterol suggests that it is desirable in early life.

Whole cow's milk. Although at one time there was considerable support for the use of whole homogenized unmodified milk in infant feeding, it is now evident that whole milk can cause gastric bleeding in infants up to 1 year of age. For that reason whole milk should not be used unless the protein has been denatured or altered by the use of high-temperature processing such as used in preparing evaporated milk. Additionally, the high sodium and protein content of whole milk causes an increased renal solute load that taxes the kidneys.

Nonfat or skim milk feedings. For some time nonfat milk was used in infant feeding on the theory that it would restrict weight gain and the tendency toward obesity and would eliminate any intake of cholesterol.

It is now evident that nonfat milk (less than 0.5% fat) feeding is undesirable in the first year of life, primarily because of its low caloric density of 35 kcal/dl of milk compared to 67 kcal in human milk. Although infants on this feeding regimen increase their intake of milk and solids and do gain some weight, they still cannot increase their energy intake to 90 kcal/kg of body weight, the level necessary to prevent the loss of significant fat reserves. This is reflected in decreased skinfold thickness.

If they do eat enough to meet their caloric requirements, the amount of protein and sodium ingested is so great that it produces a high renal solute load. In addition, the absence of linoleic acid, an essential fatty acid, results in dermatitis and growth retardation. The lack of dietary cholesterol is also considered undesirable. It is questionable whether infants are able to synthesize the lipid needed for myelin formation. Since skim milk is not fortified with iron or copper, its use increases the chance of developing anemia. In summary, the use of nonfat milk is considered inappropriate in infant feeding. The use of milk with 2% fat has many of the same disadvantages.

A comparison of some of the characteristics of milks used in infant feeding are given in Table 17-1.

Psychological. Many mothers experience psychological blocks concerning breast-feeding. These range from considering it a bovine function to considering it a form of "uneating." Others are unwilling to risk breast-feeding for fear that their figures may become permanently distorted, that breasts will remain enlarged, and that it will take longer to return to their prepregnancy weight. None of these beliefs has been confirmed. If the mother lacks the desire to breast-feed, the chances of it succeeding are greatly reduced. Positive maternal attitudes are highly correlated with successful lactation. Some studies found that mothers chose bottle-feeding because they needed to see the amount of milk the child was consuming.

Economic. According to a report of the U.S. Department of Agriculture, the cost of the increased amount of food required by the mother to provide the recommended 750 kcal, 0.4 g of calcium, and 20 g of high-quality protein needed over and above that suggested for the nonpregnant, nonlactating woman may be higher or lower than the cost of the formula needed by the infant. On a moderate-cost diet it is believed that the addition of a liter of milk, 178 ml (6 oz) of orange juice, 2 slices of whole-wheat bread, 14 g (½ oz) of butter, and an egg would provide the added nutrients at a 1978 cost of 53 cents daily. On a low-cost food budget the report considered the use of 0.1 kg of nonfat milk solids, 60 ml (2 oz) of cooking oil, 28 g (1 oz) of enriched cornmeal, 0.15 kg (⅓ lb) of turnip greens, and a vitamin supplement every other day at a total cost of 18 cents. By comparison, as shown in Table 17-2, the cost of formula can range from $2.81 a week for a formula of whole milk and sugar to $19.70 a week for ready-to-use formula in disposable sterilized individual bottles. Equipment such as bottles and sterilizers has not been included. With inflation of food costs, absolute amounts will increase but relative cost should not change appreciably.

Social. For many mothers the freedom and flexibility for professional and social life that bottle-feeding affords is an overriding consideration in the choice. In fact, among fifty-five mothers who had had a satisfying breast-feeding experience, the loss of freedom and restriction of their social life were considered disadvantages by twenty-nine. Most of these mothers had found, however, that an occasional bottle could be substituted with no adverse reaction from the child, although the

Table 17-1. Comparison of caloric distribution and other nutritional factors in milk and formula

	Breast milk	Formula	Whole cow's milk	2% cow's milk	Nonfat milk
Energy (kcal/fl oz)		20	20	18	11
Carbohydrate (% calories)	42	41	30	41	57
Protein (% calories)	7	9-11	22	28	40
Fat (% calories)	51	48	35-55	31	3
Lipid (%)	3.7	3.6	3.6	2.0	0.1
P/S ratio	0.4-0.8	2-4.5	0.4	0.4	—
Cholesterol (mg/L)	140-200	20-40	110	80	30
Iron (mg/L)	0.8	12	Trace	Trace	Trace
Potential renal solute load (mOsm/100 kcal)	13	20	46	60	86

Table 17-2. Relative costs per week of breast- and bottle-feeding

Breast-feeding mother's food and supplement over nonlactating	
Thrifty food plan	3.00
Liberal food plan	5.00
Bottle-feeding	
Whole fluid milk and sugar	2.81
Evaporated milk and sugar	2.88
Concentrated liquid formula (13 oz)	4.77
Powdered formula (1 lb can)	5.01
Ready-to-use formula	
Large can (32 oz)	6.50
Serving size bottle	13.00
Disposable serving size bottle	19.50

*From Peterkin, B., and Walker, S.: Food for the baby—cost and nutritive value considerations, Family Economics Review, Fall, 1976.

mother sometimes experienced physical discomfort from the engorgement of the breast.

ADEQUACY OF MILK DIET

The NRC recommended allowances for infants are shown in Table 17-3. A diet composed solely of human or modified cow's milk consumed at a level of approximately 850 ml a day will provide recommended amounts of all the nutrients needed except fluorine and vitamin D up to 3 months of age. At 3 to 6 months when fetal iron reserves are depleted, milk is incapable of providing sufficient iron to maintain hemoglobin level even when copper is adequate. At that time an iron supplement or the use of iron-fortified formula is recommended.

Ascorbic acid is a limiting factor only for bottle-fed infants whose formula is subjected to high heat during processing. These infants

Table 17-3. Recommended dietary allowances for infants*

Nutrient	Age (mo)		
	0-6	6-12	12-36
Kilocalories	wt (kg) × 117	wt (kg) × 108	1300
Protein (g)	wt (kg) × 2.2	wt (kg) × 2.0	23
Calcium(g)	0.36	0.54	0.8
Iron (mg)	10	15	15
Iodine (μg)	35	45	60
Zinc (mg)	3	5	10
Magnesium (mg)	60	70	150
Vitamin A (IU)	1400	2000	2000
Vitamin D (IU)	400	400	400
Vitamin E (IU)	4	5	7
Ascorbic acid (mg)	35	35	40
Folacin (mg)	0.05	0.05	0.1
Niacin (mg)	5	8	9
Riboflavin (mg)	0.4	0.6	0.8
Thiamin (mg)	0.3	0.5	0.7
Pyridoxine (mg)	0.3	0.4	0.6
Vitamin B_{12} (μg)	0.3	0.3	1.0

*From Food and Nutrition Board: Recommended dietary allowances, ed. 8, Washington, D.C., 1974. National Academy of Sciences—National Research Council.

should receive a supplementary source of ascorbic acid or an enriched formula by the tenth day of life. After the discovery of antiscorbutic properties of oranges, orange juice was fed as a source of vitamin C, starting with 1 teaspoon of juice diluted with an equal amount of water and building up to about 2 tablespoons of juice. With an increasing number of reports of allergic reactions, apparently from the oil of the orange rind that was extracted with the juice, there was a trend toward the use of a synthetic source of ascorbic acid that minimized any sensitizing reaction. This is a general practice in the first few months of life, after which the child can be given a fruit juice high in ascorbic acid. Evidence exists that infants born to mothers who had an extremely high ascorbic acid intake during pregnancy have a conditioned need for a high level of the vitamin.

The amount of vitamin D in either human or cow's milk to some extent is a function of the diet of the mother or cow but even under ideal conditions it does not approach the 400 IU recommended by the Food and Nutrition Board of the National Research Council. Thus unless a child has regular exposure to sunlight it is necessary to provide a supplement of 400 IU vitamin D, preferably by 5 days of age. Cod-liver oil, the most popular source after the discovery of its antirachitic properties in promoting normal calcification of bones and teeth, has been replaced by water-miscible preparations to avoid the danger of lipoid pneumonia from the aspiration of the oily particles of cod-liver oil into the lungs. If, however, a bottle-fed infant is given a prepared formula or a formula made with evaporated or homogenized milk, which is normally fortified with 400 IU of vitamin D per liter, no supplementation is necessary. In the light of current reports of toxicity associated with the use of diets high in vitamin D such supplementation is likely undesirable.

With the discovery of a water-soluble form of vitamin D in breast milk it is possible that supplementary vitamins will not be needed as long as the child is breast-fed. For the bottle-fed child who does not have regular exposure to sunlight supplementary vitamin D is provided either through fortified milk or formula.

Except for infants fed a formula that has been diluted with naturally or artificially fluoridated water, a fluorine supplement of 0.25 to 0.5 mg in the first year is necessary to facilitate the calcification of bones and teeth. Because of the possible hazards from excessive ingestion of fluorine, such supplements are available only by prescription.

The small amount of iron in human milk is well utilized, with 50% being absorbed. The high ascorbic acid, vitamin E, and copper content of human milk facilitates iron absorption. Although this would permit an infant to meet his needs for iron from human milk alone, it is recommended that a ferrous sulfate supplement be given, beginning at 4 months of age. After the child is weaned an iron-fortified formula is recommended. For bottle-fed infants the use of iron fortified formula is being recommended throughout the first year of life to prevent a drop in hemoglobin levels below 11 g/dl of blood.

In one study it was found that the use of a formula supplemented with vitamins and iron (12 mg/950 ml) produced no differences in growth and development, in number of illnesses, or in hemoglobin, hematocrit, or serum iron levels up to 3 to 3½ months of age. The blood values were higher after this time when the iron-fortified formula was used. Another extensive study of the use of iron-enriched formula from birth suggested that its use does provide protection against subsequent drop in hemoglobin levels by maintaining levels 1 to 1.5 g higher at 9 months of age. It appears that the infant's mechanism for regulating iron absorption is sufficiently sensitive to prevent the uptake of excess iron that leads to iron overload when it is fed prior to a time of need. About 60% of infant formulas contain added iron.

Temperature of milk

The question of the temperature of a milk feeding has been raised. Several investigators have contended that formula from the refrigerator is well tolerated by 50% of young infants and 75% of older infants and gives as good a growth response as that which has been warmed to body temperature. Research indicated that feeding ice-cold milk lowered gastric temperature for at least an hour, decreased the activity of proteolytic enzymes, and hence delayed digestion.

NUTRITIVE NEEDS OF INFANTS

Precise information on the nutritive needs of infants is available for only a few nutrients, but the National Research Council has suggested levels of intake that appear to support growth in healthy infants.

Energy. An intake of 100 to 120 kcal /kg of body weight or 54 kcal per pound appears to be adequate to meet the needs for the first six months. Since the body surface area of infants per unit of body weight is twice as great as that of adults, the insensible heat loss from the surface is also twice as great. Of energy need, 50% is used for basal energy needs, 25% for activity, and 25% for growth of 5 to 7 g a day.

A very placid infant is reported to need as few as 70 kcal/kg, whereas a crying infant may need as many as 130 kcal. By 6 months energy needs have decreased to 90 to 100 kcal/kg.

An excessive intake of calories leading to a rapid gain in weight is equally as undesirable in infants as in adults. MacKeith has suggested that a baby who weighs over 12 kg at 1 year of age is more likely to grow up to be an obese adolescent or adult than is one weighing less. This supports the concept that maximum growth is not synonymous with optimal growth. Similarly, it has been shown that weight gain in excess of 3.5 kg in each six months of early life enhances the chances of later obesity. As illustrated in Fig. 17-3, an obese infant is more likely to become an obese adult and more unlikely to become an adult of normal weight. Conversely, infants identified as light are less likely to become obese adults. The reasons for this are probably a combination of genetic, environmental, and social factors, including the early introduction of solid food.

Hirsch has postulated that the number of adipose, or fat, cells is determined early and is proportionately larger in the overfed in-

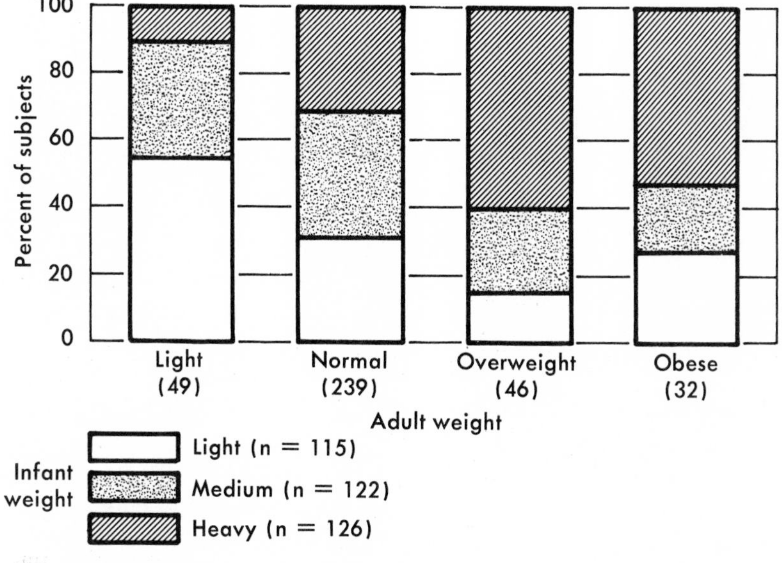

Fig. 17-3. Relationship between weight in infancy and incidence of obesity in adulthood.

fant, who has a greater need for more cells to store fat. For these infants the regulation of weight in later life is more difficult because of a tendency for these cells to remain filled with fat. There is now some question as to whether this condition is actually irreversible.

For a newborn infant, milk provides all the calories. Filer reports that by 6 months of age 70% of the energy is still provided by milk, with fruit providing 10%, and cereal, meat, egg, and vegetables each providing 5%. He, however, recommended milk as the sole energy source during that period.

Protein. The needs for protein during the period of rapid skeletal and muscular growth of early infancy are relatively high. An intake of 2.2 g of protein of high biological value per kilogram of body weight supports a nitrogen retention of about 45%, sufficiently great to allow normal growth. At 3 weeks from 60% to 75% of dietary protein is used for growth and the rest for maintenance. By 4 months of age the proportions are 45% and 55%. By 1 year the protein needs have dropped to 2 g/kg. When expressed on the basis of caloric intake, protein requirements are set at 1.8 g/100 kcal slightly more than the 1.6 g found in human milk. If protein of a lower biological value is used, the amount needed increases proportionately. Only proteins with a biological value (BV) of at least 70% to 85% should be used, however, since otherwise excessive amounts will be needed and excretion of the nonessential nitrogen will be necessary. A protein intake providing from 6.5% to 8% of the total dietary calories is capable of meeting the protein requirement, but if it should drop below this, it is very difficult for the child to get enough food to meet his requirement.

There is no evidence of advantages from protein intakes above these levels, and some evidence of disadvantages has been compiled. Infants receiving whole unmodified cow's milk, which has twice the protein of human milk, have suffered from a hypochromic macrocytic anemia caused by gastric bleeding that lead to large blood losses in the feces, apparently the result of an allergy to the cow's milk protein. The frequency with which other manifestations of a cow's milk allergy are reported indicates that the high protein content of cow's milk may lead to a protein sensitivity. High levels of protein have a depressing effect on iron absorption. Protein in excess of the body's need for growth and repair of tissue must undergo deamination in the liver so that the non-amino portion of the amino acids can be used as a source of energy. The nitrogenous NH_2 group must be converted to urea and excreted through the kidneys. Since the infant has a limited capacity to concentrate metabolites in the urine, the excretion of more wastes requires a larger volume of water. If the necessary water is not available, urea will accumulate and the infant ironically suffers from protein edema. In addition, the need for the liver to produce the enzymes (deaminases) necessary to remove the amino group may lead to an undesirable hypertrophy, or increase, in size of the liver.

It is also postulated that the higher rate of infection in infants fed cow's milk may occur because mechanisms that may normally be concerned with the formation of antibodies to protect against infective organisms are diverted to combat foreign milk protein.

In rats it was found that the animals on a high-protein diet who had suffered hypertrophy of the liver were less able to adjust to a low-protein diet than were those that had previously been on a moderate- or low-protein diet.

Studies to evaluate the relative biological value of meat and milk proteins have shown similar protein efficiency ratios (gain per unit of protein). Both meat and milk protein are well tolerated in the digestive tract, and infants appear to have adequate proteolytic enzymes to handle either if the curd tension is adequately reduced.

The amino acid requirements of infants are proportionately higher than those in adults. Histidine is required by infants at a level of 26 mg/100 kcal of diet per day, a level surpassed in both breast and bottle-feeding.

In one study of 6-month-old infants it was

found that 70% of the protein in the diet came from milk, 15% from meat, and 3% each from egg, cereal, and vegetables. There is no evidence that protein deficiency is a matter for concern among American infants. In fact, a study of over 300 infants showed protein intakes from one and a half to two and a half times recommended amounts.

Thiamin. Although studies based on the thiamin intake from human milk or formula and on urinary excretion data indicate that the minimum requirement is 0.2 mg/1000 kcal, the recommended dietary allowance has been set at 0.5 mg/1000 kcal. Breast milk is usually adequate if the mother's diet is adequate, but in a deficiency the nutritional quality rather than the quantity of the milk will be reduced. This has been observed primarily in developing countries where cereals and starchy roots are eaten, where the diet of the mother is high in carbohydrate and extremely low in thiamin and where infants are solely breast-fed for a year or more. Infants fed milk low in thiamin failed to gain weight, were constipated, and vomited frequently. In bottle-fed infants the possibility of a deficiency of heat-labile thiamin occurs when the formula is subjected to high heat.

Attempts to show that thiamin is beneficial as an appetite stimulant have failed to reveal any value in infant feeding, nor have scientists been able to demonstrate any benefit from thiamin supplementation on height, weight, manual dexterity, or retentive memory. It is conceded that once the metabolic defect caused by a thiamin deficiency has been corrected, the appetite improves.

In infants from 6 months to 2 years of age, diet records showed that those infants whose diets were adequate in thiamin were receiving enriched cereals, whereas those who did not receive adequate thiamin were not receiving enriched cereals.

Riboflavin. The recommendation that infants receive 0.5 mg of riboflavin per 1000 kcal of energy intake to maintain tissue saturation means that an infant up to 6 months of age needs 0.4 mg and by 6 to 12 months needs 0.6 mg. Human milk with 0.04 mg/dl will provide slightly below this amount in the usual 850 ml available for the newborn. The Academy of Pediatrics recommends 0.6 mg/1000 kcal.

Niacin. The recommended intake of 5 to 8 niacin equivalents for the infant can be met by human milk, which provides 0.17 mg of niacin and 22 mg of tryptophan, or a total of 0.5 niacin equivalents per deciliter of milk. This amounts to slightly more than the 6.6 equivalents/1000 kcal recommended for adults.

Pyridoxine. The National Research Council recommends an intake of 0.3 mg up to 6 months of age and 0.4 mg from 6 to 12 months. It is not concerned about the fact that human milk contains only 0.02 mg/dl by the end of the first month of life, since the infant has a sufficient store of pyridoxine at birth to protect him against a diet practically devoid of the nutrient. If the pyridoxine content of mother's milk fails to increase above 0.06 or 0.08 mg/L as will happen if the mother is undernourished, clinical and biochemical abnormalities may appear as the protein content of the diet continues to increase to the point where it overtaxes the infant's supply of pyridoxine to metabolize it.

The fact that infants are susceptible to a vitamin B_6 deficiency became evident when infants receiving proprietary preparations that had been subjected to very high heat (which destroyed the pyridoxine) developed convulsive seizures. As a result, the pyridoxine content of infant formulas is now maintained at a level to provide either 0.015 mg/g of protein or 0.04 mg/100 kcal, which will satisfy the metabolic requirements of the infant. An evaluation of commercially prepared infant foods showed that they contained a sufficient proportion of the vitamin in relation to the amount of protein that they provided.

Folacin. The National Research Council states that the infant probably needs from 0.005 to 0.02 mg of folacin a day but sets the recommended dietary allowance at 0.05 mg for the newborn and 0.1 mg for the 6- to 12-month-old baby. Since folic acid deficiency is considered rather general among pregnant women, the reserves with which the infant enters life may be minimal. Low maternal folate is associated with delayed maturation of the brain.

Vitamin B_{12}. It appears that the infant is parasitic on the mother in respect to vitamin B_{12}, since the infant at birth has blood levels approximately twice that of the mother. Although the daily intake of vitamin B_{12} from human milk is only 0.15 to 0.25 μg, the recommended dietary allowance during the first years of life is 0.3 μg a day. However, because of the reserves established during the prenatal period, little likelihood of a deficiency exists. The possibility of vitamin B_{12} deficiency in breast-fed infants of vegetarians is an increasing concern with more women seeking alternative food patterns.

There have been several reports and many claims in advertising that vitamin B_{12} acts as a growth stimulant. The Academy of Pediatrics, in reviewing the literature on the subject, found that in thirteen studies involving 546 "normal children," only two studies involving sixty-nine children reported a significant and stimulating effect on growth with either oral or intramuscular doses of vitamin B_{12}. In all cases the children were underweight at the beginning of the study.

Ascorbic acid. Infant needs for ascorbic acid have been set at 35 mg a day, although many studies suggest that a much lower level will provide protection against scurvy, and others suggest that the infant may be conditioned to need even higher levels. Breast-fed infants usually receive adequate amounts, but because of the destruction of heat-labile ascorbic acid during pasteurization, infants fed cow's milk usually rely on a dietary supplement during the first few months.

Vitamin A. It is assumed that the human infant, like the young of other species, enters life with a reserve of the fat-soluble vitamin A stored in the liver. The amount, however, will be dependent to a large extent on the vitamin A status of the mother. Since little information exists on the vitamin A requirements of infants, the Food and Nutrition Board of the National Research Council recommends that the infant receive the 1400 IU, or 420 RE, of vitamin A, the amount normally supplied in 850 ml of mother's milk—an amount that is apparently adequate to meet the needs of the first few months of life. Toxicity has been noted on intakes of 25,000 to 50,000 IU a day for thirty days, resulting in increased intracranial pressure and hydrocephalus.

Vitamin D. The need for vitamin D during infancy, when rapid calcification of bones and teeth occurs, is well documented. Although as little as 100 IU daily will prevent rickets and 300 IU daily will cure the condition, the ingestion of 400 IU a day promotes good calcium absorption and skeletal growth. Intakes above this apparently have no advantage, and at levels beyond 1800 IU a decrease in calcium utilization may occur. Since human milk does not provide the recommended level of vitamin D, a supplement should be provided in the first week of life. It is possible that as scientists learn about the amount of water-soluble vitamin D in human milk it will be established that there is no need for a dietary supplement.

For bottle-fed babies a supplement will be necessary only if the milk or formula is not itself fortified with the vitamin. In fact, there is concern that sensitive infants who consistently receives from 1000 to 3000 IU may experience such symptoms as hypercalcemia, depressed appetite, vague aches and pains, and retarded linear growth.

Vitamin E. Since little vitamin E crosses the placenta, human infants are born with low concentrations in the tissues. Although an intake of 5 IU of vitamin E is advised during the first year of life, one study revealed intakes ranging from 0.94 to 16.95 IU a day. Only when large amounts of unsaturated vegetable fats are substituted for the butterfat in formula feeding will the need for vitamin E increase. Premature infants, who have both low stores and a reduced ability to absorb vitamin E, frequently develop anemia when the membranes of the red blood cells rupture because they are without the antioxidant protection afforded by vitamin E. Diets high in polyunsaturated fatty acids (PUFA) make the situation worse.

Vitamin K. Vitamin K deficiency is most likely to occur in the first few days of life among breast-fed infants or among those suffering from malabsorption or diarrhea.

Calcium. Because of the rapid rate of calcification of bone to provide the rigidity and strength needed to support the weight of the body by the time the baby walks, a rich dietary source of calcium is needed in early infancy. Milk, the staple item in the diet at this time, is capable of providing the infant's needs, but the efficiency with which it is used is greatly enhanced when vitamin D is available simultaneously. Although some calcification of teeth has begun in the prenatal period, the availability and utilization of calcium in the postnatal period is a crucial factor in adequate tooth formation.

Breast milk provides about 60 mg of calcium per kilogram, which is apparently adequate because the high retention may amount to as much as two thirds of the intake. The recommended allowances of 400 to 600 mg daily are intended only for the bottle-fed infant who receives about 170 mg/kg of weight but retains only a third to a half of it.

Phosphorus. The calcium to phosphorus ratio of 1.2:1 found in cow's milk is considered too low for the young infant, who has difficulty excreting the relatively high amounts of phosphorus. This imbalance may result in a hypocalcemic neonatal tetany, an even greater problem if the retention of calcium is depressed. Thus it is recommended that the calcium to phosphorus ratio in an infant's diet be kept at 1.5:1, gradually decreasing in later infancy to a ratio closer to that in cow's milk. On the other hand, studies by Widdowson have shown beneficial effects on the absorption of calcium and magnesium when breast-fed infants were given supplements of 120 mg of phosphorus a day, suggesting that the calcium to phosphorus ratio of 2:1 in breast milk may limit calcification of bone and growth of soft tissue at an early age.

Iron. The infant's need for iron is determined to a large extent by his gestational age. Normally, a full-term infant has benefited from the transfer of a significant amount of iron from the mother to the fetus. If such reserves from fetal life are present, the infant will need virtually no dietary iron for at least three months. However, most pediatric nutritionists now recommend that bottle-fed infants be given formula fortified with ferrous sulfate at 10 to 12 mg/L from birth throughout the first year of life. Although only 4% of such iron is absorbed, it provides a constant and predictable source of iron sufficient to prevent the development of anemia. By that time an intake of 10 mg daily is recommended. This may be obtained from iron-fortified formula or supplements for the breast-fed infant in the next three months and after that from enriched cereal, egg yolk, and meat.

The premature infant with a shorter gestational period is deprived of these fetal reserves and will need a dietary source earlier. The same is true of twins, who must compete for maternal reserves and share that available. As much as 2 mg/kg may be needed shortly after birth by low–birth weight infants (less than 2500 g).

Dietary allowances are based on an average need of 1.5 mg/kg/day, although evidence exists that a normal full-term infant can maintain optimal hemoglobin levels on an intake of 1 mg/kg. The intake of 15 mg recommended from 6 to 12 months of age can be obtained only through the use of iron-fortified formulas and iron-enriched infant cereals. These cereals are fortified at a level of 12 mg/28 g (1 oz) with iron in finely divided particles, known as electrolytic iron, or with ferrous sulfate. In infant cereals mixed with fruit this is readily absorbed because of the acidity of the mixture. Because of the hazards from excessive supplementation, the amount given should not exceed 1 mg/kg/day or a maximum of 15 mg. There is some concern that the addition of iron to infant formulas may promote oxidation, leading to a reduction of the vitamin E content.

Breast-fed infants absorb as much as 50% of the iron in breast milk and possibly can manage without a supplement. However, a ferrous sulfate supplement between meals is recommended at age 4 months if the infant has not been weaned to an iron-fortified formula.

Zinc. Recently, studies showing that most infants are in negative zinc balance in the first weeks and possibly months of life have focused attention on the importance of zinc in early feeding. The high levels of zinc in colostrum (20 mg/L compared to 1 to 5 mg in mature milk) may represent an attempt to compensate for this. Both the well-documented role of zinc in promoting normal growth and its potential role in normal brain development now under investigation suggest a critical function for zinc during the development period. If a zinc deficiency is identified in large numbers of infants, zinc supplementation may be recommended.

Iodine. Concern over inadequate iodine intakes for infants has been reduced with the increase of iodine in food as the result of various iodine-containing additives. However, soy-based formulas for infants must be supplemented with iodine to counteract the effect of goitrogens found in soy products.

Fluorine. Fluorine assumes particular importance in the early feeding of infants, since it plays an important role in the development of teeth that are resistant to tooth decay. Since relatively little fluorine crosses the placenta from the mother to the infant, it is considered important to provide from 0.1 to 0.5 mg a day during the first five months of life and 0.2 to 1.0 mg in the rest of the first year. Analysis shows that formula diluted with fluoridated water will provide from 0.4 to 0.9 mg/L. Infants on formula alone receive 0.32 mg a day during the first four weeks of life and by 4 to 6 months of age, when a variety of baby foods have been added, are ingesting 1.2 mg. Because the amount a bottle-fed baby receives is dependent on the fluorine content of the water used in the formula and food preparation and because mother's milk will have fluorine only if she is using fluoridated water, a fluorine supplement available on prescription should be provided for infants whose intake is likely to be marginal.

Other trace elements. Estimates of the requirement for other trace elements during infancy have been based largely on information on the amount present in breast milk. Since these values vary considerably among mothers, depending on the amount in their diets and frequently vary within the same mother at different times, recommendations for daily intakes can only include a range of values. The best current estimates of need are presented in Table 17-4.

Water or fluid. Although the intake of water is crucial at all stages in the life cycle, it receives a little more attention in infancy than at other times because the demands are relatively greater then. The surface area per unit of body weight is twice that of the adult, which leads to a heat and water loss through the skin at a rate almost double that of the adult. Because of the high basal metabolic rate (two times that of an adult) proportionately more metabolic wastes accumulate, which calls for more water so that the kidneys can adequately excete them. This, coupled with the fact that the kidneys of an infant do not have the ability to concentrate urine to the extent that a mature kidney does, means that relatively more water is required in the

Table 17-4. Provisional recommendations for trace element intake (mg) for infants

	Birth to 6 months	6 to 12 months
Copper	0.5-0.7	0.7-1.0
Manganese	0.5-0.7	0.7-1.0
Fluorine	0.1-0.5	0.2-1.0
Chromium	0.01-0.04	0.02-0.06
Selenium	0.01-0.04	0.02-0.06
Molybdenum	0.03-0.06	0.04-0.08

elimination of the same amount of metabolites. The metabolic waste is higher on a diet high in protein, when the nitrogen from the deamination of amino acids in excess of needs for growth must be eliminated. More water is also required if the diet contains excess electrolytes such as sodium and potassium.

An infant receiving a diet of human milk requires 20 ml of water per kilogram of body weight to provide a sufficient amount for the kidneys to handle excretory products. If undiluted cow's milk is used, 87 ml is required, and if cow's milk formulas, with a third of the calories coming from added carbohydrate, is used, 61 ml is required. At a normal room temperature of 21° C, any one of these formulas would provide enough water, but at 34° C the cow's milk would not provide enough when proportionately more water is lost through the skin. If normal excretion of metabolic waste is to occur, additional water should be given. Even with a formula providing the usual 20 kcal/30 ml, parents should offer the child additional water when the environmental temperature is high. Formula should not have a calorie density greater than 30 kcal/30 ml. Body water will be reduced to 70% of normal before the renal excretion of water is reduced.

Since a thirsty baby acts like a hungry baby, it is not uncommon to find parents giving a baby food when they should be offering water. This only increases the need for water and hence thirst.

Many nutritional requirements of infants may be influenced by the use of drugs. There is convincing evidence that anticonvulsant drugs increase the need for both vitamin D and folic acid. Antibiotics influence the availability of several nutrients such as vitamin B_{12}, carotene, and iron and the synthesis of vitamin K.

INTRODUCTION OF SOLID FOODS

At the turn of the century, pediatricians were recommending that the milk diet of infants be supplemented with a food such as meat or cereal after 1 year of age. By 1917 Dr. Emmett Holt was suggesting that a meat broth could safely be introduced at 8 or 9 months of age but that solid foods should be withheld until 1 year. By 1956 the pendulum had swung so far in the opposite direction that some pediatricians were recommending that an infant be put on solid foods and be expected to adhere to three meals a day by 2 or 3 weeks of age.

The Academy of Pediatrics, recognizing a trend in infant feeding practices toward progressively earlier introduction of solid foods in the absence of any evidence of a nutritional or physiological need, surveyed practicing pediatricians to determine their recommendations and the bases for them. It found that the physicians were indeed suggesting the use of cereal by 3 to 6 weeks of age, followed by other foods so that by 4 or 5 months the child received a full diet of meat, eggs, fruit, vegetables, and cereal. Their reasons for this practice reflected their response to the demands of parents that they follow this "progressive" procedure rather than any belief that the infant needed the solid food.

The pendulum has now swung back with current recommendation that milk be the sole source of nourishment in the first six months of life and the primary source during the rest of the first year. This recommendation reflects a rational approach to the question of the timing and sequence of additions to the infant's diet. Considerations of the nutritional needs of the infant, his physiological readiness to use foods other than milk, his physical capacity to handle them, and the relative advantages and disadvantages of adding semisolid or solid foods all entered into this recommendation.

Nutrition. From a nutritional standpoint it is now recognized that the nutritive needs of an infant can be readily met by a milk diet supplemented with iron and fluorine and in some cases ascorbic acid and vitamin D. Since these can be added by fortification of milk or formula or as supplements, there is no need to introduce foods other than milk before age 6 months. The addition of foods other than milk has been termed "beikost." Although current recommendations are to wait until age 6 months to introduce beikost, in actual practice it is still being given at 3 to 4 months. Regardless of whether or not food is added at 3 to 4 months or at 6 months of age, the sequence and principles are the same.

By 6 months of age a milk diet alone is not capable of providing the calories necessary for the increased needs of the growing infant. At that time infant cereal is usually added to the diet. It is mixed with milk to a consistency that can be swallowed but not sucked from the spoon. After several cereals have been introduced individually for about one week at a time each to maximize the possibility of identifying a cereal allergy, the child is offered a variety of strained fruits, again one at a time for several weeks. The addition of sugar to fruit is unnecessary from a nutritional standpoint but is added in small amounts in some commercial products to assure a consistency in flavor by standardizing the natural variation in sweetness from batch to batch. Bananas that are fully ripened so that the starch is changed to sugar are a very acceptable fruit for infants. Fruits are followed by vegetables in the same pattern, one at a time. These solid foods contribute an increasingly large proportion of the infant's energy requirement with cereals providing 8% to 10% of the calories and other baby foods 30% to 40% by 9 months of age.

The protein needs of the infant also exceed that provided by milk alone and the diet must be supplemented by a source of protein. Egg yolk with 33% protein, meat with 20%, and cottage cheese with 17% are considered suitable additions to the diet. Egg, which is allergenic, should be avoided for infants in families with a history of food allergy.

As additional foods are introduced it is desirable to maintain the distribution of calories from protein at 7% to 16%, from fat at 35% to 55% and from carbohydrate at 29% to 58%, proportions close to those in human milk. The percentage of calories from various energy sources in selected types of baby foods is given in Table 17-5.

Physical development. Infants vary in the rate at which the normal rooting, sucking, and extrusion reflexes inherent at the time of birth are replaced by the ability to swallow; as these changes occur, an infant must learn to use them in the eating process, just as he learns to walk or talk. The lower jaw is very poorly developed and fat pads are located in the cheeks to facilitate sucking. As the infant matures, the contour of the jaw changes and the fat pads disappear, leaving the infant

Table 17-5. Caloric density, cost, and distribution of calories in infant foods

	kcal/100 g	Protein (%)	Fat (%)	CHO (%)	Cost (cents/100 kcal)
Egg yolk	192	21	76	3	—
Meats	106	53	46	1	—
Fruits	85	2	2	96	13.2
Soups and dinners	58	16	28	56	20.2
Vegetables	45	14	6	80	26
Human milk	67	6	56	38	—
Nonfat milk	35	40	3	57	8.5
Whole milk	67	22	48	30	5.5

with the capability of chewing and swallowing rather than sucking food.

The swallowing reflex involves sufficient innervation of the tongue to enable it to form any solid food placed at the tip of the tongue into a ball and throw it to the back of the mouth, where first gravity and then the peristaltic action of the esophagus take over to convey it to the stomach. This ability usually develops at 3 months of age, but before this the extrusion reflex that causes the infant to forcibly reject food or objects placed at the front of the tongue must diminish in strength. Since the ability to move food from the tip of the tongue to the throat normally develops at 2½ to 3 months of age, any effort to feed solid or semisolid foods prior to that time means that the food is conveyed to the esophagus by some method other than swallowing. Either it must be placed sufficiently far back in the mouth that it can reach the esophagus by gravity, or the consistency of the product must be so thin that the infant is able to suck from the spoon as a liquid, rather than using a swallowing mechanism. Many times the infant who cannot manipulate the tongue to swallow cannot use it to reject objects or food placed in his mouth either. Thus it is not uncommon to have parents report that infants who had apparently accepted solid food at 3 to 6 weeks of age appear to reject it at 10 to 12 weeks. Developmentally, few infants are ready to handle anything but liquid food until 10 to 12 weeks of age. Any effort to force them earlier may result in a frustrating and unhappy feeding experience for both the parent and the child.

Physiological development. The ability to handle foods other than milk also depends on the physiological development of the infant. All the secretions of the digestive tract contain enzymes especially suited to the digestion of the complex nutrients of human milk but few needed for other foods.

For instance, the secretion of the salivary glands is minimal at birth but increases in volume until it becomes sufficiently copious to cause drooling by 2 or 3 months. This is evident in the infant who has not developed the innervation of the outer part of the lips necessary to prevent it. Since salivary enzymes are involved only in the digestion of the complex starches, they are unnecessary as long as the child is receiving only milk with the disaccharide lactose as the only carbohydrate. The appearance of salivary amylase in the saliva occurs at the time the infant is given more complex carbohydrates such as the starch in cereals.

The proteolytic enzymes are present in adequate amounts to digest milk protein as long as it is sufficiently dilute to produce a soft flocculent curd on which the enzymes can act. As the child matures, the secretion of proteolytic enzymes in the intestinal juice increases this capacity of the infant to digest nonmilk proteins. By 4 to 6 months of age, most infants are able to handle most proteins.

The kidney function of the full-term infant is not completely mature. The well-developed glomeruli satisfactorily filter the blood presented to the kidneys, but the tubules, which are functionally less mature, are unable to resorb water and some solutes adequately. The tubules become efficient by 6 to 8 weeks, after which there is less concern over the use of a high-protein, high-sodium diet. Because of the poorly developed kidney function, it is important not to give the kidneys too much solute (renal solute load) to excrete. For this reason protein beyond that needed for growth and extra sodium usually given as sodium chloride should be avoided. This is especially important when the infant suffers excessive loss of fluid such as in a hot climate or with diarrhea or when foods of high caloric density are fed.

Low gastric acidity due to the limited secretion of hydrochloric acid in early infancy has implications for the use of vegetables such as beets, spinach, or broccoli, which contain nitrates. In the absence of gastric acidity they are more readily converted to nitrites that in turn react with amines in the intestine to produce nitrosamines, which are potential carcinogens. Alternatively, absorbed nitrites cause the conversion of hemoglobin to methemoglobin with a reduced oxygen-carrying capacity. For these reasons these vegetables should be avoided in feeding young infants and nitrites should be consumed only when used to control botulism in some foods.

When solid foods are introduced at an extremely early age, so little is consumed and they make such an insignificant contribution to the nutrient intake that one questions whether the extra work and cost and the risk of contamination can be justified. If solid foods are taken in addition to milk, there is a concern about the effects of overeating; if they replace milk, the effect of the reduced calcium intake is cause for concern.

Other considerations. Many reasons have been advanced either to support or to reject the introduction of solid foods from 2 to 8 weeks of age. The belief of many parents that they can hasten the time at which the infant sleeps through the night has not been corroborated by experimental data when the criterion of 8 consecutive hours of sleep was considered "sleeping through the night."

One must also consider that if the infant does sleep through the night at an early age, he must either experience a reduction in total food intake or consume larger amounts at each of the remaining feedings, thus taxing the capacity of the stomach. Some scientists have expressed the fear that such a pattern of overeating at an early age may persist throughout life and be a possible factor in obesity of children and adolescents. Such obesity of early onset is one of the most difficult types to treat.

Since the nutritive value of the solid food consumed in the first few months is usually of minimum significance, the major argument in favor of its use is that the child becomes accustomed early to a wider variety of flavors and textures of food and continues to accept these as he matures. Beal found that the age at which a child accepted solid foods did not parallel an advancement in the age at which the food was offered. As a result, she reported a period during which the child and mother experienced an unpleasant feeding relationship, with the mother trying to feed an infant who was not yet ready for the food. She believed that the forcible feeding of semi-solids before the ninth to twelfth weeks tended to increase the incidence of feeding problems and food dislikes in the infant. The relationship between the age of introduction

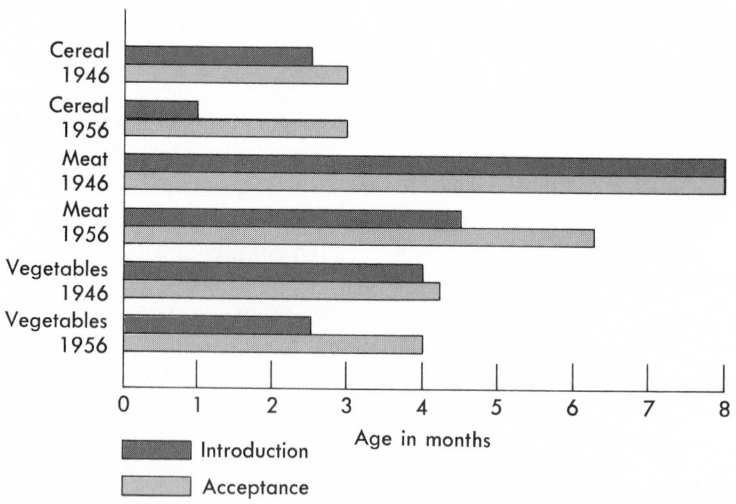

Fig. 17-4. Comparison age of introduction of solid food and acceptance between 1946 and 1956. (Based on Beal, V. A.: Pediatrics **20**:448, 1957.)

of solid foods and their acceptance is shown in Fig. 17-4.

Although findings in the literature are not consistent, many studies report an increased incidence of food allergy among infants who are introduced to a variety of foods at an early age. This is an especially important consideration among infants with a family history of allergy. For these, allergists suggest delaying the time of initial introduction of solid foods and choosing foods that are minimally allergenic, such as vegetables, fruits, and rice cereal. They also advise feeding each food for a relatively short time and then switching to another to avoid the sensitization that may arise from prolonged exposure to one food.

György recognizes that the extrusion or "thrust" reflex is innate to normal infants, but that it may be suppressed by prolonged spoon-feeding. He suggests that the inhibition of this natural defense mechanism might lead to frustration and mental insult, finally manifesting itself in a neurotic adjustment.

In addition to an immaturity of secretion of digestive enzymes, the young infant has low levels of many cellular enzymes. One that has been known for some time is phenylalanine hydroxylase, which is required for the metabolism of phenylalanine. A diet high in protein in the neonatal period will tax the infant's ability to tolerate the amino acid phenylalanine.

Concern over the safety of food additives in infant foods has focused on the use of salt (sodium chloride) and monosodium glutamate. Both have been added to many commercially prepared infant foods, primarily to make them more palatable to the mother who is feeding them, rather than to the child who is eating them. Since no physiological or nutritional reason exists for adding them, and as long as the question on their safety remains unresolved, in 1970 the National Academy of Sciences recommended to the Food and Drug Administration that the level of salt in infant foods be restricted to 0.25% in contrast to the 1% previously found in many commercially prepared products. Since then, several food processors have discontinued the use of added salt in baby foods and have issued a label statement asking the parents not to season it to their taste at feeding time. Concern about the use of salt centers around the theory that the young infant with immature kidneys cannot cope with the increased electrolyte that must be excreted and retains it, with the resultant increase in fluid volume and the potential of becoming predisposed to hypertension. The earlier a child begins eating solid foods, the earlier his intake will reach high levels. Studies of the preferences of infants showed that they ate the same amount of food regardless of whether or not salt was added. In the case of monosodium glutamate, a flavor enhancer, the concern arises from reports that mice fed high intakes developed brain tumors. So far there is no evidence of potential danger in the amounts consumed by the young infant, but commercially there has been voluntary withdrawal of the use of monosodium glutamate. Also, sugar is now used only to adjust the natural sweetness of fruit, and 2% to 4% added starch is used to adjust texture.

Additions to the diet. In spite of current trends in feeding practices, which show that 90% of infants in the United States are fed solid food before 3 months of age, the Academy of Pediatrics, after a careful consideration of all the factors involved, recommends that the optimal time for introducing solid foods into the infant's diet is 5 to 6 months of age. They agree that no nutritional or psychological benefit results from any earlier introduction.

Once the child is physically and physiologically capable of handling solid foods, the sequence and timing with which they are introduced should be determined by the nutritional needs of the child. Single-grain cereals are frequently used first because of their iron content, their ease of preparation and storage, minimal allergenic potential, and relatively low cost. This is usually followed by a variety of strained fruits and vegetables, with care being taken to avoid those that may be irritating to the gastrointestinal tract either through roughage or the production of gas. Egg yolk, which provides vitamin A, iron, and riboflavin, is frequently used as an early source of protein. Next most infants will also receive meat. The order of use of foods is not crucial, as is evidenced by the number of patterns on which children thrive. More important is the provision of the nutrients needed to supplement a milk diet in a form suited to the digestive capacities of the child and the formation of a set of eating habits that will lead to good nutrition throughout childhood.

In most infants the eruption of the first teeth and the physical readiness to chew both occur at approximately 5 to 6 months of age. It is very important that the infant be given an opportunity to chew at this critical time in order that this capacity by developed. Dry bread is the most acceptable food to stimulate chewing. Caution should be exerted to avoid the use of hard flintlike materials such as crisp bacon and certain commercial biscuits, which may irritate the throat.

As the infant's digestive capacities develop, the strained foods of early infancy can be replaced by less finely chopped foods,

Text continued on p. 465.

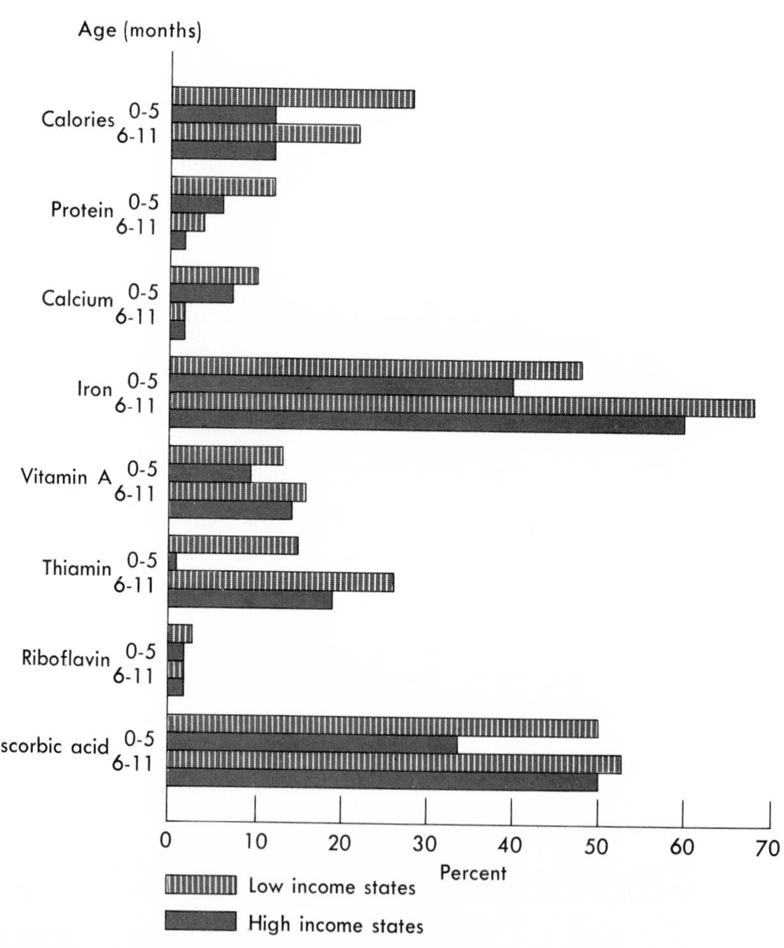

Fig. 17-5. Percentage of infants with dietary intakes below two-thirds of the RDA by age and income level. Data based on results of Ten-State Nutrition Survey (1968-1970).

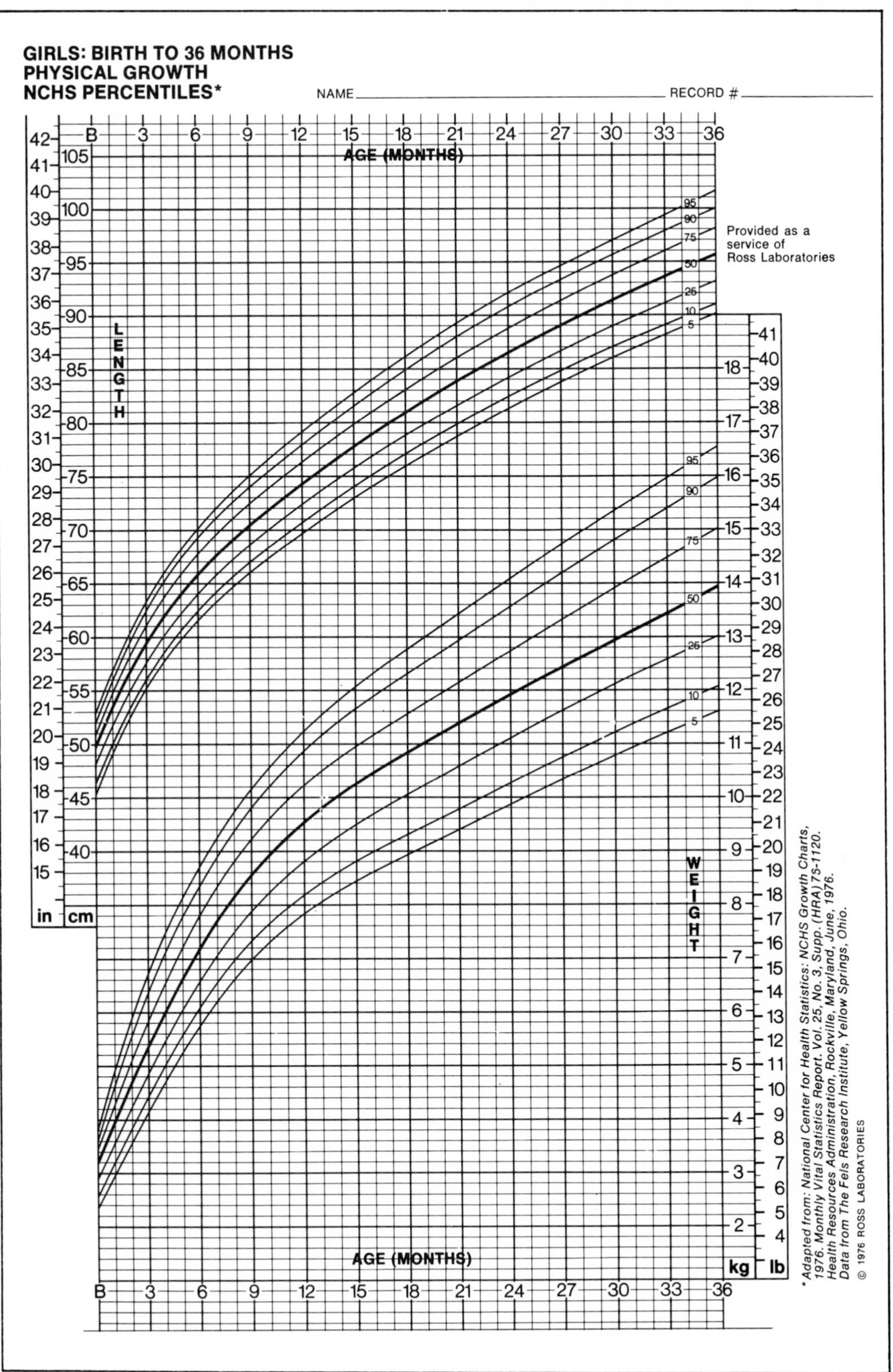

Fig. 17-6. Weight and height for age for girls from birth to 36 months. (Courtesy Ross Laboratories.)

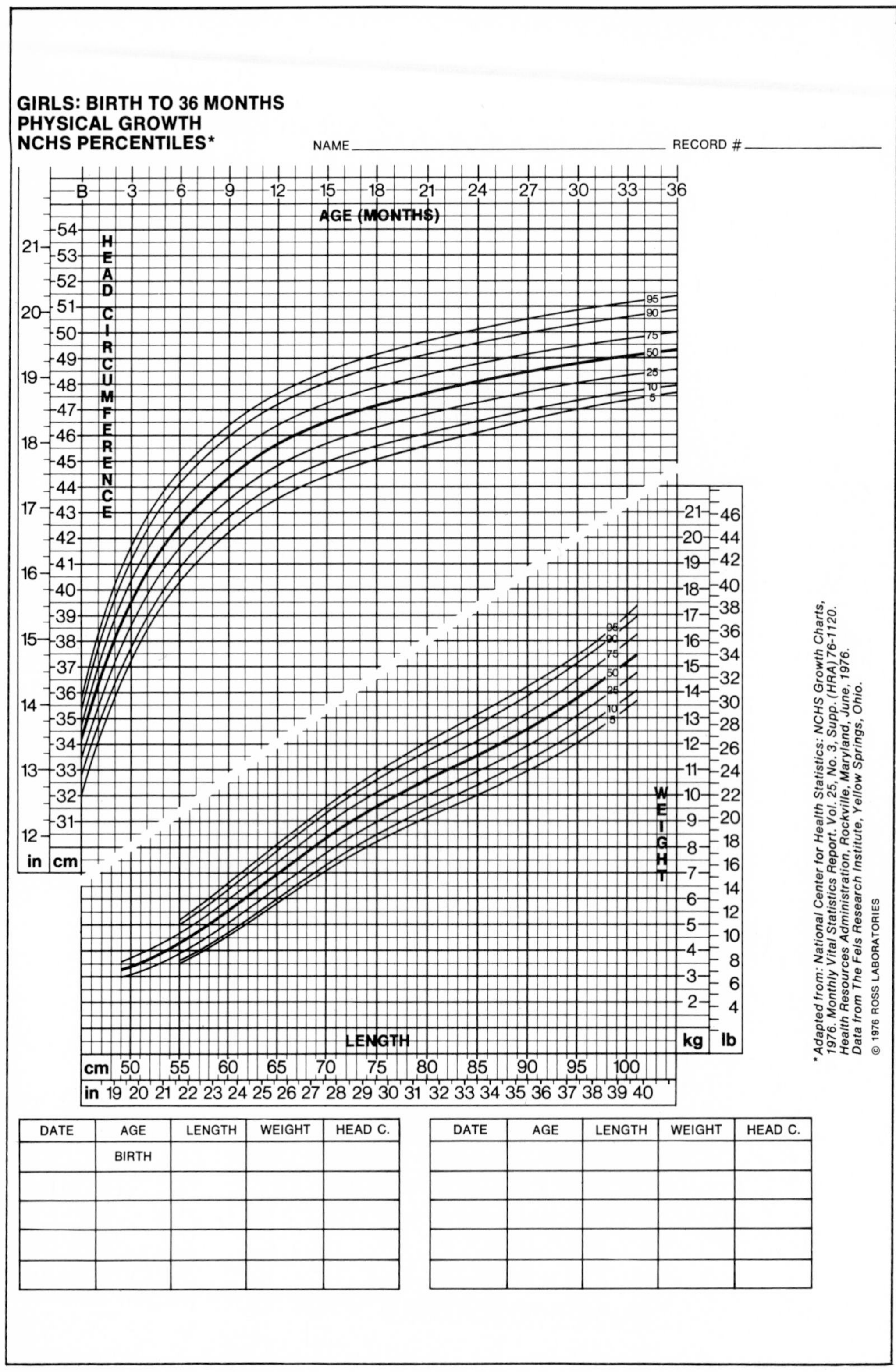

Fig. 17-7. Weight for length and head circumference for age for girls from birth to 36 months. (Courtesy Ross Laboratories.)

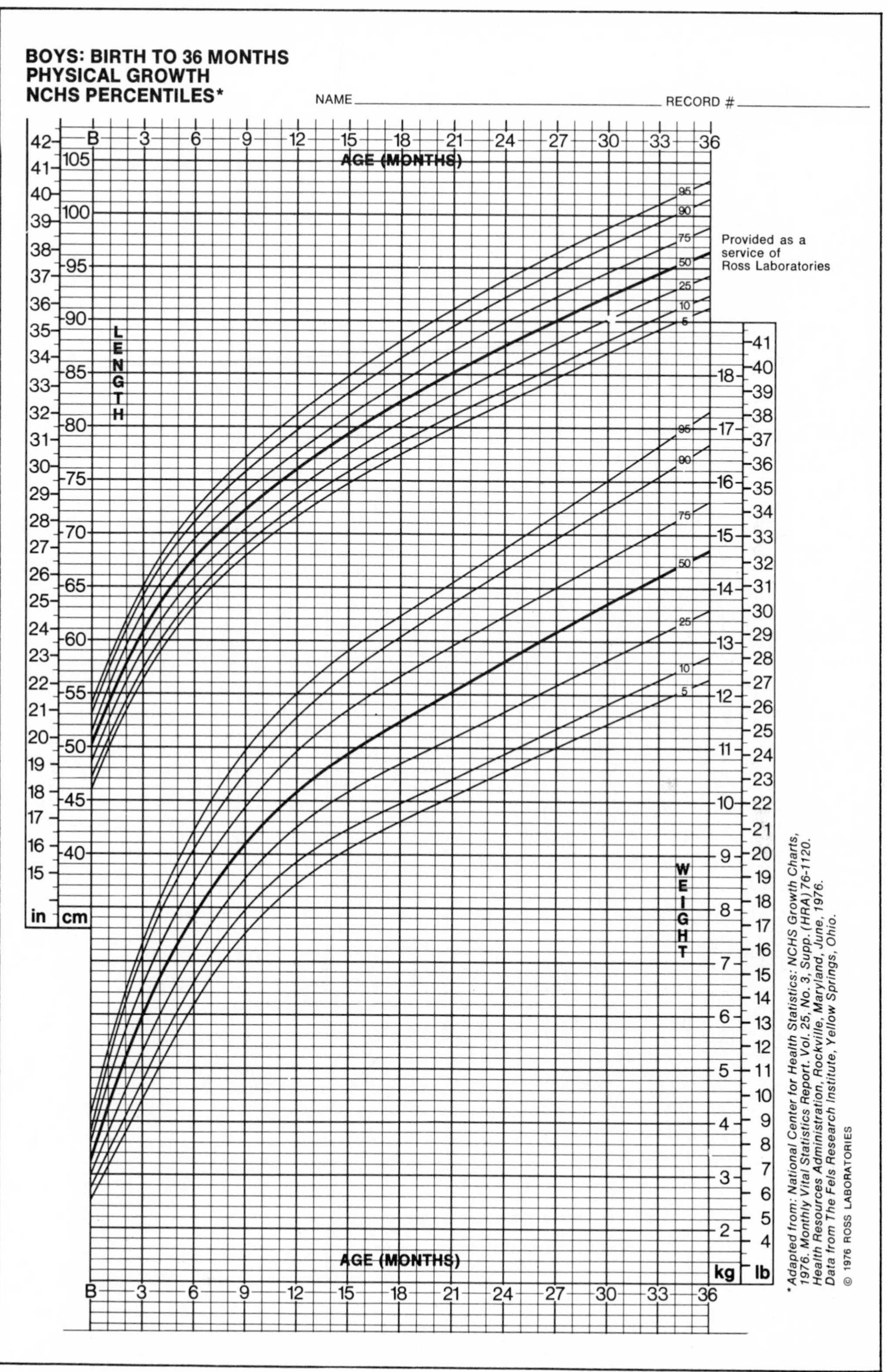

Fig. 17-8. Weight and height for age for boys from birth to 36 months. (Courtesy Ross Laboratories.)

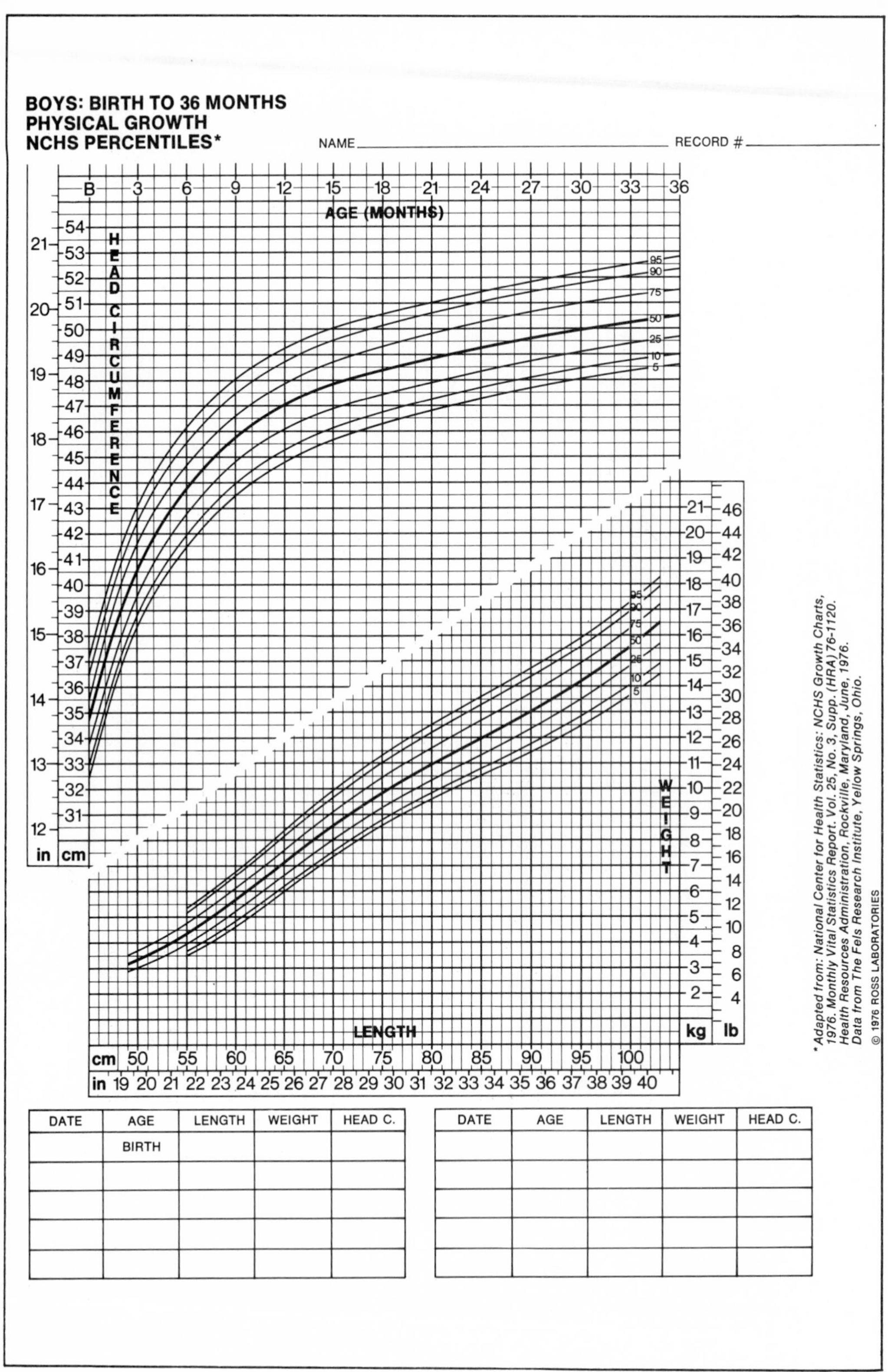

Fig. 17-9. Weight for length and head circumference for age for boys from birth to 36 months. (Courtesy Ross Laboratories.)

with a final transition to table foods. A wide range is found in the age at which this transition is made in a normal child.

EARLY FEEDING AND LATER DEVELOPMENT

In spite of the fact that it is often difficult to obtain adequate data, several investigators recently have been concerned about the effect of early feeding practices on later development. Interest has centered primarily on the question of whether infant feeding practices may predispose the child to later degenerative diseases. There is now suggestive evidence that the number of fat cells is determined in the first year of life and that overfeeding may lead to the formation of an excessive number of cells. Infants who form larger numbers of fat cells have a greater capacity to store fat and hence have a tendency toward obesity throughout life. Similarly, atherosclerosis, a major cause of death in males, is a condition in which high blood cholesterol levels and the deposition of lipid in the wall of the artery are risk factors that may be influenced by early feeding. Complete elimination of cholesterol from the diet of the young is, however, undesirable because the child apparently then loses the ability to excrete cholesterol and to regulate synthesis in later life. If polyunsaturated fats are substituted for saturated fats as a way of decreasing cholesterol levels, the amount of vitamin E must be increased. The use of high levels of salt before the child's kidneys are mature enough to excrete the excess sodium may increase the risk of hypertension (high blood pressure) in adulthood, although this may be conditioned by many other factors. It is also postulated that demyelinating disease may be the result of a disorder of carbohydrate metabolism in early life. In all cases the effect of early diet assumes more importance for infants with a family history of any one of these conditions.

Adequacy of the diets of infants

Relatively few studies have assessed the nutritive intake of infants. The National Nutrition Survey, however, did obtain information on 258 infants under 6 months of age and on 340 infants between 6 and 11 months of age. These data are presented in Fig. 17-5 and show clearly that intakes of iron are most likely to fall below recommended levels and that ascorbic acid intakes are frequently low in this age group. The mean intakes for all nutrients except iron exceeded the recommended levels.

The amount of calcium per kilogram of body weight and per 1000 kcal declined rapidly with age, reflecting the shift from milk to other foods with a lower content of calcium.

The adequacy of the diets of infants is best assessed by the rate and pattern of growth and absence of illness. To help assess growth, the National Center for Health Statistics has developed growth charts representing expected patterns at varying percentiles for both boys and girls from birth to 3 years for height for age, weight for age, weight for height, and head circumference for age. Some representative charts are reproduced in Figs. 17-6 to 17-9.

Failure to thrive in infants who fall below the 5th percentile in both height and weight is due primarily to an inadequate food intake. This may reflect an increased need related to an illness, failure to absorb food, or a variety of social factors such as child abuse or vegetarianism.

BIBLIOGRAPHY

Andelman, M. B., and Sared, B. R.: Utilization of dietary iron by term infants, Am. J. Dis. Child. **111**:45, 1966.

Athreya, B. H., Coriell, L. L., and Charney, J.: Poliomyelitis antibodies in human colostrum and milk. J. Pediatr. **64**:79, 1964.

Bakwin, H.: Erotic feeding in infants and young children, Am. J. Dis. Child. **126**:52, 1973.

Bakwin, H.: Feeding programs for infants, Fed. Proc. **23**:66, 1964.

Beal, V. A.: Breast- and formula-feeding of infants, J. Am. Diet. Assoc. **55**:31, 1969.

Beal, V. A. : On the acceptance of solid foods and other food patterns of infants and children, Pediatrics **20**:448, 1957.

Brown, R. E.: Breast feeding in modern times, Am. J. Clin. Nutr. **26**:1973.

Call, J. D.: Emotional factors favoring successful breast feeding of infants, J. Pediatr. **5**:485, 1959.

Cameron, M. E.: The effect of the addition of foods to human milk on the protein value of the infant's diet, Proc. Nutr. Soc. **27**:8A, 1968.

Committee on Nutrition, American Academy of Pediatrics: On the feeding of solid foods to infants, Pediatrics **21**:685, 1958; Trace elements in infant nutrition, Pediatrics **26**:715, 1960; Infantile scurvy and nutritional rickets, Pediatrics **29**:646, 1962; The prophylactic requirement and toxicity of vitamin D, Pediatrics **31**:512, 1963; Vitamin D intake and the hypercalcemic syndrome, Pediatrics **35**:1022, 1965; Proposed changes in Food and Drug Administration regulations concerning formula products and vitamin-mineral dietary supplements for infants, Pediatrics **40**:916, 1967; Iron balance and requirements in infancy, Pediatrics **43**:134, 1969; Salt intake and eating patterns of infants and children in relation to blood pressure, Pediatrics **53**:115, 1974; Should milk drinking by children be discouraged? Pediatrics **53**:576, 1974; Iron supplementation for infants, Pediatrics **58**:765, 1976; Nutritional aspects of vegetarianism, health foods and fad diets, Pediatrics **59**:460, 1977; Nutritional needs of low–birth weight infants, Pediatrics **60**:519, 1977; Zinc, Pediatrics **62**:408, 1978.

Dahl, L. K., Kesanen, A., and Peltonen, T.: High salt content of western infant's diets, Nature (London) **198**:1204, 1963.

Davis, K. C.: Vitamin E: adequacy of infant diets, Am. J. Clin. Nutr. **25**:933, 1972.

Eid, E. E.: Follow-up study of physical growth of children who had excessive weight gain in the first six months of life. Br. Med. J. **2**:74, 1970.

Ferris, A. G., Viliijalmsdottin, L. B., Beal, V. A., and Pellett, P. L.: Diet in the first 6 months of infants in western Massachusetts, J. Am. Diet. Assoc. **72**:115, 1978.

Filer, L. J.: Early nutrition: its long-term role, Hosp. Prac. **13**:87, 1978.

Fomon, S. J.: What are infants fed in the United States? Pediatrics **56**:350, 1975.

Fomon, S. J., Filer, L. J., Thomas, L. N., Rogers, R. R., and Proksch, A. M.: Relationship between formula concentration and rate of growth of normal infants J. Nutr. **98**:241, 1969.

Fomon, S. J.: Infant nutrition, ed. 2, Philadelphia, 1974, W. B. Saunders Co.

Fomon, S. J., Thomas, L. N., and Filer, L. J.: Acceptance of unsalted strained foods by normal infants, J. Pediat. **76**:242, 1970.

Grunwaldt, E., Bates, T., and Guthrie, D.: The onset of sleeping through the night in infancy, Pediatrics **26**:667, 1960.

Gryboski, J. D.: The swallowing mechanism of the neonate, Pediatrics **35**:445, 1965.

Guthrie, H. A.: Effect of early feeding of solid foods on nutritive intake of infants, Pediatrics **38**:879, 1966.

Guthrie, H. A.: Infant feeding practices—a predisposing factor in hypertension? Am. J. Clin. Nutr. **21**:863, 1968.

Guthrie, H. A.: Nutritional intake of infants, J. Am. Diet. Assoc. **43**:120, 1963.

György, P.: The late effects of early nutrition, Am. J. Clin. Nutr. **8**:344, 1961.

Haddy, T. B., Jurkowski, C., Brody, H., Kallen, D. J., Czaijka-Narins, D. M.: Iron deficiency with and without anemia in infants and children, Am. J. Dis. Child. **128**:787, 1974.

Hansen, A. E., Wiese, H. F., Boelsche, A. N., Hoggard, M. E., Adam, D. J., and Davis, H.: Role of linoleic acid in infant nutrition, Pediatrics **31**:171, 1963.

Heiner, D. C., Wilson, J. F., and Lahey, M. E.: Sensitivity to cow's milk, J.A.M.A. **189**:563, 1964.

Heseltine, M. M., and Pitts, J. L.: Economy in nutrition and feeding of infants, Am. J. Public Health **56**:1756, 1966.

Holt, L. E., and Snyderman, S. E.: Protein and amino acid requirements of infants and children, Nutr. Abstr. Rev. **35**:1, 1965.

Jensen, R. G., Hagerty, M. M., and McMahon, K. E.: Lipid in human milk and infant formulas: a review, Am. J. Clin. Nutr. **31**:990, 1978.

Jelliffe, D. B.: World trends in infant feeding, Am. J. Clin. Nutr. **29**:1227, 1976.

Jusko, W. J. Khanna, N., Levy, G., Stern, L., and Yaffe, S. J.: Riboflavin absorption and excretion in the neonate, Pediatrics **76**:549, 1970.

Lapatsanis, P., Makaronis, G., Vretos, C., and Doxiadis, S.: Two types of nutritional rickets in infants, Am. J. Clin. Nutr. **29**:1222, 1976.

Mata, L.: Breast-feeding: main promoter of infant health, Am. J. Clin. Nutr. **31**:2058, 1978.

Mathews, D. J., et al.: Prevention of eczema, Lancet **1**:321, 1977.

Mathews, R. H. and Workman, M. Y.: Nutrient content of selected baby foods, J. Am. Diet. Assoc. **72**:27, 1978.

McMillan, J. A., Landaw, S. A., and Oski, F. A.: Iron sufficiency in breast-fed infants and the availability of iron from human milk, Pediatrics **58**:686, 1976.

Meyer, H. F.: Breast feeding in the United States, Clin. Pediatr. **7**:708, 1968.

Naismith, D. J., Deeprose, S. P., and Ma, M. C. F.: The linoleic acid requirement of the human infant, Proc. Nutr. Soc. **35**:65A, 1976.

Nammacher, M. A., Willemin, M., Hartmann, J. R., and Gaston, L. W.: Vitamin K deficiency in infants beyond the neonatal period, J. Pediatr. **76**:549, 1970.

Neumann, C. G., and Alpaugh, M.: Birth weight doubling time: a fresh look, Pediatrics **57**:469, 1976.

Owen, G. M.: Modification of cow's milk for infant formulas. Current practices, Am. J. Clin. Nutr. **22**:1150, 1969.

Pipes, P.: Nutrition in infancy and childhood, St. Louis, 1977, The C. V. Mosby Co.
Pipes, P.: When should semisolid foods be fed to infants? Nutr. Ed. **9**:57, 1977.
Purvis, G. A.: What nutrients do our infants really get? Nutr. Today **8**:28, 1973.
Smith, N. J., and Rios, E.: Iron metabolism and iron deficiency in infancy and childhood, Adv. Pediatr. **21**:239, 1974.
Rios, E., Hunter, R. E., Cook, J. D., Smith, N. J., and Finch, C. A.: The absorption of iron as supplements in infant cereal and infant formulas, Pediatrics **55**:686, 1975.
Robson, J. R. K., Konlande, J. E., Larkin, F. A., O'Connor, P. A. and Liu, H. Y.: Zen macrobiotic dietary problems in infancy. Pediatrics **53**:326, 1974.
Roender, L. M., and Chow, B. F.: Maternal undernutrition and its longterm effects on the offspring. Am. J. Clin. Nutr. **25**:812, 1972.
Rothman, D.: Folic acid in pregnancy, Am. J. Obstet. Gynecol. **108**:149, 1970.
Salber, E. J., and Feinlieb, M.: Breast feeding in Boston, Pediatrics **37**:299, 1966.
Schubert, W. K.: Fat nutrition and diet in childhood, Am. J. Cardiol. **31**:581, 1973.
Smith, C. A.: Prenatal and neonatal nutrition, Pediatrics **30**:145, 1962.
Smith, N. J., and Rios, E.: Iron metabolism and iron deficiency in infancy and childhood, Adv. Pediatr. **21**:239, 1974.
Snyderman, S. E., Boyer, A., Roitman, E., Holt, L. E., Jr. and Prose, P. H.: The histidine requirement of the infant, Pediatrics **31**:786, 1963.
Stearns, G. : Nutrition status of mother prior to conception, J.A.M.A. **168**:1655, 1958.
Stevens, H. A., and Ohlson, M. A.: Nutritive value of the diets of medically indigent pregnant women, J. Am. Diet. Assoc. **50**:290, 1967.
Teel, B. F.: Adaptations of digestive tract during reproduction in the mammal, World Rev. Nutr. Diet. **14**:181, 1972.
Tsang, R. C., Gigger, M., Oh, W., and Brown, D. R.: Studies in calcium metabolism in infants with intrauterine growth retardation. J. Am. Diet. Assoc.
Vobecky, J. S., Vobecky, J., Shapcott, D., and Blanchard, R.: Vitamin E and C levels in infants during the first year of life, Am. J. Clin. Nutr. **29**:766, 1976.
Walravens, P. A. and Hambidge, K. M.: Growth of infants fed a zinc supplemented formula, Am. J. Clin. Nutr. **29**:1114, 1976.
Wiatrowski, E., Kramer, L., Osis, D., and Spencer, H.: Dietary fluoride intake of infants, Pediatrics **55**:517, 1975.
Widdowson, E. M.: Effect of giving phosphate supplements on the absorption and excretion of calcium, strontium, magnesium and phosphorus to breast-fed babies, Lancet **2**:1250, 1963.
Will a fat baby become a fat child? Nutr. Rev. **35**:138, 1977.
Woodruff, C. W.: The science of infant nutrition and the art of infant feeding, J.A.M.A. **240**:657, 1978.

18

Nutrition from infancy to adulthood

The period from infancy to adulthood is characterized by periodic growth spurts interspersed with periods of relatively slow increase in body size. Many such periods are characterized by nutritional stresses, which require increased intakes of specific nutrients. In addition to the physiological stresses, many social, economic, and cultural variables influences nutritional needs and intakes.

In discussing the nutritive needs during infancy in Chaper 17, we dealt with the character of the diet and the gradual change in both variety and quality of the dietary intake that occurs as the child's nutritive needs and his ability to handle a greater variety and complexity of foods increase during the first year of life. The age at which an infant makes the transition from bottle-or breast-feeding and from pureed or chopped baby foods to drinking from a cup and eating selected items from the regular family diet varies greatly from one child to another. Some make the adjustment as early as 8 months of age, whereas others may not reach this stage of maturity until 2 years of age or later. Aside from encouraging the child to chew when the ability to do so is established and to feed himself when he has the manual dexterity to manipulate a spoon, there is little reason to push the change. Indeed, some evidence suggests that the infant should not be denied the work of sucking from either the breast or bottle at too early an age, as this may predispose to thumb-sucking in early childhood or to poorly developed jaws with attendant problems of crowded dentition.

This chapter will deal with the nutritive needs and special considerations in adapting food to the child's needs after the pattern of feeding of early infancy has been modified to include the use of table foods.

CHILDHOOD

Although growth occurs at a varying rate throughout childhood, there appears to be a generally increased need for all nutrients. The pattern of increase, however, varies for different nutrients.

The dietary standards proposed by the Food and Nutrition Board of the National Research Council represent the level of intake it believes will provide optimal health benefits to practically all children in each age group. The recognition that growth of children occurs in spurts—a period of rapid increase in skeletal height followed by a slow increase in height but a more rapid increase in weight—should suggest that these values may represent an excessive margin of safety at one time and a realistic goal at another. They do remain, however, the standard against which to assess dietary adequacy and the nutritional goal used in planning food intakes. Although the total nutritional need increases with age, the requirement on the basis of body weight declines.

Fig. 18-1 represents the percentage change in nutritive needs over a base of two to three years that occurs with increasing age. It is obvious that the suggested increment varies from one nutrient to another. Fortunately, in terms of ease of diet planning the increment for calories in the majority of cases is at least as large as the increment for other nutrients.

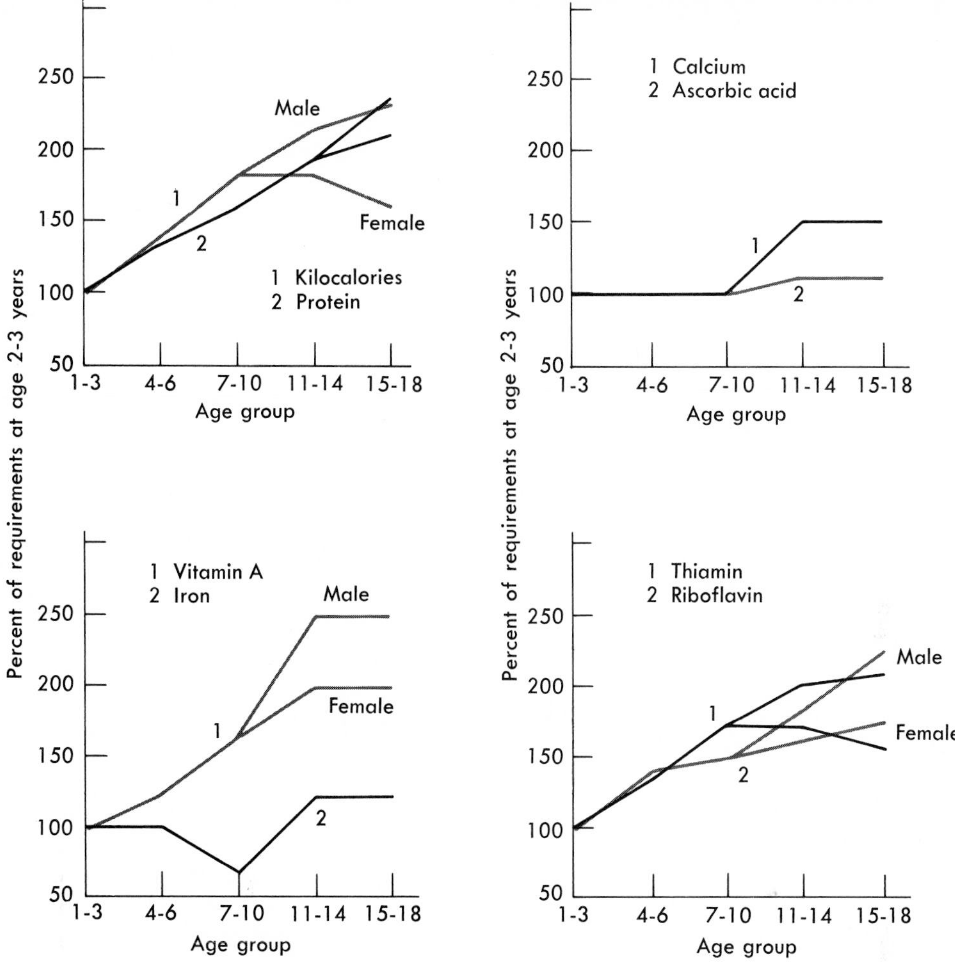

Fig. 18-1. Increase in nutritive needs during growth from age 2-3 years to 18 years. (Based on Recommended dietary allowances, ed. 8, Washington, D.C., 1974, National Academy of Sciences, National Research Council, Food and Nutrition Board.)

As one would expect, the increase in energy needs represents the amount of energy needed for basal metabolism, activity, and the amount stored as new muscle or adipose tissue. Requirements for basal metabolism and activity will increase proportionately with body size, whereas those for growth will vary with the rate of growth and deposition of new tissue.

Since many of the water-soluble vitamins, such as thiamin, niacin, and pantothenic acid, are involved primarily in energy metabolism, it is not surprising to find their requirements increasing in proportion to total energy needs. Pyridoxine, involved in the utilization of dietary protein and in the synthesis of tissue protein, will be required in greater amounts during periods of rapid muscle growth. Any increase in muscle mass that must accompany bone growth requires a positive nitrogen balance that is met by protein intakes of 1.5 to 2 g/kg of body weight. The increase in total body size necessitates a larger vascular system to transport nutrients to the tissues and waste products away, thus making demands for nutrients needed in blood formation—iron, protein, and folacin. Bone growth creates a need for protein, calcium, phosphorus, fluorine, and vitamin D. Although the biological roles of vitamin A and ascorbic acid have not been elucidated, adequate evidence indicates that the amount needed increases with body size.

Although it is known that the overall need for nutrients increases throughout the growth period, there will be periods when growth is slow, with needs for certain nutrients reduced proportionately. Children frequently reflect these fluctuations in need by fluctuations in appetite, a phenomenon that may be the cause of much anxiety to the parents. It is common and natural for a child who has a hearty appetite to go through a period in which both the appetite and food intake are noticeably reduced. Unless such a period is very prolonged and is accompanied by signs of undernutrition, such as lethargy, fatigue, and increased susceptibility to infection, it should be no basis for concern. The unnecessary concern of some parents over their children's food habits is exemplified in a study in Minnesota that showed that several

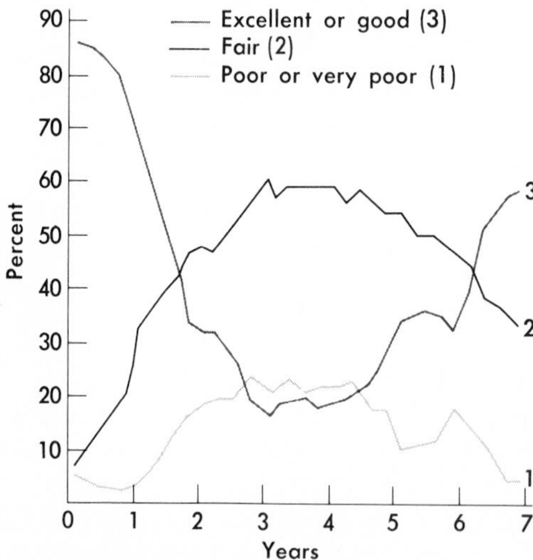

Fig. 18-2. Percentage of children 6 months to 7 years whose appetites were rated excellent, fair, or poor by their mothers. (From Beal, V. A.: Pediatrics **20:**448, 1957.)

mothers rated their children's food habits as poor even though they met all criteria for nutritionally adequate meals. Fig. 18-2 represents the fluctuations in appetite with age as reported by mothers of Colorado children.

In response to concern over appetite variations, promoters of dietary supplements have recommended both thiamin and vitamin B_{12} to stimulate appetite and growth in children, but experimental evidence indicates that thiamin is of value for only the most severely deprived human and that vitamin B_{12} is of no value as an appetite stimulant. Both, however, play significant roles in metabolism.

Transitional foods

In supervising the change from an infant diet to a regular adult-type diet, several factors about a child's reaction to food should be kept in mind to facilitate the transition and to minimize the trauma of the experience for both the parents and the child. Lowenberg, on the basis of extensive observations of the reaction of children to food, suggests that their acceptance of food represents a favorable reaction to the color, flavor, texture, and temperature of the food as well as the size of the servings and the attitude and atmosphere in which it is presented. A rejection of food often may be attributed to an unfavorable reaction to one of these. She advises that the wise parent will try to analyze the reactions and determine their cause.

Children generally favor foods that are soft in texture and are less accepting of foods that are dry or flintlike, have tough or stringy parts, or are too thick. For instance, they prefer thin to thick puddings, celery with the strings removed, stewed tomatoes with the fibers cut, soft mashed potatoes to baked potatoes, moist ground meats to dry fish, and soft bread to coarse bread. This preference for moist foods may reflect the absence of a copious supply of saliva to provide a natural lubricant for the food.

In terms of temperature they prefer foods

that are lukewarm to those that are very cold or very hot. By serving a child's food first, one finds that it is at the right temperature by the time others at the table are served. Removing milk from the refrigerator sufficiently long before serving to warm it slightly increases it acceptance. The tendency of a child to dawdle over ice cream until it is semisolid reflects his distaste for very cold foods.

Children are considered sensitive to flavors, reacting to off-flavors that may go undetected by adults. Experimental evidence, however, does not support the notion that children are more sensitive to flavor variations than their parents are. Their sensitivity to flavor has been observed when they reject milk with a slight taint or recognize when food has been only slightly scorched. In the case of vegetables, children will often refuse vegetables of the cabbage or onion families when they are cooked in such a way as to maximize the retention of nutrients and flavor but will accept them when cooked in a larger amount of water or when served with a cream sauce to modify the flavor. Once the mild flavor of the vegetable has been accepted it can be presented gradually in a more intensified form until it approaches normal flavor concentration, which also maximizes the retention of nutrients.

The quantity of food offered a child at one time influences his reaction to it. It is more satisfactory from a psychological point of view to offer a child less than the parent anticipates he will eat and have him return for more than to present him with such a large quantity that he is defeated before he begins to eat it. The use of 180 ml (6-ounce) glasses that can be easily grasped in the child's chubby hands is preferable to a large 240 to 300 ml glass that overtaxes his manual dexterity and the capacity of his stomach. Allowing the child to serve himself so that he can determine the amount of food on his plate or serving food in bite-size pieces may produce greater acceptance of the meal.

Visually, the child is responsive to a colorful meal whether the color is provided by the plate and setting, the combination of foods, or the judicious use of edible garnishes. Care should be exercised to avoid unnatural food shapes, inedible material, or colors not normally found in food, such as blue or purple, in an attempt to give the meal eye appeal.

Young children in their curiosity about their environment like to experience the feel of food. They also find that many foods are more easily manipulated with the hands than with utensils. Thus the preparation of strips of meat, wedges of lettuce, or raw vegetables as finger foods allows the child to sense the feel of foods and is certainly justified if it encourages their consumption.

The age at which a child develops sufficient manual dexterity to handle the utensils to manipulate food is again an individual matter, but until the child reaches the stage of motor development when he is skilled in their use, food should be presented in a way that requires a minimum of manipulation for its enjoyment. It should be kept in mind that children are just as individual and variable in their reactions as are adults. Thus it is to be expected that there are many children whose food preferences do not conform to the patterns that are suggested in the above generalizations.

Snacks. Snacks in the diet of young children have been encouraged by some and condemned by others. During periods of high nutritive needs the small child may be unable to take in sufficient food to satisfy his needs in three meals without overtaxing the capacity of his stomach. On the other hand, if snacks of high satiety value are taken too near regular meal hours, they may reduce the food intake at mealtimes. Munro found that snacks given 2½ hours before lunchtime had no effect on the appetite for lunch. They did, however, reduce the caloric intake at lunch, although the combined intake from lunch and snacks was greater than from lunch alone. Since adults can control the nature of snacks through control of food purchases, they have ultimate responsibility for seeing that snacks contribute to the total nutritive needs of the child. A cogent argument in favor of well-chosen snacks is provided by research showing that smaller, more frequent meals are utilized in such a way that depresses the formation of adipose tissue, as desirable during growth as in the prevention of obesity.

Food jags. Although it is deemed desirable to educate children to accept a wide variety of foods and to develop an accepting attitude toward new foods, it is common for young children to go on food jags in which they accept a very limited number of foods and reject all others. Should the accepted foods represent a nutritionally adequate, albeit monotonous, diet, as is often observed, there is little evidence that these preferences should provoke undue concern unless the foods used in excess contain additives or high amounts of salt. These habits seldom persist for prolonged periods nor is there evidence that they lead to bizarre food habits in adulthood. It has been observed, however, that the quality of the diet of 12- to 14-year-old

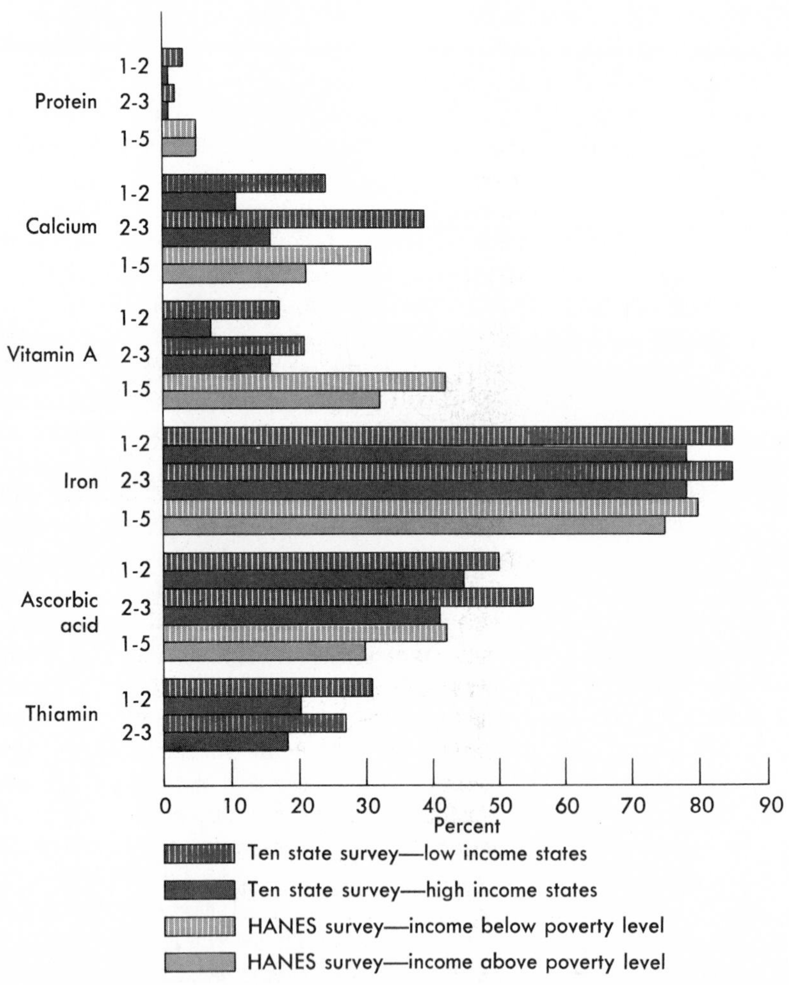

Fig. 18-3. Percentage of preschool children with intake below two-thirds RDA by age and income level. Data based on results of Ten-State Nutrition Survey (1968-1970) and Health and Nutrition Examination Survey (HANES) (1971-1974).

girls was positively correlated with the number of different food items eaten during the day, thus emphasizing the importance of encouraging the use of a variety of foods during the years when food habits are forming.

Adequacy of diets of infants and children

The results of the National Nutrition Survey confirm the findings of earlier, more limited studies that protein and riboflavin are the nutrients most often provided in adequate amounts in the diets of preschoool children and that iron is the nutrient least often provided in recommended amounts. Three fourths of the children had diets that provided less than two thirds of the RDA for iron. A third of the children had similarly low intakes of vitamin C, and a fourth had low intakes of calcium. The finding of both the Ten-State Nutrition Survey and the HANES study are presented graphically in Fig. 18-3.

Concurrent biochemical and physical assessment of these children failed to reveal any symptoms that could be diagnosed as frank deficiency conditions. The physical symptoms of nutritional deficiency tended to be nonspecific. Biochemical data did reveal a high incidence of anemia as indicated by hemoglobin levels below 10g/dl of blood.

Food preferences

Several studies to determine food preferences of children, which represent their reaction to the taste, texture, and temperature of food, have all led to similar conclusions. Only 37% to 41% of the children studied like vegetables, whereas over two thirds liked fruits. The fact that vegetables are generally unpopular may reflect the many and possibly unsatisfactory ways in which they are prepared and the generally negative reaction of adults to vegetables. Meat, milk, and bread ranked next to fruit in popularity. Food likes of youngsters appear to be related to those of other family members, especially the father, whose food preferences influence the frequency with which specific foods are served and hence the extent to which the child is familiar with them.

One of the problems in developing a liking for a particular food has been in persuading the child to taste it initially and then sufficiently frequently that the liking is reinforced. Psychologists have suggested that the application of the principles of behavior modification to the feeding situation may be effective. This involves an immediate reward for the desired behavior (vegetable eating) and the absence of any reinforcement of the undesirable behavior (not tasting the food). The reward must be something meaningful presented to the child sufficiently soon after the desired behavior has been demonstrated that it will shape his behavior. Once the eating pattern has been shaped, then the rewards can be given intermittently and finally withdrawn. For some children praise in itself may be sufficiently rewarding to mold their behavior; for others some more tangible reward may be necessary. Food, however, should not be used as a reward.

EVALUATION OF NUTRITIONAL STATUS

Since childhood is a period of active growth and a well-nourished child can be expected to have a growth pattern characterized by predictable increments in both height and weight, physical growth has become a readily available standard on which to assess nutritional status. Children in this generation are achieving a more rapid rate of growth and are reaching maturity at an earlier age than did those a few decades ago. This is a function not only of improved nutrition but also of favorable environmental factors and the advances in medical science that have reduced or eliminated many of the diseases that depressed growth in the earlier period.

It is important that any growth standard used in evaluating nutritional status be one derived from recent data. The National Center for Health Statistics has prepared charts showing curves for the 5th, 10th, 25th, 50th, 75th, 90th, and 95th percentile for height for age, weight for age, weight for height, and head circumference for age for both males and females, based on cross-sectional data in United States populations in the last ten years. Representative charts are presented in Figs. 15-4 to 15-7. It should be recognized that although data from standards will give a smooth curve, those from individuals will be characterized by peaks and valleys.

The assessment of body composition has also proved useful in evaluating growth in children. The percentage of body weight represented by fat declines up to 7 years of age. For girls the proportion of body weight as fat increases steadily until maturity, whereas for boys it declines from puberty until maturity. Techniques for measuring both cell number and cell size are making it possible to assess the nature of growth and the effect of specific deficiences on the composition of tissues, but these techniques are not appropriate in routine testing.

Nutritional-related problems in childhood

Severe malnutrition in childhood in the United States is seldom encountered now because of the availability of medical services and nutrition intervention programs to practically everyone and the improvement of techniques for identifying abnormalities before they develop into a full-fledged deficiency syndrome. Pellagra and beriberi are virtually unknown, and only an occasional case of scurvy is recorded. However, the National Nutrition Survey has revealed some evidence of growth retardation. As many as 18% of the children enrolled in Head Start programs fall below the third percentile on height and weight standards. Such a growth retardation is associated with high morbidity and some increase in mortality rates. Of all manifestations of malnutrition, anemia and obesity are the most common. In addition there are varying degrees of subclinical deficiency states. Dental caries incidence may also reflect nutrient intake.

Anemia, primarily the result of a lack of dietary iron, is encountered most often among children in lower socioeconomic groups, in whom the reported incidence of hemoglobin levels below 10g/dl of blood ranges from 20% to 40%. The lack of dietary iron may be the result of parental ignorance of the importance and sources of iron, poverty, which restricts the amount and variety of foods available, or the difficulty of providing recommended levels of iron in the diet under the best of circumstances. In some cases the situation is aggravated by the presence of intestinal parasites. A few instances are recorded of anemia resulting from the exclusive use of a milk diet, which is low in iron, after the first six months of life.

Treatment of anemia of childhood usually involves the therapeutic use of iron salts at levels providing from 30 to 100 mg of iron a day, often in conjunction with ascorbic acid, until the hemoblobin levels have been restored to normal levels. This is followed by the use of a diet high in iron-rich foods such as meat, green leafy vegetables, and enriched cereals. The child who suffers from anemia is usually lethargic, fatigues easily, and is highly susceptible to infection.

Obesity, a form of overnutrition, represents the other end of the nutritional spectrum. Childhood or juvenile onset obesity is a particular problem because it is extremely refractory to treatment and tends to persist into adulthood. This increasing problem may be attributed to several factors. Many parents, in their concern over the child's food habits, unwittingly establish a pattern of overeating when they introduce solid foods at a very early age, equate weight gain with good health, or use food as a reward for good behavior. The situation is further complicated by inactivity, as discussed in Chapter 20. The syndrome of the pale, flabby child who spends his summers in an air-conditioned house, immobilized in front of a television set and drinking beverages of low nutrient density to keep cool is frequently observed and is a cause for concern. The importance of preventing obesity in childhood through an education program involving both sound food selection and exercise cannot be overstressed. Encouraging the child to adopt a pattern of eating that allows him to "grow into his weight" has met with more success than attempting to bring about an actual weight loss. In addition, every effort should be directed at determining the underlying cause of obesity. This is especially important to the child whose parents are obese and who likely has a predisposition to obesity. Those children with features of body build identified as endomorphic should be given special guidance.

Nutrition and dental health

During childhood, dietary factors may influence dental health through their effect on both tooth formation and the character of the oral environment. Before tooth decay will occur, three conditions must be present—a caries-susceptible tooth, a fermentable carbohydrate, and microorganisms to ferment that carbohydrate. The susceptibility of the tooth to decay may be determined genetically, but few children are endowed with caries-resistant teeth. Beyond this, the integrity of the tooth structure may be a function of the nutrients that are available at a critical point in tooth formation. Vitamin A is necessary for the formation of the enamel layer; Vitamin C for the dentin layer; and calcium, phosphorus, and vitamin D for the process of calcification. In addition, the availability of fluorine during the time the tooth is calcifying will greatly decrease the susceptibility of the tooth to decay. Once the tooth has erupted, the presence or absence of a sticky carbohydrate to adhere to the tooth surface is the major dietary factor influencing tooth decay. It is not the nutrient content of the diet but rather the extent to which candy and other carbohydrates are consumed under conditions that allow them to become embedded on the tooth surface that determines the cariogenic character of the diet. Of all dietary factors associated with control of tooth decay, fluorine has the greatest effect as a preventative, and the consumption of sucrose in a form that adheres to the tooth surface is considered detrimental.

ADOLESCENCE

The period of transition from childhood to adulthood, commonly called adolescence, is a relatively short stage in the life cycle characterized by accelerated physical, biochemical, and emotional development. The observation that the age of menarche and the initiation of the rapid growth characteristic of adolescence is more related to weight (or possibly body composition) than to age suggests that nutritional status may be an important determinant of physiological maturity. The timing of the adolescent growth spurt depends on the child attaining a certain critical weight, which in the United States is considered to be approximately 30 kg (66 pounds). This represents a critical body composition of 10% body fat and usually occurs at 9½ years of age. Menarche occurs about three years later, following the period of rapid weight gain when weight reaches about 47 kg and fat stores have doubled to 20% to 24%. Menarche does not begin until body fat represents at least 17% body weight and ovulation ceases any time it falls below this level. A body composition of 22% body fat is required to maintain regular ovulation.

Since growth rate and hence nutrient needs vary widely from one adolescent to another, it has been suggested that it would be more meaningful to relate nutritional needs to a sexual maturity rating (SMR) based on the appearance of secondary sex characteristics rather than to age.

The changing life-style of an adolescent has marked effects on his food habits. As he becomes more independent and mobile he eats fewer meals at home, more meals outside the home where there is little guidance on his food choices, shares more food with his peers, learns new food preferences and discards old food habits.

Adolescence influences both nutritional needs and the absorption and utilization of nutritive intake. This period witnesses a rapid enlargement of organs and tissues and changes in physiological functions in response to hormonal changes. As reflected in the National Research Council recommended dietary allowances, this phase of the life cycle is the one of highest nutritive needs in the life of a male and for females is surpassed only during pregnancy and lactation. These allowances represent the needs for the increase in body size and the maturation of organs. Since the 13- to 19-year-olds numbered 24 million in the United States in 1970 and since they are at a vulnerable age when the dietary patterns and attitudes they develop toward food are going to influence the health of their children and dictate the food patterns of the next generation, teenagers are a prime and challenging target for nutrition education programs.

Adequacy of diets

Evaluations of the nutritive adequacy of the diets of young adults between 12 and 18 years of age in various regions in the United States have all yielded essentially the same results, although differences in degree are

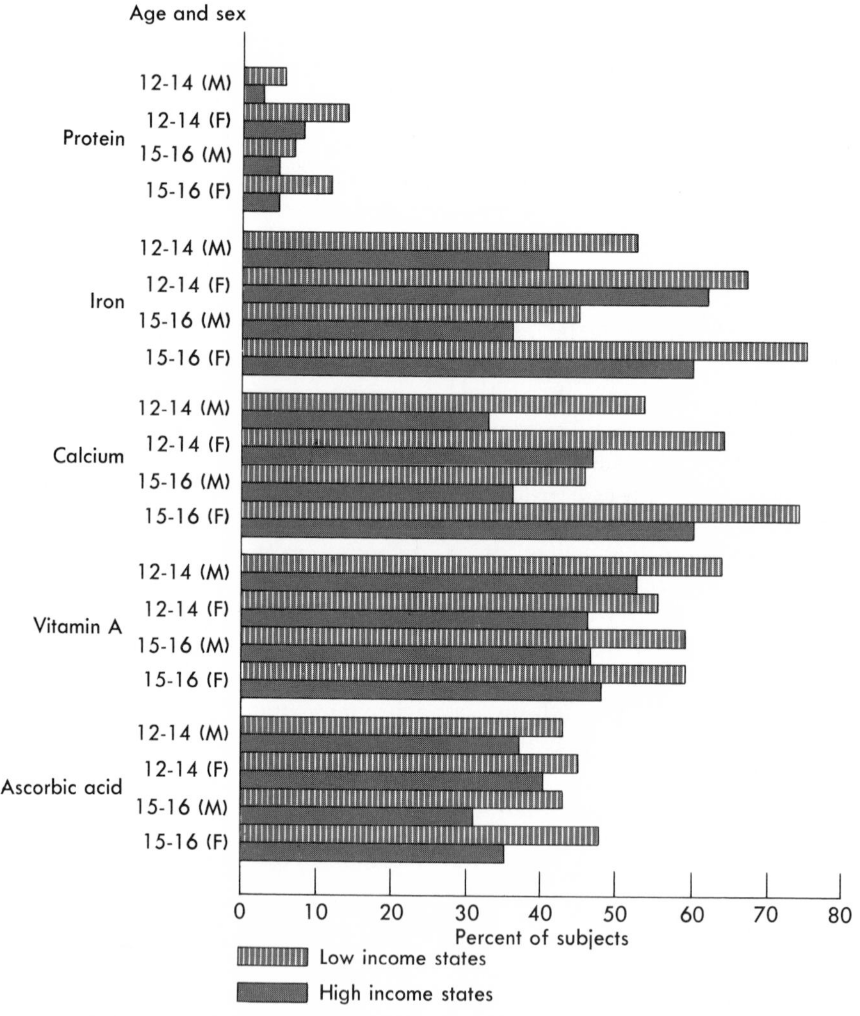

Fig. 18-4. Percentage of adolescents (ages 12 to 16) in the United States with dietary intakes below two-thirds RDA by age, sex, and income level. Data from Ten-State Nutrition Survey (1968-1970).

found. In all instances it was observed that the diets of boys were more adequate and less variable than were those of girls. This can be explained in part by the fact that the quantity of food required to provide the 900 extra kilocalories of energy needed for boys dictates at least a minimal level of other nutrients, whereas girls, with lower caloric intakes, are forced to make more judicious choices of foods to meet the needs for all other nutrients. In general, the diets of girls provided a higher proportion of their needs for ascorbic acid and calories than did those of boys, although ascorbic acid was often low for both. Girls' diets were generally low in iron, but this was not accompanied by a higher incidence of anemia. Calcium was more frequently low in the diet of girls than of boys, and vitamin A was low in both, a reflection of a general rejection of vegetables. Protein and niacin intakes, which paralleled the use of meat, were most often adequate.

Fig. 18-4 presents data on the percentage of adolescents in the National Nutrition Survey whose intake of different nutrients fell below two thirds of the NRC recommended dietary allowances. In general, the subjects with the poorest diets were those who skipped more meals, ate smaller quantities of food at meals, and ate fewer snacks.

In using the findings of dietary studies, one should bear in mind the edition of the recommended dietary allowances on which the evaluation was based. Since the recommendations have shown a downward trend for all nutrients except calcium, which has been unchanged, and iron, which has been increased in recent revisions, diets that were assessed as inadequate on earlier standards may now be considered adequate. In the case of iron, a reevaluation of the data may show an even higher incidence of suboptimal intakes.

Factors influencing food habits

Few attempts have been made to determine the attitudes that influence the selection of a diet. Young girls who were concerned about their health, who were emotionally stable and conforming, and who came from homes characterized by good family relationships chose better than did those motivated by considerations of group status, sociability, independence from parental control, or enjoyment of eating. Criticism of their eating patterns led girls to skip meals more frequently, and skipping breakfast was found to be common. Better meals were selected in winter than in summer because of the regularity of schedules. The more meals eaten away from home, the less likely an adolescent is to consume meals of adequate nutritional content, which no doubt represents a response to the habits of the peer groups. This is especially true when lunch money is used to buy lunches outside the school, a practice that is becoming less frequent with the trend toward short lunch periods in high schools and lack of freedom to leave the school building.

School lunches that qualify for federal and state subsidies are selected to provide a fourth to a third of the nutritive needs of the child. Packed lunches are found to be somewhat less adequate, and those purchased outside the school are poor. It is obvious that many factors contribute to the poor food habits observed during teen years, but the most frequently observed causes are failure to eat breakfast (or less frequently some other meal of the day), lack of time or companionship for regular meals, drinking no milk (which may be a rebellion against parental influence), lack of supervision in the selection of meals eaten away from home, an overriding fear of obesity, especially among girls, and a concern that certain foods will aggravate adolescent acne.

Obesity

Studies indicate that 30% to 35% of teenagers are overweight, although not necessarily obese. Many teenagers, especially girls, are either fat, believe they are fat, or are fearful of becoming fat. Because they idolize the fashion model in a size six dress, girls often adopt an unrealistic and unhealthy standard of body size to which they aspire. Hence they embark on self-directed program of weight reduction that can easily be hazardous to health because of inadequate levels of nutrients at a time when there are still high nutrient demands for growth and when they should be accumulating reserves for the reproductive period. The problem is even greater when weight reduction is carried out spasmodically, with a period of weight loss followed by one of weight gain.

As will be discussed in Chapter 20, the major cause of caloric imbalance among adolescents is a depressed level of activity rather than an excessive food intake. Whether the cause of this inactivity is physiological or psychological or both has not been determined. It has been observed that obese youngsters have significantly lower serum iron with normal hemoglobin levels than do nonobese youngsters. The low serum iron levels could be indicative of low levels of myoglobin and other iron-containing pigments, which may cause an unconscious reduction in activity when the oxygen available to the cells is reduced. This situation, characterized by reduced activity, can be better handled by a program of consistent moderate exercise than by one of spasmodic vigorous activity. The activity patterns that are developed in late adolescence often prevail throughout adulthood. Therefore, developing habits of active exercise at an early age becomes important in terms of preventing obesity in adulthood. Equally important is the observation that the earlier a person learns to respond to satiety signals, the more likely he is to be able to adjust his food intake to correspond to his needs in response to a sensitive satiety mechanism.

Breakfast

The importance of breakfast for any group is well documented, and there is likely no nutritional substitute for a good breakfast. Having a good breakfast has two major advantages. First, it generally provides nutrients, especially ascorbic acid, calcium, and riboflavin, that may not be provided in adequate amounts by the foods typically consumed at other meals. Second, the availability of a readily utilizable carbohydrate results in a rapid increase in blood glucose levels and the concurrent decrease in reaction time so that performance is improved and accident rate declines.

Since adolescence is a time when skipping breakfast hits a peak and a time during which dietary habits that may persist for life are formulated, this is a period when attention should be directed toward the problem. Studies show that the calcium and ascorbic acid intakes of persons who omit breakfast are reduced by about 40% and the intakes of iron and thiamin by 10%. It was also found that 17- to 19-year-old college women who skipped breakfast obtained 18% of their energy intake from snacks, whereas those who ate breakfast snacked less frequently and obtained only 7% of their energy intake from snacks. Since the snacks chosen were characteristically high in calories relative to other nutrients, those who snacked more had diets that were less adequate nutritionally than those of persons who had breakfast.

Boys report eating breakfast more frequently and eating breakfasts that provide more nutrients than do girls. Many rationalizations are presented for failure to eat breakfast, including lack of time, lack of appetite, preference for sleep, spending time over personal appearance, or fear of becoming fat.

In one study it was observed that the availability of someone with whom to eat breakfast, someone to prepare it, the availability of prepared foods, and the acceptance of the breakfast-eating habit in the peer group all influenced the extent to which breakfast or a preschool snack was eaten.

It should be pointed out that breakfast need not be the conventional fruit, cereal, toast, and beverage pattern but can be any combination of foods, either liquid or solid, that provides its nutritional equivalent, at least 300 kcal, and sufficient protein and fat to provide a sense of satiety until the next meal and has a nutrient density that will make a reasonable contribution of other nutrients.

Concern over teenagers' diets

Nutritionists express concern over the nutritional habits of the 12- to 19-year-old group for many reasons. This is a period marked by a level of physical and emotional growth that often results in stress and anxiety, which in turn influence physiological, psychological, and social behavior. All of these factors affect nutritional behavior.

The incidence of dietary inadequacies is higher during adolescence than at any other stage of the life cycle. This is a stage at which the results of nutrient lack are far reaching, especially for girls. Many relationships between physical abnormalities and dietary practice have been observed.

The incidence of tuberculosis is highest in adolescence, and some evidence suggests a relationship between nutritional status and onset of tuberculosis, speed of recovery, and rate of reinfection.

Emotional instability, noted especially among girls who mature early, influences the utilization of nutrients. Negative nitrogen and calcium balances have been observed among both young girls and older persons who are under extreme emotional stress.

With 53% of girls between 15 and 19 years of age married, the possibility that a girl will bear a child before she has fully matured herself is a reason to focus special attention on her nutritional status. One out of four mothers bearing her first child is less than 20 years old, and 6% of all deaths among 18- to 19-year-old girls result from complications of pregnancy. If the nutritive intake of a girl has been inadequate prior to conception, she is less able to cope with the added physical stress of pregnancy and the demands of the growing fetus and is unable to make up for her own nutritive deficits. As a result, babies of teenagers are more often born prematurely, have more congenital defects, and have inadequate nutritive stores to carry them through the initial period of extrauterine life. In all respects the malnourished mother is a poor obstetrical risk. Whether a concern over the welfare of their yet unconceived children will provide sufficient motivation to teenage girls to modify their food habits remains to be tested, but the concern of nutritionists over the present status of the diets of adolescents has prompted a concerted effort to reach this group.

ROLE OF SNACKS IN DIETARY INTAKE

Until recently nutritionists tended to stress the importance of three "good" meals a day and to ignore the possibility that snacks could provide anything other than foods of low-nutrient density. With the recognition that smaller, more frequent meals may have many physiological and nutritional advantages, and that snacking is a way of life with teenagers, there has been concern about improving the quality of snacks. Data on food intake patterns show that snacks are eaten by over 75% of all adolescents and provide from a fourth to a third of their caloric intake. The extent to which snacks contribute to the intake of other nutrients is a function of the nature of the snacks.

An analysis of the nutritive contribution of snacks reported by both boys and girls between 12 and 16 years of age in the National Nutrition Survey showed that, in general, they provided much more than empty calories. In the case of protein, riboflavin, and ascorbic acid snacks provided at least as much per 100 kcal as recommended in the Recommended Dietary Allowances. The relationship between calories and nutrients in snacks is shown in Table 18-1.

Once the adult has accepted the fact that snacking is not necessarily detrimental and need not spoil the appetite for well-planned meals, he can do much to see that snacks are beneficial by monitoring the kinds of foods that are available. The most likely places for the adult to make his influence felt are through access points such as the school lunch program, the home refrigerator, and the offerings of vending machines.

From a nutrition education standpoint it may be better to make snacks with a full

Table 18-1. Mean nutrient intake per 100 kcal from between-meal foods and total nutrient intake per 100 kcal for males and females ages 12 to 16 years, based on data from Ten-State Nutrition Survey, 24-hour recalls*

Nutrient	Males†			Females†		
		Mean intake per 100 kcal§			Mean intake per 100 kcal§	
	RDA per 100 kcal‡	Between-meal foods	24-hour total	RDA per 100 kcal‡	Between-meal foods	24-hour total
Protein (g)	2.0	2.3	3.8	2.2	2.2	3.7
Calcium (mg)	50.0	39.1	44.6	55.3	34.3	41.0
Iron (mg)	0.64	0.33	0.55	0.77	0.34	0.53
Vitamin A (IU)	178.0	128.0	193.5	212.0	117.4	196.0
Thiamin (mg)	0.05	0.03	0.05	0.05	0.03	0.06
Riboflavin (mg)	0.04	0.07	0.09	0.06	0.06	0.09
Ascorbic acid (mg)	1.7	2.6	2.8	2.0	3.9	2.9

*From Thomas, J. A., and Call, D. A.: Eating between meals—nutrition problem among teenagers? Nutr. Rev. **31**:137, 1973. Source of data: Tables 4-7, pp. V-312-V-314, Ten-State Nutrition Survey, Vol. V, Dietary. Atlanta, U.S. Department of Health, Education, and Welfare, 1972.

†Number of teenagers reporting snacking on day covered by recall: 1351 males, 1460 females.

‡Based on RDA for kcal of 2800 for males and 2350 for females.

§Based on calorie intake from between-meal foods of 634 kcal for males and 495 kcal for females, and total intake of 2770 kcal for males and 2157 kcal for females.

range of nutritional qualities available, including less nutritious snacks, and give the child the information on which to base an informed decision, than to ban "nonnutritious" foods in vending machines so that the child can only select nutritious foods. In this case he does not learn to cope in real life situations. Studies have shown that as long as the teenager had three meals a day, little difference in nutrient intake was found with increased frequency of meals.

Snacking can be encouraged when it becomes an integral part of the total eating pattern but must be condemned if it constitutes overeating in disregard of the total food pattern. Snacking that is confined to the evening hours in what is described as the "night-eating syndrome" has been implicated a factor in obesity.

SCHOOL LUNCH

With 25 million of the nation's school children participating in the National School Lunch Program, it can be considered an important factor in the nutrient intake of schoolchildren. The program was originally conceived to "safeguard the health and well-being of the nation's children and to encourage the domestic consumption of nutritious agricultural commodities and other foods."* From its inception in 1946 the School Lunch Act required that a type A lunch provide a third or more of the daily nutrient intake of the 10- to 12-year-old child with adjustments made for both younger and older children. To encourage the preparation of nutritious lunches the U.S. Department of Agriculture

*National School Lunch Act, Public Law 396, Seventy-ninth Congress, June 4, 1946.

Table 18-2. School lunch pattern requirements—amounts of foods listed by food components to serve children of various ages*

Food components	Preschool children		Elementary school children		Secondary school children
	Group I (1-2 yr)	Group II (3-5 yr)	Group III Grades K-3 (6-8 yr)	Group IV Grades 4-6 (9-11 yr)	Group V Grades 7-12 (12+ yr)
Meat and meat alternates‡	1 oz equiv.†	1½ oz equiv.	1½ oz equiv.	2 oz equiv.	3 oz equiv.
A serving (edible portion as served) of cooked lean meat, poultry, or fish, *or* meat alternates					
Following meat alternates§ may be used to meet the meat/meat alternate requirement:					
Cheese (1 oz. equals 1 oz. cooked lean meat)					
Eggs (1 large egg may replace 1 oz cooked lean meat)					
Cooked dry beans or peas‖ (½ cup may replace 1 oz cooked lean meat)					
Peanut butter (2 tbsp may replace 1 oz cooked lean meat)					

*From School lunch pattern requirements, Federal Register Vol. 43 No. 163, 1978.
†Equivalents will be determined and published in guidance materials by FNS/USDA.
‡It is recommended that in schools not offering a choice of meat/meat alternates each day, no one form of meat (ground, sliced, pieces, etc.) or meat alternate be served more than three times per week. Meat and meat alternates must be served in a main dish or in a main dish and one other menu item.
§When it is determined that the serving size of a meat alternate is excessive, the particular meat alternate shall be reduced and supplemented with an additional meat/meat alternate to meet the full requirement.
‖Cooked dry beans or dry peas may be used as part of the meat alternate or as part of the vegetable/fruit component, but not as both food components in the same meal.

Continued.

Table 18-2. School lunch pattern requirements—amounts of foods listed by food components to serve children of various ages—cont'd

Food components	Preschool children		Elementary school children		Secondary school children
	Group I (1-2 yr)	Group II (3-5 yr)	Group III Grades K-3 (6-8 yr)	Group IV Grades 4-6 (9-11 yr)	Group V Grades 7-12 (12+ yr)
Vegetables and fruits‖	½ cup	½ cup	½ cup	¾ cup	¾ cup
Two or more servings consisting of vegetables or fruits or both. A serving of full-strength vegetable or fruit juice can be counted to meet not more than half the total requirement.					
Bread and bread alternates¶	5 sl or alt/wk	8 sl or alt/wk	8 sl or alt/wk	8 sl or alt/wk	10 sl or alt/wk
A serving (1 slice) of enriched or whole-grain bread; *or* a serving of biscuits, rolls, muffins, etc., made with whole-grain or enriched meal or flour #; *or* a serving (½ cup) of cooked enriched or whole-grain rice, macaroni, or noodle and other pasta products**					
Milk, fluid	½ cup	¾ cup	¾ cup	½ pint	½ pint
Two types of milk must be offered, one of which must be unflavored fluid low-fat milk, skim milk, or buttermilk.††					

¶One-half or more slices of bread or an equivalent amount of bread alternate must be served with each lunch with the total requirement being served during a five day period. Schools serving lunch six or seven days per week should increase this specified quantity for the five day period by approximately 20% (one fifth) for each additional day.

#Bread alternates and serving sizes will be published in guidance materials by FNS/USDA.

**Enriched macaroni products with fortified protein may be used as part of a meat alternate or as a bread alternate, but not as both food components in the same meal.

††Half pint of milk may be used for all age groups if the lesser specified amounts are determined by school food authority to be impractical.

provided subsidies in the form of technical advice, surplus agricultural commodities or those purchased as part of the price support programs, and a cash subsidy if the food service adhered to certain requirements. Specifically, the School Lunch Act required that each participating school operate on a nonprofit basis, serve meals at a regular meal hour, provide lunches free or at reduced cost to those unable to pay, and serve meals meeting specified nutritional standards. In addition, each state was required to match each dollar of federal money with \$3 from sources within the state. In 1978 about 20%, or 8.9 million, of the children participating received free or reduced-price lunches. A 1970 amendment has authorized schools to make contracts with food service management companies to provide school lunches. They must, however, keep records available for inspection and must use federally donated commodities only for the benefit of the participants. To qualify for reimbursement, a school must serve as a plate lunch a meal containing foods as indicated in Table 18-2.

To cope with the recognized problem of excessive plate waste, junior and senior high-school students are now given the option of selecting three of the five designated items on the Type A lunch and still have the meal qualify for reimbursement. The effect of this policy on nutrient intake has not yet been assessed.

An evaluation of the adequacy of school lunches in relation to recommended dietary allowances has led to concern that the lunches are failing to provide a third of the requirement for magnesium and pyridoxine. There are proposals to modify the Type A lunch pattern to assure desirable intakes of these nutrients. The act has been modified to allow for satellite feeding operations in which food is provided to several schools from a central facility, not necessarily a non-profit organization. The necessity of providing a hot lunch for every child is also being questioned, especially in this era of well-heated schools and school buses. Evidence shows that cold lunches can be equally nutritious and acceptable.

The Special Milk Program supplements the School Lunch Program and provides a subsidy for each 240 ml (½ pint) of whole milk served in a school.

Under the Child Nutrition Act of 1966 some pilot school breakfast programs have been instituted. The selected schools participating in this part of the feeding program are primarily those with many needy pupils or pupils who travel great distances from their homes. About 63% of the 1.8 million children participating in 1974 received free or reduced-price breakfasts. Schools provide at cost one serving of fruit or juice, 240 ml of whole milk, and one serving of cereal prior to the regular school hour. This program has been promoted as a means of dealing with the nutritional deficits more common in the lower socioeconomic groups in the country. Although the evidence is subjective, it is suggestive of better school performance and improved attention among children who have this breakfast before school.

In 1977 the Child Nutrition Act was amended to mandate that the federal government allocate to each state 50 cents per student for nutrition education. Following an assessment of the needs in each state, the state director of nutrition is to have responsibility for implementing a program. In most cases it will be coordinated with the school lunch program.

Other innovative intervention programs are being investigated as a possible means of improving the nutritional intake of the nation's schoolchildren, especially those from economically deprived groups.

ATHLETES

Although the principles of good nutrition are the same for athletes as they are for others, adolescent athletes participating in varsity and intramural sports frequently receive confusing dietary advice. This advice represents the many theories that exist regarding the role that nutrition may play in maximizing the performance of the athlete. Many athletes, preoccupied with winning, prestige, and social or peer approval, are ready to accept any advice that they believe will give them a competitive advantage. Diet, however, is no substitute for aptitude, training, and motivation.

Contrary to general opinion, muscular exercise does not require an increased intake of protein but rather involves only an expenditure of energy. The energy requirements of an athlete vary with the same factors as the nonathlete—body size, age, sex, and degree of activity. They are, however, usually much higher with 60% of the athletes requiring over 3000 kcal and 6% over 6000. As with anyone else the caloric intake that leads to the maintenance of desirable body weight is the proper level. A major problem for athletes is a failure to adjust their intake during the off-season and in postcompetitive years when energy intakes may be substantially reduced. The incidence of obesity in ex-football players and wrestlers is considerably above that of the rest of the population and may be a factor in their reduced life expectancy.

The capacity for prolonged strenuous exercise is enhanced when the carbohydrate stores of glycogen are large. Research has shown that the normal reserve of about 800 to 1000 kcal in the form of glycogen in the liver and muscle can be almost doubled by a dietary regimen in which the athlete consumes a diet low in carbohydrate and high in fat and protein for several days prior to the meet while in training. Then for two days before the contest the diet is switched to one high in carbohydrate, which is preferentially stored in the liver at a level up to 700 g, almost double that which normally occurs. This type of regimen may be especially useful for those, such as marathon runners or soccer players, who must sustain a high level of energy expenditure for a prolonged period. The formation of glycogen requires the retention of water, which in some results in a feeling of heaviness and stiffness. On a high-carbohydrate diet an athlete may exercise longer before becoming exhausted. With the widespread practice of carbohydrate loading, some evidence of adverse effects on kidney and heart functions among older athletes is accumulating.

Fat is the major source of energy for prolonged exercise of lower intensity. Even the leanest athlete with low fat reserves has sufficient stores to meet this need.

Protein intakes of 1 g/kg of body weight easily meet any increased requirements for protein and are generally provided by a normal diet, as are the needs for 2 g/kg for the growing athlete. Not only does the use of protein supplements fail to stimulate muscle growth, it also places an unnecessary burden on the kidneys, which must excrete the urea formed from the deamination of the excess amino acids. In addition, protein supplements are a very expensive source of either protein or energy. It is, however, common practice for coaches to arrange a pregame meal relatively high in protein, which includes almost invariably a generous serving of meat. This serves a psychological rather than a physiological purpose.

Coaches are concerned about the digestibility of the pregame meal when the athlete is under emotional stress. Many are recommending a liquid pregame meal. It is less expensive, can be taken closer to game time, and is associated with reduced incidence of pregame vomiting and muscle cramps. By feeding a meal that is completely digested by game time, the competition between the muscles and the digestive system for simultaneous use of the blood pool is reduced. Such competition could result in a compromised efficiency of both. The pregame meal is usually eaten 3 to 5 hours before competition. High levels of protein or fat should be avoided to be sure that the food is digested by the time of competition. Gas-producing foods and foods high in bulk are usually considered undesirable.

There has been much concern over the effect of milk on athletic performance. Although many enthusiastically recommend it, others recommend that it be eliminated, mainly on the basis of some unfounded beliefs. Some controlled studies of the effect of varying levels of milk on performance showed that there were no differences in training response or all-out performance when an intake of 1.5 liters of milk per day and 1 liter of ice cream per week was compared to a diet without any milk.

The American Medical Association is concerned over the hazards of indiscriminate and excessive weight reduction to which adolescents are frequently subjected to meet a specific weight requirement for participation in various athletic competitions. Required weight loss can be accomplished through food restriction, water deprivation, the use of hot boxes, rubberized or plastic clothing, diuretics, and induced vomiting, none of which are recommended. Since premature fatigue is associated with even a minimal water loss of 3% of body weight, such a fluctuation in weight may be accompanied by a depressed muscle strength and level of performance that will undo the benefits of training. Dehydration is less serious if it is confined to 2 to 3 hours before weigh-in and is followed by immediate rehydration. The practice of withholding water and inducing severe dehydration over several days may cause serious problems such as the excretion of a reduced and highly concentrated urine, deposits of calculi (stones) in the kidneys, the retention of urea (uremia), lower blood volumes, reduced efficiency of the heart, and problems of temperature regulation. These same problems occur among athletes competing in hot humid environments who may also suffer from dehydration.

Many substances believed to be ergogenic (strength producing) have been recommended, but their effectiveness has not been demonstrated. Any value seems to be psychological rather than physiological. Similarly, there is no evidence that any vitamin or mineral taken in excess of needs has any effect in improving performance, nor do the procession of special dietary items such as bee pollen, gelatin, or wheat germ that are represented as having beneficial effects on performance.

To compensate for the salt loss that accompanies water loss and sweating, many coaches are using flavored electrolyte solutions containing salt, other electrolytes, and sugar. The products currently on the market provide the equivalent of 1 g of salt (the amount in two salt tablets) per liter of solution and will compensate only for low sodium losses. Salt supplements are likely unnecessary until water losses exceed 3 liters (6 pints).

ANOREXIA NERVOSA

This condition is best described as a state of emaciation that has been brought on by voluntary starvation. It is seen primarily in adolescent girls from middle- and upper-class families. Unless it is recognized before it has advanced too far, it is very difficult to treat, since the individual refuses to eat. Instead of being lethargic and apathetic as one would expect in undernutrition, victims of this condition have a drive to be active. Although most cases have a psychological basis, they represent a form of malnutrition far more severe than that resulting from lack of available food.

IMPROVING NUTRITIONAL HABITS

It has been well documented that nutrition knowledge is not necessarily reflected in food habits. The key to the application of sound nutritional principles to eating patterns appears to be motivation. In adolescence the most effective motivation is the hope for vitality, good looks, and popularity. Concern over long-term effects of malnutrition or undernutrition on health has relatively little impact on the high school student or even the college student. Of the various methods attempted, the use of group sessions during which the group accepts certain standards of eating and then helps provide the incentive and backing to implement them has been most effective. In some cases it is necessary to "unlearn" sets of habits, but in others it is merely a case of modifying or improving current habits. A positive approach that builds on desirable habits rather than on correcting a negative one is preferable and more effective. It is important to start with the present habits of the individual, reinforce the good aspects and replace the poor with new habits and to recognize that good diets do not just happen but are planned.

BIBLIOGRAPHY

Childhood

Breckenridge, M. E.: Food attitudes of five-to twelve-year-old children. J. Am. Diet. Assoc. **35**:704, 1959.

Bryan, M. S., and Lowenberg, M. E.: The father's influence on young children's food preferences, J. Am. Diet. Assoc. **34**:30, 1958.

Cheek, D. B., Shulz, R. B., and Parra, A.: Over growth of lean and adipose tissues in adolescent obesity, Pediatr. Res. **4**:268, 1970.

Committee on Nutrition, American Academy of Pediatrics: Appraisal of the use of vitamins B_1 and B_{12} or supplements promoted for the stimulation of growth and appetite in children, Pediatrics **21**:860, 1958.

Committee on Nutrition, American Academy of Pediatrics: Childhood diet and coronary heart disease, Pediatrics **49**:305, 1972.

Committee on Nutrition, American Academy of Pediatrics: Should milk drinking by children be discouraged? Pediatrics **53**:576, 1974.

Dierks, E. C., and Morse, L. M.: Food habits and nutrient intakes of preschool children, J. Am. Diet. Assoc. **47**:292, 1965.

Garza, C., and Scrimshaw, N. S.: Relationshop of lactose intolerance to milk intolerance in young children, Am. J. Clin. Nutr. **29**:192, 1976.

Head, M. K., and Weeks, R. J.: Conventional vs. formulated foods in school lunches. II. Cost of food served, eaten and wasted. J. Am. Diet. Assoc. 71:629, 1977.

Herbert-Jackson, E., Cross, M. Z., and Risley, T. R.: Milk types and temperature—what will young children drink? J. Nutr. Ed. **9**:76, 1977.

Huenemann, R. L.: Environmental factors associated with preschool obesity. J. Am. Diet. Assoc. **64**:580, 1974, **64**:588, 1974.

Institute of Food Technologists: Diet and hyperactivity: any connection? Nutr. Rev. **34**:151, 1977.

Kerrey, E., Crispin, S., Fox, H. M., and Kies, C.: Nutritional status of preschool children., I. Dietary and biochemical findings, Am. J. Clin. Nutr. **21**:1274, 1968.

Knittle, J. L.: Obesity in childhood: a problem in adipose tissue cellular development, J. Pediatr. **81**:1048, 1972.

Kolata, C. B.: Childhood hyperactivity. A new look at treatment and causes, Science **199**:515, 1978.

Lantis, M.: The child consumer—cultural factors influencing his food choices, J. Home Economics **54**:370, 1962.

Lowenberg, M. E.: Food preferences of young children, J. Am. Diet. Assoc. **24**:430, 1948.

Martin, H. P.: Nutrition: its relationship to children's physical, mental, and emotional development, Am. J. Clin. Nutr. **26**:766, 1973.

Metheny, M. Y., Hunt, F. E., Patton, M. B., and Heye, H.: The diets of preschool children. I. Nutritional sufficiency findings and family marketing practices, J. Home Economics **54**:297, 1962.

Mooty, J., Ferrand, C. F., and Harris, P.: Relationship of diet to lead poisoning in children, Pediatrics **55**:636, 1975.

Munro, N.: How do snacks affect total caloric intake of preschool children, J. Am. Diet. Assoc. **33**:601, 1957.

Norman, F. A., and Pratt, E. L.: Feeding of infants and children in hot weather, J.A.M.A. **166**:2168, 1958.

Owen, G. M., Kram, K. M., Garry, P. J., et al.: A study of nutritional status of preschool children in the United States, 1968-1970, Pediatrics **53**(suppl.):597, 1974.

Owen, G. M., Garry, P. J., Lubin, A. H., et al.: Changes in levels of hemoglobin and hematocrits among children and youth registrants between 1968 and 1971, Clin. Pediatr. **14**:445, 1975.

Seelig, M. S.: Are American children still getting an excess of vitamin D? Clin. Pediatr. **9**:380, 1970.

Sims, L. S.,and Morris, P. M.: Nutritional status of preschoolers, J. Am. Diet. Assoc. **64**:592, 1974.

Sobotka, T. J.: Hyperkinesis and food additives: a review of experimental work, FDA By-lines **8**:165, 1978.

Weil, W. B.: Current controversies in childhood obesity, J. Pediatr. **91**:175, 1977.

Winick, M.: Childhood obesity, Nutr. Today **9**:6, 1974.

Woodruff, C.: Nutritional anemias in early childhood, Am. J. Clin. Nutr. **22**:504, 1969.

Adolescence

American College of Sports Medicine: Position stand on weight loss in wrestlers, Sports Med. Bull. **11**:1, 1976.

American Medical Association Committee on Medical Aspects of Sports: Wrestling and weight control, J.A.M.A. **201**:541, 1967.

Astrand, P.: Something old and something new—very new, Nutr. Today **3**(2):9, 1968.

Bergstrom, J., and Heltman, E.: Nutrition for maximal sports performances, J.A.M.A. **221**:999, 1972.

Christakis, G., Sajecki, S., Hillman, R. W., Miller, E., Blumenthal, S., and Archer, M.: Effect of a combined nutrition educational program and physical fitness program on the weight status of obese high school boys, Fed. Proc. **25**:15, 1966.

Conzalazio, C. F., and Johnston, H. L.: Dietary carbohydrate and work capacity, Am. J. Clin. Nutr. **25:**85, 1972.

Delgado, H., Habicht, J. P., Yarbrough, C., Lechtig, A., Martorell, R., Malina, R. M., and Klein, R. E.: Nutritional status and the timing of deciduous tooth eruption. Am. J. Clin. Nutr. **28:**216, 1975.

DePaola, D. P., and Alfano, M. C.: Diet and oral health, Nutr. Today **12:**6, 1977.

Everson, G. J.: Bases for concern about teenagers' diets, J. Am. Diet. Assoc. **36:**17, 1960.

Food and Nutrition Board, NAS—NRC, Committee on Nutritional Misinformation: Water deprivation and performance of athletes, Nutr. Rev. **32:**314, 1974.

Frisch, R.: Weight at menarche: similarity for well-nourished and undernourished girls at differing ages, and evidence for historical constancy, Pediatrics **50:**445, 1972.

Gaines, E., and Daniel, W., Jr.: Dietary iron intakes of adolescents, J. Am. Diet. Assoc. **65:**275, 1974.

Gallagher, J. R.: Weight control in adolescence, J. Am. Diet. Assoc. **40:**519, 1962.

Head, M. K., and Weeks, R. J.: Conventional vs. formulated foods in school lunches, J. Am. Diet. Assoc. **71:**629, 1977.

Heald, F. P., and Khan, M. A.: Teenage obesity, Pediatr. Clin. North Am. **20:**807, 1973.

Hueneman, R. L., Hampton, M. C., Behnke, A. B., Shapiro, L. R., and Mitchell, B. W.: Teenage nutrition and physique, Springfield, Ill., 1974, Charles C Thomas, Publisher.

Jakobovits, C., Halstead, P., Kelley, L., Roe, D. A., and Young, C. M.: Eating habits and nutrient intakes of college women over a thirty-year period, J. Am. Diet. Assoc. **71:**405, 1977.

Kaufmann, N. A., Posnanski, R., and Guggenheim, K.: Eating habits and opinions of teenagers on nutrition and obesity, J. Am. Diet. Assoc. **66:**264, 1975.

Leverton, R. M.: The paradox of teen-age nutrition, J. Am. Diet. Assoc. **53:**13, 1968.

Lewis, S., and Gutin, B.: Nutrition and endurance, Am. J. Clin. Nutr. **26:**1011, 1973.

Nutrition for athletes, Washington, D.C., 1971, American Association for Health, Physical Education and Recreation.

Ohlson, M. A., and Hort, B. P.: Influence of breakfast on today's food intake, J. Am. Diet. Assoc. **47:**282, 1965.

Peckos, P. S., and Heald, F. P.: Nutrition of adolescents, Children **11:**27, 1964.

Richardson, B. D., and Pieters, L.: Menarche and growth, Am. J. Clin. Nutr. **30:**2088, 1977.

Roth, A.: The teenage clinic, J. Am. Diet. Assoc. **26:**27, 1960.

Rowe, N. H., Garn, S. M., Coark, D. C., and Guire, K. E.: The effect of age, sex, race and economic status on dental caries experience of the permanent dentition, Pediatrics, **57:**457, 1976.

Sims, L. S., and Morris, P. M.: Nutritional status of preschoolers. An ecological perspective, J. Am. Diet. Assoc. **64:**492, 1974.

Slovic, P.: What helps the long-distance runner run? Nutr. Today **10:**18, 1975.

Stahl, S. S.: Nutritional influences on periodontal disease, World Rev. Nutr. Diet. **13:**277, 1971.

Steele, B. F., Clayton, U. U., and Tucker, R. E.: Role of breakfast and of between-meal foods in adolescents' nutrient intake, J. Am. Diet. Assoc. **28:**1054, 1952.

Tanner, J. M.: Growing up, Sci. Am. **229:**35, 1973.

Thomas, J. A., and Carl, D. L.: Eating between meals—a nutrition problem among teenagers? Nutr. Rev. **31:**137, 1973.

Tipton, C. M., and Tcheng, T. K.: Iowa Wrestling Study, J.A.M.A. **214:**1269, 1970.

Webb, T. E., and Oski, F. A.: Iron deficiency anemia and scholastic achievment in young adolescents, J. Pediatr. **82:**827, 1973.

White, H. S.: Inorganic elements in weighed diets of girls and young women, J. Am. Diet. Assoc. **55:**38, 1969.

19

Nutritional considerations in aging

With the growing number of individuals surviving to enjoy their "renaissance years," there has been a considerable increase in interest in assessing nutritional needs in these mature years. These needs are influenced not only by the physical state and activity of the individual but also by long-standing food habits and the many social, environmental, emotional, and physiological stresses to which a person is subjected throughout growth and maturity. Many social programs have been developed to help senior citizens achieve nutritional adequacy to maximize their health status.

Geriatrics, the branch of medicine dedicated to the care of the aging as well as the aged, is concerned with prolonging the prime of life, delaying the onset of the severely degenerative aspects of aging, and treating the diseases of the aged. Gerontology is the broader branch of science dealing with the psychological, sociological, economic, and physiological as well as the medical aspects of aging. Both fields of study have witnessed a surge of activity in the last three decades. This increasing concern over the problems of the aging population has been the result of the increase in both the total numbers and proportion of the population who are living beyond retirement age. Advances in medical technology, environmental hygiene, and nutrition have meant that more persons are living longer with greater freedom from disease and in many cases better health for a longer period of time. The extension of life has meant also that more of the complications of aging, both physiological and psychological, have become evident, calling for more thorough studies of the problem.

The current (1978) population of 32 million individuals over 60 years of age represents 15% of the total United States population. Predictions are that both the number and proportion will continue to increase and that there will be an even greater increase in the proportion over 70 years of age. As indicated in Table 19-1, however, life expectancy at birth is no longer increasing but continues to be greater for women than for men. This suggests that environment factors over which there is some control, including air and water quality, the use of drugs, alcohol, and tobacco and proper nutrition, are only a few of the factors that determine health and longevity.

The study of the nutritional needs of the aging is complicated by the fact that the older a person is, the more complex he is from both a physical and physiological point of view. Thus the elderly constitute a heterogenous group because of normal genetic differences compounded by all the varying stresses, injuries, emotional and physical traumas, and nutritional imbalances to which they have been subjected throughout growth and maturity and that influenced their development. Although wide variations in the ability of the elderly to ingest, digest, absorb, and utilize nutrients make it difficult to generalize about nutritional needs, studies on a few subjects do make it possible to provide guidlines for the nutrition of the elderly.

Table 19-1. Life expectancy at birth

Year of birth	Life expectancy (years)
1850	40
1900	47
1940	63
1950	68
1960	70
1970	70

The importance of good nutrition in later years is evident from the number of intervention programs with an emphasis on nutrition that have been developed as part of government efforts to enhance the quality of life for the elderly.

Since the nutritional status of an individual at any age is a reflection of his previous as well as his present dietary habits, Shock has suggested that the best preparation for a healthy old age begins in the office of the pediatrician. As with any biological process, aging occurs at different rates in different individuals even under similar environmental conditions. A person with a chronological age of 80 may have a biological age of 50 and vice versa. One factor believed to be responsible for delaying the onset of the senile process is a high but not excessive level of nutrient intake in the presenile years in the presence of adequate but not excessive caloric intake.

Although it has been impossible to test it with humans, there is evidence from animal studies to show that calorie restriction in early life results in an increase in the life span, whereas similar restrictions during adult life actually hasten the death of cells associated with aging. Conversely, there is evidence that overfeeding in early life hastens maturity and shortens life, whereas overfeeding after maturity increases the incidence of degenerative diseases associated with aging.

In aging, as at any other time, the state of nutrition of the body is determined by the state of nutrition of the individual cells. Cells will be less than adequately nourished under conditions of dietary deficiencies or excesses, impaired digestion, incomplete absorption, inefficient distribution and utilization of nutrients, and accumulation of waste products. Many of these conditions are likely to occur as the body ages.

The stresses that affect aging may be subtle and insidious, but over a period of years, they become cumulative and detrimental. This can be most vividly illustrated by a caloric imbalance of as little as 10 kcal a day, which at the end of a year amounts to a gain or loss of 0.5 kg of weight. When accumulated over a forty-year period this represents an appreciable change in the body size. Similarly, rather small stresses in individual cells or organs that accumulate over the years may become sufficiently great to cause impaired cellular functioning.

Physiologists have been seeking an answer to the question of the nature of the degenerative changes that occur with aging. Aging, in theory, begins with conception, but during the period of growth the anabolic, or building-up, processes exceed the catabolic, or degenerative, changes; therefore the net result is one of growth and increased functional capabilities of the organs and tissues of the body. Once the body has reached physiological maturity, the process is reversed, slowly at first, until the rate of degenerative changes outweighs the growth changes. Along with this comes impaired functioning of many organs of the body.

The difficulties of studying one person through the fifty or sixty years of aging are obvious. So far scientists have relied on data from cross-sectional studies on many different persons at different ages, but there is at least one longitudinal study designed to assess the biochemical and physiological changes that occur in a group of men to be studied for twenty years. Such an investigation should shed considerable light on the biochemistry and physiology of the aging process.

There is general agreement that the decrease in physiological function in aging is the result of a progressive loss of cells rather than of poorly functioning cells, but there is likely no single cause of aging. Among the many theories that have been advanced to explain the biochemical and physiological basis of the aging process are (1) the "clinker theory," which attributes loss of cell function with aging to the accumulation of waste in the cell; (2) the wear-and-tear theory, which relates aging to chemical and mechanical exhaustion of the cells; (3) the somatic mutation theory, which suggests that somatic (growing or dividing) cells are inactivated; (4) the autoimmune theory, which suggests that antibodies, which normally attack bacteria and foreign cells, start attacking and destroying normal body cells; (5) the cross-linkage theory, which maintains that collagen molecules are immobilized by cross-linking by free radicals; and (6) the lipid peroxidation theory, which suggests that the oxidation of lipid in the cell membrane destroys its integrity and leads to destruction of the cell and the accumulation of lipofusin granules (oxidized lipoproteins) in the cell. Additionally, it is postulated that with aging the cells form defective RNA from DNA, which appears to be damaged with age. The defective RNA then calls for the synthesis of defective enzymes, which are not capable of performing normal cellular functions. This, of course, leads to death of the cell. When many cells fail to reproduce effectively, the number of cells of an organ and hence its size and functional capacity are reduced, although each remaining cell is functional. Some researchers, however, have reported a 15% decrease with age in the number of mitochondria, the site of energy metabolism, in cells from heart and liver tissue suggesting that the capacity of a cell to release energy may be diminished.

In addition to the decrease in the number of cells of the body in aging, there are structural changes associated with collagen, the noncellular protein substance that binds the cells together. Collagen, in which the rate of protein turnover is slow, becomes less elastic and more fibrous as the cell ages. Some evidence appears to show that the connective tissue replaces some of the more active cells lost from an organ; thus the decline in functional capacity of an organ may be greater than that represented by the decrease in organ weight. In muscle tissue, muscle fibers may be replaced by connective tissue. The accumulation of collagen in the skin is believed to contribute to the aging appearance of the skin. Although complete agreement does not exist on the cause of aging, it is agreed that, generally speaking, the changes are irreversible.

Table 19-2. Percentage of tissues remaining in a 75-year-old man compared to a 30-year-old man*

Tissue	Percent remaining in 75-year-old man
Brain weight	56
Number of glomeruli in kidneys	69
Number of nerve trunk fibers	63
Number of taste buds	36
Body water content	75

*Modified from Shock, N. W.: Sci. Am. **206:**100, 1962.

The percentage of various tissues remaining in a 75-year-old man compared to those in a 30-year-old man is shown in Table 19-2.

The rate of decline in the functioning capacity differs in various systems of the body. A decline in kidney function of about 0.6% per year results in a decrement of 10% to 15% in cellular function, which in turn leads to decrements of 40% to 60% in organ function.

Shock has studied and measured the change in 50- and 70-year-old men compared to a 30-year-old man. Some of his results are summarized in Fig. 19-1. The effects of these and other physiological changes in the utilization of nutrients will be discussed later.

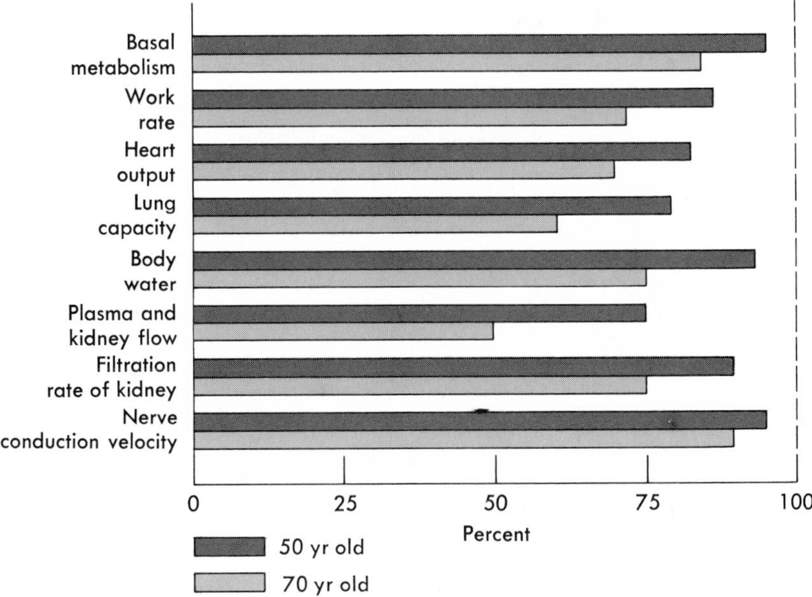

Fig. 19-1. Percentage of certain physiological functions remaining at ages 50 and 70 compared to age 30 (100%). (Modified from Shock, N. W.: Sci. Am. **206:**100, Jan., 1962.)

NUTRIENT INTAKE

The factors that influence the nutritional requirements and intake of older individuals can be classified as those which affect intake, digestion, absorption, storage, and metabolism of nutrients, and elimination of waste products.

Factors affecting the ingestion of nutrients

Long-standing dietary habits. Patterns of eating are established early in life, and there is evidence that persons tend to prefer the type of foods they learned to eat when young. This is especially true under stressful conditions such as illness or loneliness.

Nutrition education has had relatively little impact on the food habits of mature individuals; thus we find an older person is likely to choose and enjoy the foods he has eaten throughout his life. To him they may represent a certain form of security. Since many experiences with food are pleasant ones, the use of a specific food may conjure up pleasant memories.

Many individuals now in their later years were forming their habits in an era when the kinds and variety of foods available the year round were much different from and fewer than those available in the markets fifty years later. As a result, these older persons do not readily make use of the new marketing techniques that increase the variety of food available, and they may eat in the same way they learned to eat when the selection was more limited.

An examination of dietary intakes of older persons reveals that vitamin A and ascorbic acid are the nutrients most likely to be lacking. These, it will be recognized, are provided through ample use of fresh fruits and vegetables that were available only seasonally, unless home preserved, sixty to seventy years ago.

In old age, as in other stages of life, one of the major deterrents to promoting optimal nutrition is the established eating habits of the individual. Because the many meanings food has for older persons may be deeply ingrained, it is likely unwise to insist on any abrupt change in dietary habits without a thorough knowledge of the individual's feelings about food. A slower, more subtle approach in which modifications are made within the framework of the individual's food preferences is more likely to be successful. When abnormal metabolic conditions, such as diabetes, ulcer, or obstruction of the bile duct, dictate regulated dietary patterns, the medical necessities of the changes are of primary concern and leave no alternative but a sudden modification of eating habits.

Loss of teeth. The longer one lives, the more likely he is to lose his teeth, and the lower his socioeconomic status, the less likely he is to replace them with satisfactory dentures. The American Dental Association estimates that of every hundred 70-year-olds, 28 men and 45 women have lost all their teeth; 80% of these either fail to replace them or replace them with ill-fitting dentures. Some of these dental problems are attributed to the loss of the supporting jaw bone in periodontal disease. One cause of this is low calcium/phosphorus ratio in the diet which results in osteoporosis in 25% of women over 50. Regardless of the cause, the absence of a satisfactory method of chewing food leads to many modifications in eating patterns.

Food that is inadequately chewed is difficult to swallow. Thus those with unsatisfactory teeth tend to substitute foods requiring little chewing for those requiring more. When foods high in cellulose such as fruits and vegetables are eliminated from the diet, the bulk of the diet is reduced, with the resultant decrease in gastrointestinal motility and problems of elimination. A reduced intake of meat—one of the most available sources of iron—will possibly have a depressing effect on hemoglobin levels, which in turn may influence behavior. If fluoridation of the water supply by reducing dental caries decreases the number of edentulous senior citizens, its benefits may be even greater in later years than in childhood.

Diminished sense of taste and smell. The noted decline in the number of taste buds at age 70 to 36% of those at age 30 may explain the observation that a decreased interest in food often develops with increase in age. With a diminished number and sensitivity of taste buds, it is understandable that much of the pleasure of eating is removed. There is some evidence that the ability to recognize flavors is not affected, but the ability to discriminate higher concentrations is lost. A zinc deficiency may be a compounding factor, since it too results in decreased taste sensitivity. Recent evidence shows that the ability to taste salt declines with age while sensitivity to sweet is not diminished. Many older persons complain of an unpleasant taste in their mouth that reduces their enjoyment of food. This has been attributed to the excretion of a fluid from around the teeth during chewing.

Loss of neuromuscular coordination. The ability to maintain fine neuromuscular coordination declines with the aging process, frequently manifesting itself as an inability to manipulate eating utensils. Rather than risk the embarrassment that would come with spilled food or inability to cut meat or eat soup, a person will avoid all such foods. This may lead to marked dietary changes and often nutritional inadequacies.

Persons whose ability to coordinate their movements has deteriorated recognize the hazards of working with boiling water or gas ranges. As a result, to avoid the danger associated with cooking food for themselves, they choose foods that do not need cooking.

Physical discomfort. The discomfort that often accompanies ingestion of certain foods is more pronounced in older persons. Some may cause heartburn, others cause gastric distention, and still others are incompletely digested. Efforts to avoid the offending foods may lead to the elimination of nutritious foods from the diet.

Economic considerations. The economic pressures to which many older persons are subjected play an important role in determining dietary adequacy. When it is recognized that 50% of persons over 65 years of age had an income of less than $1480 per year and 25% had less than $1000 in 1974, it is not surprising that they have restricted amounts for food expenditures. The necessity of living on a meager income to remain financially independent forces many older individuals to choose the least expensive foods that provide them with energy and satisfy their hunger. This frequently means substituting the relatively inexpensive carbohydrate foods, bread, and cereal products, which are often low in the protective nutrients, for the more expensive meat, milk, and fresh fruits and vegetables, which are normally dependable sources of protein, minerals, and most vitamins. The ease with which carbohydrates are obtained and stored enhances their appeal.

A study of the food consumption of older persons in Rochester, New York, showed that less than half the households had diets that furnished full amounts of NRC recommended dietary allowances for all nutrients, and a fourth had diets that failed to meet two thirds of this standard for one or more nutrient. When the nutritive adequacy was related to the amount spent for food, it was found that 80% of those who spent more than the cost of the U.S. Department of Agriculture's liberal-cost food plan met the recommended allowances in full, whereas those who spent less than its estimate for the cost of a low-cost food plan failed to meet two thirds of the recommended allowance for one or more nutrients. It should be pointed out that the recommended allowances may be increasingly generous the older the person grows, since all persons over 51 are grouped together. This recommendation has persisted in spite of considerable evidence that most needs decline after that age.

The disappearance of the corner groceries from the older residential and downtown areas and their replacement with large supermarkets in suburban shopping plazas have compounded the problem of the older citizen, who characteristically chooses to live in the more familiar, central, less expensive part of town. To take advantage of the lower prices at the larger market he must either pay for public transportation to and from the store or must become dependent on friends with cars. Once in the store, he may become overwhelmed and confused by the choices with which he is confronted and in the end may shop rather ineffectively or he may return to the smaller delicatessen or service store at which prices are higher but where familiar personnel provide service. Shopping in supermarkets is rendered even more difficult for a person with faulty vision who is unable to read the labels or for the short or physically unstable individual who is unable to reach food on high shelves.

The elderly suffer from a pervading fear that they may become ill and be unable to look after themselves or bear the cost of medical care. This renders them ready prey for the food faddist or purveyor of natural food and food supplements who promises them excellent health, eternal youth, increased vitality, and assurance that they will avoid the debilitating diseases so feared in old age. All too frequently they are persuaded by door-to-door salesmen to invest a significant part of their income in all-but-worthless products, greatly overpriced, that cannot provide the protection they seek against conditions for which no cure is known. Of even greater concern than the waste of money is the possibility than in relying on the nostrums of the salesman they may delay seeking medical help until the condition has deteriorated to a point where legitimate therapy is much less likely to succeed and where treatment will be even more costly.

Social factors. A person who preserves his independence by living alone may find that this in itself leads to modification of his eating pattern. Lack of motivation to cook regular meals leads to the use of snack-type foods at irregular times, resulting in a poorly balanced meal nutritionally. Inexpensive living quarters may lack adequate cooking and refrigeration facilities. Swanson has observed that it is not unusual to find an older person showing a very erratic eating pattern—a day of nibbling followed by a day of overeating. In one instance she found a woman's daily intake varying from 800 to 3700 kcal accompanied by loss of nitrogen except on days when the intake was above 3000 kcal and 100 g of protein. Others have found that many older persons eat more and with greater pleasure when they have company.

Psychological factors. Conditions of emotional stress or deprivation often lead to modifications in attitudes toward food and in food habits as well as changes in utilization of nutrients. Persons who are anxious may experience loss of appetite and resultant undernutrition or, on the other hand, may indulge in compulsive nibbling, which leads to overnutrition. Their interest in food may represent emotional poverty or lack of other interests. Some older persons who find their living situation intolerable escape it by relying on the sedative effect of a large meal. In spite of this tendency to overeat, obesity is rarely a problem in old age. The use of foods as an attention-getting device is common. The older person who is completely self-sufficient is often neglected by his relatives and friends. On the other hand, the person who does not eat adequate meals becomes a cause of concern and is often the recipient of attention and invitations. The nutritional implications of this are evident from studies showing that the same diet consumed under the emotionally unhappy condition of living alone compared to the pleasant atmosphere of companionship leads to a loss of nitrogen over a period as short as thirty days.

Factors affecting digestion and absorption

Changes in digestive secretions. With the degeneration in the size of the salivary glands that has occurred by age 60 there is a decrease in the secretion of saliva. The effect of this on carbohydrate digestion is minimal, since other enzymes are capable of complete carbohydrate digestion. However, the loss of saliva as a lubricant for food may have a more profound effect. With the decline in saliva, a trend develops toward the use of softer, more moist foods, such as creamed dishes, mashed potatoes rather than baked potatoes, and thinner starch-thickened products, possibly a means of compensating for the natural lubricants in the saliva.

The secretion of most digestive enzymes shows a decline with aging, but the extent of the decrease and the age at which it occurs have not been fully established. Depending on the extent of the decrease, food may be less completely digested or will require a longer time for complete digestion. Impaired liver function with a loss of bile secretion has been shown to influence fat digestion. An earlier report that a decline in hydrochloric acid secretion of 9% to 35% occurred in aging has been refuted in more recent work that failed to show a decline. Should hydrochloric acid secretion decline it will have an adverse effect on the absorption of both calcium and iron and the utilization of protein. A decline in calcium absorption after age 65 has been observed but it may be due to factors other than gastric acidity.

Factors affecting metabolism and excretion

Decline in physiological function. Many of the changes associated with aging occur in functions that require a coordination among various organ systems that decline at varying rates. The rate at which nerve impulses are conducted varies only slightly, but there is a greater decline in the amount of blood the heart can pump and the capacity of the lungs, which limits the amount of physical exercise an older person can tolerate.

The rate of blood flowing through the kidneys is decreased to 50% of the normal adult capacity. This means that less blood is presented to the filtering system of the kidneys, through which the waste products of metabolism are eliminated and the nutrients are returned to the general circulation. In addition, an older person has a reduced capacity to form either a more concentrated or more dilute urine. As a result, there is a decline in the ability to handle either large amounts of waste products or of water.

The composition of the fluid surrounding individual cells is normally maintained within very narrow limits. However, the speed with which older persons are able to compensate for alterations in blood and hence intercellular fluid composition due to the ingestion of excess acid-forming or base-forming substances may be four times as slow as in younger persons. This is only one example of changes in the rate at which the body can adjust to stress.

Alterations in the blood vessels, such as the narrowing of the lumen, loss of elasticity, thickening of the wall, and replacement of elastic muscle fibers with nonelastic material, reduce the capacity of the blood vessels to effectively nourish all parts of the body.

Hormonal secretions. Changes in hormonal secretions that exert a regulatory effect on a wide range of physiological processes have a direct or indirect effect on the nutrition of the cells and hence of the whole organism. By regulating the diameter of blood vessels, the endocrine glands regulate the amount of blood and hence the nutrients reaching the tissues. In aging persons there is a greater restriction in the size of the blood vessels leading to the kidneys than in the size of those leading to the brain, thus assuring more adequate blood supply to the more vital centers.

The adrenal gland, which normally responds to stimulation by the pituitary hormone during stress, does not respond as rapidly in older persons. In contrast, the thyroid gland retains its ability to synthesize and secrete thyroxin.

Following are factors that influence the nutrient intake and nutritional status of the elderly:

Physical

- Decreased activity
- Physical weakness
- Loss of neuromotor coordination
- Loss of teeth

Physiological

- Depressed kidney function
- Decreased taste sensitivity
- Use of drugs
- Decreased digestive efficiency
- Constipation
- Lactose intolerance

Psychological

- Depression
- Amnesia
- Food preferences
- Long-standing food habits

Social

- Income
- Living facilities
- Food beliefs
- Susceptibility to food fads
- Loneliness

Nutritive needs

The information available on the nutritive needs of persons over 40 years old is scanty and is based primarily on studies of the intake of healthy persons, rather than on experimental balance studies designed to determine their needs. Some allowances are extrapolated from data on younger persons and others are based on estimates of necessary losses from the body. In general, it is suggested that the nutritive intakes proposed for early adulthood be maintained throughout life. The National Research Council has reflected this by grouping all persons over 51 years together in establishing Recommended Dietary Allowances. Except for calories, there is little evidence that needs either diminish or increase.

Energy. The National Research Council has recognized the change in activity patterns and energy needs that occurs with aging. The trend from active sports to spectator sports, the decline in activity accompanying retirement, the decrease in the amount of housework, and the decline in basal metabolic needs as the number of cells in the body decreases with the loss of tissue mass—all contribute to this. They suggest that the energy allowances for persons over 50 years of age be reduced to 90% of that of mature adults.

On the other hand, FAO/WHO suggest no

change in energy intake up to age 39 but after that recommends a decrease of 5% per decade to age 59, 10% from 60 to 69, and an additional 10% after age 70. Regardless of the recommended level, the intake that results either in weight maintenance or a desired weight adjustment is the proper energy intake. The diet must, however, be chosen from foods that meet other nutrient requirements.

Studies on nutritive intake of older persons have shown intakes below 1400 kcal, representing either efforts to reduce weight, inability to buy or eat more, failure to eat regularly, or inability to chew food. In addition to failing to meet the needs for energy, such diets invariably are inadequate in some other nutrients, such as calcium, iron, and several vitamins. Even though the suggested amount of protein may be provided, much that should go into the synthesis of body proteins is diverted to be used as a source of energy, leading to a negative nitrogen balance. Experimentally diets of less than 1800 kcal resulted in negative nitrogen balance.

Failure to consume adequate calories and with it adequate levels of other nutrients may account for the fatigue, lassitude, and lack of interest in life so often experienced by elderly persons. The lassitude and fatigue may depress activity to the extent that the need for calories is reduced, leading to weight gain even on a low energy intake. It is conceivable that the use of nutritionally suboptimal low-calorie meals may be related to the premature signs of aging.

One study of 100 women 40 to 70 years of age established a relationship between caloric intake and general level of health. Those whose health was rated good consumed from 1650 to 1825 kcal, whereas those whose health was rated as poor were consuming from 1125 to 1475 kcal. This study confirmed that the number of symptoms and the likelihood of other nutrient deficiencies increased when the energy value of the diet was lower. It is difficult to separate cause and effect in such a situation, however. The contribution of various food groups to the caloric intake of elderly women compared to younger women is shown in Fig. 19-2.

Protein. The National Research Council recommends that an intake of 0.6 g of high quality or 0.8 g of protein of mixed quality per kilogram of body weight be maintained throughout adulthood. This approximates the 0.57 and 0.52 g/kg of body weight for males and females recommended by FAO/WHO. Since the total amount of protein synthesized daily declines only slightly with age, an intake greatly in excess of this is considered undesirable because of the added burden of excreting the urea from the deamination of protein by the less efficient kidneys. On the other hand, evidence that calcium absorption is enhanced at higher protein intakes and that various illnesses in the elderly result in decreased absorption and increased losses are considered reasons for recommending higher intakes of 1 g/kg of body weight.

Studies showed that average intakes of elderly persons are in the neighborhood of 45 g daily. This may occur for many reasons. A low protein intake almost always occurs with a low caloric intake. Inability to chew properly reduces the intake of protein-rich meat, and the rejection of milk as a food suitable only for infants or because of lactose intolerance eliminates another potentially good source of protein. Protein-rich foods are the most expensive and their use may well be reduced for considerations of economy.

Some evidence has been established that the elderly have amino acid requirements that differ from those of younger adults. Specifically, the need for lysine and methionine is thought to increase, whereas trytophan and threonine needs are unchanged.

The emotional state of a person influences nitrogen balance, with emotional instability depressing nitrogen and calcium retention.

In the adult, protein is used primarily for maintenance of cells and for the synthesis of enzymes needed for digestion and cellular matabolism. If cellular enzymes are not produced, the cell cannot function properly and ultimately dies, leading to a loss of cell mass

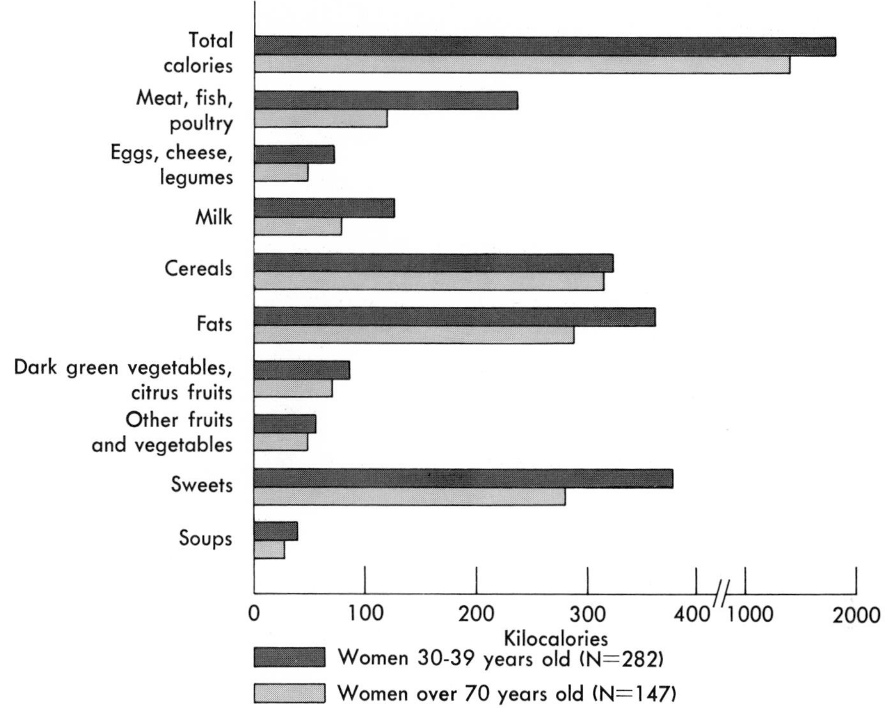

Fig. 19-2. Caloric contribution of various food groups in 30- to 39-year-old women and women over 70 years of age as related to age—spring, 1965. (From Agricultural Research **56:**728, 1964.)

reflected in decreased organ size and reduced organ function. This may be one explanation for the observation that as the amount of protein decreased, the number of symptoms reported went up.

Since iron, thiamin, riboflavin, and niacin occur together in many foods high in protein, a deficiency of protein will lead to a deficiency of these other nutrients as well. A reduction in thiamin to critically low levels depresses appetite, which further reduces total food intake and compounds the problem of dietary inadequacy.

Calcium. Early in the study of bone and tooth metabolism it was believed that these tissues were metabolically inert and that once they were formed, the need for a dietary source of calcium was drastically reduced. Although subsequent research has clearly established that bones are metabolically dynamic tissues calling for a constant source of dietary calcium, it has been very difficult to convince older individuals that they do not outgrow their need for calcium. The loss of 100 mg of calcium a day, which can occur on a diet providing 400 mg or less, would lead to a loss of 30% of the skeleton in ten years. Such a loss would result in osteoporosis, a condition characterized by a decrease in bone mass but no change in bone quality. Osteoporosis occurs in about 30% of persons over age 65 and affects women four times as often as men. It is characterized by a loss of both bone matrix and about 30% of body calcium due to an increased rate of bone loss rather than decreased rate of bone formation. It shows up in a reduction of normally calcified bone mass per unit volume of bone, a narrowing and separation of the trabeculae, decreased tensile strength (reflected in susceptibility to fracture), compression of bone, low back pain, and decreased stature. Calcification of the lower arm and the neck of the femur (the leg bone that inserts into the hip socket) are most adversely affected in osteoporosis and thus are most susceptible to fracture. It is estimated that 5 million women a year have spontaneous fractures as a result of osteoporosis. In many cases of osteoporosis bone such as that in the jaw, which normally supports teeth, completely disappears to become a major factor in periodontal disease.

Although factors other than diet are implicated in this condition, evidence exists than an intake of calcium that leads to the formation of bones with a maximum density at maturity, coupled with an intake of 800 to 1000 mg during adulthood, is the best protection against the development of osteoporosis in old age. Once osteoporosis has developed, one can only hope to inhibit its progress. Increased calcium intake for six to twelve months results in positive calcium balance and increased bone density in some but not all persons with osteoporosis. Intakes of vitamin D as high as 1000 to 5000 IU have been shown to restore positive calcium balance. The ingestion of fluorine at levels of 1 ppm in water throughout adult life is believed to have a beneficial effect in retarding the course of osteoporosis. Intakes of fat above 200 or below 50 g also inhibit calcium absorption. An inadequate intake of calcium rather than poor absorption, however, is likely to be the cause of the lowered retention. The decreased use of milk products and the resultant decrease in calcium intake is evident from Fig. 19-3, based on data from a 1965 survey of food consumption in households in the United States.

Phosphorus. There is considerable evidence that in addition to low calcium intakes throughout adulthood, high phosphorus intakes associated with the extensive use of carbonated beverages and processed foods to which various phosphorus compounds are added, causing a decreased ratio of 1:4 may be a contributing factor in the bone loss in osteoporosis.

Iron. The need for iron does not change for men, but the postmenopausal women, who no longer suffer iron losses in monthly menstrual flow, the recommended allowances drop back to 10 mg from 18 mg. In spite of this reduced requirement, iron deficiency and resulting anemia occur frequently among low-income elderly. This has been attributed to consumption of a diet low in iron associated with decreased caloric and protein intake and increased blood losses, poor absorption, and poor utilization.

Vitamins. Since some nutrients such as thiamin and niacin are required primarily for energy metabolism, the requirement for these will fluctuate with energy needs. The changes in vitamin requirements with aging are so poorly documented that it is difficult to quantify their effect on nutrient needs.

Pyridoxine. Although some reports indicate that the need for pyridoxine increases with age, this is most likely the result of the effect of some medications such as isoniazid or penicillamine used in treating infections.

Vitamin B_{12}. Several investigators have shown that when vitamin B_{12} is given the elderly, symptoms of fatigue disappear and the sense of disorientation and confusion may be alleviated.

Folic acid. Although as many as 80% of elderly persons have been shown to have low blood folate levels, they have a relatively low incidence of megablastic anemia usually associated with a folacin deficiency. Certain mental disorders common in the elderly also tend to occur in persons with a folate deficiency. Since folic and ascorbic acid tend to be found in the same foods, it is not surprising that folate deficiency occurs more often among those whose diets are also low in ascorbic acid. It is also more frequent among those taking anticonvulsant drugs.

Ascorbic acid. The intake of vitamin C among older persons is frequently reported to be extremely low. Often long-standing food habits have not established the practice of using fresh fruits and vegetables. The relatively high cost of these foods and the bulk that many provide may be some of the other

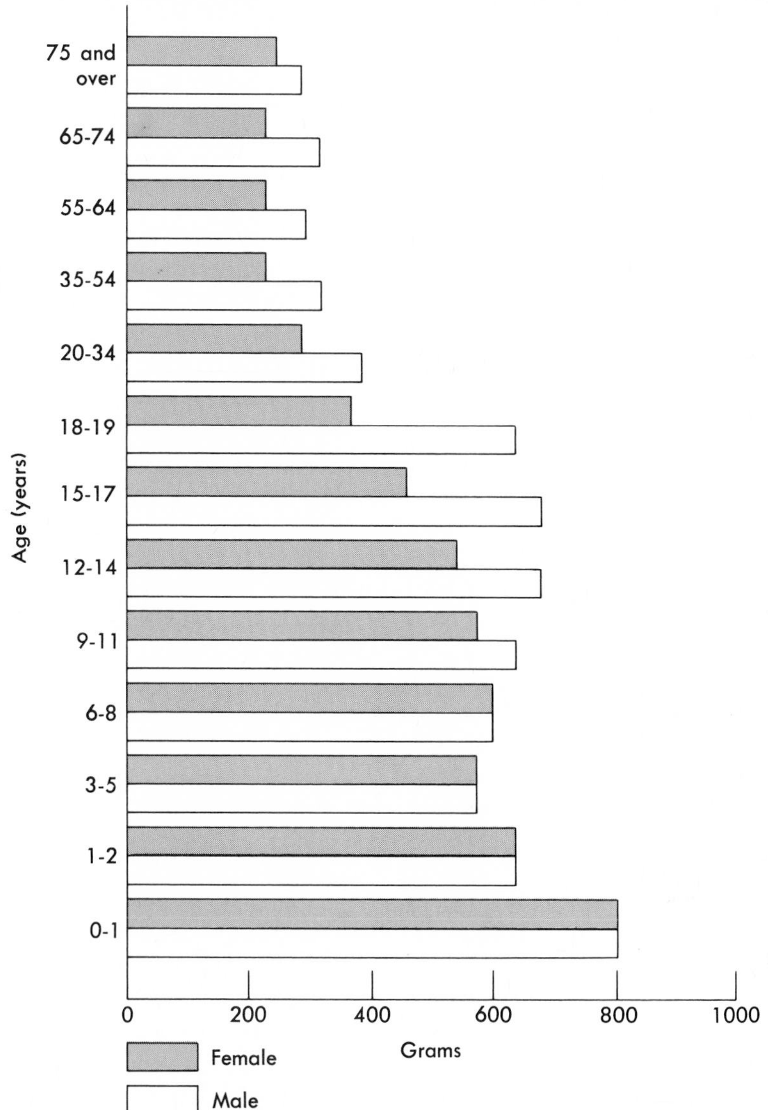

Fig. 19-3. Consumption of milk and milk products (calcium equivalent, quantity per person per day) as related to age—spring, 1965; 28 g = 1 oz. (From Agricultural Research Service, U.S. Department of Agriculture, 1969.)

factors contributing to a restriction in their use. A beneficial effect from ascorbic acid (as replacement for hydrochloric acid in older individuals) on the absorption of calcium and iron has not been substantiated.

Fat-soluble vitamins. There is little specific information on the need for fat-soluble vitamins among the elderly. Vitamin A absorption may be depressed by a lack of dietary fat, depressed bile secretion, and the use of laxatives and antibiotics. Vitamin E needs increase when the proportion of fat as polyunsaturated fat increases, an especially important consideration in light of the fact that oxidation products of fat have been implicated in the aging process.

Fat. Because of a possible relationship between high fat and excessive calorie intake and the development of atherosclerosis and heart disease, it is suggested that older persons, especially those who may be overweight, restrict their fat intake to a level providing 30% to 35% of the calories. Age per se does not affect tolerance for fat.

Water. The need for fluid is often overlooked in assessing dietary intake. Because of reduced kidney function, an older person needs at least 1.3 liters of water a day to maintain fluid balance.

Adequacy of diets

The assessment of adequacy of diets of aging persons is complicated by the difficulty in obtaining subjects. In one study only 13% of those contacted agreed to participate, raising the question how representative they were of the original group. In spite of the difficulties of obtaining the cooperation of a sufficiently large group of aging individuals, several studies have been successfully completed to give some picture of prevailing dietary patterns. Although the majority have been confined to persons in institutions because of ease in data collection, some have been carried out on groups of individuals living in their own homes.

Swanson, comparing the nutrient intake of Iowa women at 30 to 39 years of age with those of women over 70, reported a decrease in intake of calories, protein, ascorbic acid, and calcium. The relative and absolute amounts of meat, fish, and poultry, of sweets, of fats, and of milk products accounted for this decrease. The relationship between calories contributed by these groups in the two age groups is shown in Fig. 19-2. The amount of cereal products in the diet remained constant but constituted a higher proportion of the total calories as aging persons reduced their total caloric content.

In a study of food selection of 114 older Michigan women, low intakes of calcium and ascorbic acid as well as vitamin A were observed. A higher mortality rate among those getting less than 40% of the recommended allowances of one or more nutrients was also reported. A large number of the subjects complained of tiredness, pains in joints, shortness of breath, constipation, and other signs of general malaise.

Fry and co-workers, in a study of thirty-two women over age 65, found their diets to be reasonably adequate, with iron, calcium, and vitamin A the most likely limiting factors. But only 12%, 16% and 9% of the women, respectively, showed these specific deficiencies. Similarly, a study of low- and moderate-income elderly persons in rural Pennsylvania showed vitamin A and calcium intakes below two thirds of RDA for 66% of the subjects and caloric, thiamin, riboflavin, and vitamin C intakes below two thirds for over 40%. Iron and protein were most often taken above this level. Those on low incomes had significantly lower iron and protein intakes than those on moderate income.

A study of 283 households in which homemakers were over age 60 and were dependent on Old Age Survivors and Disability Insurance showed 44% with diets evaluated as good and 25% with poor diets defined as containing less than two thirds of the recommended allowances for one or more nutrients for both high- and low-income individuals. Fig. 19-4 shows that low income was associated with less adequate diets. Diets low in protein were low in at least four other nutrients. Thiamin, which was lacking in the diets of 40% of the households, and calcium and ascorbic acid, low in 30% of the cases, were the nutrients most often limiting.

Steinkamp and co-workers were able to follow a group of 577 aging persons in California over a fourteen-year period. They found that the mean intake met the standards for all nutrients except calories for men, calcium for women, and ascorbic acid for both. However, a fourth of the men and half of the women had less than two thirds of the recommended calcium allowances, and a fourth of both sexes had equally low intakes of ascorbic acid. The subjects showed a slight down-

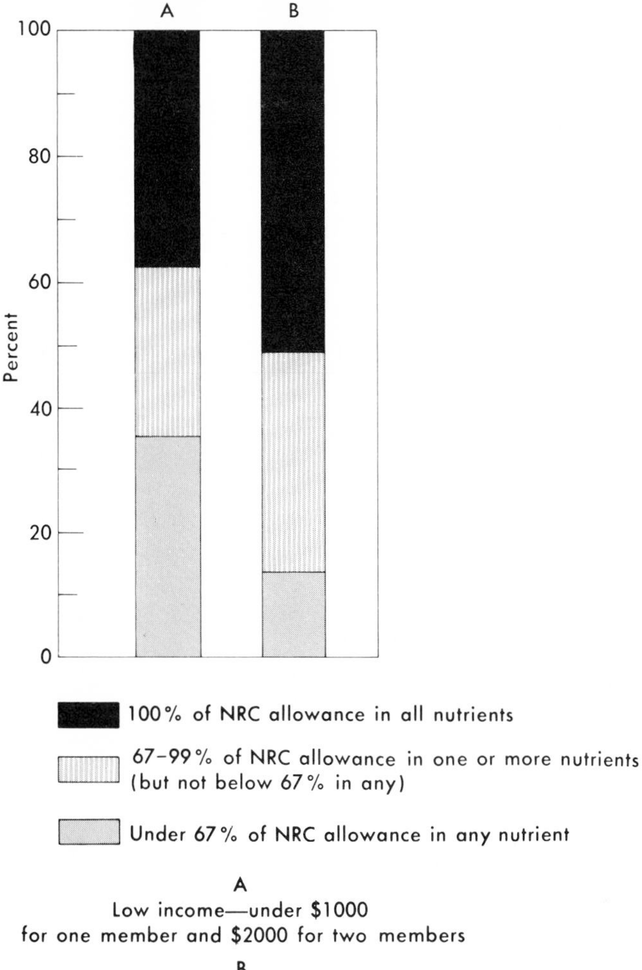

Fig. 19-4. Diet quality as related to income among older households in Rochester, New York. (From LeBovit, C., and Baker, D. A.: Food consumption and dietary levels of older households in Rochester, New York, Home Economics Research Report No. 25, Washington, D.C., 1965, U.S. Department of Agriculture.)

ward trend for all nutrients with age, and a sharp downward trend after age 75. The investigators found that the decrease in calories was associated with a general decrease in the amount of food consumed, rather than a decrease in a particular food or food group.

The most extensive studies of the dietary habits of the elderly have been the Ten State Nutrition Survey and the HANES study. In the former 895 persons were evaluated and in the latter 1515 persons over 60 years of age were studied. Results are shown in Fig. 19-5. From these data it is evident that intakes of a large percentage of the elderly fall below recommended standards. While undoubtedly many would benefit from increased intakes of many nutrients, it is also possible that the

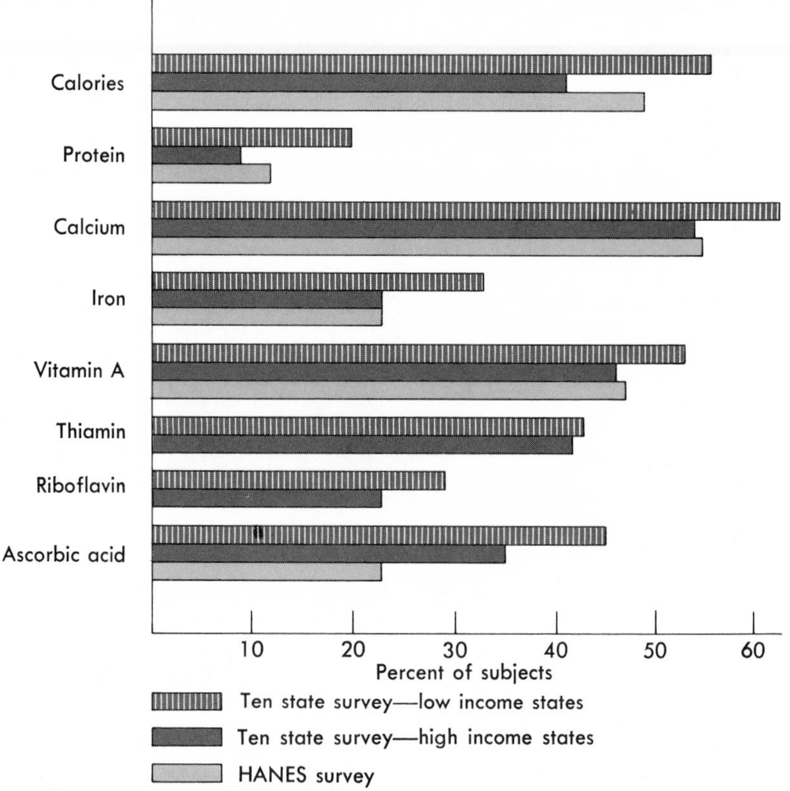

Fig. 19-5. Percentage of persons over 60 years of age with dietary intakes below two-thirds RDA for selected nutrients. Data based on results of the Ten-State Nutrition Survey (1968-1970) and the first Health and Nutrition Examination Survey (HANES) (1971-1974).

dietary allowances, which are based on very little experimental data, are unrealistically and unnecessarily high.

NUTRITIONAL STATUS

Attempts to evaluate the nutritional status of the elderly through the assessment of nutrient and metabolite levels in the blood and urine have been confined almost exclusively to the Ten-State Nutrition Survey and the HANES survey. In the former it was established that low biochemical levels in two or more blood and urine measures occurred in less than 8% of white persons over age 60 but in 25% of blacks and Spanish-Americans. Over 60% of the former and 50% of the latter had satisfactory levels in all measures. The HANES study found that 29% of blacks over age 60 had low hemoglobin levels, confirming the fact that this group is nutritionally vulnerable.

A similar survey in Canada revealed that low serum folate levels were the most prevalent nutritional problem. These low levels were found in 60% of men and 61% of women over age 65 surveyed. Urinary thiamin values were low in about 30% of the males and 12% of the females studied.

Other less comprehensive studies have revealed 70% of a group of elderly with delayed prothrombin times, indicative of vitamin K deficiency associated with liver disease or the use of salicylates (aspirin) or antibiotics.

DIETARY SUPPLEMENTS

The fact that older persons are concerned about their health and are highly motivated to take any steps that they believe will help maintain a sufficient level of health for them to retain their independence means that the use of dietary supplements—especially multivitamin and mineral capsules—is widespread. In Rochester, New York, it was found that 37% of the households of people 55 or older were using supplements, 29% of which were ordered by a physician. Of these 104 persons, forty-eight were consuming diets adequate in all nutrients and needed no supplements, and fifty-six with fair or poor diets would have benefited from the correct supplement. However, only twelve of this group used supplements that provided all the nutrients lacking in their diets, thirty-one used products providing some but not all of the nutrients they needed, and thirteen supplemented their diets with nutrients they were already getting in adequate amounts in their regular diet but not with the nutrients they needed. A similar situation was noted in a study of men and women over 50 years of age in California. Steinkamp and co-workers found that 35% were using mineral, vitamin, or other food supplements. Of those taking vitamin supplements, 37% had diets already adequate in the vitamins taken. Of the sixty-three diets found low in vitamin A, twelve diets were supplemented; of forty-three low in ascorbic acid, eleven; for niacin, eight of forty-five; for riboflavin, four of twenty-nine; and for thiamin, three of eleven. In the case of minerals only three of eighty-nine persons with suboptimal intakes of calcium took supplements including calcium, and none of the twenty-three needing iron received it. Since the amount spent on supplements may represent an appreciable proportion of the money available for food, one would hope that more guidance could be available to help those who would profit from supplements to choose the correct ones and to counsel those whose diets are already adequate against wasting their money.

INTERVENTION PROGRAMS

Watkins has pointed out that in planning programs to improve the nutritional status of the elderly, it is important to consider (1) that each person has a unique nutritional history that has been influenced by physical, emotional, and attitudinal factors, (2) that since much malnutrition is secondary to disease or disability, diagnosis and treatment of the underlying cause must be made concurrent with efforts to improve the diet, and (3) that education in health, nutrition, and consumer issues can be effective.

Although many health problems may be the result of metabolic changes related to intake, the major concerns are negative nitrogen balance as the result of a decreased rate of protein synthesis, decreased glucose tolerance due to impaired carbohydrate metabolism, hyperlipidemias due to poor utilization of lipid, hypochromic anemia as a result of poor iron absorption, and spontaneous fractures and periodontal disease due to depressed calcium utilization.

Concern over the inadequacy of food intake among the elderly, whether for social, economic, or emotional reasons, has led responsible community and government groups to develop intervention programs to help alleviate the problems of inadequate food intake. Among these are Meals-on-Wheels and Congregate Meals Programs. In the former a hot meal is delivered to the recipient's home three to seven days a week depending on the funding and personnel of the program. In some cases food to be refrigerated for the evening meal and possibly also for breakfast is delivered at the same time. This program is designed for those elderly who have inadequate cooking facilities or who are unable to shop for and prepare food. The Congregate Meals program, on the other hand, is designed to meet the social as well as the nutritional needs of the participants. The elderly are provided with transportation to a centrally located "diners' club" where, in addition to receiving an appetizing and nutritionally adequate meal in the company of others, they are able to participate in a variety of recreational, social, and educational experiences. Both programs are designed to meet the needs of older persons regardless of income. Those who can pay the full cost do so; others receive their meals at reduced or no cost and are given the opportunity to use food stamps as payment. While these are the two types of programs receiving the most financial backing, others that attempt to attack the problems of hunger and social isolation of the elderly with stable incomes in a spiraling economy are being investigated.

BIBLIOGRAPHY

Anderson, W. F.: Nutritional problems of the elderly, Proc. Nutr. Soc. **27**:185, 1968.

Berry, W. T. C.: Protein status of the elderly, Proc. Nutr. Soc. **27**:191, 1968.

Black, K., and Guthrie, H. A.: Dietary practices of the elderly in Bedford County, Pennsylvania, Gerontologist **12**:330, 1972.

Brink, M. F., Speckmann, E. W., and Bailey, M.: Current concepts in geriatric nutrition, Geriatrics **23**:113, 1968.

Brown, P. T., Bergan, J. G., Parsons, E. P., and Krol, I.: Dietary status of elderly people. Rural, independent living men and women vs. nursing home residents, J. Am. Diet. Assoc. **71**:41, 1977.

Calloway, N. O.: A critical ratio of aging: water loss—heat production. J. Am. Geriatr. Soc. **19**:306, 1971.

Carlson, L. A., editor: Nutrition in old age; Symposium of Swedish Nutrition Foundation, Upsala, 1972, Almquist & Wiksell.

Clarke, M., and Wakefield, L. M.: Food choices of institutionalized vs. independent-living elderly, J. Am. Diet. Assoc. **66**:600, 1975.

Curtis, H. J.: Biological mechanisms underlying aging process, Science **141**:686, 1963.

Davidson, C. S., Livermore, J., and Anderson, P., and Kaufman, S.: Nutrition of a group of apparently healthy aging persons, Am. J. Clin. Nutr. **10**:181, 1962.

Elwood, T. W.: Nutritional concerns of the elderly. J. Nutr. Ed. **7**:50, 1975.

Esposito, S. J., Vinton, P. W., and Rapuano, J. A.: Nutrition in the aged. Review of the literature, J. Am. Geriatr. Soc. **17**:790, 1969.

Fry, P. C., Fox, H. M., and Linkswiler, H.: Nutrient intakes of healthy older women, J. Am. Diet. Assoc. **42**:218, 1963.

Garry, R. C.: Symposium. Nutrition and the elderly, Proc. Nutr. Soc. **19**:107, 1960.

Greger, J. L., and Sciscoe, B. S.: Zinc nutriture of elderly participants in an urban feeding program, J. Am. Diet. Assoc. **70**:37, 1977.

Harrill, I., and Cervone, N.: Vitamin status of older women, Am. J. Clin. Nutr. **30**:431, 1977.

Howell, S. C., and Loeb, M. V.: Nutrition and aging, monograph for practitioners, Gerontologist **9**:1, 1969.

Kupers, E. C.: Feeding the elderly heart, J. Am. Geriatr. Soc. **22**:97, 1974.

Leaf, A.: Getting old, Sc. Am. **229**(2):44, 1973.

LeBovit, C.: The food of older persons living at home, J. Am. Diet. Assoc. **46**:285, 1965.

Leeming, J. T.: Skeletal Disease in the elderly, Br. Med. J. **4**:472, 1973.

Lutwak, L. : Continuing need for calcium throughout life, Geriatrics **29**:171, 1974.

Lutwak, L.: Nutritional aspects of osteoporosis, J. Am. Geriatr. Soc. **17**:115, 1969.

Mayer, J.: Aging and nutrition, Geriatrics **29**:57, 1974.

Pelcovitz, P.: Nutrition in older Americans, J. Am. Diet. Assoc. **58**:17, 1971.

Pelcovitz, J.: Nutrition to meet the human needs of older Americans, J. Am. Diet. Assoc. **60**:297, 1972.

Shock, N. W.: Physiologic aspects of aging, J. Am. Diet. Assoc. **54**:491, 1970.

Steinkamp, R. C., Cohen, N. L., and Walsh, H. E.: Resurvey of an aging population—fourteen-year followup, J. Am. Diet. Assoc. **46**:103, 1965.

Stiedman, M., Jansen, C., and Harrill, I.: Nutritional status of elderly men and women, J. Am. Diet. Assoc. **73**:132, 1978.

Tappel, A. L.: Will antioxidant nutrients slow aging processes? Geriatrics **23**:97, 1968.

Watkins, D. : Aging—Symposium, Am. J. Clin. Nutr. **26**:1095, 1973.

Watkins, D. M.: The impact of nutrition on the biochemistry of aging in man, World Rev. Nutr. Diet. **6**:124, 1966.

Watkins, D. M.: New findings in nutrition of older people, Am. J. Public Health **55**:548, 1965.

Watkins, D. M.: A year of developments in nutrition and aging. Med. Clin. North Am. **54**:1589, 1970.

Weinberg, J.: Psychologic implications of the nutritional needs of the elderly, J. Am. Diet. Assoc. **60**:293, 1972.

Wheeler, M.: Osteoporosis, Med. Clin. North Am. **60**:1213, 1976.

20

Weight control

Obesity, recognized as a major health problem in the United States affecting from 10% to 30% of any age group, must be considered a condition of multiple origins. Although weight accumulates only when energy intake exceeds energy expenditure, the possibility of this occurring is influenced by physiological, physical, social, cultural, and genetic factors. An excess of 3500 kcal of energy results in an increase of 0.5 kg of body weight. A caloric deficit of the same magnitude is needed to bring about a weight loss of 0.5 kg of body weight.

Weight control is a term generally applied to efforts to maintain body weight within the limits compatible with maximum level of health or to adjust body weight to conform to these established standards. For the vast majority of adults this control is readily achieved with little or no conscious effort. This is impressive when one considers that most individuals consume one million kcal a year and that a daily error of 10 kcal (0.5% of the caloric intake of a sedentary adult female) will accumulate to represent a change in body weight of 0.5 kg a year, and a daily 100 kcal error, a change of 5 kg. For a relatively small group suffering from caloric undernutrition (Fig. 20-1) the problem is one of keeping weight up to desired levels; for a somewhat larger group, estimated as high as 25% of the population, the problem is one of restricting weight gain (Fig. 20-2).

Although the health hazards of being underweight may be equally as great as those of being overweight, persons in the latter group are the subject of vastly more research and are more ready targets for promoters of all types of weight-reducing aids and books ready to capitalize on their desire for a panacea for weight problems. The underweight individuals who may be even more motivated to achieve a normal weight are, comparatively speaking, totally ignored. This discussion will reflect the situation by drawing rather extensively on the vast literature available to discuss obesity and dealing with the problems of the underweight individual in a few paragraphs. This must not be interpreted to imply that the underweight individual does not warrant attention.

OBESITY

Obesity is generally defined as a condition in which there is an abnormal accumulation of fat in body tissue. When 20% of body weight of a man and 28% to 30% of the weight of a woman is composed of fat (normal values are 12% to 18% and 18% to 24%, repectively), the amount of fat is judged to be abnormally high, and the individual is described as obese. An increase in fat to these levels means the body cells that normally contain some fat have become saturated with fat. In addition, to accommodate the fat that must be formed to store energy intake in excess of expenditures, there are special fat, or adipose, cells capable of holding as much as 62% fat. These specialized cells are formed primarily in perinatal life or in adolesence. Connective tissue cells are possibly converted into fat cells also. This increase in body fat usually corresponds to a weight at

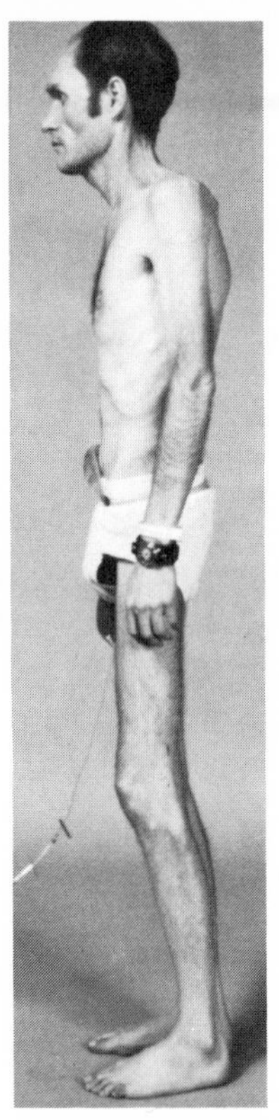

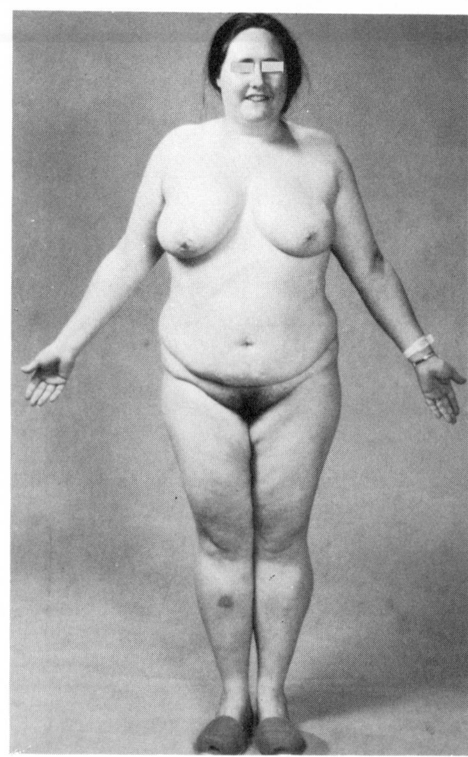

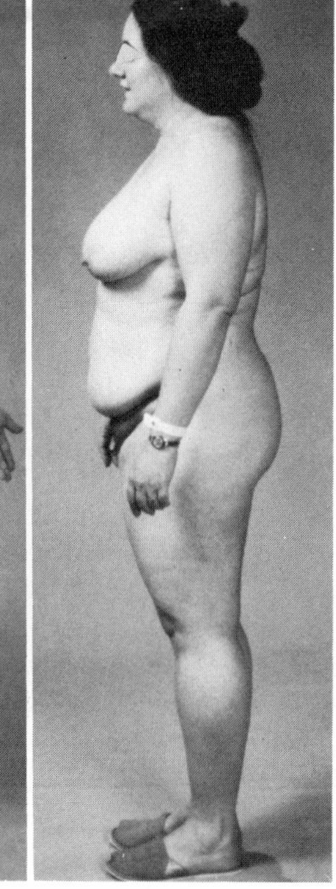

Fig. 20-1 **Fig. 20-2**

Fig. 20-1. Typical case of undernutrition. (Courtesy Dr. Lyn Howard, Albany Medical Center.)

Fig. 20-2. Case of extreme obesity representing high percent of body fat. (Courtesy Dr. Lyn Howard, Albany Medical Center.)

least 15% above ideal or desirable weights and is evidenced by an increase in the bulk or size of the body, which may be either localized or distributed throughout the body.

Since obesity can occur only when energy intake has exceeded energy expenditure, it was formerly described as simple obesity. The condition is now recognized as a symptom of one or more disturbing influences—either physiological, psychological, or pathological. It is indeed a condition of multiple origins. Treatment likewise must be multifaceted to reflect the multiple causes and the individualized responses to treatment.

In addition to the segment of the population who can be theoretically described as obese, there is another group designated as merely overweight, whose body weight is above the level believed to be compatible with the optimal level of health but not sufficiently high to represent an excess accumulation of fat. Overweight individuals, of course, are likely to become obese unless preventive measures are taken when the increments in weight begin.

Bruch suggests that the body may have a preferred weight that bears no relation to an accepted standard but one that the individual tends to maintain or to revert to after an attempt at weight adjustment. For those indi-

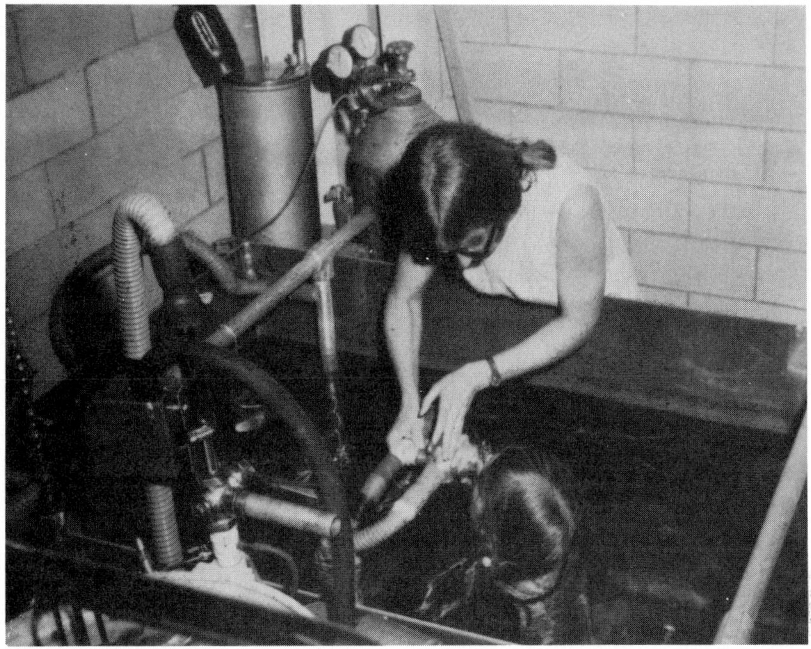

Fig. 20-3. Underwater weighing for the determination of body density. (Courtesy Dr. E. S. Buskirk, Pennsylvania State University.)

viduals for whom this is true, attempts at weight loss may almost certainly be doomed to failure.

Diagnosis

The absence of any single feasible and effective technique for measuring body fat on which to base a diagnosis of obesity has led to the use of many methods, only some of which correlate even relatively well with the direct methods of inferring body fat from measures of body density and lean body mass.

Determination of lean body mass. Three major techniques are available to determine the relative amounts of fat and lean body mass comprising body weight, but all require trained workers and expensive equipment. The measurement of specific gravity involves comparing the weight under water (corrected for residual air in the lungs) to the weight in air (Fig. 20-3). When the proportion of fat is in the range of 15% to 20% body weight, the ratio of weight in water to weight in air, or specific gravity, will be approximately 1, indicating a normal distribution of musculature and fat. As the proportion of fat increases, the specific gravity decreases, since fat, with a specific gravity of 0.92 compared to 1.1 for the rest of the body, is lighter per unit of volume than lean body mass. The lower the specific gravity, the greater the proportion of fat in the body.

Since the amount of water in the body is known to be approximately 72% of lean body mass, knowledge of the amount of water in the body can be used to compute the amount of lean body mass. This in turn could be subtracted from the total body weight to determine the amount of body fat.

The technique for measuring body water involves injecting a known amount of either of the chemicals antipyrine or deuterium oxide into the blood and removing a sample of blood after a prescribed period to determine the extent to which body water had diluted the chemical. From this determination of the amount of the chemical in a measured volume of blood total body water, then lean body mass, and finally body fat can be calculated.

A technique known as the *whole body counter* is based on the theory that potassium represents a fixed percentage of lean body mass or protoplasm and that potassium 40, a radioactive form of potassium, is a fixed percentage of the potassium in food consumed and hence of the potassium in body tissue. By measuring the radioactivity of potassium 40 in the body using a whole body scintillation counter, it is possible to measure the amount of this substance in the body, and from this to calculate the total amount of potassium and then the lean body mass. Subtracting this from total body weight, one then calculates the amount of body fat. Although the equipment is initially expensive and requires a skilled operator, the 40-minute test subjects the individual to no discomfort or hazards and may have potential as a diagnostic tool.

Appearance. Diagnosis of severe obesity can be made reliably on the basis of physical appearance, but this criterion is less useful in identifying cases of borderline obesity, since it does not allow a distinction between body size caused by an accumulation of fat and that caused by an accumulation of water or muscle. On the basis of appearance some persons such as muscular athletes may be judged to be obese at a body weight that cannot be considered unhealthy.

Skinfold measurements. Efforts to assess subcutaneous fat, which represents 50% of the total body fat, by measuring the thickness of skinfolds in one or several places on the body have been only moderately successful. Many believe that a single skinfold measurement on the triceps, located at the back of the right upper arm midway between the elbow and the shoulder, is adequate for diagnostic purposes. Others, however, maintain that there are difficulties in using this one site and that measurements must be made of the subscapular or iliac fatfolds, also.

Measurements must be made with a constant-pressure caliper (usually 10 g per square millimeter) (Fig. 15-3). These measurements must then be compared to an established standard for obesity or used as components in a formula to yield an obesity index. Generally, the relation of skinfold or fatfold thickness to body fat is independent of height. The major drawback to these methods is the difficulty of getting reliable measurements not only from different technicians but also from the same technicians on separate occasions. The wide variation noted under normal conditions is another complicating factor. For instance, in 12-year-old boys the median measurement of triceps skinfold was 9 mm, with a range of 4.5 to 22 mm.

X-ray measurement of body fat. A relatively new technique in which the thickness of fat is measured in various parts of the body as it shows up on an x-ray plate is useful in clinical studies but is of limited value for routine diagnostic purposes because of its high cost and the relative hazard of widespread use of x-ray technique.

Comparison of body weight to an established standard. In spite of the limitations of a comparison of the weight of an individual to established standards of weight for specific age and height, this remains the most widely used criterion available. Practically all standards for adults are based on figures made available by insurance companies and are the ones associated with the lowest mortality rates. The current standards described as "desirable weights" at age 25, released by the Society of Actuaries, are reproduced in Appendix F. These weights are made with normal clothing, and heights are taken with 5 cm heels for women and 2.5 cm heels for men. Nude weights are 3 to 4 kg less for men and 2 to 3 kg less for women than are weights with clothing on. The individual using these tables must arbitrarily classify himself in one of three body frame types—small, medium, or large. This makes it possible for an individual to place himself in the category that best suits his needs as he perceives them or to choose the one that represents his present status in the most favorable light.

The use of standard height-weight tables

to determine presence or absence of obesity, considered 15% to 20% above desirable weight, can be very misleading if weight is composed of an unusually high proportion of either fluid or muscle. The newer standard growth curves for infants and children up to 18 years of age represent recent data from a cross section of the population and allow one to judge weight compared to others of the same height or age. They do not, however, specify a weight associated with obesity, but an individual with a weight above the 75th percentile should certainly be considered at high risk of becoming obese if he is not already. Additionally, a trend toward heavier weights for height or age in successive measurements should be interpreted carefully.

Other techniques. The search for a simple method of recognizing obesity has led to the development of many relatively unscientific criteria of limited usefulness.

Prevalence

The difficulty of arriving at a suitable criterion for diagnosing obesity has led to confusing reports on its incidence, even when one recognizes that marked differences may exist in various segments of the population. For example, public health statistics suggest an incidence of 10% to 13%, insurance statistics based on a selected population is 6% to 7%, and statistics from a study of Iowa women an incidence of 25%. A weight at least 20% above standards, which represents a doubling of fat reserves, is found in millions of Americans, representing 3% of the population over 30 years of age. *The Build and Blood Pressure Study* reports that 5% of the males (one in twenty) and 11% of women (one in nine) are at least 20% over the desirable weights suggested by life insurance statistics as most conducive to longevity. The incidence reported in other studies ranges from 8% to 40% with a study of 110,000 people in Manhattan showing seven times the incidence of obesity in the lower socioeconomic groups as in the middle and upper groups. The former continued to gain weight after 35 years of age, whereas the latter groups did not.

Many of the apparent discrepancies can be attributed to differences in the social, cultural, and economic environments.

Practically all studies agree that obesity becomes a progressively greater public health problem as the ability to regulate exercise and intake decreases after age 20 with the gradual decline in energy requirements. At birth the infant requires 50 kcal/kg of body weight for basal metabolism, at 5 years a child needs 45 kcal and at age 15 an adolescent needs 40 kcal after which needs decline steadily at a rate approximating 2% per decade. After 60 to 70 years of age the incidence of obesity declines somewhat, reflecting the higher mortality rates among younger obese persons in the population.

Disadvantages

Before a person is motivated to correct a condition such as obesity, which calls for considerable willpower and perseverance over a long period and is often fraught with disappointment, he must be convinced that the disadvantages of the condition are sufficiently great to warrant the self-discipline involved. There are many disadvantages from a health standpoint as well as physically, physiologically, economically, and socially.

Health hazards. Although there has been a long-standing belief that mortality from a wide range of health problems is higher among moderately overweight individuals than persons of normal weight and increases progressively with higher levels of obesity, there is now evidence that the hazards are minimal until weight exceeds the standards by 20% to 30%. At that point the ponderal index (height/weight$^{1/3}$) (Fig. 20-4) falls below 12.3 and is associated with a marked increase in mortality rates. This index reflects body shape rather than body size with the lower values found primarily among endomorphs. The fact that the moderately overweight individual is very likely to continue to gain and reach the level of obesity associated

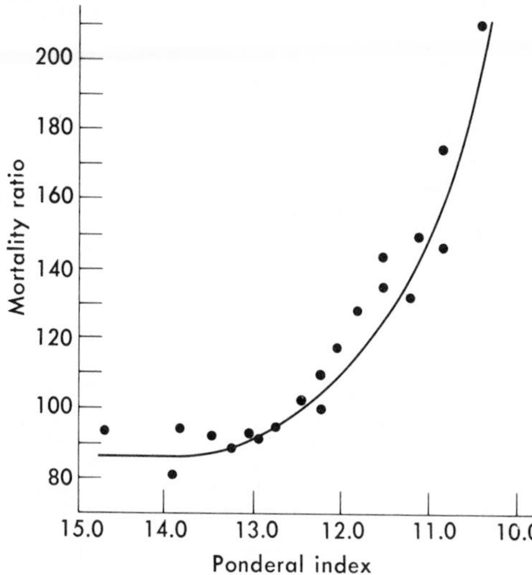

Fig. 20-4. Association of mortality ratio with ponderal index for men, issue ages 40 to 49. Ponderal index = height in inches divided by cube root of weight in pounds; mortality ratio = actual/expected deaths. (Data derived from Build and blood pressure study, 1959; from Seltzer, C. C.: N. Engl. J. Med. **274:**254, 1966.)

with increased mortality does place him at a higher risk.

The relationship between the degree of obesity and mortality rates from specific diseases is shown in Fig. 20-5. It is obvious that the risk of diabetes, digestive diseases, and coronary artery diseases such as stroke and hypertension are greater among the obese and that of suicide and respiratory diseases among the underweight. Only in some cases, however, is there evidence of a causal relationship. For diabetes there is ample evidence that reducing weight is an effective treatment but the evidence for a similar effect on coronary heart disease and hypertension is scant.

The relationship between obesity and diabetes may not be one of cause and effect, since current theories suggest that obesity may be an early sign of adult-onset diabetes and may be caused by essentially the same metabolic defect. Obesity may be a stress factor that precipitates diabetes in susceptible individuals.

Although the presence of some fat surrounding vital organs such as the kidneys, heart, and lungs is desirable, excessive fat accumulation interferes with their mechanical efficiency.

Social disadvantages. The obese person frequently finds himself caught in a vicious circle from a social point of view. Often the initial weight gain is a reflection of an unhappy social adjustment. The resultant obesity leads to social rejection, which in turn leads to more overeating, to increased weight, and to continued or more profound rejection. Adolescents in particular are victims in this chain of events. Excessive weight precludes their effective participation in many active sports, such as tennis, badminton, or swimming, and in social activities, such as dancing. The reduced activity often accompanied by a nibbling pattern of eating makes weight gain easier, again contributing to the vicious circle. There is evidence that obesity can be considered a deterrent to advancement on the socioeconomic scale, since more emphasis is placed on appearance in the higher groups.

Economic disadvantages. The obese individual finds that certain occupations, such as airline stewardess, dietitian, nurse, salesperson, receptionist, and other jobs in which public impressions are important or mobility essential are closed to him. Some employers are reluctant to hire persons who are obviously health risks. This not only limits the vocational choices but also curtails advancement in many occupations. In addition, the obese person may find that the cost of special clothes, furniture, or transportation will increase his cost of living well above normal. In considering economic factors, one may also consider the amount that may well be spent in potential cures or weight-reducing panaceas, the cost of excessive food intake, and the cost of various forms of self-indulgence associated with the unhappy social status.

Psychological disadvantages. Although it has been impossible to attribute any particular personality traits to obese individuals, several studies have revealed some interest-

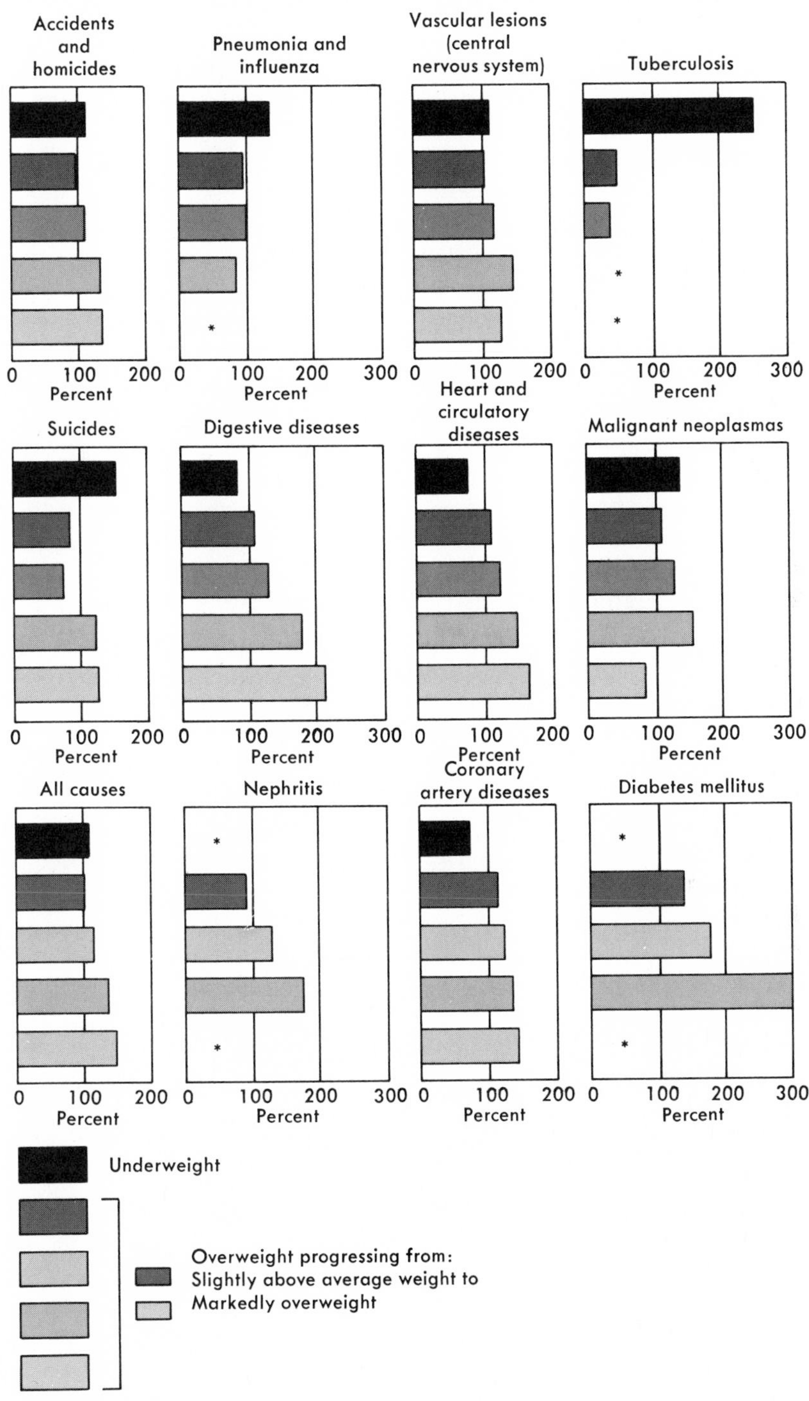

Fig. 20-5. Relationships of body weight to mortality from specific diseases in men. (From Weir, E.: Human Nutrition Report No. 2, Washington D.C., 1971, U.S. Department of Agriculture.)

ing relationships. It is difficult to determine if psychological factors are a cause or effect of obesity, but it may be easy to underestimate the psychological effects of obesity on an obese individual, especially an adolescent girl. Obese girls have been found to possess personality characteristics—self-blame, withdrawal, passivity, inferiority feelings, and sensitivity about one's status—often found in other groups rejected by society. Lack of family support exposes obese adolescents to greater tension. Obese persons have been found to have "distorted body images," a preoccupation with weight, and a tendency to blame all failures and disappointments on their weight. It is possible that social pressures on obese juveniles affect their personalities permanently. It should be pointed out, however, that some obese individuals may indeed have a good life adjustment and are truly "jolly fat people."

Causes

The development of the concept that obesity is a disease of multiple origins or a syndrome rather than a single disease entity does not represent any rejection of the long-established concept that fat will accumulate only when the intake, or consumption, of energy (measured in kilocalories) exceeds the output, or expenditure, of energy. It does, however, propose that the cause of a failure to make a successful adjustment in caloric intake may be found in diverse areas, genetic, metabolic, endocrinologic, or nutritional as well as social, racial, economic, and ethnic and even suggests that perhaps not all persons should reduce. It still holds true that when caloric intake exceeds caloric expenditure, the excess cannot be excreted and will be stored as body fat once the limited glycogen reserves of liver and muscle have been saturated. Nor is there any reason to believe that body fat arises spontaneously. It arises only as a storage form of energy. In the growing individual, however, energy will also be used in the increase in body musculature and bone. In short, the law of conservation of energy still holds. Calories do count. In general, the factors that influence the individual's ability to adjust caloric intake to expenditure will be classified as environmental, psychological, genetic, cultural, and physiological.

Environmental factors

Availability of food. Obesity is a significant problem for large segments of the population only in countries where the food supply exceeds the demand. It is, in essence, a disease of plenty. The middle and upper socioeconomic classes in less affluent countries have always had plenty of food and hence have been the ones who have tended to become obese. This is depicted in medieval paintings in which the corpulent rich man is shown being waited on by lean servants. In many societies today a plump, well-fed wife reflects the success of her husband.

Consumers are constantly being induced to buy more food both at home and away. At the same time weight-reducing aids for those who have bought and consumed too much food are promoted with equal fervor. If food is not available or not consumed in excess, it cannot contribute to the obese state.

Comfort of environment. Well-heated houses and warm, lightweight clothing have reduced the amount of energy needed to maintain normal body temperature in temperate climates. At the same time the human energy expenditure of procuring food have been decreasing constantly with the mechanization of the food and agriculture industries, the increase in convenience foods, and the development of labor-saving devices for food preparation.

Food and hospitality. The use of food and beverages as an expression of hospitality plays an important role in the energy intake of the population by making food more constantly available. Persons are offered food and drink in almost all social situations from the early-morning coffee klatsch to the late-evening buffet supper and midnight snack. Failure to offer food in a social situation may be interpreted as a lack of hospitality, and failure to accept food on the part of the guest may be interpreted as a rejection of hospitality. The more important the occasion, the greater the amount of food and drink offered. Although foods of high calorie density seem to predominate in such situations, it is the amount consumed that is the important factor. In many cultures even the very poor feel compelled to save or borrow for a special festive occasion such as a wedding or baptism to save face by providing a feast.

Family food habits. Long-standing family food habits, many of which were established when existence involved more strenuous physical activity with less protection against extremes of weather, have been retained in the current push-button, air conditioned era. Modern homemakers serve the same kind of meal to their families that their parents served several decades earlier in spite of marked changes that have occurred in family energy needs. Studies on obesity in biological and adoptive children show a strong familial as well as genetic pattern.

The pattern of food intake is a significant factor among overweight persons. In one group 75% consumed most of their food between 4 PM and midnight (night-eating syndrome). Only 17% of the subjects reported eating only three meals a day. There may be some advantages to smaller, more frequent meals, as long as the total intake is not increased.

Decreased activity. A decrease in the amount and intensity of physical activity tends to occur with increasing age. For homemakers often the activity associated with housework decreases. Not only do they exercise less in looking after the needs of their children and home but also expect the children to take over some of the household tasks they formerly did themselves. The increased availability of labor-saving devices and more readily available transportation has resulted in lower energy expenditures among succeeding generations. For instance, power steering in a tractor reduces the energy expenditure by 20% compared to regular steering. Secretaries working 6 hours a day on an electric typewriter expend 450 kcal less per week than their counterparts using a standard typewriter. Similarly, it has been estimated that the average man expends 210 kcal in walking 1.6 km (1 mile), 171 kcal in cycling the same distance, and 17 kcal in driving an automobile. The telephone company claims that the installation of an extension in the home will save 112 km of walking a year. This could account for 0.65 kg of weight a year. If traditional meal patterns are not adjusted accordingly, the likelihood of an undesirable weight gain is increased.

Mayer, in studying the activity patterns of obese and nonobese children, found that the obese exercised significantly less each day with less enthusiasm than did the nonobese. Even when they reportedly participated in an activity for a comparable period of time, their actual time of activity was as little as one third that of the nonobese. They also ate less, but the adjustment was not sufficiently large to compensate for the lower caloric requirements. Because of their larger weight load, obese individuals are often less skilled in sports and may limit their participation even more. Mayer also observed that adolescent obesity usually began in the winter, traditionally a period of reduced activity in the temperate climate. For some persons, periods of forced immobility coupled with admonitions to eat to keep up strength may initiate an excessive weight gain. The widespread use of school buses in transporting children to and from school further deprives young people of a mild but consistent form of exercise. To compensate for such things, these students must make a conscious effort to increase their activity, since prescribed periods of physical activity in schools are much too short to substitute for this, It has been shown similarly that obese women walked only half as much as controls or 32 km less during a week. In many cases they sought ways of reducing activity, such as using elevators, efficient schedule planning to reduce activity, or choosing a mode of living that called for a minimum energy expenditure.

Response to external stimuli. Schachter observed that in contrast to nonobese persons, the obese ate in response to external stimuli, rather than to internal sensations of hunger. They were more likely to eat in response to the time on a clock, the physical availability of food, or stress than in response to hunger sensations associated with physiological needs. In contrast to the nonobese they bought just as much food when they shopped after eating as before; they would stop in a delicatessen moments after completing a full restaurant meal and would eat all the sandwiches on a plate within reach but would not get up to get them. When food is available, the obese apparently cannot distinguish between being hungry and not hungry.

Patterns of infant feeding. The tendency of parents to consider large weight gains in early infancy as highly desirable and to compare the eating habits of their infants to those of other infants leads them to introduce solid foods at an early age, to feed high caloric density milks, and to encourage the consumption of large quantities of food. Bakwin attributes some of the problems of obesity in adolescence to a pattern of eating in which the individual is trained to eat beyond the point where he experiences normal satiety signals to the point where he is overeating. He believes that such a situation can be conditioned by patterns of feeding in early infancy.

The parents of a bottle-fed infant, who can see how much a child is getting, are able to encourage the child to eat to satiety, although it is unlikely that the child can be forced to consume more than he wants.

Some infants have been encouraged to eat as much as they want as frequently as they want; at the same time, physical activity is often minimized. Eid has demonstrated that children who double or triple their birth weights earlier than usual are more likely to become obese adolescents. Others, however, have found that such a relationship is hard to quantify. There is substantial evidence that during periods of rapid cell division (the first year of life and adolescence) fat cells will also increase in number if there is an excessive caloric intake, which requires that more fat cells be available to store the energy. Once these cells are formed, they apparently "demand" a caloric intake that will allow them to store a certain amount of fat. As a result, such individuals have great difficulty adjusting their food intake to a lower caloric level (set point) and continue to store excess amounts of fat and maintain an obese or overweight state.

Psychological factors

Investigations to determine whether psychological factors are causative or perpetuating in obese persons were begun in the late 1940s and have not yet identified any personality factors common to persons who experience difficulty in making a satisfactory weight adjustment. The psychological makeup of the individual influences not only the intake of food but also the level of activity and hence the energy expenditure.

An extensive review of the relationship between specific psychological factors and the incidence of obesity is well beyond the scope of this discussion, but some of the more established relationships will be discussed.

Although obesity is compatible with normal personality factors, some characteristics occur more frequently in obese than nonobese subjects. According to Bruch, overeating may be a balancing factor in adjustment to life. If overeating is to be stopped, the individual must be helped to find some other form of emotional support. Failure to do so may result not only in unsuccessful weight reduction but may also produce trauma far worse than the obesity it was designed to cure. The threat of earlier mortality from many diseases is not a motivating factor for many. To them the prospect of dying early and happy is much less threatening than is the prospect of an unhappy life adjustment that comes with an inability to reduce in the face of continuing efforts. Indeed, without his pattern of overeating the obese person may be in danger of developing a form of mental illness. The need for individual therapy is evident. From a psychological point of view, overeating may be a response to nonspecific emotional tensions or a symptom of underlying emotional tensions, or it may represent an addiction to food.

Anxiety. An anxious person deprived for one reason or another of an outlet in physical activity may seek solace in food, the consumption of which represents a pleasureful pastime. The greater the level of anxiety, the more likely weight gain is to occur.

Substitute for love and security. To at least some obese individuals, overeating a pleasant experience, is used as a substitute for love and affection or as an expression of self-pity. Overprotective parents may overfeed their children to reinforce their love for them. For others the strength symbolized by a large body is apparently a source of security representing a bulwark against an unfriendly world.

Tenseness or frustration. In some persons food is a response to, compensation for, or defense against tension and frustration.

Genetic factors

Characteristics of an individual that determine his level of intake and pattern of utilization of food may be determined by heredity. Such factors may explain the different responses in different individuals in common environments or similar responses among identical twins in markedly different environments.

Somatotype. The anthropological classification of somatic body types as endomorphic (plump and round), mesomorphic (muscular), and ectomorphic (linear and fragile) is based on genetically determined traits. The endomorph is likely to become obese, whereas the individual with few of the endomorphic characteristics tends to remain slim, as does the individual with a high ectomorphic component in his body build. The mesomorph will become obese if his build includes more of an endomorphic then ectomorphic component.

The endomorph tends to gain weight easily, whereas the ectomorph seldom does. Obese girls have been demonstrated to have broader, shorter hands than nonobese, which further points to a relationship between the fragile bony structure of the ectomorph and the absence of obesity.

Level of enzyme activity. There is evidence that the rate of production of enzymes involved in either fat storage or fat mobilization affects not only the formation of fat but also the ease with which it can be used as a source of energy. An efficient or active enzyme system involved in fat formation (lipogenesis) may remove glucose from the bloodstream so rapidly that the normal satiety signals to reduce food intake do not operate quickly enough to regulate food intake, leading to an increased food intake and hence fat formation. This rate of lipogenesis in obese persons may be as much as five times greater than normal. Once fat has been deposited in adipose tissue, primarily as triglycerides, it must be broken down into fatty acids and glycerol (lipolysis) before the fat can be released from the storage site to be transported in the bloodstream for use as a source of energy in tissues requiring energy. This lipolysis depends on the presence of a fat-splitting enzyme—a lipase. In obese individuals the level of activity of this enzyme may be low or inhibited; thus they do not mobilize or release stored fat rapidly enough to meet the body's demand for a source of energy. To meet the need, the individual is forced to consume more food. It has also been established that once fat has been deposited in adipose tissue, the cell will again store fat more readily after its removal. Thus it is easier for a person who has been obese to become obese again than it is for one who has never been overweight.

Although each gram of carbohydrate or protein has the potential of yielding 4 kcal in the body and each gram of fat 9 kcal, many enzymes are involved in the many steps in their conversion to carbon dioxide, water, and energy in the form of ATP. Since there is evidence of biochemical individuality in many enzyme reactions in the body, it is logical to assume that wide individual differences exist in the degree of efficiency with which energy will be released from these potential sources and with which it will be converted to mechanical, chemical, osmotic, or electrical energy for vital body functions. Such differences are undoubtedly genetically determined and are encoded in the DNA of the cell nucleus. An individual with a low lipase activity or a very inefficient enzyme system for the release of energy may have more difficulty regulating his weight. Conversely, a person with an adequate lipase activity and a high efficiency rate in the release of energy will make a much more adequate weight adjustment. Aerobic metabolism is more efficient than anaerobic metabolism, in which it is necessary to expend energy to resynthesize glycogen. It is possible that the tendency toward aerobic metabolism, the more efficient type, may be genetically determined, leaving more energy to be stored. Such differences are well known to animal breeders; they choose animals whose genetic characteristics allow them to gain the most weight on the smallest amount of food or which facilitate the production of wool, milk, or eggs.

Genetically determined characteristics also influence a person's athletic aptitude and hence his participation in active sports and his energy output.

The sensitivity of the appetite-regulating center of the brain, the hypothalamus, appears to be genetically determined. A sensitive hypothalamus responds quickly to an elevated level of arterial blood glucose relative to venous blood glucose and depresses appetite. A less sensitive hypothalamus will respond more slowly and will allow the individual to eat more before a feeling of satiety is reached. A sensitive hypothalamus will respond more quickly. The neurotransmitter dopamine acts to inhibit food intake and counteract the effect of another transmitter, norepinephrine, which stimulates eating behavior.

Studies to determine the incidence of obesity in children of obese parents have shown that if both parents are obese, the chance is 73% that the children will be; if one parent is obese, the chance is 50%; and if neither parent is obese, the chance is only 9% that the children will be. In addition, obese children of two obese parents have fatfold thicknesses three times as great as obese children of two lean parents. When the children are reared in the same environment as the parents, the relationship is undoubtedly partially environmental and partially hereditary. However, Mayer, in studying the effect of environment on the incidence of obesity, found that infants adopted into families with one or more obese parents did not become obese, whereas those born into similar families did become obese.

Once genetic factors are recognized as determinants, it would be reasonable from a public health standpoint to encourage persons with a hereditary predisposition to obesity to participate in a preventive program based on a regimen of activity and a regulation of food intake begun at an early age. Genetically determined differences among individuals may be impossible to detect with the sensitivity of present analytical methods, but if even small differences accumulate, they become appreciable.

Cultural factors

The meaning of body size varies from one cultural group to another and influences attitudes toward obesity. To many groups a large body represents success; the man with the plump wife is one who is sufficiently successful to provide her with adequate food. The stereotype of the plump, successful nineteenth century businessman, an object of envy to his less successful contemporaries, is gradually being replaced by that of the sleek, well-dressed, efficient young executive. In certain primitive tribes young girls will be kept in, fed, and fattened into attractive young women. In many royal courts the women carried about on litters vie with one another to be the fattest and hence the most attractive to royalty. In contrast, in western society young women are under constant pressure to maintain a trim figure if they are to remain attractive and have a likelihood of succeeding.

Food assumes special meanings in various life situations; it is frequently offered in times of sickness or death; it is basic to the feasts used to celebrate births, marriages, and deaths in many cultures.

Physiological factors

Decreased basal energy needs. The need for energy to carry on the vital body functions, known as basal metabolism, declines gradually with age. Although the difference in needs between one year and the next may be imperceptible and may call for no conscious adjustment in energy intake, failure to make a satisfactory adjustment of intake to needs over a period of years can lead to an appreciable positive caloric balance in old age.

Secretion of endocrine glands. The basal metabolic rate is determined by the level of thyroxin secreted by the thyroid gland. In most individuals this is maintained within a normal range, but a small segment of the population may find their energy needs depressed because of a depressed secretion of thyroxin. Such persons experience an easy accumulation of fat and may find it easier to achieve caloric balance if either thyroxin or the closely related compound thyronine is administered. Because of the hazards from unsupervised use of the hormone, it is available only on prescription after clear evidence is established that secretion is depressed.

Insulin, the secretion of the pancreas that is necessary for the uptake of carbohydrate by the cells and hence the utilization of carbohydrate as a primary source of energy, can influence the rate at which adipose tissue is formed.

Some endocrine secretions influence the distribution of fat in various parts of the body, and abnormal distributions represent an abnormal endocrine balance.

Adaptation. A severe caloric restriction for a period of time activates an adaptive mechanism that leads to a lowered basal metabolic rate and a greater efficiency in energy expenditure, thus conserving the energy available.

Regulation of food intake. The mechanisms by which the amount of food a person eats is regulated are still subject to much study, but it now appears that there is both a short-term and long-term regulation.

Short-term regulation. The meal-to-meal or short-term, regulation of intake is controlled by the appetite-regulating center of the brain, the hypothalamus. The glucostatic theory proposed that there was satiety center in the ventromedial section of the hypothalamus that responded to blood glucose or fatty acid levels to inhibit eating, which was stimulated by a feeding center in the lateral part of they hypothalamus. This theory has not been confirmed. It is now believed that the posterior part of the hypothalamus has nerve fibers which are destroyed by the chemical norepinephrine to produce a sensation of satiety and that the fibers in the hypothalamus respond to the chemical dopamine to stimulate eating.

Long-term regulation. The long-term regulation of food intake is governed by the reserves of fat in the adipose tissue cells of the body. It is hypothesized that a type of feedback mechanism operates whereby the desire for food on one day reflects the intake of the previous days, with hunger being stimulated when low intakes have led to a depletion of fat reserves.

Persons who have difficulties in reducing weight have low levels of free fatty acid in the blood after fasting compared to those in persons whose obesity responds to reduced caloric intake. This suggests a difference in their ability to mobilize fat reserves to supply energy during caloric restriction. These same persons respond slowly to the presence of a fat-mobilizing substance such as epinephrine. It may be the result of a metabolic defect that limits the breakdown of body fat stores or one that hastens the reformation of fatty acids and glycerol into fat depots or the presence of a lipase inhibitor.

Classification

Obesity can be classified on several bases. One classification chooses to differentiate between *juvenile onset obesity,* which usually develops before the child is 10 years old, and *adult onset obesity,* which develops later in life. The former is generally more severe than the latter, is more difficult to treat, has a poor response to therapy, and occurs twice as frequently in girls as boys. Frequently, it is associated with a low intelligence and occurs among those with relatively little schooling. In some respects it may be an inherited condition caused by either more efficient use of energy or greater efficiency in energy expenditure. In contrast, adult onset obesity is characterized by a constant food intake in conjunction with a slowly declining energy expenditure both for basal metabolism and for activity. It is the result of the slow insidious weight gain of as little as 0.25 to 0.5 kg a year, which may occur with aging but may go unrecognized until it is well advanced. Sometimes the reduction in cell mass that occurs with reduced activity masks the accumulation of fat, which signals the onset of obesity.

In another classification based on pathogenesis, obesity has been identified as either *regulatory,* in which there is either a psychological or physiological defect in the regulation of food intake in relation to energy expenditure, or *metabolic,* in which there is an underlying metabolic defect in the handling of either carbohydrate or lipid that can be enzymatic, hormonal, or neurological in nature. It is suggested that juvenile onset obesity and metabolic obesity are the same and that adult onset and regulatory obesity are the same.

Bruch, whose experience is primarily with persons seeking psychological help, has suggested that *constitutional obesity* can be distinguished from *reactive obesity.* In the former, which is due primarily to the physiological causes, the person has a healthier personality adjustment to obesity and may suffer some form of maladjustment if forced to reduce. Reactive obesity is most common in adults in whom overeating is a response to tension or frustration. This form is often accompanied by decreased physical activity. Episodes of grief or depression frequently correspond to weight gains. Persons with reactive obesity can experience a night-eating syndrome or a higher level of eating corresponding with periods of depression. These two forms, Bruch believes, are different from *developmental obesity,* which is common in children whose emotional development centers around eating as much as they want, at the same time avoiding physical activity and social contacts.

In general, the basis on which the classification is made reflects the perspective of the investigator. It may be that physiological factors mediate the psychological trauma that leads to overeating.

Treatment

The treatment of obesity involves the successful reversal of the positive caloric balance that caused the condition; that is, a caloric intake less than caloric expenditure. Because of the multiple origins of obesity and the many meanings of food to individuals, it is often difficult to find the cause of obesity. Until the cause is known, efforts to correct the condition are discouraging.

Although the effectiveness of treatment depends on many factors, the motivation of the patient and the establishment of a realistic goal are of prime importance. In most cases the obesity is the result of a small caloric surplus over a long period of time. A small error in intake when accumulated over a period of years is reflected in a sizable weight gain. Conversely, a constant intake of 100 kcal less than daily expenditure will result in a 4.5 kg weight loss in one year. A loss of 0.5 kg a week requires a daily energy deficit of 500 kcal.

The patient launching a weight-reducing regimen should be aware that there may be no drop in body weight for perhaps two or three weeks regardless of strict adherence to a diet known to be deficient in calories. The explanation is that as fat is withdrawn from storage sites, water enters the cells to replace fat and remains there for a period of time, after which it may be released rapidly. Unfortunately, this phenomenon occurs at the stage in weight reducing when a person is most in need of some evidence of success. Usually when weight loss is looked at over a longer period of two to three months, the predicted weight loss will be observed. It is common for a person to experience periods of weight loss followed by a plateau, even with constant caloric intake and expenditure. This pattern of weight loss reflects the composition of the tissue used to provide for the energy deficit, being greater when protein or glycogen, with a higher water content, are used instead of fat.

Studies on the prognosis of treatment have shown that success is more likely in adult onset than in juvenile onset obesity, in males than in females, in younger persons than in older, in married persons than in widowed, separated, or divorced, in single persons (especially women under 30), in the higher socioeconomic groups, in those making their first attempt than those making subsequent attempts, among those less than 60% overweight, among emotionally mature and well-adjusted rather than anxious or depressed persons, and among those with a medical problem that is complicated by obesity. It should also be emphasized that success will be greater if attempts are made in early stages and if done under supervision of a physician who concerns himself with the underlying causes, rather than with a quack, charlatan, faddist, pseudoscientist, or well-meaning but misguided friends. Under any circumstances long-term success in weight reduction has been very discouraging with a 5% success rate common.

The reversal of the caloric balance involves setting the total caloric intake at a level less than that required to meet energy needs. This may be accomplished by either decreasing the intake or increasing activity or preferably both. The level of caloric intake that will accomplish this varies greatly from one person to another because of the many individual factors that contribute to the situation.

Behavior modification. Achievement of weight adjustment either through increased activity or decreased food intake or both has captured the attention of social scientists with expertise in behavior modification. These investigators are reporting short-term success in a program in which the individual is guided through a process of analyzing the conditions under which he usually eats or is not active. He then agrees to a set of rules in which he receives a reward to encourage the desired behavior (i.e., either not eating or being more active) and/or an adversive stimulus from the behavior that should be discouraged. For example, a person who watches a television program without nibbling will reward himself credits toward a desired goal while the person who fails will lose credits. While this approach to weight control can be very costly if it necessitates a one-to-one counselor-client relationship, the use of autotutorial self-instructional, written material shows promise of being reasonably effective. As with most other approaches the long-term effects of the behavioral approach have been discouraging.

Decreased caloric intake. Decreased caloric intake may be achieved by a strict diet that prescribes a specific number of calories from specific foods or by a prudent diet in which an individual maintains his customary eating patterns but selects smaller portions and avoids foods of high caloric value. Although popular literature abounds in diets designed to lead to a painless loss of weight, few have stood the test of time, and the search for the panacea continues.

Experimental evidence shows that weight loss is a function of caloric intake regardless of the source of calories. The distribution of total calories throughout the day can influence the relative amount of muscles and fat deposited. If a large number of calories is consumed at one time in a condition described as *nutrient overload,* some calories that might have been used in muscle growth or in tissue repair are diverted to fat depots because of the demand suddenly placed on one metabolic pathway. The same number of calories distributed in smaller, more frequent feedings leads to decreased fat and increased muscle increments. Thus some evidence appears in support of the nibbling habit in weight reduction, provided, of course, the amount of food eaten does not exceed the needs of the individual.

In addition to a restriction in the total caloric intake, certain other considerations may be important in dieting success. Understanding guidance and support from physician or friends or family is crucial. A rigid diet may be anxiety-producing for some, whereas for others only such a very clearly prescribed regimen will provide the motivation necessary for adherence to the diet. Eating slowly, tasting food thoroughly, using a smaller than average plate, and including such carbohydrates as potatoes because of their satiety value may contribute to a successful weight-reducing program. Even more important is developing a set of eating patterns in which the caloric intake is restricted and can be maintained to replace the eating pattern that led to the weight gain. For some persons this may involve a reeducation of their concept of serving size. Some research shows that the overweight person's concept of an average serving of food is a much larger quantity than that of a person of normal weight.

Starvation diets. Complete starvation diets may be effective in part because they lead to the accumulation of ketone bodies in the bloodstream, which in turn depress the appetite. The hazards involved in overtaxing the body's capacity to counteract excess ketones or to excrete them dictate that such regimens be employed only in extreme obesity that has been refractory to all other conventional methods and that they be undertaken with strict medical supervision. Persons on such diets are usually hospitalized and are kept in bed because of the extreme weakness and fatigue accompanying the loss of sodium and water that occurs in the absence of dietary carbohydrate and as water is needed to excrete the urea resulting from the metabolism of protein and the ketones formed from the incomplete oxidation of fat. The short-term effects of such programs have been dramatic, but the long-term effects have been discouraging, with very few patients maintaining, let alone continuing, their weight loss. Part of the rapid initial weight loss can be attributed to an initial loss of sodium with the concurrent loss of water and the fact that protein has been deaminated to provide sufficient glucogenic amino acids to obtain the glucose needed to maintain the energy supply for the central nervous system and erythrocytes. This is reflected in negative nitrogen balance. Since protein is a less concentrated storage form of calories than fat tissue is, much more must be catabolized or broken down, to provide the same number of calories. The extensive loss of protein in starvation diets is manifest not only by a negative nitrogen balance but also by loss of body potassium. The catabolism of 0.5 kg of muscle tissue yields about a sixth as many calories as 0.5 kg of fat tissue. Concern over the loss of body nitrogen on this starvation diet led to the concept of a protein-sparing fast in which 60 to 80 g of protein were fed as milk, soy, or egg protein to prevent nitrogen loss and protect body protein stores. Clinical success led to the appearance in drugstores of liquid protein diets, which consisted solely of hydrolyzed collagen with added tryptophan and other amino acids. Warnings that it be used only under medical supervision were generally unheeded with the result that after about one year of growing use with apparent success, many deaths associated with refeeding were reported. This led the FDA to require even more forceful warnings and raised serious doubts about allowing such products to be freely available. Deaths were attributed primarily to heart attacks but there was no apparent explanation of the cause. Powdered protein supplements, designed to help the obese individual regulate his food intake, appear to be safe, but their effectiveness is due to a reduced caloric intake rather than to any unique metabolic role of protein.

Intermittent fasts of one to twelve days' duration showed promising results initially, giving the patient a feeling of well-being and cheerfulness, but have proved no more satisfactory than a continuous reduction in caloric intake in the long run. Persons who have been on a fasting regimen usually eat less immediately afterwards and experience satiety with less food. This has led to the hypothesis that during fasting the satiety center in the hypothalamus may become more sensitive to satiety signals.

High-protein, high-fat, low-carbohydrate diets. The unrestricted protein and fat, minimal or no carbohydrate diets have appeared and reappeared over a period of time under different sponsorships. Most recently it was in vogue as Dr. Atkin's Diet Revolution, but it has previously been promoted as the Drinking Man's Diet, the Air Force Diet, Dr. Taller's Calories Don't Count Diet, Dr. Stillman's Diet, and the Pennington Diet. Undoubtedly, it will surface again several times in the next twenty years. It is obvious that if such an approach provided a permanent acceptable form of weight loss it would have survived the test of time rather than being reincarnated periodically. As yet no one has found a way of repealing the first law of thermodynamics that energy can be neither created or destroyed. Energy for the body is still obtained from food and lost only as heat, excreta, and metabolic and physical work. Permanent loss of body fat can occur only when energy intake is less than expenditure. The loss of ketones, the intermediary products of fat metabolism, which occurs in the urine on low-carbohydrate diets, amounts to a maximum equivalent of 20 g with a caloric equivalent of 4.5 kcal/g. When coupled with the insignificant amount of ketone (1 g) lost in respiration, the caloric equivalent of lost ketones is a maximum of 100 kcal (418 kilojoules).

The weight loss experienced on a low-carbohydrate diet is attributable in part to the fact that if a person restricts his carbohydrate intake to 50 g he probably will not consume sufficient additional fat and protein to make up the calorie deficit—which of course is reflected in a weight loss. Aside from the fact that they may be relatively ineffective in bringing about a permanent weight loss, high-fat, high-protein diets have the additional hazard of leading to high blood levels of triglycerides and cholesterol, both of which are risk factors in coronary heart disease and atherosclerosis. High blood uric acid levels characteristic of gout and hypotension (an undesirable drop in blood pressure when changing from a reclining to an upright position) also occur. Diets that attempt to achieve a calorie deficit by restricting intake to a limited number of foods may be successful for short periods of time but are too monotonous to be considered more than a short-term solution.

Criteria for evaluating diets designed for caloric restriction are discussed in Chapter 5.

Increased activity. The effectiveness of an increased level of activity in establishing caloric equilibrium has been alternately overrated and underrated. As illustrated in Chapter 5, the 3000 to 3500 kcal represented by 0.5 kg of stored body fat is sufficient energy for many hours of such vigorous activity as tennis. However, a few minutes of the same activity every day for a longer period will help maintain the fine daily caloric balance necessary for weight control without undue stimulation of the appetite. Thus, while a 60 kg (132-pound) woman will have to walk for 30 hours at an energy cost of 2 kcal/kg/hr to use the energy stored in 0.5 kg of body fat, if she walks 0.8 km a day at a rate of 5 km/hr, after 180 days she will have used the equivalent amount of energy. Such a mild degree of exercise can represent the loss of 1 kg per year.

Sometimes the initiation of a program of moderate exercise not only increases caloric expenditures sufficiently that a weight loss will occur on a diet that previously maintained weight but also improves muscle tonus, stimulates circulation, and creates a general sense of well-being. Strenuous exercise, on the other hand, may lead initially to a loss of appetite but may later stimulate the appetite to counter-balance any advantages of the regimen.

A study to determine the effectiveness of a

Table 20-1. Energy equivalents of food calories expressed in minutes of activity

Food	kcal†	Activity				
		Walking‡ (min)	Riding bicycle§ (min)	Swimming‖ (min)	Running¶ (min)	Reclining# (min)
Apple, large	101	19	12	9	5	78
Bacon (2 strips)	96	18	12	9	5	74
Banana, small	88	17	11	8	4	68
Beans, green (1 cup)	27	5	3	2	1	21
Beer (1 glass)	114	22	14	10	6	88
Bread and butter	78	15	10	7	4	60
Cake (1/12, 2-layer)	356	68	43	32	18	274
Carbonated beverage (1 glass)	106	20	13	9	5	82
Carrot, raw	42	8	5	4	2	32
Cereal, dry (½ cup) with milk and sugar	200	38	24	18	10	154
Cheese, cottage (1 tbsp)	27	5	3	2	1	21
Cheese, cheddar (1 oz)	111	21	14	10	6	85
Chicken, fried (½ breast)	232	45	28	21	12	178
Chicken, "TV" dinner	542	104	66	48	28	417
Cookie, plain (148/lb)	15	3	2	1	1	12
Cookie, chocolate chip	51	10	6	5	3	39
Doughnut	151	29	18	13	8	116
Egg, fried	110	21	13	10	6	85
Egg, boiled	77	15	9	7	4	59
French dressing (1 tbsp)	59	11	7	5	3	45
Halibut steak (¼ lb)	205	39	25	18	11	158
Ham (2 slices)	167	32	20	15	9	128
Ice cream (1/6 qt)	193	37	24	17	10	148
Ice cream soda	255	49	31	23	13	196
Ice milk (1/6 qt)	144	28	18	13	7	111
Gelatin, with cream	117	23	14	10	6	90
Malted milk shake	502	97	61	45	26	386
Mayonnaise (1 tbsp)	92	18	11	8	5	71
Milk (1 glass)	166	32	20	15	9	128
Milk, skim (1 glass)	81	16	10	7	4	62
Milk shake	421	81	51	38	22	324
Orange, medium	68	13	8	6	4	52
Orange juice (glass)	120	23	15	11	6	92
Pancake with syrup	124	24	15	11	6	95

*From Konishi, F.: Food energy equivalents of various activities, J. Am. Diet. Assoc. **46:**186, 1965.
†To convert to kilojoules multiply by 4.2, to joules by 4200.
‡Energy cost of walking for 70 kg individual = 5.2 kcal/min at 3.5 mph.
§Energy cost of riding bicycle = 8.2 kcal/min.
‖Energy cost of swimming = 11.2 kcal/min.
¶Energy cost of running = 19.4 kcal/min.
#Energy cost of reclining = 1.3 kcal/min.

Table 20-1. Energy equivalents of food calories expressed in minutes of activity—cont'd

Food	kcal	Activity				
		Walking (min)	Riding bicycle (min)	Swimming (min)	Running (min)	Reclining (min)
Peach, medium	46	9	6	4	2	35
Peas, green (½ cup)	56	11	7	5	3	43
Pie, apple (1/6)	377	73	46	34	19	290
Pie, raisin (1/6)	437	84	53	39	23	336
Pizza, cheese (1/8)	180	35	22	16	9	138
Pork chop, loin	314	60	38	28	16	242
Potato chips (1 serving)	108	21	13	10	6	83
Sandwiches						
Club	590	113	72	53	30	454
Hamburger	350	67	43	31	18	269
Roast beef with gravy	430	83	52	38	22	331
Tuna fish salad	278	53	34	25	14	214
Sherbert (1/6)	177	34	22	16	9	136
Shrimp, french fried	180	35	22	16	9	138
Spaghetti (1 serving)	396	76	48	35	20	305
Steak, T-bone	235	45	29	21	12	181
Strawberry shortcake	400	77	49	36	21	308

program of nutrition education and exercise on the course of obesity in 13- to 14-year-old boys more than 30% overweight in the beginning of the program showed that obese boys in the experimental group gained 5.8 pounds during the 18-month study period, whereas those in the control group who did not receive nutrition education and who did not participate in a program of physical activity gained 13.5 pounds. These results suggest that a program of nutrition education coupled with one of prescribed physical activity can be an effective method of controlling adolescent obesity. The energy costs of activity in relation to the energy value of representative foods is shown in Table 20-1.

Group approaches. Group self-help approaches to weight control such as the currently popular groups TOPS and Weight Watchers combine sound dietary advice with the social pressures that a group can exert. They work on the premise that if an overweight individual reports regularly to a group with similar problems and goals he will be shamed into regulating food intake.

Again, they are characterized by short-term success, but an evaluation of their long-range effectiveness indicates that they have no advantage over now conventional approaches.

Dietary aids

A discussion of weight control would not be complete without some mention of the types of dietary aids, representing a $100 million business, with which the adult public is constantly confronted. Fig. 20-6 gives the reader an appreciation of the range of approaches used. The magnitude of this enterprise likely reflects the fact that many obese persons cannot adhere to a diet without supportive measures. It also represents the constant search of the overweight for some easy, painless, and quick road to weight loss. Since

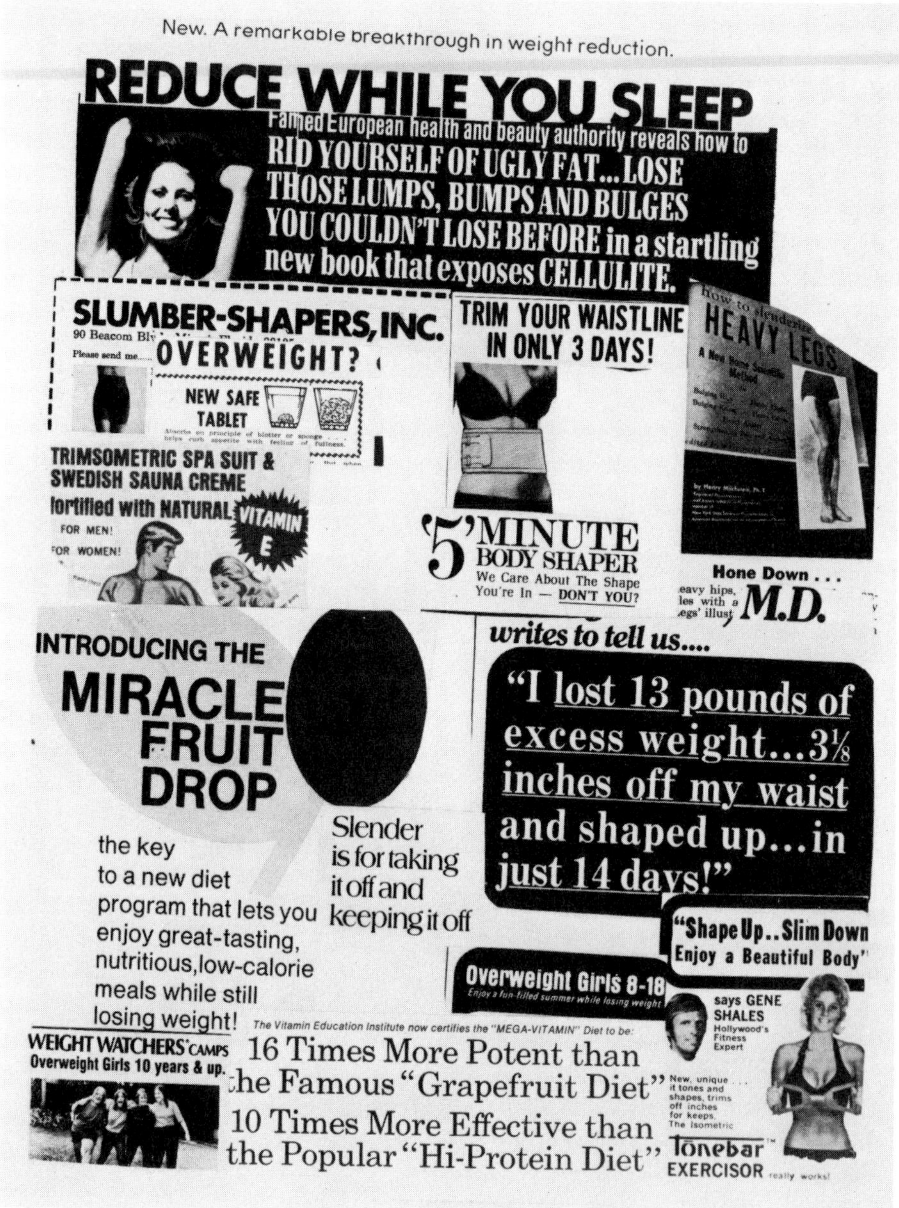

Fig. 20-6. Examples of weight control aids advertised in popular magazines.

few of these aids stand the test of time and remain on the market for more than a brief period, this discussion will be confined to the general types of dietary aids.

Agents reducing food intake. Appetite depressants, or anorexigenic drugs, are the basis of many dietary aids. Pills containing sugar, milk solids, or gelatin taken about half an hour before meals act as an appetite depressant by raising blood glucose levels and depressing the appetite at mealtime. These are relatively harmless but generally greatly overpriced even when the cost of minerals and vitamins that are often added to them is considered. The same effect could be achieved with caramels from the corner grocery store if only one were taken. Fruit juices high in carbohydrate, such as grape juice or prune juice, would have a similar effect.

Stimulants. Products containing amphetamines, which are stimulants for the central nervous system, are useful in overcoming depression and the nibbling that often accompanies it. They are the basis of other products but must be used with caution, since they result in an elevated blood pressure, dryness of the mouth, a rapid heartbeat, and constipation, effects that cannot be divorced from the effect on the appetite. Dexedrine and Benzedrine, common appetite depressants, are also cardiac stimulants, as are epinephrine or ephedrine-like compounds. These stimulating drugs may be an essential crutch in the initial period of caloric restriction for the person who has become addicted to food and who eats compulsively but should be used only under strict medical supervision.

Tranquilizers as weight-reducing aids function by decreasing activity but at the same time reducing nibbling, which may have been the cause of weight gain. Their effectiveness depends on the balance of these opposing effects.

Loss of body water. Diuretics lead to a loss of body water but no loss of body fat. If extra weight is caused by an accumulation of water in the tissues, diuretics will lead to permanent weight loss, but under normal conditions such water must be quickly replaced to maintain normal electrolyte balance. Steam baths, special plastic clothing, belts, and bath salts—also designed to reduce weight by reduction in body water—will effect only transient weight loss.

Bulk-producing substances. Noncaloric substances such as methyl cellulose are advocated as appetite depressants because of their affinity for water and their tendency to increase in volume on the theory that bulk in the stomach will depress appetite. It has been experimentally demonstrated that the swelling of methyl cellulose takes place in the small intestine rather than in the stomach, thus limiting its supposed effectiveness.

Psychological aids. Testimony of individuals who have thought or prayed their way to slimness is evidence of psychologically oriented approaches to weight control. Other devices with strong powers of suggestion such as records played during sleep, pictures of the individual in slimming clothes, or messages on refrigerator doors are some of the current psychological gimmicks.

Transition diet

Once a desired weight adjustment is achieved, it is important that the individual be given guidance in the transition from a reducing diet to a maintenance diet. It is especially important that one recognize the level of intake that will maintain the desired weight and that is sufficiently different from the regular diet that led to the initial weight gain to prevent a recurrence. Although no clear explanation exists for the phenomenon, maintenance requirements for a person who has lost weight have often been found to be lower than those for a person of comparable weight who has not reduced. Any maintenance diet must be sufficiently individualized to be compatible with the cultural, environmental, and social situation in which the individual lives.

Prevention

From a public health point of view the most feasible attacks on the problem of obesity are through prevention. By learning to identify those individuals who, because of genetic makeup, personality characteristics, or environmental factors, are most likely to become obese, it should be possible to develop an educational program designed to control weight gain in the incipient stage. Such an approach could embrace a program of exercise coupled with education and training in the choice of foods and patterns of eating to minimize caloric intake. Pediatricians, with access to weight grids, which help identify deviations in growth patterns in the early stages, have an opportunity to alert parents and to encourage them to help the child acquire a set of eating patterns that will help forestall weight gain. Similarly, school health officials utilize sequential weight and height data to identify students at risk and guide them into appropriate preventive programs. Obstetricians and gynecologists working with women during pregnancy and menopause, two periods when weight gain is frequent are in a position to help them to cope with such an eventuality. Similarly, physicians dealing with middle-aged males working under any form of emotional stress who have a family history of heart disease have a unique opportunity to offer preventive therapy before weight reaches the stage where it enhances the possibility of coronary or arteriosclerotic heart disease. Persons with deviant activity patterns are just as prone to caloric imbalances as are those with deviant eating habits; thus it is important to work on both sides of the energy equation, promoting a habit of moderate but consistent exercise along with moderation in food intake.

It is becoming increasingly clear as scientists learn more about the problems of weight control that these problems are extremely complex and that many questions are still unresolved. In light of the lack of success in regulating weight gain it may be neceesary to reevaluate some current concepts and possibly reject some of them.

UNDERWEIGHT

A person whose weight is more than 15% below desirable weight, although not subjected to the same social pressures to adjust as is his overweight counterpart, is more susceptible to certain health hazards. He is almost twice as likely to succumb to respiratory disease such as tuberculosis and has greater difficulty maintaining body temperature as environmental temperature drops.

Treatment

The treatment of underweight individuals involves creating a positive energy balance by increasing energy consumption beyond energy expenditure. Just as in obesity, it is important to recognize the cause of the undernutrition if it is to be adequately treated. If a depressed appetite is involved, various techniques can be used. Thiamin-deficiency anorexia may be reversed by the use of thiamin supplements. Handling of anorexia nervosa is considerably more complex and should involve determining the underlying cause. The use of smaller, more frequent meals of lower caloric value rather than fewer larger meals may help promote and increased energy intake. The addition to regular foods of highly concentrated sources of energy such as sugar, jellies, butter, mayonnaise, sauces, or dried milk solids is a fairly successful way of increasing the energy value of a diet without an increase in bulk. Just as in weight reduction, the adjustment in weight needs to be made gradually, and it may be even more difficult, albeit more pleasant, for an underweight person to try to gain 0.5 kg/wk than for an obese person to lose it.

BIBLIOGRAPHY

Bortz, W. M., Wroldsen, A., Issekietz, B. and Rodahl, K.: Weight loss and frequency of feeding, N. Eng. J. Med. **274:**376, 1966.

Bruch, H.: Psychiatric aspects of obesity, Metabolism **6:**461, 1957.

Committee on Nutrition of Mothers and Preschool Children, Food and Nutrition Board: Fetal and infant nutrition and susceptibility to obesity, Am. J. Clin. Nutr. **31:**2026, 1978.

Council on Foods and Nutrition: A critique of low carbohydrate, ketogenic weight reduction regimens, J.A.M.A. **224:**1415, 1973.

Darling, C. D., and Summerskill, J.: Emotional factors in obesity and weight reduction, J. Am. Diet. Assoc. **29:**1204, 1953.

Drenick, E. J., and Smith, R.: Weight reduction by prolonged starvation, Postgrad. Med. **36:**A95, 1964.

Dudleston, A.K., and Bennion, M.: Effect of diet and/or exercise on obese college women, J. Am. Diet. Assoc. **56:**126, 1970.

Eid, E. E.: Follow-up study of physical growth of children who had excessive weight gain in first six months of life, Br. Med. J. **2:**74, 1970.

Fabry, P., and Tepperman, J.: Meal frequency—a possible factor in human pathology, Am. J. Clin. Nutr. **23:**1059, 1970.

Fellner, C. H., and Levitt, H.: A new approach to overweight, Am. J. Clin. Nutr. **15:**50, 1964.

Fernstrom, J. D., and Wurtman, R. J. Nutrition and the brain, Sci. Am. **230**(2):84, 1974.

Forbes, G. : Lean body mass and fat in obese children, Pediatrics **34:**308, 1964.

Goldberg, M., and Gordon, E. S.: Energy metabolism in human obesity, J.A.M.A. **189:**616, 1964.

Gordon, E. S.: New concepts of the biochemistry and physiology of obesity, Med. Clin. North Am. **48:**1285, 1964.

Halpern, S. L.: Methodology of effective weight reduction, Med. Clin. North Am. **748:**1335, 1964.

Hamburger, W. W.: The psychology of weight reduction, J. Am. Diet. Assoc. **34:**17, 1958.

Hashim, S. A., and Van Itallie, T. B.: Clinical and physiologic aspects of obesity, J. Am. Diet. Assoc. **46:**15, 1965.

Huenemann, R. L.: Environmental factors in preschool obesity, J. Am. Diet. Assoc. **64:**588, 1974.

Hunt, E. E.: Epidemiologic considerations, Adv. Psychsom. Med. **7:**148, 1972.

Krzywick, H. J., Ward, G. M., Rahman, D. P., Nelson, B. A., and Consolazio, C. F.: A comparison of methods for estimating human body composition, Am. J. Clin. Nutr. **27:**1380, 1974.

Lepkovsky, S.: Newer concepts in the regulation of food intake, Am. J. Clin. Nutr. **26:**271, 1973.

Mahoney, M. J., Moura, N. G., and Wade, T. C.: The relative efficiency of self-reward, self-punishment, and self-monitoring techniques for weight loss, J. Consult. Clin. Psychol. **40:**404, 1973.

Mann, G. V.: The influence of obesity on health, N. Engl. J. Med. **291:**178, 1974.

Mann, G. V.: Diet and obesity, N. Engl. J. Med. **296:**812, 1977.

Mayer, J.: Overweight causes, cost and control, Englewood Cliffs, N.J., 1968, Prentice-Hall, Inc.

Mayer, J.: Some aspects of the problem of the regulation of food intake and obesity, N. Engl. J. Med. **274:**610, 662, 722, 1966.

Mayer, J., and Thomas, D. W.: Regulation of food intake and obesity, Science **156:**328, April, 1967.

McCracken, B. H.: Etiological aspects of obesity, Am. J. Med. Sci. **243:**99, 1962.

Mendelson, M.: Deviant patterns of feeding behavior in man, Fed. Proc. **23**(part 1):69, 1964.

Mendelson, M.: Psychological aspects of obesity, Med. Clin. N. Am. **48:**1373, 1964.

Mok, M. S., Parker, L. N., Voona, S., and Bray, G. A.: Treatment of obesity by acupuncture, Am. J. Clin. Nutr. **29:**832, 1976.

Moore, M. E., Stunkard, A. , and Strole, L.: Obesity, social class and mental illness, J.A.M.A. **181:**962, 1962.

Research on obesity, Nutr. Rev. **35:**249, 1977.

Rodin, J.: The puzzle of obesity, Hum. Nature **1**(2):38, 1978.

Rosenberg, B. A., Bloom, W., and Spencer, H.: Obesity—treatment and hazards, J.A.M.A **186**(suppl.):43, 1963.

Ruffer, W. A.: Two simple indexes for identifying obesity compared, J. Am. Diet. Assoc. **57:**326, 1970.

Schacter, S.: Obesity and eating, Science **161:**751, 1968.

Sebrell, W. H.: Weight control through prevention of obesity, J. Am. Diet. Assoc. **34:**919, 1958.

Seltzer, C. C.: Some re-evaluations of the build and blood pressure study, 1959 as related to ponderal index, somatotype and mortality, N. Eng. J. Med. **274:**254, 1966.

Seltzer, C. C., Goldman, R. F., and Mayer, J.: The triceps skinfold as a predictive measure of body density and body fat in obese adolescent girls, Pediatrics **36:**212, 1965.

Seltzer, C. C., and Mayer, J.: Body build and obesity. Who are the obese? J.A.M.A. **189:**677, 1964.

Shipman, W. G. and Plesset, M. R.: Predicting the outcome for obese dieters, J. Am. Diet. Assoc. **42:**383, 1963.

Stein, M. R., Julis, R. E., Peck, C. C., Hinshaw, W., Sawicki, J. E., and Deller, J. J.: Ineffectiveness of human chorionic gonadotropin in weight reduction: a double-blind study, Am. J. Clin. Nutr. **29:**940, 1976.

Swendseid, M. E., Mulcare, D. B., and Drenick, E. J.: Nitrogen and weight losses during starvation and realimentation in obesity, J. Am. Diet. Assoc. **46:**276, 1965.

Tullis, I. F.: Rational diet construction for mild and grand obesity, J.A.M.A. **226:**70, 1973.

Van Itallie, T. B., and Yang, M. U.: Diet and weight loss, N. Engl. J. Med. **297:**1158, 1977.

Weil, W. B.: Current controversies in childhood obesity, J. Pediatr. **91:**175, 1977.

Weisenberg, M., and Gray, E.: What's missing in behavior modification for obesity, J. Am. Diet. Assoc. **65:**410, 1974.

Wright, F. H.: Preventing obesity in childhood, J. Am. Diet. Assoc. **40:**516, 1962.

Young, C. M.: Some comments on the obesities, J. Am. Diet. Assoc. **45:**134, 1963.

Young, C. M.: The prevention of obesity, Med. Clin. North Am. **48:**1317, 1964.

21

Alternative food patterns

As concern over the safety of the food supply mounts and an increasing number of persons question the use of animal foods, there is a trend toward the adoption of alternatives to conventional food patterns. The rationale and nutritional adequacy for each of these varies, with some based on sound nutritional principles and others leading to a variety of nutritional problems. In general, the more restrictions on the varieties of food that can be used, the greater the possibility of nutritional inadequacies.

In earlier editions of this text, this chapter was entitled "Food Faddism and Quackery," which implies a discussion only of practices characterized by fraudulence. The present title was chosen to more accurately reflect the many bases for the alternative food patterns now finding wide acceptance. Many alternative practices reflect a genuine concern over the quality of the food supply and the impact of nutrition on health; only some are the result of attempts by unscrupulous, misdirected, and/or uninformed individuals to influence food practices for monetary gain. In many cases there may be no rationale for the fervor or zeal with which the modification in dietary practices is accepted. In others, however, when the rationale is founded on accepted scientific knowledge, the practices represent acceptable alternatives although certainly not the only answer to the real or imagined limitations of conventional eating patterns.

Beal has suggested that those who follow alternative food patterns do so from a variety of motivation. They may be expressing antiestablishment sentiments, seeking "super health," notoriety, or truth, hoping for a miracle, following fashions, expressing distrust of the medical profession, or showing concern about the uncertainties in their environment. Any food behavior is the result of a complex of external influences such as friends, family, advertising, or education and internal influences including attitudes, self-concepts, values, beliefs, and biological, psychological, and sociological needs.

Regardless of the basis on which alternative food patterns are chosen, they constitute a source of concern to the nutritionist because of the potential health, economic, and social problems associated with their use. Such practices are by no means confined to the uniformed, the poor, or the suspicious. There is, however, the likelihood that those who have practiced poor food habits throughout their lives are more prone to feel the need for changed food habits and may be particularly vulnerable to accepting new food patterns that may be no improvement. It is frequently observed that as individuals who previously had poor food habits change to questionable diets that are better than those they had previously used, they erroneously attribute their increased vitality to some specific aspect of the diet, which they then promote as a magical element.

Among the various diet patterns now enjoying popularity are vegetarian, ovolacto-vegetarian, macrobiotic, single-food diets, liquid protein diets, and natural or health-food diets. The list is constantly changing but the motivation remains the same—special health-giving properties obtained through the use of certain foods or through the elimination of others that are supposed to be harmful either alone or in certain combination. An examination of trends in popular diets and beliefs reveals that there is seldom a really new approach but merely a constant and cyclic revival of old ones that have been discarded earlier. These diets are not necessarily inadequate, but as the number of foods in the diet decreases, it becomes more important to choose food with a full knowledge of its nutritive content and of human nutritional requirements. The chances of inadequacy increase as the variety in the diet decreases.

VEGETARIANISM

The early 1970s saw a surge of interest in vegetarianism as an alternative food pattern. It is estimated that millions of persons, most of whom are young and from middle- and upper-class backgrounds, espouse it to varying degrees for a variety of reasons, sometimes alone, sometimes in a communal setting. To some it represents a form of religion or spiritual release through which they hope to purify their bodies. For others, vegetarianism represents a form of rejection of many aspects of our affluent society, still others have a genuine concern over the wisdom, economy, esthetics, and safety of using animal products as a source of food, while some feel that diet can replace medicine in curing illness.

While it is possible for an ovolacto-vegetarian (who will eat eggs and milk in addition to foods of vegetable origin) to select a nutritionally adequate diet, the true vegetarian often referred to as a *vegan* has more difficulty and hence is more susceptible to nutritional inadequacies particularly vitamin B_{12}, protein, riboflavin, calcium, and iron and their consequences. Since there is no reliable plant source of vitamin B_{12} for the person who practices vegetarianism for prolonged periods, the symptoms of vitamin B_{12} deficiency, such as anemia, soreness of the tongue, back pain, and menstrual irregularity, are to be anticipated. Failure to simultaneously consume sources of all essential amino acids from a variety of vegetable protein sources will have the same effect as a diet devoid of protein. In addition, only when the diet provides sufficient calories will the protein be used for growth rather than for energy. Persons who consume no animal foods are also more prone to develop rickets due to a lack of vitamin D compounded by a calcium deficiency—especially children who are not exposed to sunlight. When unrefined cereals are used, there is a hazard of irritation in the gastrointestinal tract.

Since vegetarian diets are high in bulk, or cellulose, it is often difficult for a true vegetarian with high energy needs to eat enough food to maintain energy balance. Although most adults can thrive on a true vegetarian diet, there is concern that it is almost impossible to meet the growth needs of a young child on such a food pattern. Concern focuses on lack of calories, vitamin B_{12}, and vitamin D and the poor availability of dietary iron.

Macrobiotic diet

An extreme form of vegetarianism is the Zen macrobiotic diet, which requires its followers to proceed in seven to ten steps to reduce the number and kinds of foods in the diet until only brown rice is consumed or a balance of "strong" and "weak" foods is achieved. Followers believe there is no disease that cannot be cured by this diet. Although such a diet is lacking in vitamins, calcium, and high-quality protein, the lack of ascorbic acid seems most crucial, since scurvy has been reported among those (especially pregnant women and young children) who adhere to the regimen. The restricted fluid intake designed to spare the kidneys represents an additional hazard, since this diet is high in sodium, which increases thirst and need for fluid. The use of sea water to alleviate thirst serves only to compound the problem.

Table 21-1. Nutritive content of 28 g (1 oz) of foods featured in health-food stores

Food	kcal	Protein (g)	Calcium (mg)	Iron (mg)	Thiamin (mg)	Riboflavin (mg)	Vitamin C (mg)	Vitamin A (IU)
Brown rice	102	2.1	11	0.6	0.09	0.02	0	0
Sunflower seed	140	6.0	30	2.8	0.5	0.6	0	0
Dried apples	78	0.3	9	0.5	1.0	0.3	Trace	—*
Soya beans	130	11	73	2.7	0.4	0.2	0	30
Wheat germ	104	7.6	40.5	2.6	0.42	0.2	0	0
Pumpkin seeds	180	9.8	11	3.3	0.13	0.04	0	186
Natural seaweed	104	0.4	252	2.6	0.003	0.07	0	—
Honey	90	Trace	2	0.2	Trace	Trace	0	0
Carob flour	51	1.2	99	—	—	—	—	—
Sesame seeds	140	5.0	290	2.6	0.3	0.08	0	15
Blackstrap molasses	43	—	116	2.3	0.5	0.5	—	—
Soybean sprouts	13	1.7	13.6	0.3	0.06	—	4	22
Desiccated liver	120	28	10	6	0.2	4.4	70	0

*Indicates no data available.

Other single-food diets. Food patterns that restrict food intake to a single item or a limited number of foods are destined to lead to nutritional inadequacies. When used as the sole source of nutrients, foods such as spinach with its high oxalic acid content may prove toxic; orange juice, devoid of protein, will not support growth; milk, low in iron, leads to anemia; and nonfat milk can lead to vitamin A deficiency.

NATURAL OR HEALTH-FOOD DIETS

Frequently, but by no means always, adherents to natural or health-food diets are also vegetarians. Those who espouse this pattern of eating eat only food which they believe has been grown on soil either unfertilized or fertilized with organic fertilizers, and which has not been subjected to any treatments with chemicals either during growing or processing. Food that meets these criteria is costly to produce and sold in small retail wayside or mail-order outlets with relatively small volumes of business. As a result, the cost is high. Many unconventional food items such as papaya tea, alfalfa, sunflower seeds, carob, wheat germ, and buckwheat flour are staple items in the diet. Animal foods should come from animals fed only nonchemically treated feed who have been given no antibiotics, hormones, or other growth-stimulating chemicals. Eggs generally should be fertile and milk unpasteurized. Many of these requirements mean that shelf-life is greatly reduced with rancidity and insect infestation constant problems. The safety of food produced and processed to meet these criteria is also questionable. There is little reason to think that such food is either more or less nutritious than other food. It is invariably more expensive. For many items there is little information on nutritive content but Table 21-1 provides information for some for which data are available.

In assessing the merits of natural or organic foods, several facts should be kept in mind. First, before a plant can utilize the elements in a fertilizer they must be in an inorganic form separated from organic material. When organic fertilizer is used, separation is usually accomplished by bacteria or microorganisms in the soil. Organic fertilizers will provide only the elements excreted by the animal, which in turn got them from the food it consumed. Thus an animal grazing on crops grown on depleted soil recycles a manure that is also deficient in trace elements. Second, should it be established that organically grown food is indeed better, the country is incapable of providing the quantity of fertilizer necessary for the vast acreage devoted to food production. It is questionable if even the small amount of food now sold as organically grown could indeed have been produced this way. Since weeds and pests must be controlled by hand, labor costs are high and quality quite often low. The contention that organically grown food tastes better may often be true since it is usually sold in local markets and may be fresher than much food available through regular channels. Similarly, in many cases persons who change to eating this food frequently do feel better—the result of improved food habits rather than a function of the "organic" or "natural" foods.

When alternative food patterns or the use of specific food or nutrient supplements are the result of unscientific assessment of needs and are promoted on the basis of false promises, they are justifiably characterized as food fads and the process as food quackery.

Starvation

Many who adhere to alternative food patterns engage in intermittent fasts of one to thirty days' duration in the belief that this cleans the digestive systems, gives the organs a rest, purges the body of any toxins, and creates a heightened awareness. The adverse effects of such procedures are well documented.

FOOD FADDISM

Nutritionists are recognizing that many purveyors of food supplements with their strongly emotional appeal, exaggerated claims, and powers of persuasion, are commanding attention from a significant segment of the population and in many instances are undermining the teaching of the legitimate nutritionists. So far nutritionists have had litle success competing with the faddist because of their unwillingness to misrepresent or distort scientific knowledge in the field by making unrealistic and unsubstantiated claims. Although it is understandable how uninformed persons are easily influenced, those with ready access to sound scientific information in the field are frequently attracted to faddism also. The forces that operate to keep food faddism alive are a complex of economic, sociocultural, emotional, and educational factors.

Food fads, defined as favored or popular fashions in food consumption that prevail for a period of time, are constantly changing. Although some basic beliefs of the food faddist recur and gain wide acceptance, the form in which they are manifest changes, and they can usually be destroyed if adequately and persistently attacked. A person who follows a food fad whether good or bad becomes known as a food faddist, and the whole subject of fashions in food is known as food faddism. In many ways, food faddism can be considered a paradox of advancing medical and food technology. Only since nutritionists created an awareness of the importance of good food habits in maintaining a high level of health have the food faddists been able to capitalize on the public's concern about eating well and its reservations about the adequacy of the food supply.

Some food fads, such as coffee drinking, are merely fashions that by and large are not considered harmful. Others, such as the use of food grown only on organically fertilized soil, may lead to patterns of eating at greatly and unnecessarily inflated costs. Perhaps most serious is the possibility of nutrient deficiency and other physiological problems resulting from consumption of a limited variety of foods. In addition to attacking the problem of food fads, the nutritionist is constantly combatting food misinformation; this is often more difficult to fight, since it involves scientific half-truths, distortions, or misrepresentations of scientific information as well as outright fallacies and fancies. The food quack pretends to have information he does not possess, perpetrates his ideas or products on large groups, and is usually motivated by personal financial gain. If confronted with arguments to discredit him, he frequently abandons one food fad and espouses another with equal fervor.

EXTENT OF FOOD FADDISM AND QUACKERY

The Food and Drug Administration believes that 10 milion Americans are being bilked of at least a billion dollars each year by purveyors of nutritional supplements and special food products and vendors of books and special devices reputed to solve the nutritional ills of the country. Over 3000 stores sell only health foods, and most major chains have health-food sections. If a comparable amount were spent on improved food intakes, both the consumer and the food industry would benefit. Such a large expenditure of money on unnecessary supplementation or modification of the diet could occur only in an affluent society and reflects the health consciousness of the nation and our eternal quest for a longer and healthier life. Thus food quackery is confined to the technically developed countries that enjoy a high standard of living. It has been suggested that if the amount of money spent in the United States on dietary supplements (used by 75% of all households) is any indication of the nutritional status of the population, we must be considered the most poorly nourished nation in the world. In reality, it takes more effort to be malnourished than well nourished with prevailing food patterns in the United States. The frustration of the Food and Drug Administration in their attempts to regulate the promotion and sale of supplements of unnecessarily high and possibly unsafe potency reached its height in 1977 when a lobbying effort from health-food stores successfully supported a bill to deny the FDA this kind of regulatory power.

Jalso and co-workers, in a study of nutritional beliefs and practices in New York state, found that people who adhered to restricted food patterns had less formal education and less nutrition education than did nonfaddists and were concentrated in the older age and lower socioeconomic groups. On the basis of a personality test, they were found to have more rigid personalities than did those with more conventional food habits.

Nature of food fads

Food fads, in addition to representing mere fashions in food or the persistence of folk beliefs, follow several prescribed patterns, usually stressing a food concept rather than a nutrient concept.

Exaggeration of the virtues of a particular food. Many food fads revolve around the belief that specific foods have almost magical medicinal properties, usually in the cure of conditions over which medical science has produced no effective control or cure. Among the more common beliefs are that fruits cure cancer, carrot juice relieves leukemia, garlic reduces high blood pressure, and royal jelly extends the prime of life and leads to sexual rejuvenation. It is interesting to note that different cultures ascribe different properties to the same food. For instance, the tomato is considered poisonous by some, an aphrodisiac by others, and a cancer cure in still other situations. Similarly, the folk belief that honey and vinegar are capable of curing ailments ranging from warts to hypertension to cataracts was recently popularized in a book by a New England physician and represents a cure that has been promoted from time to time in other cultures. Of current concern is the promotion of laetrile (vitamin B_{17}), a potentially toxic cyanide compound found primarily in apricot pits, as a cancer cure.

Food quacks constantly refer to the "secret formula of a product, to which they attribute its special merits. In one case the secret formula was alfalfa, ground bones, and the germ from cereal products; in another garlic, lecithin, and wheat germ; and in still another dried nonfat mild sold at greatly inflated prices.

Omission of foods because of harmful properties. The omission of certain foods is as much a food fad as is the exaggerated use of them in the diet. The notion that any food enriched with nutrients (referred to in this context as "chemicals") is poisonous has led to the rejection of such staples in the diet as enriched white bread or milk fortified with vitamin D. The belief in a relationship between fruit and fever has led to the exclusion of fruit from the diet.

Emphasis on "natural" foods. Many natural food organizations with very impressive and authoritative-sounding names propound the basic philosophy that all mental and metabolic diseases are caused by commercially processed foods. In several cases it has been established that the president of the organization or editor of its publication is the owner of a natural-food store. Their propaganda war against all foods other than natural food is continuous and knows no bounds.

Stores devoted entirely to sale of foods reportedly grown on naturally fertilized soil do a thriving business with customers who have lost all faith in the adequacy of food bought in normal food outlets and who fear the dangers of chemicals. Such persons travel long distances and pay exorbitant prices to avoid these "contaminants" in the food supply. A list of the foods available in such outlets includes carrot juice, stone-milled buckwheat flour, unsulfured fruit, wheat germ, fertile eggs, and Irish sea moss as well as more conventional food items. All these, the customer is led to believe, have been grown on soil that has not been treated with chemical fertilizers and are sold in their natural, unprocessed form. The use of such terms as "counterfeited," "prefabricated," "worthless," "natural scandal," and "devitalized" to describe processed foods and "natural" and "vital" for unprocessed foods is described to heighten the effect.

A survey of prices at a health-food store revealed that unsulfured raisins cost six times the price of regular raisins; unenriched, unbleached flour four times as much as enriched all-purpose flour; canned tomatoes from "untreated" tomatoes five times as much as regular canned tomatoes; organic chicken three times as much as regular chickens; and apple butter from unsprayed apples ten times the cost of conventional apple butter. Food bills at such stores average from 50% to 80% above normal. The inflated prices may be a function of a low volume of business or excessive profits. They may also reflect the fact that if crops are indeed grown without the benefit of chemical fertilizers, herbicides, and pesticides, the production will be low and the per unit price high.

Natural foods are for the most part wholesome foods that are rich in nutrients and flavor and certainly should never be condemned from a nutritional standpoint, but neither are they *essential* for health. Most processed foods have not been shown to be inferior and should not be excluded.

Special devices. Many entrepreneurs also direct their attention to the types of equipment in which or on which food is prepared. Great merit has been attributed to devices for grating or shredding vegetables, to blenders often selling at twice the price of conventional blenders, or to cooking utensils (available only in large sets) that are said to be capable of conserving nutrients.

Avoidance of chemicals in food. The Delaney Clause, an amendment to the Food, Drug, and Cosmetic Act, which requires the Food and Drug Administration to ban the use of any substance in food for which there is any evidence from animal or human studies of possible carcinogenicity at any level, has resulted in a ban on items such as cyclamates and several coloring materials that had previously been considered safe. This has resulted in a general distrust of any additives in foods and a complete disregard of their essential role in maintaining the food supply. The fear is further compounded by the fact that many have awesome and mysterious names such as calcium silicate, butylated hydroxy toluene, and monosterate. These names are meaningless to most consumers but do imply something bad.

The Food and Drug Administration is constantly seeking the help of the scientific community in assessing the safety of any chemicals appearing intentionally or incidentally in the food supply. But without those that serve as preservatives, such as salt and proprionate, or nitrites that prevent botulism, or colorings that give foods an acceptable appearance, such as carotene used in butter, the food supply would be costly, much less safe, and unacceptable in color, flavor, and texture.

Although there is indeed a need to be assured of the safety of any additives, it is unrealistic to promote a total ban on their use. Instead there needs to be a constant monitoring of their safety both individually and in conjunction with other additives. Many "additives" such as nitrites used in curing meats are also formed in the body through conversion by bacteria in the digestive tract of naturally occurring nitrates found in vegetables such as beets, celery, carrots, and spinach. Either of these can react with amines in the intestinal tract to form nitrosamines, which are known carcinogens. Antioxidants may be naturally occurring substances such as vitamin E or added chemicals used to prevent rancidity and the formation of carcinogenic substances from unsaturated fats. Other additives serve to inhibit mold and bacterial growth, to increase shelf life, enhance flavor, improve color, etc. Although they have become an integral part of our food processing system, additives must be constantly evaluated. It would, however, be catastrophic to the whole food delivery system if there was widespread and indiscriminate rejection of all additives.

Dangers of food zealotry

The major concern of the government and other agencies involved in protecting the consumer against the fraudulent claims and ineffectual products of the food quack stems not only from a fear that the product he sells is in itself harmful but also from a concern over the economic and ethical aspects of his operation. There is concern that millions of people are spending money for products that cannot possibly do what they are reported to do and, more specifically, that among the victims are many who can ill afford to divert their food money to nutritional supplements or overrated food products or devices. Older individuals in whom the fear of becoming ill or dependent is ever present are particularly susceptible. In addition to the loss of money on a product that is worthless for the purpose for which is was bought, there is concern that a person in need of medical treatment will delay in seeking competent medical advice until the damage is irreparable.

Mode of operation of the quack

The food quack capitalizes on the desire for information and creates a market for his product or ideas through a variety of highly emotional appeals. He uses the overriding fear of many that they will become incapacitated through illness. For others he provides a crutch for their organic and psychic ailments. Quacks undermine the public's faith in the adequacy of the nation's food supply to provide them with the essentials for good health. Not only do they suggest that available foods may be incapable of providing the essentials, but also they claim that certain products used to increase food production, such as chemical fertilizers, herbicides, pesticides, and the chemicals used in processing, are undermining health and leading to all kinds of dire consequences. Competent scientists recognize that there can be hazards from the indiscriminate use of these substances and urge that their use be kept under surveillance so that we may have the benefits without the hazards.

By his contentions that all disease is caused by faulty diet, that the population suffers from widespread malnutrition, that food-processing destroys the nutritive value of foods, and that soil depletion is an underlying cause of faulty diets, the quack is able to create such a fear of sickness in his victim that he has little trouble selling his panacea. The imaginary illnesses he conjures up are often created by the use of vague, meaningless terms such as "roundness of corpuscles," "tired blood," and "vitagenic," all of which have scientific overtones to the gullible.

Food quacks frequently pose as members of legitimate-sounding professional organizations. It is virtually impossible for a lay person to recognize the names of the official representatives of the profession, let alone to discriminate them from others with equally impressive names. To expect the general public to recognize that the American Institute of Nutrition, the organization of recognized nutrition scientists, is different from the American Academy of Applied Nutrition or the American Nutrition Society, both of which are nonscientific organizations, is to assume a level of interest and available information that does not exist. In at least one case the telephone number listed on the letterhead of one of these pseudoscientific societies is the number of a health-food store. Many of these organizations publish their own monthly journal with "scientific" articles by their own members, most of which support the use of the type of product sold in their outlets or advertised as available by mail in their catalogue. Even reputable scientific groups have been temporarily deceived into accepting them as scientific.

Besides mentioning specific organizations, quacks also promote themselves by the use of self-conferred titles such as "world-renowned nutritionists," "dietitian," "international authority," and other convincing accolades. Indeed, several individuals who have earned degrees that qualify them to use the title of doctor have been diverted into the lucrative food faddism business. By quoting scientific data out of context or in an incomplete form or by applying findings of animal studies to humans, they are able to create an illusion of scientific know-how.

The faddist is quick to capitalize on new developments in science by taking an observation from scientific literature and by clever and timely merchandising parlaying it into a profit. The promoters of safflower oil as an aid to reducing blood cholesterol levels were able for a short time to convince the public to buy it at the drugstore in 1100 mg capsules at 6 cents each or approximately $25 per 0.5 liter when the same product was available in the grocery store at 80 cents per 0.5 liter. Similarly, persons with the unfounded belief that gelatin will improve the condition of their fingernails eagerly pay $2 per ounce for gelatin in capsule form that the grocer offers at 10 cents for the same amount. The ingredients in one widely distributed pill selling for 12 cents each were found to be the same as those in half a cent's worth of dried nonfat milk solids.

The discovery of vitamin K, naturally present in alfalfa, as necessary for blood coagulation gave food supplement promoters another product in which the margin of profit was very high. Vitamin E, for which a human deficiency has seldom been demonstrated, is a favorite promotion of the quack, who attributes to humans all the most severe deficiency symptoms ever observed in animals.

Characteristics of a quack

One can be suspicious of food quackery under any of the following conditions:

1. The promoter claims that his food has miraculous powers, usually in the cure of conditions that are still baffling medical science, such as arthritis, leukemia, and arteriosclerosis. He usually claims to have information not available through regular medical channels.

2. He claims that he is being persecuted by medical "trusts and cartels" whose livelihood is threatened by him and his product.

3. He maintains that the soil is depleted and is no longer capable of producing a food supply sufficient to meet the nutritional needs of the population. His only solutions to this are the use of food supplements or the exclusive use of the nutritious foods grown in soil fertilized with organic fertilizers.

4. He maintains that practically everyone is suffering from some degree of malnutrition that cannot possibly be corrected by foods readily available. He attributes this to the following dietary habits:

a. Use of pasteurized rather than raw milk
b. Use of nonfertile rather than fertile eggs
c. Ingestion of mixed meals of a variety of foods
d. Use of canned fruits and vegetables
e. Use of white flour rather than freshly milled whole grains or sprouted grains
f. Use of refined sugars
g. Use of plant foods of all types grown on impoverished soils
h. Use of chemically pure or synthetic vitamins
i. Use of chemically contaminated foodstuffs resulting from pesticides, etc. (addition of fluorine to water supplies is opposed)

Methods of merchandising

Food quacks can be found in almost any aspect of the food-marketing business, but they have tended to rely on the less conventional merchandising procedures. High-pressure advertising in their own publications, Sunday supplements, and some magazines in which an introductory offer with refund privileges for dissatisfied customers is offered are common. They are sufficiently astute psychologists to realize that very few disillusioned buyers are going to bother to seek a refund.

Door-to-door salesmen or "doorbell doctors" are successful in convincing consumers that the only way they can protect their own health and their families' health is through the use of whatever product he is promoting, be it special saucepans, a recipe book, vitamins, food supplements, or a potential cure for asthma. Usually these products are available at a "special low price" for quantity purchases on a cash basis. In many cases victims realize too late that to supposedly safeguard the health of their families, they have committed an unreasonable part of the family income. In some door-to-door selling situations the parent company protects itself against responsibility for the claims of its salesmen, making it difficult to take effective legal action to stop the sales. Some states have introduced legislation that allows a person who has been a victim of high-pressure sales techniques to cancel any contract within a specified time period (usually one to three days).

Public lectures, often "by invitation only," are used to lure the public. After an initial

SOYBEAN LECITHIN
Here is natural, organic soy lecithin. Rich in natural choline and inositol. Available in granules for use with water, juice or sprinkled on cereals, salads, etc., and in convenient easy to use capsule form.
CAPSULES—Fortified with Vitamin D
100—1.00 500—4.50 1000—6.90
Postage Paid*
SEA-PRO CERTIFIED* PROTEIN
*Clean Protein from Gardens-of-Sea!
ROYAL JELLY
50 MG. CAPSULES
Here is the sensational but controversial Royal Jelly, offered as a new food for human consumption in this convenient, easy to take form.
DOLO-ZYME tablets
Original Dolomite plus Sturdegest!
IRISH SEA MOSS
A rich bounty from the sea in its natural unadulterated form.
Unbleached 12 oz.—50c
Add Postage—See Back Page
CITRÒN-X TABLETS
LEMON BIOFLAVONOIDS
Research workers have been very hopeful regarding the value of some of the ingredients contained in this exciting formula as a dietary supplement.
Three Tablets Contain:
Vitamin C (From Rose Hips Extract) ....100 mg.
Lemon Bioflavonoid Complex ....100 mg.
Rutin (From Buckwheat) .... 30 mg.
Hesperidin Complex .... 30 mg.
VEGETABLE CONCENTRATES
ORGANICALLY GROWN
Here you can get the added nutritional benefits of these natural vegetables in handy, convenient tablets at a low, economical price. Add postage on items below. Shipping weight 500 tablets 1 lb., 1000 tablets 2 lbs.
CABBAGE TABLETS 500—1.95 — 1000—3.70
ALFALFA TABLETS 500—1.50 — 1000—2.15
CELERY TABLETS 500—1.90 — 1000—3.25
DULSE TABLETS 500—2.25 — 1000—3.50
RICE POLISH TABLETS 500—1.70 — 1000—2.60
WATERCRESS TABLETS 500—2.80 — 1000—4.90
OKRA TABLETS 500—1.95 — 1000—3.70
11 VEGETABLE TABLETS 500—2.80 — 1000—4.90
Containing Beets, Carrots, Celery, Endive, Kale, Lettuce, Alfalfa, Parsley, Spinach, Tomato, Kelp and excipients.
GARLIC PARSLEY
TABLETS
Millions of these Garlic Parsley tablets have been sold to satisfied, happy users. Thousands can't be wrong. If
C-RUTIN
Three tablets contain 100 mg. of Vitamin C derived from Rose Hips and 50 mg. Rutin derived from Buckwheat which contains subnutritional amounts of factors called by some investigators Vitamin P. Plus excipients.
Vegetable Broth
NATURAL BRAND
A combination of natural dehydrated vegetables for making a tantalizing delicious vegetable broth.
8-oz.—1.00 1-lb.—1.65
Add Postage—See Back Page
Alfalfa Seeds
Here are finest quality Alfalfa Seeds money can buy. Carefully selected to meet Natural Sales Company's high quality standards.
1-lb.—70c 5-lbs.—3.25
Add Postage—See Back Page
SUNFLOWER SEEDS
HULLED — ORGANICALLY GROWN
If you have not already enjoyed this wonderful food, order today. Rich in bone forming Calcium. Excellent source of B-1 and Niacin. High in protein. Delicious as a cereal or added to other foods.
1-lb.—1.10 — 5-lbs.—5.25
Add Postage—See Back Page
'FROM-THE-SEA' No. A-134
KELP·ALL
Derived entirely from natural rich Pacific Kelp. Provides a fine all natural source of Iodine and minerals in trace amounts to supplement daily diet. Small tabs, easy-to-take. Note extra special buy!
AMO TABS
AMINO ACID TABLETS
A source of essential Amino Acids obtained from the enzymatic predigested protein of yeast.
Unsaturated Fatty Acids
(VITAMIN F)
Now Natural Sales Company's low cost purchase plan makes it possible for you to obtain these valuable Natural, Unrefined Protective Food Oils at a sensible price.
Each capsule contains 168 mg. of Unsaturated Fatty Acids (Vitamin F) from Linseed Oil. Principally Lenoleic and Linolenic Acids.
CAROB POWDER
An alkaline food to substitute for cocoa. High in natural sugar. Ideal for chocolate-like drinks, pies, cakes and other confections.
PAPAYA B-PAPS
Contains Papaya, Papain and Natural Vitamin B-1, Vitamin B-2 and Niacin. An aid in the digestion of protein.
ROSE HIPS
Here is the same Rose Hips you have read and heard so much about. An excellent natural source of Vitamin C. Specially selected and picked for Natural Sales Co. these Rose Hips are sun-dried and cleaned without artificial processing. Once you try Natural brand Rose Hips you'll prefer them always, just as many thousands of others do.
SUPREME
ROSE HIPS REGULAR
TEA
POWDER
MORVITE
Fabulous New Food Supplement. 20 Food Factor Supplying 34 Natural Vitamins and Minerals.
DESICCATED LIVER
This is pure — very highest quality, defatted Liver.
Dried at low heat to retain all the beneficial factors. Finest
Sensational New Nutritional Development
MIRACLE WAFERS
Delicious Candy-Like Wafer, chuck full of Delightful Ingredients:
YOGHURT LICORICE
WHEY MOLASSES
BANANA FLAKES ROYAL JELLY
WHEY
Superior quality. Rich in milk minerals and lactose — the intestinal floral sugar that combats putrefaction and excess protein decomposition.
NATURAL-ORGANIC
PAPAYA ENZYME
ACIDOPHILUS PLUS
Exclusive With Natural Sales!

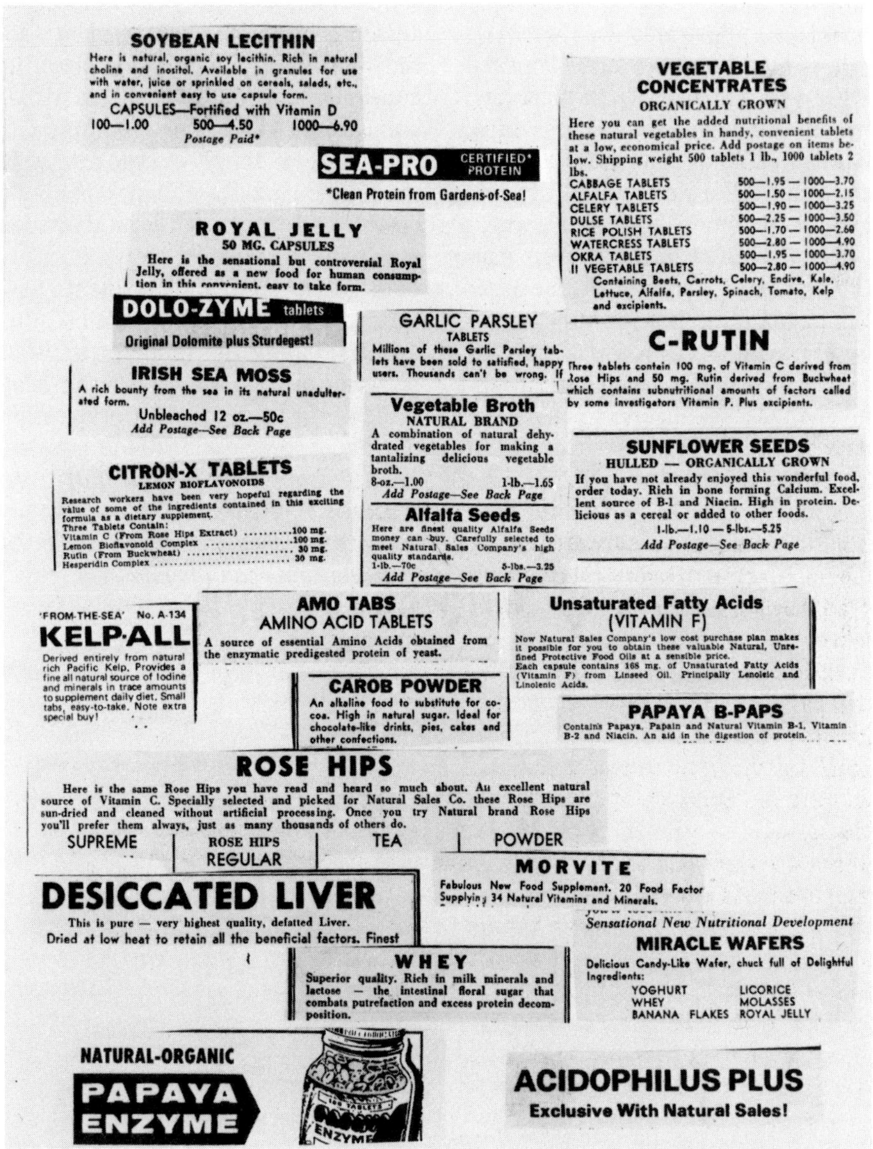

Fig. 21-1. A composite of items offered for sale in the catalogue of a health-food store.

period in which some fairly plausible nutritional information is given, the lecturer launches into a train of thought designed to lead the audience to only one conclusion—that their only hope of salvation is to rely on the product for which he will be glad to take orders. Radio and television time are also purchased and used in much the same way.

Health-food stores thrive in the densely populated areas of large cities, especially when they offer food grown on organically fertilized soil. As illustrated in Fig. 21-1, their inventory includes several hundred items, such as carrot powder, papaya tablets, alfalfa and alfalfa concentrates, rose hips, miracle wafers, amino acid tablets, royal jelly, millet, special-formula tablets of natural vitamins and minerals, bone meal, wheat germ, brewer's yeast, dessicated liver, fish-liver oil, kelp, parsley, and iron. At the other end of the merchandising continuum are the health-food farms located in a pastoral setting uncontaminated by herbicides, pesticides, and chemical fertilizers; to these the devotee may travel for the privilege of paying two to three times regular grocery prices for the same products. Practically all these outlets also offer mail-order service. While many condemn the use of chemicals to nourish plants, they promote a wide range of pills (chemicals) to nourish humans.

The labeling on a product may also purposefully be misleading. For instance, 10 mg capsules of gelatin bore a listing of the percentage of the total protein represented by seventeen different amino acids, the names of which would give the average consumer the impression that the product was highly nutritious. The fact that the whole capsule provided about 0.0014% of the day's protein requirement was not mentioned.

Books on nutrition have been a source of much misinformation and half-truths for the consumer and a source of tremendous income for the successful writer, especially one who can legitimately use the title M.D. Since the food quack is not limited in his claims by established findings, he is able to make a much stronger and more emotional appeal than is the legitimate scientist, who often tends to be overly cautious in his attempts to avoid violating the limits of knowledge. A perusal of the following titles of chapters in some of the more popular publications gives the reader some notion of the approach used: *"Are poisons making you old?" "Help for prostates," "Learn to live without an ulcer," "Skin problems are more than skin deep,"* and *"Arthritis can often be relieved!"* Others

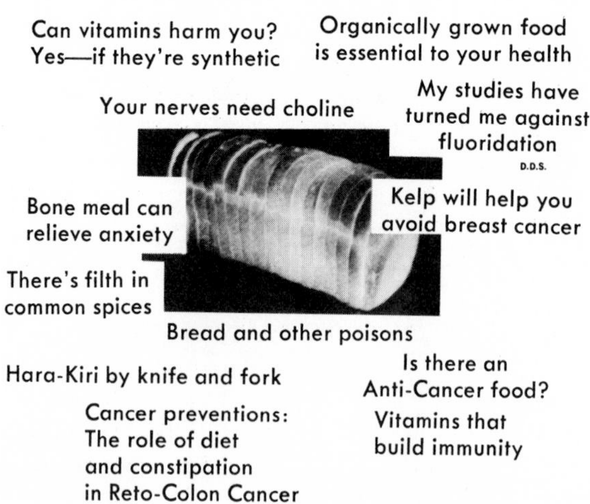

Fig. 21-2. Samples of titles of articles in publications of health-food stores or organizations.

are shown in Fig. 21-2. Again, much of the information is based on sound basic principles of nutrition, but in their zeal to sell books the authors frequently distort facts to achieve a strong emotional appeal. The sale of half a million copies of a book can earn the author a quarter of a million dollars and the publisher half a million, and so the motivation to appeal to a wide audience is great. By the time the fraudulent nature of the contents is exposed the book has earned the author a sizable royalty and he is not upset by adverse publicity. In fact, he often republishes the book under a new title for new profits.

Special equipment for food preparation has been another lucrative approach of the food quack. This is often demonstrated at fairs, summer resorts, arcades, department stores, or invitational parties in private homes. The promoter relies heavily on impulse buying. He attributes a wide range of merits to the equipment, such as increasing the consumption of fruits and vegetables, eliminating poisons from foods, conserving vitamins, or incorporating oxygen in food.

Types of products

"Shotgun" formula. Products characterized by "shotgun" formulas may list as many as fifty different nutrients on the label and are designed to impress the gullible consumer who is awed by the range of items included. Some of these are nutrients for which recommended daily allowances have been established; others are those known to be essential but for which no requirements have been established; and still others are harmless but of no known nutritional significance. Of those known to be required, some will be present at many times the recommended level, whereas others will be present in insignificant amounts. For instance, one product in the recommended daily dose contains 400% of the U.S. RDA of vitamins A, D, C, B_1, and B_2 and about 2% of the daily requirement of potassium. This same product lists 10 mg of unsaturated fatty acids, which represents about 0.1% of the 1% of the calories from linoleic acid recommended in the adult diet. The mixture is obviously irrational from a nutritional and physiological point of view but completely rational from the point of view of the uninformed consumer. Recent legislation requiring that information be given in relation to requirements should alleviate this problem.

"Loaded" formula. The term *"loaded" formula* is applied to the high-potency product that competes by providing more of a nutrient than its competitor. Thus consumers find a spiraling in trade competition, with one company adding more of a nutrient for a very insignificant difference in price than does his competitor. The average consumer does not realize that he merely excretes the excess amounts of water-soluble vitamins and may develop toxic reactions from excessive levels of the fat-soluble vitamins.

The Food and Drug Administration attempted in 1973 to enact legislation to limit the number of nutrients that could be used in dietary supplements to those for which need in the American population has been demonstrated. In addition, it tried to establish the upper limits of nutrient content at 150% of the RDA to assure an effective but not toxic dose of any nutrient.

Unfortunately a powerful lobby headed by the National Health Federation succeeded in attaching an amendment to the Heart and Lung Bill that prohibited the FDA from limiting the potency, number, combinations, or variety of any synthetic or natural vitamin, mineral, or other nutritional substance or ingredient of any nutritional supplement unless the amount recommended is found to be injurious to health. After passage Congress modified the bill to allow the FDA to limit the amount in nutrient supplements for children under 12 and for pregnant and lactating women to include from 50% to 150% of the U.S. RDA and to require that multinutrient supplements contain all of a list of nutrients. These standards, which went into effect January, 1978, are reproduced in Table 10-3. There is, however, no control over the number or amount of nutrients in supplements for adults. Foods or supplements for children and pregnant and lactating women containing over 150% of the U.S. RDA are considered drugs and available only on prescription.

Natural organic products. Natural organic foods are reportedly grown in organically fertilized soil without the addition of insecticides and herbicides or chemical fertilizers.

Miracle products. Miracle products include such products as garlic pills to relieve high blood pressure, honey and vinegar for arthritis, wheat germ for sterility, and lecithin for coronary disease.

Unnecessary supplements. The sale of protein supplements to the American population may well be questioned, especially at suggested prices. One firm created doubts about the adequacy of protein in the American diet to soften the market for its protein pills, each of which contained 728 mg of protein. To obtain the equivalent of the 20 g of protein in one serving of meat it would require 28 pills at a cost of 25 cents of one type of supplement and 100 pills for $1.00 of another. More recently, liquid protein diets made from hydrolyzed collagen provide protein at a cost of 30 cents per 20 g portion compared to 12 to 69 cents from conventional food sources that are more palatable and provide other nutrients. Reports of deaths following the use of these products has resulted in label warnings that they can be dangerous. Powdered protein supplements composed primarily of casein or soy protein are not hazardous but are equally unnecessary.

Useless products. Seawater, which enterprising persons living in coastal areas were shipping all over the country, would be placed in the category of useless products. When the cost of shipping used up some of the profit, they reverted to dehydrated seawater to further enhance their earnings! Many products that may be beneficial in significant amounts are useless at the levels at which they are sold.

Megavitamin therapy. Passage of the Proxmire Amendment limiting the power of the FDA to regulate the potency of nutrient supplements for adults has encouraged the use of megavitamin therapy, in which massive doses of vitamins and excessively high intakes of minerals are promoted to cure a whole range of human illnesses. These range from the common cold to senility and schizophrenia to sexual impotence. Since vitamins act primarily as coenzymes in the release of energy or in the synthesis or degradation of body compounds, the amount needed is limited by the extent to which these reactions are taking place. Any excess must either be stored, excreted, or used for some nonvitamin function. In the latter case it must be considered a drug rather than a nutrient once the needs for growth and the synthesis of essential body compounds has been met; minerals are needed in even smaller amounts to maintain body stores and to catalyze metabolic reactions. In this case excesses may lead to serious internal imbalances and reduced rather than improved functioning.

Although unfounded claims for the merits of a product cannot be made at the point of purchase, either on the label or within 9 m of the product, there is no restriction on articles in the popular press and trade magazines or the content of radio and television talk shows where most claims of the reported value of megadoses of nutrients are made. In addition, some persons in health professions support the use of megavitamin or orthomolecular therapy in the treatment of disease. Although in most cases ineffective, if done under supervision, such therapy is much less dangerous than widespread self-medication with massive doses of nutrients. It is just as likely, however, to produce a whole range of debilitating side effects. The possibilities of even more harmful interacting effects when many nutrients are taken simultaneously has not been investigated at all.

COMBATTING MISINFORMATION AND FOOD FADDISTS

Efforts to protect the public against unscrupulous purveyors of misinformation and nutritional supplements in the name of nutritional science and to prevent exaggerated claims of the efficiency of food products are the concern of several government and community agencies.

Better Business Bureaus in many communities attempt to police, restrict, or regulate the activities of peddlers of health foods, special cooking devices, or nutrition supplements within their regions. They also require the registration of all persons giving public lectures, and on the basis of information available from one community to another are able to deny lecture privileges to those with a reputation for abusing these privileges. They describe their efforts to combat food misinformation as preventative, corrective, and educational.

The Food and Drug Administration (FDA) is constantly concerned with protecting the consumer against mislabelling and harmful, contaminated, and worthless products but is faced with an overwhelming job, considering the resources available. When personnel and funds are limited, it is frequently necessary to restrict its activities to those aspects that present immediate dangers to the population. It takes time to prove that labelling is misleading or that the product is injurious to health. After the FDA believes it has sufficient evidence to press charges, court proceedings are extremely slow and costly to both parties. In some instances by the time enforcement agencies are prepared to take action, the defendant has already realized sufficient profit that he does not contest the action. Regulations enacted in 1963, which require that a company present evidence that the product it proposes to sell is safe for human consumption, have done much to lighten the load of this agency, which previously had to prove that a product was harmful before its sale could be restricted. A reluctance on the part of the public to initiate charges against a firm by which they have been victimized also hampers the operation of enforcement agencies. To admit that one has been "taken" is to admit a human frailty that many persons prefer not to publicize.

The FDA is responsible for formulating and enforcing regulations regarding the processing and sale of food products and dietary supplements. On their recommendation the amount of folic acid that can be included in nutritional supplements was restricted to 0.1 mg in a daily dose; the addition of vitamin D was limited to milk and infant formula at a level to provide no more than 400 IU in the recommended daily dose, and the use of the term *low-calorie* is allowed only for foods providing less than 40% of the energy normally expected. The FDA has legislated that the quantities of vitamins and minerals in nutritional supplements for children and pregnant and lactating women be limited to amounts that are nutritionally useful and that only nutrients for which a deficiency is likely to occur be allowed.

The American Medical Association has recognized the threat that quackery and faddism poses for the health of the nation and has launched a counterattack in the form of an exposè of the tactics and claims of the quack and faddist. It has developed films for use in nutrition education programs with supporting literature; it prepares periodic statements of its stand on prevailing practices and products; and it publishes a popular magazine that frequently includes articles pertaining to the use of nutritional supplements and special health foods or devices. In spite of the efforts of this professional group to promote sound information, occasionally one of its own members, under the protection and aura associated with his degree, publishes a book on nutrition-related topics about which he is not adequately informed or qualified to speak. The American Medical Association also maintains a Bureau of Investigation that answers inquiries about specific persons or products and promotes an active campaign against quackery.

Other professional groups such as the American Public Health Association, The Nutrition Consortium, The American Dietetic Association, The Institute of Food Technology, and the American Home Economics Association all have active programs designed to combat food faddism and misinformation and are constantly attempting to inform the public in an effort to help them separate fiction from fact. The Society for Nutrition Education focusses its efforts on educating the public from elementary schoolchildren to adult groups on the principles of nutrition so that they function as informed decision makers on nutrition issues.

The Federal Trade Commission is involved in the fight against food quackery in its responsibility to protect the American public against false and misleading advertising. Cases involving charges of false advertising may take several years to try and will involve hundreds of hours of testimony. Some of its cases have concerned the superiority of vitamins from natural sources over synthetic vitamins, the need for delivery of garden-fresh vitamins, the need for time-released vitamin-mineral capsules, and claims that juices prepared in special blenders have miraculous curative powers.

Since 1975 it has been developing regulations pertaining to nutrition information in advertising. These regulations have involved defining terms such as nutritious, nourishing, and rich or excellent sources of nutrients and establishing the conditions under which foods can be compared on the basis of their nutrient content.

The U.S. Postal Service, which regulates the use of the mails to defraud, also performs a watchdog function to protect the public against nutritional hoaxes.

On the theory that an informed public is a less gullible public, nutrition education should be one of the most effective ways of combatting food fads and quackery, especially with the potential of all the media available to disseminate sound information. When even the well-educated and scientifically enlightened are prey to the wiles of the faddist and the quack, one wonders what level of education is necessary to protect consumers from becoming victims of the promoter who claims his product will cure everything from corns to sterility to leukemia. To combat faddism, it is necessary to recognize the emotional and psychological influences that perpetuate it. Thus an educational campaign aimed at combatting it must be multifaceted, attacking as many of the forces that support it as possible.

Only through a constant flow of legitimate nutrition information can progress be made in combatting the high-pressure salesmanship of the quack. It appears that for each person involved in merchandising sound nutritional information, several hundred are merchandising their own pet schemes. Several nutritionists who write regular syndicated columns for daily or weekly newspapers utilize this opportunity to fight faddism and to help enlighten the public. Dietitians in some larger cities operate a service known as Dial-a-titian in which persons with questions related to nutrition may call the service and have their query referred to the person most qualified to answer it. Nutrition information and resource centers are being established in various cities.

The difficulties in combatting misinformation in the press are much more formidable than those on labels or advertisements for products.

The final chapter in the saga of food faddism is far from written. One can only hope that it can be brought under reasonable control before the health of too many persons is jeopardized by the use of products promoted through unsubstantiated claims. On the other hand, one should not overlook the fact that the faddists have done much to dramatize the importance of nutrition and have created a nutrition consciousness in a larger segment of the population. The challenge to nutritionists is to tap this interest and divert the attention of the concerned to more reasonable and appropriate solutions.

BIBLIOGRAPHY

Academy of Pediatrics: Nutritional aspects of vegetarianism, health foods and fad diets, Pediatrics **59:**460, 1970.

Academy of Pediatrics: Megavitamin therapy for childhood psychoses and learning disabilities, Pediatrics **58:**910, 1976.

Anderson, M. A., and Standal, B. R.: Nutritional knowledge of health food users on Oahu, Hawaii, J. Am. Diet. Assoc. **67:**116, 1975.

Barrett, S., and Knight, G.: The health robbers—how to protect your money and your life, Philadelphia, 1976, George F. Stickley Co.

Beal, V. A.: Food faddism and organic and natural foods, paper presented at National Dairy Council Food Writers' Conference, Newport, R.I., May, 1972.

Beeuwkes, A. M.: Food faddism and consumer, Fed. Proc. **13:**785, 1954.

Bernard, V. W.: Why people become the victims of medical quackery, Am. J. Public Health **55:**1142, 1965.

Brown, P. T., and Bergan, J. G.: The dietary status of "new" vegetarians, J. Am. Diet. Assoc. **67:**455, 1975.

Bruch, H.: The allure of food cults and nutrition quackery, J. Am. Diet. Assoc. **57:**316, 1970.

Calvert, G. P., and Calvert, S. W.: Intellectual convictions of "health" food consumers, J. Nutr. Ed. **7:**95, 1975.

Coon, J. M.: Natural toxicants in foods, J. Am. Diet. Assoc. **67:**213, 1975.

Council on Foods and Nutrition: Iron in enriched white flour, farina, bread, buns, and rolls, J.A.M.A. **220:**855, 1972.

Council on Foods and Nutrition: Problems of antibiotics in food, J.A.M.A. **170:**139, 1959.

Council on Foods and Nutrition: Safe use of chemicals in food, J.A.M.A. **178:**749, 1961.

Deutsch, R.: Nuts among the berries, New York, 1972, Ballantine Books, Inc.

Deutsch, R.: The new nuts among the berries, New York, 1977, Ballantine Books, Inc.

Dwyer, J. T., Mayer, D., Dowd, K., Kandel, R. F., and Mayer, J.: The new vegetarians: the natural high? J. Am. Diet. Assoc. **65:**529, 1974.

Elwood, P. C.: The enrichment debate, Nutr. Today, **12:**18, 1977.

Erhard, D.: Nutrition education for the "now" generation, J. Nutr. Ed. **2:**135, 1971.

Food facts talk back, Chicago, 1967, The American Dietetic Association.

Frankle, R. T., and Heussenstamm, F. K.: Food zealotry and youth: new dilemmas for professionals, Am. J. Public Health **64:**11, 1974.

Frankle, R. T., McGregor, B., Wylie, J., and McCann, M. B.: Nutrition and life style, J. Am. Diet. Assoc. **63:**269, 1973.

Graham, D. M., and Hertzler, A. A.: Why enrich or fortify foods? J. Nutr. Ed. **9:**166, 1977.

Henderson, L. M.: Nutritional problems growing out of new patterns of food consumption, Am. J. Public Health **62:**1194, 1972.

Henderson, L. M.: Programs to combat nutritional quackery, J. Am. Diet. Assoc. **64:**372, 1974.

Hertzler, A. A., and Owen, C.: Sociologic study of food habits—a review. I. Diversity in diet and scalogram analysis, J. Am. Diet. Assoc. **69:**377, 1976.

Hertzler, A. A., and Owen, C.: Sociologic study of food habits—a review II. Differentiation accessibility and solidarity, J. Am. Diet. Assoc. **69:**381, 1976.

Institute of Food Technology: Sulfites as food additives, Nutr. Rev. **34:**58, 1976.

Jalso, S. B., Burns, M. M., and Rivers, J. M.: Nutritional beliefs and practices, J. Am. Diet. Assoc. **47:**263, 1965.

Jukes, T. H.: Current concepts in nutrition: food additives, N. Engl. J. Med. **297:**427, 1977.

Layrisse, M.: Martinez-Torres, C., and Renzi, M.: Sugar as a vehicle for iron fortification: further studies, Am. J. Clin. Nutr. **29:**274, 1976.

Larrick, G. P.: The nutritive adequacy of our food supply, J. Am. Diet. Assoc. **39:**117, 1961.

Let's talk about food, Chicago, 1974, American Medical Association.

McBean, L. D., and Speckman, E. W.: Food faddism: a challenge to nutritionists and dietitians, Am. J. Clin. Nutr. **27:**1071, 1974.

Majumder, S. K.: Vegetarianism: fad, faith or fact, Am. Sci. **60:**175, 1972.

Mills, E. R.: Psychosocial aspects of food habits, J. Nutr. Ed. **9:**67, 1977.

Milstead, K. L.: Science works through law to protect consumers, J. Am. Diet. Assoc. **48:**187, 1966.

Olson, R. E.: Food faddism—why? Nutr. Rev. **16:**97, 1958.

Register, U. D., and Sonnenberg, L. M.: The vegetarian diet—scientific and practical considerations, J. Am. Diet. Assoc. **63:**253, 1973.

Roe, D. A.: Nutrient toxicity with excessive intake, New York J. Med. **66:**1233, 1966.

Rynearson, E. H.: Americans love hogwash, Nutr. Rev. **32** (suppl. 1), 1974.

The role of nutrition education in combatting food fads, New York, 1959, The Nutrition Foundation.

Schafer, R., and Yetley, E. A.: Social psychology of food faddism: speculations on health food behavior, J. Am. Diet. Assoc. **66:**129, 1975.

Schwartz, L.: Groups ask USDA to ban nitrites, nitrates in meat, Supermarket News, Nov. 21, 1977.

Sherlock, P., and Rothschild, E. O.: Scurvy produced by a Zen macrobiotic diet, J.A.M.A. **199:**794, 1967.

Sims, L. S.: Communication characteristics of recommended and nonrecommended nutrition books, Home Econ. Res. J. **6:**2, 1977.

Stare, F. J.: Your food and your health, Garden City, N.Y., 1969, Doubleday & Co., Inc.

Strong, F. M.: Toxicants occurring naturally in foods, Nutr. Rev. **32:**225, 1974.

Subcommittee on Food Technology: Technology of fortification of foods, proceedings of a workshop, Washington, D.C., 1975, National Academy of Sciences.

Todhunter, E. N.: Food habits: food faddism and nutrition, World Rev. Nutr. Diet. **16:**287, 1973.

Wagner, M.: The irony of affluence, J. Am. Diet. Assoc. **57:**311, 1970.

Walker, A. R. P.: Problems in nutritional supplementation and enrichment, Am. J. Clin. Nutr. **12:**157, 1963.

Williams, R. J.: Nutrition in a nutshell, Garden City, N.Y., 1962, Doubleday & Co., Inc.

Wolff, R. J.: Who eats for health? Am. J. Clin. Nutr. **26:**438, 1973.

22

Nutrition—a national and an international concern

Nutritional inadequacies may result from either a lack of food or a failure to select those foods which result in a nutritionally balanced diet. Nutritional scientists have sought the help of politicians, sociologists, agriculturalists, geneticists, psychologists, economists, and planners in attempts to minimize the possibility of nutritional deficits due to either a failure to produce enough food or a lack of an adequate system to distribute it.

Interest in nutrition as a national and an international concern has come into focus only in the last twenty-five years. At the international level, concern stems from an analysis of the increase in world population relative to the capacity of the world to provide adequate amounts of food for an expanding population. Since 60% of the current population and 70% of its children are judged to be undernourished, the problem is not only one of improving the level of nutrition but also of providing this more desirable level for a large population increase. The magnitude of the problem became evident with the recognition in 1950 that a protein deficiency resulted in kwashiorkor, a major cause of infant mortality in developing countries. Other effects include permanently retarded physical growth, increased susceptibility to infection, and, if it occurs early enough in life, depressed development of the central nervous system. High-quality protein is an expensive nutrient in terms of the productivity of the land, since an acre will yield twenty-five times as much protein from soybeans and ten times as much from rice as from beef. Under conditions of high land pressures it is evident that other protein sources such as vegetable protein mixtures and legumes rather than animal proteins must be developed and exploited to narrow the protein gap.

More recently those concerned with world food problems have been focussing their attention on increasing the energy value of the food supply on the theory that if calories are adequate even a limited amount of protein can be used for its primary purpose of building and repairing tissues. This shift is reflected in the use of the term energy protein deficit (EPD) to replace the term protein calorie malnutrition (PCM) to describe the major nutritional problem facing the developing countries.

Recognition of malnutrition as a national concern for developed countries is an even more recent phenomenon. In the United States the publication *Hunger USA* by the Citizens Board of Inquiry into Hunger and Malnutrition in 1968 and the CBS television program *Hunger in America,* both charging that hunger in the midst of plenty was a national disgrace, shocked the nation. This was followed by the Senate hearings on Nutrition and Human Needs from 1968 to 1977, the White House Conference on Food, Nutrition, and Health in December, 1969 and a follow-up conference in 1974. All presented evidence not only that malnutrition was much more prevalent than previously suspected but that relatively little information on the nutritional status of the American population has been compiled.

Thus we now find that nutrition has become both a national and international concern, with many agencies dedicated to alleviating it and Congressional leaders staking their political careers on legislation dealing with nutritional issues. It is the subject of much research effort not only by nutritionists, agronomists, and biochemists but also by social scientists—economists, sociologists, psychologists, and anthropologists. The following discussion will focus on current knowledge of some of the factors that are contributing to the problem. Although the foregoing chapters have been concerned primarily with the physiological and biochemical aspects of nutritional inadequacies, this chapter will concentrate on the social, economic, and psychological aspects of nutritional diseases as they pertain to causes and solutions of the problem.

A NATIONAL CONCERN

Until 1968 attempts to evaluate the nutritional status of the American population had been confined to small, geographically isolated groups selected to meet the criteria of individual investigators. The findings of many of these were summarized in *Nutritional Status USA,* a compilation of studies supported by the U.S. Department of Agriculture, published in 1960. A subsequent compendium of similar studies appeared in 1969. These studies showed that the quality of nutrition was generally related to economic status and level of education. Infants and children from families of lower socioeconomic levels tended to be below average in height and weight. From 15% to 20% of adolescents were found to be obese, and older persons tended to be overweight. Iron deficiency was common in pregnant women and infants but not among adolescents. Ascorbic acid, vitamin A, calcium, and iron were the nutrients most commonly consumed at levels below the recommended dietary allowances, but biochemical evidence of vitamin deficiencies was rare.

The U.S. Department of Agriculture has regularly assessed food consumption of households every ten years and is now planning to repeat the study every five years.

The most recent survey to be reported was completed in the spring of 1965 and included 7500 households drawn to be representative of all housekeeping households in the United States. Data from a similar study conducted in 1978 and 1979 will provide comparable information on consumption by the household and by individuals, with adjustments for meals eaten away from home. The 1965 study showed that half the households had diets rated good on the basis that they provided the recommended levels of all nutrients. One fifth of the families had diets rated poor, since they provided less than two thirds of the recommended levels for one or more nutrients. Diets were most often inadequate in calcium, vitamin A, and ascorbic acid. Intakes of protein, iron, thiamin, and riboflavin met the recommended standards for 90% of the families. Dietary adequacy improved as income increased, although an adequate income provided no assurance of a good diet, since 9% of households with incomes over $10,000 had poor diets.

Analysis of 24-hour dietary recall records of food eaten at home and away from home for 14,500 individual members of the household as reported by the homemaker showed that calcium and iron were the nutrients most often taken at levels below recommended allowances. Individuals in families with incomes below $3000 also had diets with less than recommended amounts of ascorbic acid and vitamin A.

The first comprehensive attempt to assess the nutritional status of the American people was launched in 1968 and has been identified as the National Nutrition Survey. This study was designed to examine the dietary practices and nutritional status of a representative sample of persons identified by the 1960 census data in the lower quartile on the basis of income. Most families had incomes below $3000 per year. Ten states—Louisiana, North Carolina, Washington, New York, California, Texas, Kentucky, Michigan, West Virginia, and Massachusetts—were chosen to provide representation of the various ethnic and social groups within the total U.S. population. Nutritional status was assessed on the basis of physical and anthropological measurements, biochemical determinations on blood and urine, and a dental examination. Dietary intake was evaluated on the basis of a 24-hour dietary recall by the homemaker and selected nutritionally vulnerable members of the household.

An evaluation of the dietary data indicates regional differences, but, as shown Fig. 22-1, in all areas vitamin A, ascorbic acid, and iron were the nutrients most often taken in less than recommended amounts. Low hemoglobin levels were encountered in 11% of the total population and in 30% of the black population. Low vitamin A levels were found in the serum of children (particularly Spanish-Americans); low serum levels of vitamin C occurred in mothers, and there was some evidence of growth retardation in children. Obesity in adult women was reported in 50% of the survey group. Poor dental health was associated with poor nutrition.

Another federally sponsored nationwide study of the dietary practices and nutritional status of preschool children in all socioeconomic strata of the American population has been completed. This age group has been singled out for attention because it represents a nutritionally vulnerable group.

In 1970 the Department of Health, Education, and Welfare announced plans for continuing surveillance of the nutritional status of the population through an examination of 30,000 individuals every two years. This study, known as HANES (Health and Nutrition Examination Survey), focused on people from 1 to 74 years of age from sixty-five primary sampling units in the United States. Preliminary data on 10,216 persons from thirty-five sampling units have appeared throughout this text. For most age groups the mean intake for calcium, vitamin A, ascorbic acid, and protein either met or exceeded the recommended levels. However, for vitamins A and C, over 50% had intakes that fell below the standard used in evaluation, and for calcium, except among children, over 30% were low. The intake of iron failed to meet established standards for females and for children under 17 years of age. Biochemical data revealed that although 15% of the males and 2% of the females had low hematocrit values, hemoglobin, serum iron, and transferrin values fell below accepted levels for a smaller portion of the population. Both the dietary and biochemical findings are summarized in Tables 22-1 and 22-2.

Although undernutrition and malnutrition are not confined to any one social, economic, cultural, or ethnic group, available studies show several groups within the United States for whom these are special problems. These include the Indians, migrant workers, Eskimos, Spanish-Americans, the poor, and the elderly. In many respects these groups are difficult to reach with either assistance or education, since they neither belong to organized groups nor tend to seek help. In general, it has been suggested that their nutritional status may be a function of their cultural backgrounds, their inadequate knowledge of the nutritive value of foods, the economic problems resulting from low and often irregular incomes, the pressures of large families, and the trauma of high morbidity rates. Some of the specific factors involved for each particular group will be considered briefly.

American Indians, numbering fewer than half a million, live on 53 million acres of barren, dry, unproductive land, and have restricted freedom to roam for food and limited opportunities to earn income. The animals and fruit on which they formerly depended for food are vanishing. Meat is less available at higher prices, which leads Indians, whose incomes average less than $1000 per year, to consume a less expensive high-carbohydrate diet. Infant mortality rates of 140 per 1000 live births compared to a national average of

Low-income—ratio states:
Kentucky, Louisiana,
South Carolina, Texas, West Virginia

Ethnic group	Age	Sex	Iron	Protein	Vitamin A	Vitamin C	Riboflavin	Thiamin	Iodine	Growth and development	Obesity
Black	0-5 years	Both	●	O	●	O	●	O	O	●	—
	6-9 years	Both	●	•	•	O	●	O	O	●	—
	10-16 years	Females	●	•	•	O	●	•	O	•	•
		Males	●	O	•	O	●	•	O	•	•
	17-59 years	Females	●	•	O	•	●	O	O	—	●
		Males	●	O	O	●	●	O	O	—	O
	Over 60 years	Females	●	•	O	O	●	O	O	—	●
		Males	●	•	O	●	●	O	O	—	O
White	0-5 years	Both	●	O	•	O	•	O	O	●	—
	6-9 years	Both	●	O	•	O	•	O	O	●	—
	10-16 years	Females	●	O	•	O	•	•	O	•	•
		Males	●	O	•	O	•	•	O	•	●
	17-59 years	Females	●	O	O	O	O	O	O	—	●
		Males	●	O	O	●	O	O	O	—	•
	Over 60 years	Females	●	O	O	O	O	O	O	—	●
		Males	●	O	O	●	O	O	O	—	O
Spanish-American	0-5 years	Both	●	O	●	O	●	O	O	●	—
	6-9 years	Both	●	O	●	O	●	O	O	●	—
	10-16 years	Females	●	•	●	O	●	O	O	•	—
		Males	●	O	●	O	●	O	O	•	—
	17-59 years	Females	●	•	●	O	•	O	O	—	—
		Males	●	•	●	O	•	O	O	—	—
	Over 60 years	Females	●	•	●	O	•	O	O	—	—
		Males	●	•	●	●	•	O	O	—	—
Pregnant and lactating women			●	●	—	—	—	—	—	—	—

Continued.

Fig. 22-1. Relative importance of nutritional problems in the Ten-State Nutrition Survey (1968-1970).

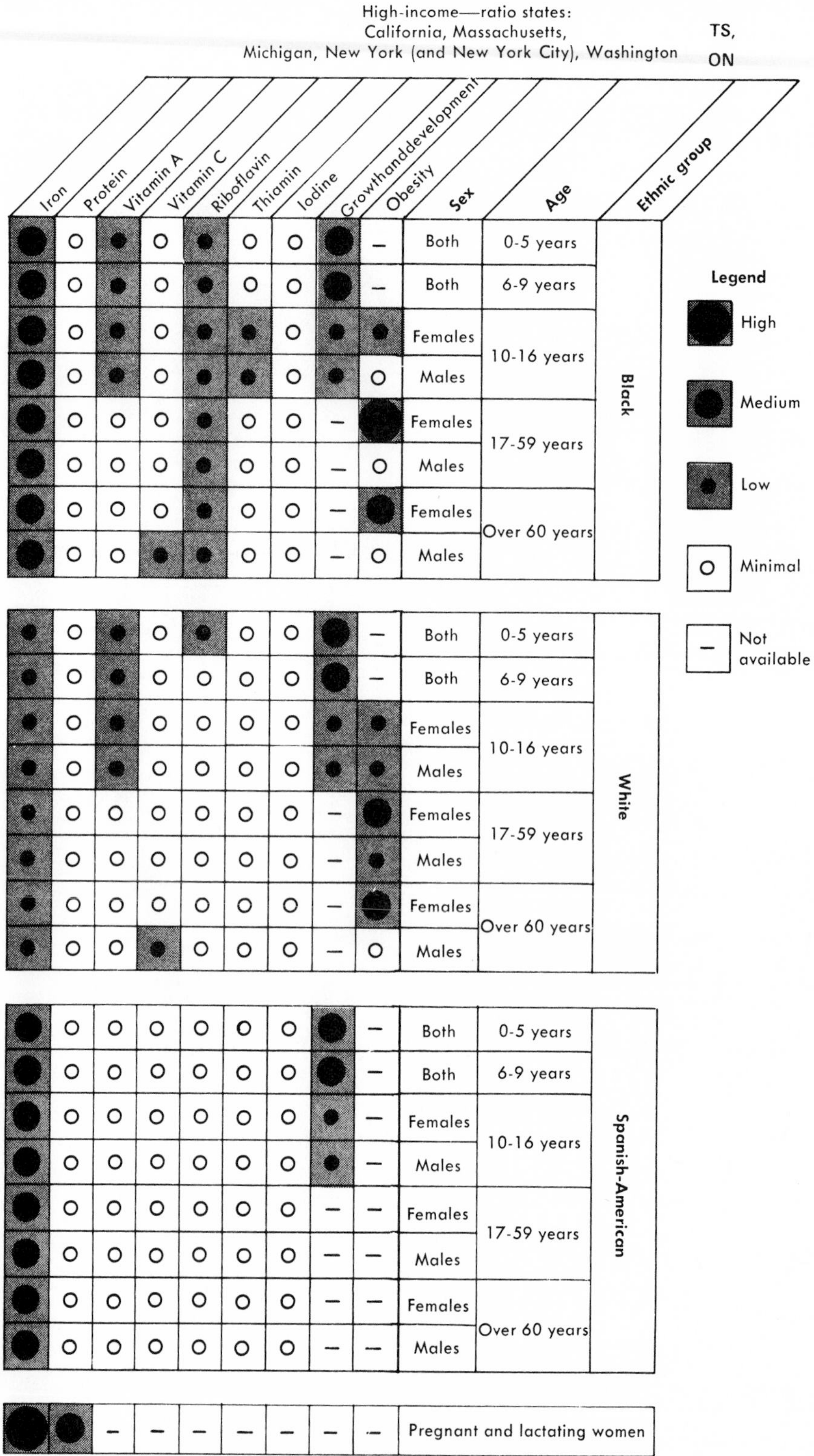

Fig. 22-1, cont'd. For legend see p. 547.

Table 22-1. Mean nutrient intake for some representative age groups surveyed in HANES, 1971-1974*†

	All ages	2-3	8-9	15-17	25-34	35-64
Number of subjects	20,749	1170	644	1019	2700	1267
Calories	1994 (87)‡	1489 (122)	2015 (86)	2394 (78)	2163 (87)	1710 (80)
Protein (g)	77.8 (139)	54.4 (225)	73.1 (195)	90.4 (127)	86.1 (123)	70.3 (105)
Calcium (mg)	867 (175)	865 (192)	1079 (240)	1123 (182)	845 (181)	670 (142)
Iron (mg)	11.9 (98)	7.7 (52)	10.5 (105)	13.0 (72)	13.4 (110)	11.6 (116)
Vitamin A (IU)	4774 (150)	3541 (177)	4290 (172)	4740 (135)	4815 (137)	5956 (170)
Vitamin C (mg)	86.3 (167)	78.3 (196)	81.1 (203)	87.0 (170)	82.7 (143)	97.0 (170)
Thiamin (mg)	1.28 (160)	1.02 (1.73)	1.29 (160)	1.48 (150)	1.35 (155)	1.17 (170)
Riboflavin (mg)	1.92 (175)	1.73 (211)	2.15 (193)	2.29 (173)	1.95 (163)	1.70 (180)

*From Dietary intake findings, United States, 1971-1974, Family Health Series 11.76.202, Washington, D.C., 1977, National Center for Health Statistics.
†Standards for evaluating dietary intake were presented in Table 15-1.
‡Figures in parentheses represent the percentage of the standard based on age and sex.

21.4 and a tuberculosis rate eight times the national average are evidence of poor health conditions. Studies of dietary adequacy among the Indians indicate that low intakes of ascorbic acid and vitamin A are the most prevalent nutritional inadequacies.

Migrant workers, dependent on agriculture for a living, have virtually no financial security. Because of the mobile nature of their existence, they have limited and irregular opportunities for education and their housing is marginal, often lacking facilities for the preparation and storage of food and for adequate sanitation. The latter increases the possibility of infection, to which resistance is low because of poor nutrition and possible intestinal parasitism. In many cases the mother who must work in the field all day is home to cook at most two meals a day. Older children care for younger ones and thus cannot attend school. Dietary studies indicate that diets of migrant families are low in vitamins C and A, calcium, and riboflavin, reflecting limited use of fruit and vegetables and milk.

Eskimos traditionally consumed a diet obtained largely by hunting and fishing, high in fat and protein, and low in carbohydrate.

Table 22-2. Biochemical determinations for persons 12 to 17 years of age by sex and income levels: number of persons, mean, median, and percent with low values, United States, 1971-1972 (HANES Preliminary)*

Biochemical test	Male	Female	Income below poverty level†	Income above poverty level†
n	517	528	264	732
N	12,508	12,239	3,626	19,694
Hematocrit (%)				
Mean	43.13	40.74	40.73	42.14
Median	42.65	40.94	40.82	41.86
Percent with low values	15.46	2.42	16.54	7.86
Hemoglobin (g/dl)				
Mean	14.77	13.33	13.70	14.39
Median	14.74	13.73	13.63	14.34
Percent with low values	7.39	1.91	11.58	3.56
Serum iron (μg/dl)				
Mean	112.50	104.24	103.43	109.25
Median	110.76	102.09	101.72	106.36
Percent with low values	2.80	1.12	3.70	1.75
Transferrin saturation (%)				
Mean	33.63	30.48	30.46	32.31
Median	32.33	29.09	29.80	31.00
Percent with low values	7.66	5.29	9.22	6.36

NOTE: n = examined persons, N = estimated population in thousands.
*From Preliminary findings of the First Health and Nutrition Examination Survey, United States, 1971-1972, Dietary intake and biochemical findings, Washington, D.C., 1974, Department of Health, Education, and Welfare.
†Excludes persons with unknown income.

They have migrated to the city in search of a steady income. At the same time, they have lost their food-gathering skills and resources. The result has been a shift to a high-carbohydrate diet, with a concurrent increase in dental caries.

The poor have been identified in many nutritional surveys as a group with generally less than adequate diets. This is attributed in part to their limited resources for all necessities of life, including food, and in part to the fact that low-income families in general have less education and less sound nutritional knowledge on which to base their food choices. Their problem is compounded by the fact that in an era of rising food costs the cost of less expensive foods eaten by the poor, who spend 37% of their income on food, is rising faster than that of more expensive foods usually consumed in larger quantities by the more affluent.

The nutritional practices of the elderly are discussed in Chapter 19, in which it is pointed out that psychological as well as social factors such as low income, long-standing food habits, loneliness, poor housing, lack of adequate storage and preparation facilities, lack of transportation to stores, and indifference to or ignorance of adequate food habits are involved. Physiologically they suffer from decreased ability to absorb and transport nutrients, increased excretion of nutrients, and thus relatively increased need.

Nutritional problems are by no means confined to these groups. Many others, such as adolescent girls and pregnant women, are often underfed. Another significant group, the overfed, suffer from obesity and may represent up to 20% of some population groups. Although the causes may be multiple, nutrition is one factor in the etiology of atherosclerosis, responsible for premature death of a large number of middle-aged men.

Improvement of nutritive intake in the United States

National programs to improve nutrient intake and to alleviate malnutrition in the United States have included the National School Lunch Program, the Special Milk Program, and the School Breakfast Program, the Expanded Nutrition Education Program, the Child Care Food Program, the Food Donations Program, the Food Stamp Program, the Supplemental Food Program for Women, Infants and Children, and Congregate Meals Program.

The National School Lunch Program, discussed in detail in Chapter 18, makes lunches available free or at reduced prices for 9 million children participating. With over half a billion dollars in federal funds being allocated to the School Lunch Program, participation is expected to increase. In addition, several states are making nutrition education an integral part of the School Lunch Program and are urging that it be incorporated into other academic programs. The Child Nutrition Act was amended in 1977 to mandate that 50 cents per child be allocated in each state for nutrition education. The impact of such a program will be evident only after it has been fully implemented.

The School Lunch Act also provides support for the Special Milk Program. Under this plan the United States Department of Agriculture reimburses schools and child care institutions for part of the cost of providing a special milk service as snacks or at mealtime to children not participating in the lunch program. Up to 0.5 liter (1 pint) of milk per day is provided free to needy children in a program that costs $155 million in 1978 for over 2 million children.

The Child Nutrition Act passed in 1966 provided funds for the purchase of equipment for schools in districts wishing to establish, maintain, and expand school food service programs to participate in the School Lunch Program. In addition, it provided for a pilot study of a School Breakfast Program to initiate, maintain, and expand nonprofit breakfast programs in schools and authorized the use of federal school feeding funds for feeding preschool children. The pilot School Breakfast Program has been extended; in 1977, 1 million of the 1.8 million participants received free breakfast in a program costing over $201 million. In 1974 over 3600 schools, 90% of which also had a School Lunch Program, participated. Only 5% of the schools with a lunch program also have a breakfast program, however.

In 1972 the Child Nutrition Act of 1966 was amended to provide through state and local agencies a supplemental food program for pregnant and lactating women and infants and children up to 4 years of age who are considered to be nutritional risks. This includes mothers from populations with known inadequate nutritional patterns, unacceptable high incidence of anemia, high prematurity rates, and inadequate patterns of growth; children from low-income populations known to have inadequate diets and deficient patterns of growth are also included. The program known as WIC (Women, Infants, and Children) is administered by the Department of Agriculture and is designed to provide foods with high-quality protein, calcium, iron, vitamin A, and ascorbic acid. Infants are provided with iron-fortified infant formula, infant cereal with at least 90 mg of iron per 100 g of dry cereal, and fruit juice with at least 30 mg of ascorbic acid per deciliter. Vitamin D-fortified milk, iron-enriched cereal (30 mg/100 g), vitamin C rich fruit or vegetable juice, cheese, and eggs are provided for children and pregnant and lactating women.

The effectiveness of the program is still being evaluated but in a pilot project in Washington, D.C., infant mortality decreased from 7.4 to 1.7 from 1970 to 1972 when a similar food supplementation program was in effect. In 1978, these projects, funded at $560 million, were providing food to 1.2 million women, infants, and children with the expectation that participation would continue to increase.

In 1969 funds for the Expanded Nutrition Education Program were allocated by the United States Department of Agriculture. The Extension Service supervises the training of nutrition aides with the responsibility of working on a one-to-one basis with low-income homemakers to help them with homemaking skills and to provide nutrition education. Most of the aides are recruited from the same socioeconomic group as those with whom they will be working. In 1970 the funds were increased, with a provision that 25% of available resources must be allocated for work by youth professionals in the inner city. These persons are to integrate nutrition education in other programs for the young.

The Congregate Meals Program designed to meet both the social and nutritional needs of the elderly, is providing meals for groups up to five days a week in centrally located "diners' clubs" at a cost of $30 million (Chapter 19).

Child Care has provided a feeding program along with medical, psychological, educational, and social services for children enrolled in their program. By 1974 this program reached 2 million children at a cost of $39 million. Little information has been collected on the nature and extent of hunger and malnutrition among this group nor on the effectiveness of the nutrition component of the project.

The Food Donation Program was introduced with a dual purpose of improving the nutrient intake of families with limited incomes and at the same time providing an outlet for domestically produced agricultural products. In 1960 when the primary emphasis was on providing a few surplus foods, only lard, rice, dried milk, flour, and cornmeal were available. With a change in emphasis toward providing a more adequately balanced diet, up to fifty-nine foods, many nutritionally improved, are available. The choice within any one district is the decision of local officials and is determined in part by availability in relation to demand. The facts that food was usually distributed only once a month and often at a center remote from the recipient's home, coupled with problems of transporting and storing large quantities of food, were deterrents to the success of the program. In 1974, although 2 million persons received food commodities, only a third of the eligible families were participating in the program. Eligibility of individual households, which must be certified every three months, is based on income relative to the number in the family and total cash assets. In addition to providing food for individual families, the Commodity Distribution Program made food available to schools, feeding programs for the elderly, nonprofit institutions, and nonprofit summer camps for children. In 1970 donated foods amounted to about 1 billion kg, over half of which went to needy families. Additional commodities are also available through maternal and child health centers to expectant and nursing mothers and young infants in an attempt to decrease the risk to these nutritionally vulnerable groups.

The Food Stamp Program, begun as a pilot program in 1961 and initiated under the Food Stamp Act of 1964, has been rapidly replacing the Commodity Distribution Program. In 1977 all but one of the eligible counties in the United States were participating in either program. Practically all had elected the Food Stamp Program, which was used by 17 million persons. This program is designed to improve the diets of low-income households and at the same time to expand the market for domestically produced food. Basically, the program increases the purchasing power of the eligible family by allowing the purchase of sufficient food stamps to provide food for an adequate diet for the family based on the cost of the low-income food plan prepared by the U.S. Department of Agriculture. The cost of the stamps varies on the basis of income and represents a reasonable amount to spend for food. Thus a family of 5 with an income of $120 per month is able to purchase $216 worth of food stamps for $33, whereas a similar family with an income of $300 pays $84 for the same value in stamps. In 1978 the face value of stamps used by a family of four was $182 per month with a total program cost of $5.8 billion. Stamps can be purchased twice a month at the bank and are used as cash at participating and approved grocery stores. This program is currently being expanded and modified to provide for more equitable use of funds. The program is directed by the state agency responsible for administering other federally aided assistance programs. Consideration is now being given to "cashing-out" the program to give participants a cash subsidy rather than requiring them to buy stamps at a reduced price.

Many other innovative programs are being introduced to improve food habits, especially among low-income groups for whom nutritional intakes are least adequate. For instance, one city housing authority is providing after-school snacks for 1500 children in housing developments. The Department of Agriculture sponsors a summer recreational feeding program in a low-income area to provide up to three meals and two snacks a day for 1 million children at a cost of $50 million. Feeding programs in migrant camps are increasing in number. Several cities have introduced noon feeding programs for older persons. All these programs are utilizing donated commodities, and, in many cases, labor and equipment costs are borne by the federal government.

Enrichment. Enrichment of food products has been an effective way of correcting some aspects of undernutrition, especially since many synthetic nutrients have become available at a low cost. Compulsory enrichment of bread and flour introduced in 1940 remained in effect during the national emergency of World War II. At the end of that period, jurisdiction for enrichment policies reverted to the individual states. Currently thirty-four states require the enrichment of bread and flour, with thiamin, riboflavin, niacin, and iron mandatory and calcium optional within prescribed limits. Since most wheat is milled in three or four large milling centers, 90% of the bread and cereal sold in the United States is enriched Some states require the addition of these same nutrients to cornmeal, corn grits, farina, and macaroni and noodles and the addition of thiamin, niacin, and iron to rice.

Iodization of salt, although not compulsory, has contributed to a reduction in the incidence of goiter in the United States. Fortification of fresh whole and evaporated milk with vitamin D, nonfat milk with both vitamins A and D, and margarine with vitamin A is a general practice. Iron enrichment of infant cereals is not governed by any state or federal regulation other than that it be adequately labeled but has contributed to the control of iron-deficiency anemia in infants. Although many other forms of enrichment are used by the food industry, they have not received endorsement of nutritionists for several reasons: nutrients may be used in foods that are not effective carriers, or demonstrable deficiency of the nutrient may not have been found in the population consuming the product, or the nutrient may be unstable under normal conditions of preparation. With the possibility of toxicity from the excessive intake of fat-soluble vitamin D, there is concern about the indiscriminate practice of food enrichment and fortification.

In an effort to discourage ineffective and unnecessary enrichment of food products the Food and Nutrition Board endorses the addition of nutrients to foods when all of the following conditions are met:

a. The intake of the nutrient(s) is below the desirable level in the diets of a significant number of people
b. The food(s) used to supply the nutrient(s) is likely to be consumed in quantities that will make a significant contribution to the diet of the population in need
c. The addition of the nutrient(s) is not likely to create an imbalance of essential nutrients
d. The nutrient(s) added is stable under customary conditions of storage and use
e. The nutrient(s) is physiologically available from the food
f. There is reasonable assurance against intake sufficiently in excess to be toxic

Specifically, the following practices in the United States continue to be endorsed: The enrichment of flour, bread, degerminated corn meal, corn grits, whole grain corn meal, white rice, and certain other cereal grain products with thiamin, riboflavin, niacin, and iron; the addition of vitamin D to milk, fluid skim milk, and nonfat dry milk; the addition of vitamin A to margarine, fluid skim milk, and nonfat dry milk; and the addition of iodine to table salt. The protective action of fluoride against dental caries is recognized and the standardized addition of fluoride to water in areas in which the water supply has a low fluoride content is endorsed.*

Because of the confusion resulting from the terms **enrichment,** generally used to refer to the addition of nutrients to cereals and **fortification,** generally used to refer to the addition of nutrients to other foods, and *restoration* used when nutrients are added to replace those lost in processing, it has been suggested that the term **nutritionally enhanced** be used to identify all foods that have been modified in an attempt to increase their nutritive value.

In 1977 the Senate Select Committee on Nutrition and Human Needs proposed the following set of dietary goals* for the United States population that it felt would lead to the highest level of health:

1. To avoid overweight, consume only as much energy (calories) as is expended; if overweight, decrease energy intake and increase energy expenditure.
2. Increase the consumption of complex carbohydrates and "naturally occurring" sugars from about 28% of energy intake to about 48% of energy intake to account for 55% to 60% of the (caloric) intake.
3. Reduce overall fat consumption from approximately 40% to 30% of energy intake.
4. Reduce saturated fat consumption to account for about 10% of total energy intake; and balance that with polyunsaturated and monounsaturated fats, which should account for about 10% of energy intake each.
5. Reduce cholesterol consumption to about 300 mg a day.
6. Reduce consumption of refined and processed sugars by about 45% to account for about 10% of total energy intake.
7. Decrease consumption of salt and foods high in salt content.

The goals suggest the following changes in food selection and preparation:

1. Increase consumption of fruits and vegetables and whole grains.
2. Decrease consumption of animal fat and choose poultry and fish, which will reduce saturated fat.
3. Decrease consumption of foods high in total fat and partially replace saturated fat with polyunsaturated fat.
4. Except for young children, substitute low-fat and nonfat milk for whole milk and low-fat dairy products for high-fat dairy products.
5. Decrease consumption of butterfat, eggs, and other high cholesterol sources. Some consideration should be given to easing the cholesterol reduction goal for premenopausal women, young children, and the elderly

*From Food and Nutrition Board: Proposed fortification policy for cereal-grain products, Washington, D.C., 1974, National Academy of Sciences.

*From Dietary Goals for the United States, ed. 2, Washington, D.C., 1977, Senate Select Committee on Nutrition and Human Needs.

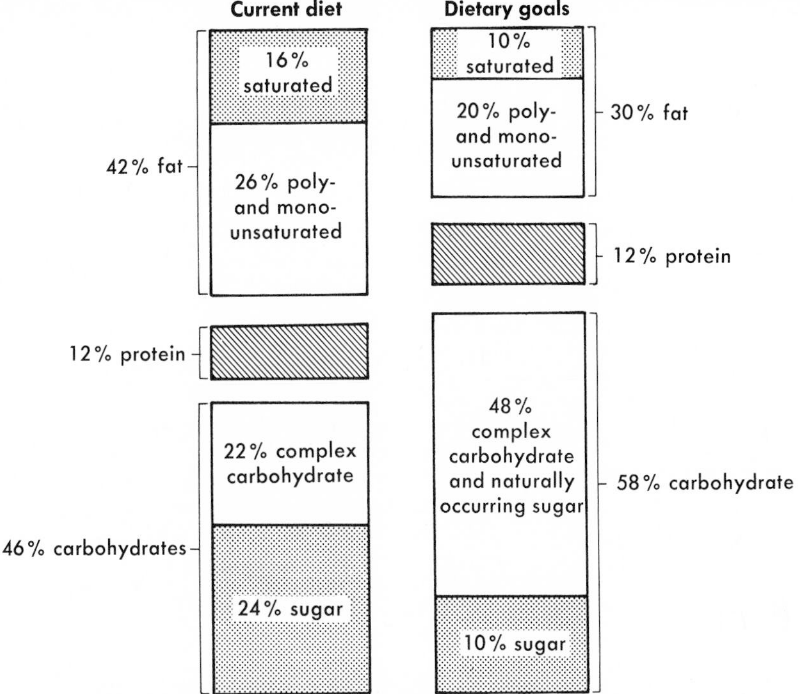

Fig. 22-2. Comparison of current U.S. diet with that proposed in U.S. dietary goals. (From Dietary Goals for the United States, ed. 2, Washington, D.C., 1977, Senate Committee on Nutrition and Human Needs.)

to obtain the nutritional benefits of eggs in the diet.

6. Decrease consumption of refined and other processed sugars and foods high in such sugars.
7. Decrease consumption of salt and foods high in salt content.

A comparison of the goals with current dietary practices is presented in Fig. 22-2. Implementation of the goals would require an increased consumption of whole grains, fruits and vegetables, poultry, fish, and polyunsaturated fats, a marked reduction in the use of sugar and sugar-rich foods, salt and foods high in salt, butterfat, eggs, and other cholesterol-containing foods, meat, and foods high in fat. The implications of these for food guides, nutrition intervention programs, and individuals are significant and far reaching. As a result they are the subject of extensive and often acrimonious debate among nutrition scientists and educators, some of whom support the goals and many of whom believe they were based on inadequate evidence, cannot be implemented, or may even be counterproductive. They also question the wisdom of a government body setting goals. Whether these goals or further modifications will ever be accepted is an open question, but these proposals have served a useful purpose in stimulating debate and a serious assessment of the state of nutrition knowledge.

AN INTERNATIONAL CONCERN

At the global level, efforts toward improving the nutritional status of the world's population have centered on the possibility of balancing the increase in population with an increase in food production. At the present rate of increase of up to 2% per year, world population will double in 36 years. Unfortunately, this increase is not occurring evenly in all areas of the world. The largest increases are occurring in the poor, ill-fed areas with the most limited potential for food production. Fig. 22-3 presents graphically the variation in calories and protein available in different countries.

The immediacy of the problem was recognized in late 1974 with the convening of the World Food Conference in Rome under sponsorship of the United Nations. It focussed on ways to save the 500 million people threatened with starvation the next year because of the deficit of 6 to 10 million metric tons of grain as the result of flood, drought, and fertilizer shortage. The conference made

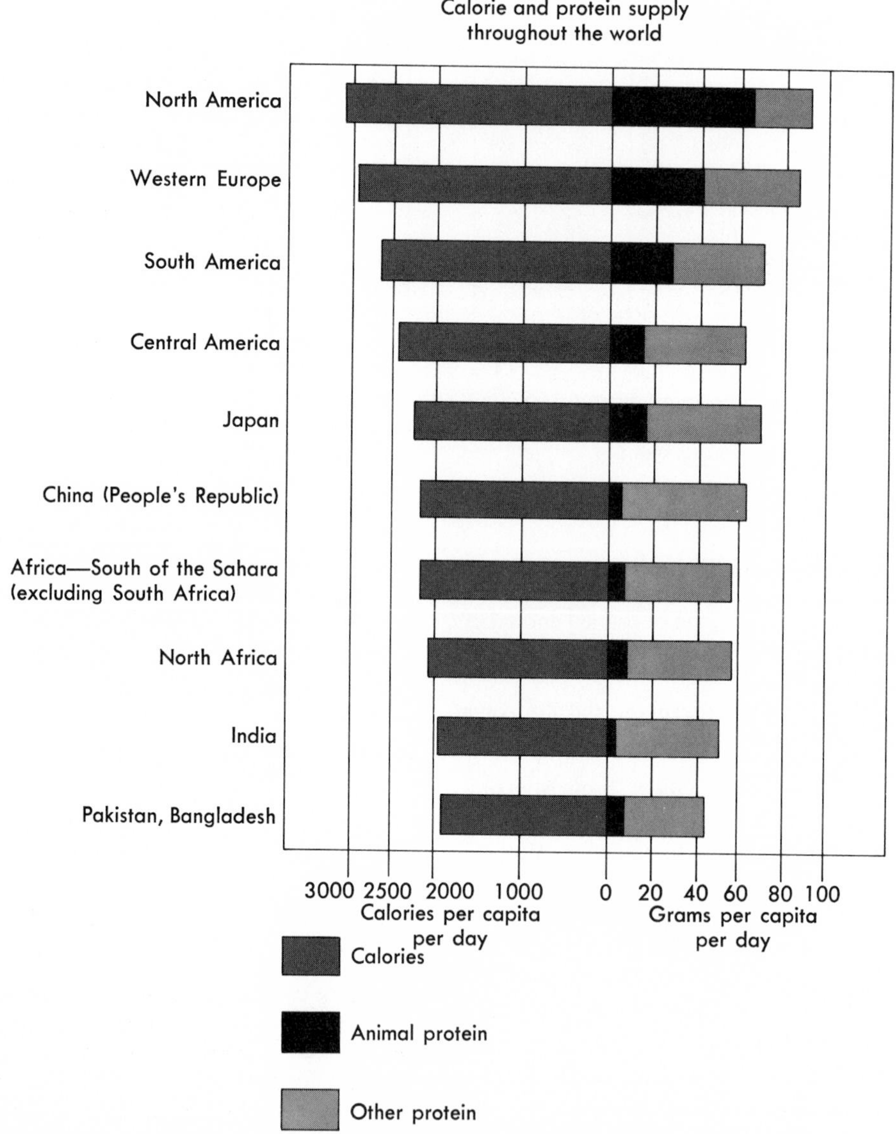

Fig. 22-3. Calorie and protein supply throughout the world. (From Cloud, W.: Science **13**[8]:6, 1973.)

plans for establishing an international grain reserve and a World Food Council in efforts to minimize the chances of such catastrophic conditions arising again.

This was followed in 1977 with a report from the National Academy of Sciences entitled "World Food and Nutrition Study: the Potential Contributions of Research" which involved the effort of 1500 experts on fourteen study teams over a two-year period to recommend research strategies to alleviate the chronic shortages of food and the debilitating effects of malnutrition. The report dealt with crop and animal productivity, aquatic food resources, food and health interventions, and nutrition education. It depicted the complex interrelationships of a nutrition intervention as shown in Fig. 22-4.

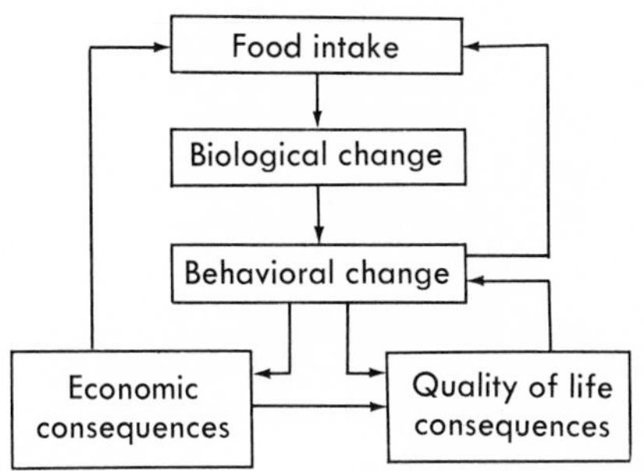

Fig. 22-4. Chain of effects of a nutrition intervention. (From World Food and Nutrition Study, Washington, D.C., 1977, National Academy of Sciences.)

At present the food-deficit areas of Asia, Africa, and Latin America have 50% of the world's population, 25% of the world's food supply, 12.5% of the income, and 50% of the arable land. On the other hand, Europe, Oceania, and North America, with 20% of the population, have 59% of the food and 80% of the income. Fig. 22-5 shows recent and predicted changes in population for various parts of the world. If these predicted population trends materialize, it is estimated that to maintain present nutrient intake, food supplies must increase 123% by the year 2000 over the levels for 1965. This calls for an increase of 3.9% annually compared to the current rate of 2.7%. To improve nutritional status, the Food and Agricultural Organiza-

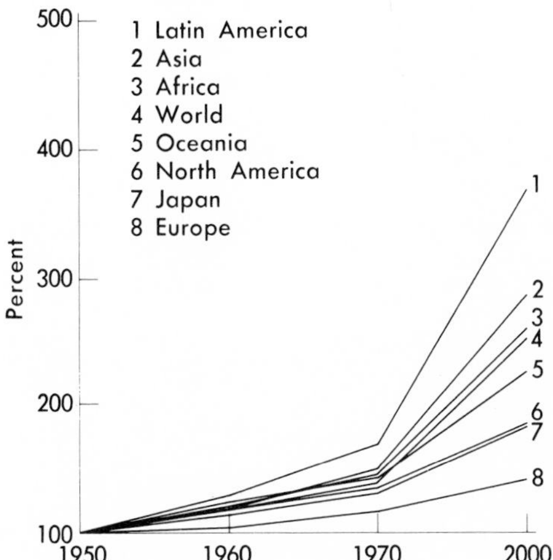

Fig. 22-5. Population trends and projections based on population in selected areas of the world, 1950. (Modified from Freedom From Hunger Campaign: Basic Study No. 7, Population and food supply, Rome, 1963, Food and Agricultural Organization.)

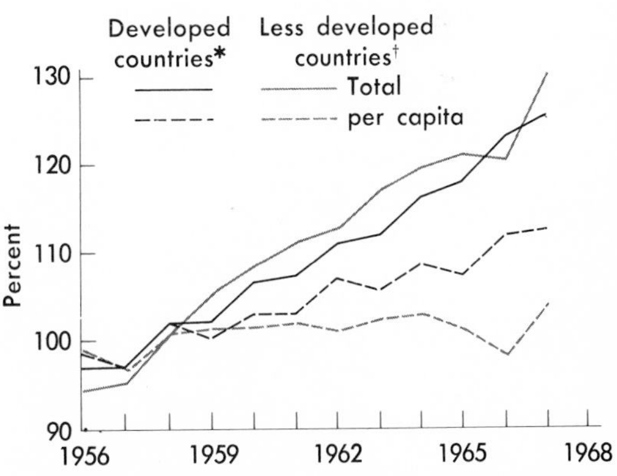

Fig. 22-6. Trends in total and per capita agricultural production in developed and developing countries. *United States, Canada, U.S.S.R., Japan, Europe, Australia, New Zealand, and South Africa. †Latin America, south Asia, east Asia, west Asia, and Africa. (From Editorial: A year of action, War on Hunger No. 2, p. 3, Feb., 1969.)

tion estimates comparable needs would be a 274% increase for the world and 393% for the less-developed countries.

Current trends in food production in relation to population are shown in Fig. 22-6. The Indicative World Plan (IWP) for Agricultural Production forecasts a food demand in developing countries in 1985 two and a half times current production. Since even the most optimistic view of the potential for increased food production does not foresee an increase of this magnitude, it is obvious that efforts must be made simultaneously to reverse or to slow down the population trend. Should this not be accomplished, the possibility of the malthusian correctives of famine, pestilence, and war is ever present.

Efforts to increase world food production must include increasing the yield of land currently under cultivation, increasing the amount of land under cultivation, making maximum use of land not suitable for agriculture for the grazing of animals, exploiting the sea as a potential source of food, and capitalizing on the capability of advancing food technology to provide nonconventional food sources. The success of these efforts will depend to a certain extent on the application of agricultural technology in the form of improved plant and animal breeding; the use of herbicides, pesticides, fertilizers and irrigation; and social changes in the form of an available market and credit and efficient transportation and distribution systems. Each must be evaluated in relation to its energy cost. These approaches will be effective, however, only when introduced with an understanding of the social and cultural framework of society. Such influences as traditional value systems, social organization, land ownership and tenure relationships, and political climate are equally as important as technology in the success of innovations in agricultural production and marketing. For a more complete understanding of the complexity of the problem a consideration of the ecology of nutritional disease is in order.

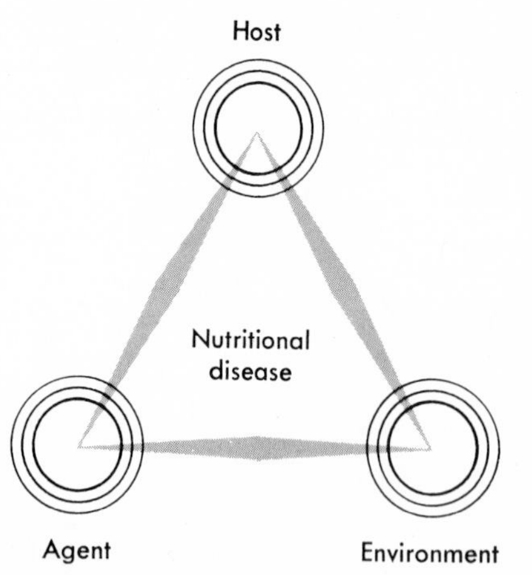

Fig. 22-7. Epidemiological triad depicting relationship among agent, host, and environment as factors in in nutritional disease.

Ecology of nutritional disease

Epidemiologists have traditionally considered disease to be the result of a complex interaction between *host, environmental factors,* and *agent*, as depicted in Fig. 22-7. The use of this model provides a meaningful basis for a discussion of factors contributing to nutritional disease. Such considerations help explain the varying incidence of nutritional disease under seemingly similar patterns of food consumption—differences that may be a function of time, place or person.

Host. The nature of the nutritional needs and the extent to which the available nutrients are utilized are known to vary from one individual to another. The factors affecting needs include age, sex, prior nutritional state, health, rate of growth, stage of maturity, current emotional and physical stress, and genetic background. In general, the needs for nutrients are relatively high during periods of rapid growth and decline gradually with age after maturity. Differences attributed to sex are due not only to variations in body composition and in rate of growth and the effect of different endocrine secretions, but also to different patterns of activity. That the needs and utilization of nutrients vary as a result of genetically determined characteristics has been well established. In his discussion on biochemical individuality, Williams demonstrates a wide range of normal requirements of specific nutrients—a consideration that has been recognized in formulating dietary allowances for healthy individuals.

Whether or not a certain dietary intake will be nutritionally inadequate is influenced by the extent to which the individual is able to adapt to, or to compensate for, suboptimal intakes. For instance, persons accustomed to low-calcium diets are able to use the calcium more effectively than those accustomed to higher intakes. Similarly, when sodium intake is restricted or sodium needs are increased, a series of hormonal changes occurs that lead to increased retention and decreased excretion of the nutrient. The lethargy so common in the undernourished may represent a conservation of energy to compensate for the energy deficit.

The physiological state of the person—pregnancy, lactation, or growth—will account for varying nutritional needs. Such stress factors normally result in an increased need for nutrients, but at the same time, physiological adjustments increase the efficiency with which a nutrient can be utilized. Similarly, the stress of infections, such as tonsillitis, measles, tuberculosis, or pneumonia and of parasitic infestations increases the nutrient need and in cases of marginal intake is often regarded as responsible for precipitating a nutrient inadequacy. Such a synergism between malnutrition and infection is considered a major cause of the high mortality and morbidity rates among preschool children in developing countries.

Environmental factors. The role of environmental factors in nutritional disease is the result of their effect on the availability of nutrients, the nutritional requirements of the host, and the intake of nutrients. The environment includes not only the important physical and biological environment but also the social or cultural environment.

The availability of nutrients for both a population and an individual will vary with the season. The phenomenon of seasonal hunger in which food intakes hit a low point just before harvest season and a peak after harvest is well known in developing countries. For persons dependent on sunshine as a source of vitamin D, the rainy season will lead to a marked reduction in the amount of the nutrient available. Similarly, the practice in many cultures of protecting infants from exposure to sunlight deprives the child of a supply of the nutrient at a time of maximum need. Seasonal fluctuations in employment such as those experienced by migrant workers, with the resultant fluctuations in income also account for seasonal variations in availability of nutrients.

Agricultural productivity, especially in economically underdeveloped areas with poorly developed transportation and storage facilities, is an obvious determinant of availability of food. This in turn is dependent on the nature and fertility of the soil, the climate, the topography of the land, and the prevalence of natural disasters, such as floods, droughts, and storms. These determine the type of plant or animal that can be raised in the area and the nutritive value of the food produced. For instance, cassava and soybeans can be grown on marginal land, whereas rice and wheat require more productive soil. The trace mineral content of the soil determines the mineral content of the plants produced, and this in turn influences the growth of animals feeding on the crops or the nutrient intake of persons eating plant foods directly.

Even where the physical and biological environment would be conducive to agricultural productivity, social factors are also determinants. Education of the farmer in effective agricultural practices and the provision of adequate incentives to increase production are of prime importance. These in turn may be a function of the effectiveness of mass communication or the availability of a resource person who can inspire the confidence of the farmers. Adequate irrigation systems, terracing of hillsides, land tenure policies, availability of credit for seed at planting time and for herbicides and pesticides during cultivation, adequate food storage and distribution systems, and price-support policies are all socially and often politically determined factors that can influence agricultural practices and hence productivity.

The capacity of the farmer to produce food is influenced by the condition of his health. A malaria or a tuberculosis victim has reduced work capacity. A farmer with intestinal parasites experiences a blood loss, with a resultant decrease in hemoglogin level and a concomitant apathy. The reduced work capacity reduces his food production and income, which in turn reduce his food intake and his ability to resist intestinal parasites and infectious agents. Thus he finds himself caught in a vicious circle that must be broken if his situation is to improve.

Nutrient requirements also fall under the influence of environmental variables. Climate as it affects heat and water and hence electrolyte losses accounts for variations in nutrient requirements. Loss of nutrients through perspiration in a hot climate may be a precipitating factor in nutritional deficiency diseases. In highly developed countries the ubiquitous nature of laborsaving devices reduce the requirements for calories and for nutrients involved in energy metabolism. Dietary practices, themselves an element in the environment, can influence nutrient requirements. For instance, a high-carbohydrate diet calls for an increase in thiamin; a diet high in polyunsaturates, more vitamin E; a goitrogenic diet, more iodine; and a vegetarian diet, a supplementary source of vitamin B_{12}.

The intake of nutrients is determined to a large extent by both the physical and social environment. In the cold arctic climate only 20% of dietary calories are derived from carbohydrate, whereas in the tropical regions about 80% are from the carbohydrate sources, which grow well there at a high yield per acre.

Long-standing food habits are a function of the availability of food. To a certain degree they are also culturally determined. Food taboos, such as the Hindus' avoidance of meat and the Jew' avoidance of pork, are religious in origin. Superstitions, such as fish causing worms, eggplant causing the skin to be dark, eggs causing sterility, and a combination of cherries and milk causing illness, have their orgins in folk beliefs. The association of milk intake and diarrhea originally attributed to inadequate sanitation has been found to have a sound physiological basis for those persons who fail to produce the enzyme lactase necessary to digest milk sugar.

Lack of income has been identified as a significant factor in undernutrition. It has led older persons to adopt a high-carbohydrate diet, parents to feed diluted milk to their children, the poor to exist on a monotonous and inadequate diet of rice and beans, and persons in developing countries to use insignificant amounts of relatively expensive animal protein of high biological value. Although availability of money is no guarantee of an adequate diet, when income falls below a certain point, the chances of obtaining an adequate nutrient intake decrease as income decreases.

Food intake is influenced by many physiological factors. The inability to chew, the loss of neuromuscular coordination, or the inability to tolerate certain foods because of allergy, gastric distress, or heartburn lead to marked changes in the character of the diet, often with resulting nutritional inadequacies. The Chinese restaurant syndrome, in which the consumption of monosodium glutamate has been implicated in a series of adverse physical symptoms, has provided further evidence of an environmental factor influencing food consumption. Loss of appetite may accompany emotional states such as fear or anxiety, whereas overeating may be a compensatory mechanism to combat unhappiness or loneliness.

In developed countries particularly, one of the major determinants of food intake may be food faddism. Practices advocated by faddists often result in diets completely devoid of a particular nutrient. Scurvy has occurred among adherents to the Zen macrobiotic diet, which may be based solely on brown rice. Vegetarians put themselves on a vitamin B_{12}–deficient diet, with the possibility of precipitating pernicious anemia. Any diet that restricts consumption to one or two food groups increases the likelihood of a nutrient deficiency.

Agent. The third member of the epidemiological triad, the agent, is a relative lack of a nutrient. As has been discussed, the need for a nutrient varies with host and environmental variables. Diets also vary in their nutritive content. In addition, many factors, such as method of food processing and storage, cooking procedures, and distribution of nutrients in a day's meals, affect the amount actually available. When nutrient stores have been depleted or cannot be mobilized and when the amount of the available nutrient is inadequate relative to the need, a nutrient deficiency develops. The nature and severity of the symptoms vary with the specific nutrient, as does the speed with which deficiency symptoms manifest themselves. The detection of the biochemical changes in the blood and urine that usually precede physical symptoms is of prime importance in prevention.

Increasing the world food supply

As just pointed out, the causes of malnutrition may be multiple and interrelated. By the same token, the cure or prevention of malnutrition involves the identification of the basic cause or causes and their interrelationships and the promotion of means of counteracting them. Thus an increase in availability and utilization of food for the prevention of malnutrition may necessitate a modification of the social, physical, or biological environment, rather than a mere increase in food production. In this discussion some of the approaches that are being used to increase food production with a goal of increasing nutrient intake and improving nutritional status will be considered.

Increased agricultural productivity has resulted from more extensive use of pesticides and herbicides. Although safe and effective when used properly, they are not without hazards, since their indiscriminate use may result in environmental contamination that adversely affects the life of animals, themselves an important source of food. Similarly, animal food production has been increased through the use of antibiotics and some hormones. Again, controls are necessary to prevent misuse so that levels in animal tissues as used for human consumption do not exceed established safe standards.

Selective breeding of plants has resulted in high-yielding crops particularly suited to the area. The Maize and Wheat Improvement Center in Mexico has produced a strain of wheat especially suited to the climatic and soil conditions of Central and South America. The International Rice International Rice Institute in the Philippines was responsible for so-called miracle rice (1R8) that is high yielding, responds well to fertilizer and irrigation, and has a shorter maturation period making it possible to produce more crops each year. This product has been responsible for a large increase in rice production throughout southeast Asia—a development that has been characterized as a Green Revolution. The Institute for Tropical Agriculture in Nigeria and one in Taiwan concentrating on vegetable production are expected to stimulate similar advances for crops such as sorghum, millet, and corn. Purdue University plant geneticists have perfected a high-yielding corn with high disease resistance and a content of the amino acid lysine sufficient to raise the normally low biological value of corn protein from 1.3 to 2.3, a level approaching that of casein. Similar advances will undoubtedly follow for other staple crops.

Animal breeders have also contributed. The International Center fo Tropical Agriculture in Colombia will concentrate on improving tropical livestock production. By developing a cow that thrives in the tropics, is resistant to tropical diseases, and can range on rough marginal land, the potential supply of animal protein in such areas where only

20% to 30% of the animal protein is now produced has been increased. Nonprotein nitrogen sources such as urea, which can be manufactured from carbon dioxide and ammonia, can be used as at least a partial source of nitrogen in feeding some animals. The development of a rapidly maturing chicken with a high protein efficiency ratio in converting food into protein and an early maturing pig with an increased proportion of its body weight as protein are other examples of the potential of animal breeding techniques. The raising of rapid-turnover species such as poultry and hogs is also encouraged. In addition, the "farming" of animals not now extensively used for food, such as the elephant, antelope, hippopotamus, or frog, is being investigated for countries with large game lands, for example, those in Africa. The use of these animals by cultures that prohibit the use of more conventional domestic animals, such as the cow, for human food has great potential.

The addition of fertilizer in areas of food deficiency could result in a marked increase in food supply from current acreage. At the present time only 15% of the fertilizer is used in the area of the world that feed 50% of the world's population. To increase the use of fertilizer, it will be necessary not only to develop fertilizer manufacturing plants close to the areas where it is needed and to make credit readily available at the time of planting but also to make available information on its proper and effective use. Since a sizable financial outlay is involved, subsistence farmers who operate on a small margin with virtually no cash reserves need to be convinced that the returns will justify the risk. Demonstrations of its effectiveness, especially by farmers identified as more progressive, have been feasible methods of increasing its acceptance. Current increases in the cost of fuel essential for fertilizer production may, however, make the use of fertilizer excessively costly.

Adequate irrigation systems have increased the productivity of land and have made it possible to utilize much unproductive land. The use of either atomic or solar energy to run plants to desalinate ocean water is being explored as a means of using salt water for land irrigation. Recognition of the importance of a water supply is evident in the inheritance patterns of many primitive societies in which the water rights to land are considered as important as the land itself.

Scientific animal-feeding techniques that include the use of cut forage crops, urea, oilseed cakes, by-products of the sugar industry, and other foods not used by humans are being promoted. Since the energy value of food from animal sources is only one third that of the vegetable crops fed, the use of animal foods is economically unsound under conditions of land pressures unless animals eat food that could not otherwise be used for human consumption or graze on lands that are suitable for grazing only. Control of animal diesases, such as hoof-and-mouth disease, rinderpest, hog cholera, and tuberculosis, is now possible, but losses from these causes still account for 15% to 20% of annual animal food production.

The potential of the sea, which now provides 1% of calories and 3% of protein in the world food supply, as a source of food has been considered, but opinions vary as to its feasibility. Those who maintain that it represents an untapped resource point to the fact that the sea is capable of yielding over 126 million metric tons of fish per year compared to the current production of 55 million metric tons and a projected need of 96 million metric tons in 1985. They also point to the feasibility of harvesting small fish otherwise unfit for human food that can be utilized in the production of fish protein concentrate (FPC), a powder containing 90% protein. This product (deodorized and defatted) has been suggested as an addition to basic cereal products, such as noodles, breads, and pasta, in which the FPC is incorporated with the basic cereal to provide a product with protein of enhanced biological value.

Those less optimistic about the potential of the sea as a source of protein point to the role of small fish in the food chain and suggest that by removing the small fish, we will eventually decrease the size of the herd of large fish—a more acceptable source of protein. They also point to the restrictions that have already been placed on the size of the catch of big fish to preserve the larger species. In addition, they indicate the need for considerable advances in food technology if we are to utilize the potential of the sea.

Aquaculture is now recognized as a separate field of agriculture, and this discipline is concentrating on the development of new species and methods that can be employed to maximize the potential of the sea as a source of food. The Food and Agricultural Organization has promoted the development of fish ponds in which either brackish water or freshwater can be used for the cultivation of freshwater fish. Yields as high as 4.5 metric tons per acre have been reported from properly fertilized ponds. Even higher yields are obtained if flowing water prevents the buildup of wastes and oxygen depletion.

Supplementation of food either with synthetically produced nutrients or with concentrates of natural foods holds promise. The enrichment of rice with thiamin, riboflavin, niacin, and iron; the iodization of salt; the enrichment of wheat and rice with the amino acid lysine; the addition of FPC to cereal products; and the addition soybean hydrolysates to infant foods are examples although each has its inherent limitations. The effectiveness of an enrichment program depends on its use with a staple food product that is bought from major production sources, rather than produced in many small places, and that can be purchased by all economic segments of the population. Decentralization of rice milling and an unfavorable taxation system have been a deterrent to the success of rice enrichment in the Philippines. Similarly, in India the value of adding lysine to milled wheat has been minimal because it has been impossible to provide the machinery and control necessary in a multitude of small mills. There are many investigations into the feasibility of employing salt, a universally used product that even the very poor must buy, as a carrier for enrichment nutrients, such as fluorine, vitamin A, or iron.

Incentives for increased food production must be present. These must be great enough to overcome the old habits, customs, and traditions on which existing food production is based. In some cases marked changes in the social structure may be involved—changes that have profound implications. In any case, increases in food production must be accompanied by comparable advances in facilities for the storage and distribution of crops.

Activities of international organizations

The World Health Organization (WHO) is primarily concerned with combatting disease and other health problems and strengthening national health services. Since nutrition plays a significant role in combating infection and reducing infant mortality and morbidity, WHO has cooperated with other agencies in seeking means of improving nutritional intakes. Much of their effort has been focused on improvement of infant and maternal nutrition, and this is undertaken primarily through the medical profession, rather than on a direct contact basis.

The Food and Agricultrual Organization (FAO), first organized under the auspices of the United Nations, has been charged with the responsibility to increase food production, to encourage agricultural practices that will increase food production and will result in a more equitable distribution of food for the world population, and to improve the nutritional status of rural populations in underdeveloped areas of the world. Working in conjunction with WHO, they have formulated practical dietary standards for energy, protein, calcium, iron, vitamin A, thiamin, riboflavin, niacin, folacin, and vitamin B_{12}. They believe that these standards are compatible with a high level of health and that it is within the potential of the world to produce this level of intake.

The United Nation's Children's Emergency Fund (UNICEF), another organization within the United Nations, has focused its attention on the nutritional needs of children. It was responsible for the distribution of protein-rich foodstuffs in infant-and child-feeding projects throughout food-deficit areas of the world. It has also promoted school gardens through the provision of seeds and tools.

Most recently the World Food Council, formed in 1974, is responsible for directing world food reserves and money to needy nations to forestall food shortages and the threat of starvation.

Many other agencies sponsored by both private and government groups have contributed to the solution of the nutritional concerns of the developing nations.

• • •

In summary, one can say that in 1979 we find ourselves at both a national and an international level with a vast fund of nutritional knowledge but with stark evidence that much of this is not being used for the betterment of human health. Many questions at the level of basic nutritional knowledge are still unanswered, but the gap between the knowledge we have and the application of this knowledge is even more disconcerting. Correction of this situation is going to call for a united effort on the part of nutritionists working with anthropologists, sociologists, and agriculturists as well as biological and physical scientists. The challenge in terms of the alleviation of human suffering is ever present.

BIBLIOGRAPHY

Altschul, A. M.: Food proteins: new sources from seeds, Science **158**:221, 1967.

Burkitt, D. P.: Economic development—not all bonus, Nutr. Today **11**:6, 1976.

Buzina, R. : Growth and development of three Yugoslav populations in different ecological settings, Am. J. Clin. Nutr. **29**:1051, 1976.

Chancellor, W. J., and Goss, J. R.: Balancing energy and food production, 1975-2000, Science **192**:213, 1976.

Cloud, W.: After the green revolution, Science **13**:6, 1973.

Coon, J. M.: Natural food toxicants—a perspective, Nutr. Rev. **32**:321, 1974.

Cottam, H. R.: The World Food Conference: "Perceptions 1974" in perspective, J. Am. Diet. Assoc. **66**:333, 1975.

Darby, W. J.: Nutrition, food needs and technologic priorities: the World Food Conference, Nutr. Rev. **33**:225, 1975.

Darby, W. J., and Heimbraeus, L.: Proposed nutritional guidelines for utilization of industrially produced nutrients, Nutr. Rev. **36**:65, 1978.

Dietary goals for the United States, Nutr. Rev. **35**:122, 1977.

Dwyer, J. T., and Mayer, J.: Beyond economics and nutrition: the complex basis of food policy, Science **188**:566, 1975.

Emery, K. O., and Iselin, C. O. D.: Human food from ocean and land, Science **157**:1279, 1967.

Ennis, W. B., Jr., Dowler, W. M., and Klassen, W.: Crop protection to increase food supplies, Science **188**:593, 1975.

Food and Drug Administration: Vitamin and mineral products—labeling and composition regulations. Fed. Reg. **41**(203):46156, 1976.

Freedom From Hunger Campaign: Basic Study No. 7, Population and food supply, 1963; No. 10, Possibilities of increasing world food production, 1963; No. 11, Third World Food Survey, 1963; No. 12, Malnutrition and disease, 1963; No. 14, Hunger and social policy, 1963; No. 15, Education and agricultural development, 1964; and No. 22, Manual on food and nutrition policy, Rome, 1969, Food and Agricultural Organization.

Goldsmith, G. A.: Nutrition and world health, J. Am. Diet. Assoc. **63**:513, 1973.

Guthrie, H. A.. : Infant and maternal nutrition in four Tagalog communities, Institute of Philippine Culture Papers, No. 7, p. 60, 1969.

Greecher, C. P., and Shannon, B.: Impact of fast food meals on nutrient intake of two groups, J. Am. Diet. Assoc. **70**:368, 1977.

Harper, A. E.: Nutritional regulations and legislation—past developments, future implications, J. Am. Diet. Assoc. **71**:601, 1977.

Harper, A. E.: Dietary goals—a skeptical view, Am. J. Clin. Nutr. **31**:310, 1978.

Hegsted, D. M.: Priorities in nutrition in the United States, J. Am. Diet. Assoc. **71**:9, 1977.

Hegsted, D. M.: Dietary goals—a progressive view, Am. J. Clin. Nutr. **31**:1504, 1978.

Hirst, E.: Food related energy requirements, Science **184**:134, 1974.

Indicative world plan for agricultural development, vols. 1 to 3, Rome, 1969, Food and Agricultural Organization.

Johnson, P. E.: Misuse in foods of useful chemicals, Nutr. Rev. **35**:225, 1977.

Jukes, T. H.: Megavitamin therapy, J.A.M.A. **233**:550, 1975.

Kallen, D.: Nutrition and society, J.A.M.A. **215**:94, 1971.

Kelsay, J. L.: A compendium of nutritional status studies and dietary evaluation studies conducted in the United States, 1957-1967, J. Nutr. **99:**119, 1969.

Lee, P. R.: Nutrition policy—from neglect and uncertainty to debate and action, J. Am. Diet. Assoc. **72:**581, 1978.

Longhurst, R. W., and Call, D. L.: Scientific consensus, nutrition programs and economic planning, Am. J. Clin. Nutr. **28:**1177, 1975.

Mayer, J.: Toward a national nutritional policy, Science **176:**237, 1972.

Mayer, J.: White House Conference on Food, Nutrition and Health, J. Am. Diet. Assoc. **55:**553, 1969.

Mertz, E. T.:Genetic improvement of cereals, Nutr. Rev. **32:**129, 1974.

Morgan, A. F.: Nutritional status USA, Interregional Research Pub., California Agricultural Experiment Station Bull. 769, University of California, Berkeley, Calif., 1959.

Mrak, E. M.: Food science and technology: past, present, future, Nutr. Rev. **34:**193, 1976.

National Nutrition Consortium: Guidelines for a national nutrition policy, Nutr. Rev. **32:**153, 1974.

Olson, R. E.: Clinical nutrition, an interface between human ecology and internal medicine, Nutr. Rev. **36:**161, 1978.

Perspective: U.S. dietary goals, J. Nutr. Ed. **9:**152, 1977.

Pimentel, D., Hurd, L. E., Bellotti, A. C., and others: Food production and the energy crisis, Science **182:**443, 1973.

Poleman, T. T.: World food: a perspective, Science, **188:**510, 1975.

Schaefer, A.: Are we well fed? The search for the answer, Nutr. Today **4:**2, 1969.

Schrimshaw, N. S.: Meeting tomorrow's protein needs, J. Am. Diet. Assoc. **54:**94, 1969.

Spurgeon, D.: The nutrition crunch: a world view, Bull. Atomic Scientists **29**(8):50, 1973.

Stare, F. J.: Nutritional improvement and world health potential, J. Am. Diet. Assoc. **57:**107, 1970.

U.S. Department of Health, Education and Welfare: First Health and Nutrition Examination Survey, United States 1971-1972, dietary intake and biochemical findings, Rockville, Maryland, 1974, Health Resources Administration.

Ward, A. G.: Safeguarding our food, Nutr. Rev. **35:**116, 1977.

Winikoff, B.: Changing public diet, Hum. Nature **1:**60, 1978.

World Food and Nutrition Study, Washington, D.C., 1977, National Academy of Sciences.

Appendices

APPENDIX A

Glossary of terms

absorption Process by which the products of digestion are transferred from the intestinal tract into the blood and lymph or by which substances in the interstitial fluid are taken up by the cells.

achlorhydria Absence of hydrochloric acid from the gastric secretion.

acid-base balance Relationship of the acid-forming and base-forming elements in the body.

acidosis Condition caused by an accumulation of excess acid (anions) in the body or the loss of base (cations).

active transport Energy-requiring process by which a substance crosses a biological membrane.

aerobic Living or functioning in air or free oxygen. Opposite of anaerobic.

alopecia Loss of hair.

amino acid Organic compounds of carbon, hydrogen, oxygen, and nitrogen. Each amino acid molecule contains one or more amino groups ($—NH_2$) and at least one carboxyl group ($—COOH$). In addition, some amino acids (cystine and methionine) contain sulfur. Many amino acids are linked together in some definite pattern to form a molecule of protein.

anabolism Process by which substances are formed or built up. It includes all the chemical reactions that nutrients undergo in the construction of body compounds, such as blood, enzymes, muscle tissue, and fat. Opposite of catabolism.

anaerobic Living or functioning in the absence of air or free oxygen. Opposite of aerobic.

anion Ion that carries a negative electrical charge and therefore goes to the positively charged anode.

anorexia Pathological absence of appetite or hunger in spite of a need for food.

antibody One of many specific substances produced in the body to react against disease-producing or other foreign materials in the bloodstream. Some antibodies remain available for many years and help to give a person permanent immunity.

antioxidant Substance capable of chemically protecting other substances against oxidation.

antivitamin, or vitamin antagonist Substance chemically similar to a vitamin that is able to replace the vitamin in an essential compound but it not capable of performing its role.

apatite Crystals of calcium phosphate that give strength to bone or tooth matrix.

apoenzyme Protein part of an enzyme.

appetite Complex sensations by which an organism is aware of desire for and anticipation of ingestion of palatable food.

arteriosclerosis Thickening or hardening of the inner walls of the arteries.

atherosclerosis Thickening of the walls of the blood vessels by deposits of fatty materials.

basal metabolism Irreducible minimum of energy needed to carry on the body processes vital to life.

bioassay Testing performed with use of an animal or microorganism.

biosynthesis The coming together of chemical building units to form new materials in the living plant or animal.

blood serum Whole blood from which the cells and the clotting factor have been removed. It is the colorless fluid portion of the blood that separates when blood clots.

buffer Substance that can help a solution resist or counteract changes in free acid or alkali concentration. Many buffers in the body help maintain the acid-base balance compatible with life.

calcification Process by which organic tissue becomes hardened by a deposit of calcium salts.

calorimeter Instrument for measuring heat changes in any system.

calorimetry Science of measuring heat.

carbon Chemical element present in all substances designated as organic. These include proteins, carbohydrates, and fats. When a compound containing carbon combines with oxygen in the body, energy is liberated and carbon dioxide is formed. Compounds that do not contain carbon are classed as inorganic.

carbon dioxide Compound that is formed when carbon combines with oxygen. It leaves the body chiefly when air is exhaled from the lungs.

cartilage Special form of white connective tissue attached to the ends of bones that are either divided into joints or united by joints. It is more flexible than but not as strong as bone. Cartilage is the first substance to form in growing bone; then calcium and phosphorus are deposited in the cartilage to change it to bone.

catabolism The breaking down in the body of chemical compounds into simpler ones, usually accompanied by the production of heat. Opposite of anabolism.

catalyst Substance that speeds up the rate of a chemical reaction but is not itself used up in the reaction.

cation Ion that carries a positive electrical charge and migrates to the negatively charged pole.

cell Smallest structural unit of living material.

cheilosis Condition characterized by lesions of the lips and corners of the mouth.

chlorophyll Magnesium-containing green coloring matter present in growing plants, which under stimulus of light is active in the manufacture of carbohydrates from carbon dioxide and water in a process known as photosynthesis.

chylomicrons Very small (micro) globules of fat of varying sizes in transport in the blood.

coenzymes Enzyme usually containing a vitamin that activates or combines with another enzyme to give a substance with enzyme activity.

collagen Protein that forms the chief constituent of connective tissue, cartilage, tendon, bone, and skin. Collagen is changed to gelatin by the action of water and heat.

colostrum Thin, watery, yellowish fluid secreted during the first few days of lactation.

combustion Combination of substances with oxygen, accompanied by the liberation of energy.

congenital Existing at or near birth.

cytoplasm Substance enclosed within the cell membrane, exclusive of the nucleus.

deamination Removal of an amino (NH_2) group from an amino acid.

decalcification Withdrawal of calcium from the bones or teeth where it has been deposited.

dehydrogenation Removal of hydrogen from a molecule.

denaturation Physical or chemical alteration of the natural properties of a substance.

dermatitis Inflammation of the surface of the skin.

digestion Process by which complex food nutrients are changed or hydrolyzed into smaller units that can be absorbed and used by the body.

eclampsia Convulsions occurring during pregnancy or at delivery.

edema Swelling of a part of or the entire body caused by the accumulation of excess water.

electrolyte Any substance that dissociates into ions when dissolved.

element Any one of the fundamental atoms of which all matter is composed.

endemic Occurring infrequently but more or less constantly in a particular region or population.

endocrine Secreting internally or into the bloodstream, as in endocrine glands, or glands of internal secretion.

endogenous Originating within or inside the cells or tissues.

endoplasmic reticulum System of membranes within the cell that permits exchange of substances among the cytoplasm, the nucleus, and the extracellular fluid.

enrichment Addition of nutrients to cereals to replace those lost during processing.

enzymatic Related to that class of complex organic substances called enzymes, such as amylase and pepsin, that accelerate (catalyze) specific chemical reactions in plants and animals, as in digestion of foods.

enzyme Protein produced by living tissue to accelerate metabolic reactions. Identified by the suffix "ase" and a prefix indicating the substrate on which it acts.

epithelial Those cells that form the outer layer of the skin or those that line all the portions of the body that have contact with the external air, such as the eyes, ears, nose, throat, and lungs.

erythrocyte Mature red blood cell.

erythropoiesis Process by which red blood cells are produced.

etiology Theory or study of the causes of a disease or a disorder.

exogenous Originating or produced from outside.

exudation Abnormal outpouring of a substance that becomes deposited in or on tissues.

fabricated foods Foods prepared principally from ingredients specifically designed to achieve a particular function not possible with common food ingredients. They may or may not be analogous to conventional or formulated foods.

fetus Unborn young or embryo of animals in the later stages of their development before birth (adj, fetal).

flora (intestinal) Bacteria and other small organisms that are found in the intestinal contents.

Food and Agriculture Organization (FAO) Branch of the United Nations concerned with problems of food supply and distribution on a worldwide basis to help provide an adequate level of nutrition for all people.

Food and Nutrition Board Group of scientists in foods and nutrition or related fields who act in an advisory capacity to the National Research Council of the National Academy of Sciences.

formulated foods Mixtures of two or more foodstuffs or ingredients other than seasonings, processed or blended together.

fortification Addition of nutrients to foods other than cereals to replace those lost during processing.

geriatrics Branch of medicine, concerned with the diseases and problems of old age and the aging.

gerontology Study of aging and of the problems (including social problems) of the aged.

gluconeogenesis Formation of glucose from noncarbohydrate substances, such as amino acids or glycerol.

goitrogen Substance that produces goiter.

health food Encompasses both natural and organic foods. Used very loosely.

hepatic Pertaining to the liver.

homeostasis Steady biochemical states in the body maintained by physiological processes.

hormone Chemical substance that is produced in an organ called an endocrine gland and is transported by the blood or other body fluids to other cells. A hormone greatly influences the functions of some specific organs and of the body as a whole.

hunger Complex of unpleasant sensations felt after prolonged food deprivation that will impel an animal or human to seek, work for, or fight for immediate relief by ingestion of food.

hydrogenation Addition of hydrogen to any unsaturated compound. Oils are changed to solid fats by hydrogenation.

hydrolysis Splitting of a substance into the smaller units of which it is composed by the addition of the elements of water. For example, when starch is heated in water containing a small amount of acid or is subjected to the action of digestive enzymes, the simpler sugar glucose is released.

hyperplasia Increase in cell number.

hypertrophy Enlargement in size.

hypervitaminosis Condition in which the level of a vitamin in the blood or tissues is high enough to cause undesirable symptoms.

ingest To eat or take in through the mouth.

isocaloric Having the same energy value.

ketogenesis Formation of ketones from fatty acids and some amino acids.

ketosis Condition resulting from the incomplete oxidation of fatty acids and consequent accumulation of ketones (compounds containing a CO grouping) in the blood.

labile Unstable; easily decomposed.

lactation Secretion of milk or the period during which milk is formed.

lactic acid Three-carbon acid produced through the anaerobic metabolism of glucose during muscle exercise or from the bacterial fermentation of lactose in milk.

lecithin Phospholipid occurring in animal and plant tissue.

lipase Enzyme that acts on fat to hydrolyze it into component parts.

lipids Broad term for fats and fatlike substances; characterized by the presence of one or more fatty acids. Lipids include fats, cholesterol, lecithins, phospholipids, and similar substances that do not mix readily with water.

lipogenesis Formation of lipid or fat.

lumen The interior of the gastrointestinal tract.

lymph Fluid circulating in the lymphatic system containing cells and lipid.

lysosome (perinuclear dense body) Organelle of the cell that contains enzymes capable of destroying the cell.

macrocyte Abnormally large red blood cell.

matrix Intercellular framework of a tissue.

membrane Thin, soft, pliable layer of animal or

vegetable tissue, usually composed of layers of protein and lipid.

metabolism All the chemical changes that occur from the time nutrients are absorbed until they are built into body substances or are excreted. This term includes both anabolism and catabolism.

micelle Microscopic particle of lipid and bile salts.

microsome Any one of the organelles of the cell.

microorganisms Very small living cells, such as bacteria, yeasts, and molds.

mitochondrion Organelle of the cell in which most of the transformation of energy occurs.

mucosa Mucous membrane in an epithelial tissue that lines the passages and cavities of the body, such as the gastrointestinal tract and the respiratory tract. It usually has the ability to secrete.

National Research Council (NRC) Group of leading scientists appointed by the National Academy of Sciences to coordinate the efforts of major scientific and technical societies of the United States to serve science and government.

natural foods Made from ingredients of plant or animal origin that are altered as little as possible and contain no synthetic or artificial ingredients or additives.

neonatal Pertaining to the newborn.

nutrient density Nutrient content expressed in terms of caloric value of a serving related to a standard such as the RDA for calories and nutrients.

nutritional enhancement Addition of nutrients to foods by fortification or restoration.

organelle Part or division of a cell that has a definite structure and function within the cell.

organic acids Acids containing only carbon, hydrogen, and oxygen. Among the best known are citric acid (in citrus fruits) and acetic acid (in vinegar).

organic foods Plant products grown in soil enriched with humus and compost on which no pesticides, herbicides, or inorganic fertilizers have been used or meat products from animals raised on "natural" foods and not treated with drugs such as hormones or antibiotics.

orthomolecular medicine Treatment or prevention of disease by altering body concentration of certain normally occurring substances.

osmosis Transfer of materials that takes place through a semipermeable membrane separating two solutions or between a solvent and a solution, tending to equalize their concentrations. The walls of living cells are semipermeable membranes, and much of the activity of the cells depends on osmosis.

ossification Process of forming bone. Cartilage is made into bone by the process of ossification. The minerals calcium and phosphorus are deposited in the cartilage, changing it into bone.

oxidation Removal of electrons in the most general sense; it may also mean the combining with oxygen or the removal of hydrogen.

parturition Giving birth to a child.

passive transport Process by which a substance crosses a biological membrane by diffusion or without the use of energy.

peristalsis Rhythmic wavelike movement of the intestinal wall, which moves food forward.

phagocyte Cell that can engulf particles or cells that are foreign or harmful to the body. Phagocytes are present in the blood and lymph and also in the lungs, liver, and spleen.

phosphorylate Chemical term that applies to the introduction of a phosphate group into a complex chemical compound.

photosynthesis Process by which the chlorophyll of green plants utilizes the energy from the sun to synthesize carbohydrate from carbon dioxide and water.

physiological Refers to the science of physiology, which deals with functions of living organisms or their parts.

pica Consumption of nonfood items.

pituitary gland Gland in the lower part of the brain that produces a number of hormones that regulate the growth of all body tissues and regulate the development and action of other endocrine glands, such as the thyroid, pancreas, and adrenal glands.

placenta Organ on the wall of the uterus (womb) to which the developing young animal is attached by means of the umbilical cord. Nourishment is transferred from the maternal organism to the fetus and fetal waste products are returned to the maternal circulation through it.

plasma Colorless fluid portion of the blood from which the cells have been removed.

portal vein Blood vessel leading from the wall of the intestine to the liver.

prosthetic group Nonprotein portion of an enzyme.

protease Enzyme that catalyzes the hydrolysis of protein into amino acids.

protein efficiency ratio (PER) Gain in body weight per gram of protein consumed. Standardized procedures are available, such as using diets containing 9.09% protein. Values are generally measured using rats.

protoplasm Living matter possessing capability for growth, repair, and reproduction. It is composed of water, inorganic salts, and organic compounds.

radical In chemistry, a group of elements joined in a set formation, which appears as a unit in a series of compounds or behaves as one piece without decomposition in chemical reactions. Examples are the glycerol radical in fats, the carboxyl group in organic acids, and the phenol radical (benzene ring) in certain amino acids. Amino acids themselves act as larger radicals in making up proteins.

Recommended Dietary Allowances (RDA) Quantities of specified vitamins, minerals and protein needed daily that have been judged adequate for maintenance of good nutrition in the United States population, developed by the National Academy of Sciences, National Research Council.

renal Pertaining to the kidneys.

restoration Addition of selected nutrients to breakfast cereals to approximate the levels of these nutrients in the finished product as were present in the whole grain before processing. Thiamin, niacin, and iron are added most commonly.

reticulocyte Young red blood cell.

reticuloendothelial system Liver, spleen, and bone marrow.

ribosome Organelle of a cell responsible for protein synthesis. It frequently occurs in groupings known as polyribosomes, polysomes, or ergosomes.

safe level of protein intake Amount of protein considered necessary to meet the physiological needs and maintain the health of nearly all individuals in a specified age/sex group.

satiety Cessation of desire for further nourishment at the end of the meal.

saturated State in which a substance holds all of another substance that it can.

serum Fluid portion of the blood that separates from the blood cells after clotting.

syndrome Medical term meaning a group of symptoms that occur together.

synthesis Process by which a new substance is formed from its individual parts.

toxicity Quality of a substance that makes it poisonous, or toxic; it sometimes refers to the degree of severity of the poison or the possibility of being poisonous.

transamination Transfer of an amino group from an amino acid to another molecule, usually to a different amino acid.

transmethylation Transfer of a methyl (CH_3) group from one molecule to another.

trimester Three months or one third of the nine months of pregnancy. The nine months of pregnancy are divided into the first, second, and third trimesters.

urinary Occurring in the urine.

U.S. Recommended Daily Allowances (U.S. RDA) A standard set of daily quantities of specified vitamins, minerals, and protein judged to be essential in human nutrition by the Food and Drug Administration. Values are taken from the Recommended Dietary Allowances developed by the Food and Nutrition Board of the National Academy of Sciences, National Research Council, as published by FDA on March 14, 1973.

vegan Individual who eats only foods of vegetable origin and share a philosophy and life-style with others.

whole-grain cereal Cereal that contains all parts of the kernel of the grain from which it is made.

APPENDIX B

Meaning of prefixes and suffixes used in nutrition terms

Prefix	Meaning	Example
a-	lack of	avitaminosis
ab-	away from	abnormal
ad-	toward	addiction
amyl-	starch	amylose
an-	negative, lack of	anemia
ante-	before, preceding	antenatal
anti-	against	antibiotic
bi-	two, double	bilateral
calori-	heat	calorimetry
co-	with	coenzymes
di-	in two parts	disaccharides
dys-	bad	dysentery
endo-	within	endogenous
epi-	upon, on, over, above	epithelium
ex-	out	exogenous
heme-	iron-containing	hemoglobin
hepato-	pertaining to the liver	hepatitis
hyper-	excessive, above	hyperactive
hypo-	under	hypothyroidism
iso-	the same	isocaloric
lacto-	pertaining to milk	lactose
lip-	fat	lipid
leuko-	white	leukocyte
mono-	one	monosaccharide
neo-	new	neonatal
os-	bone	osteoblast
pan-	all, entire	panacea
peri-	around, on all sides	pericardium
poly-	many	polyneuritis
post-	after, behind	postnatal
ren-	kidney	renal
syn-	with, together	synthesis
tachy-	rapid	tachycardia
thio-	containing sulfur	thiamin
tox-	poison	toxemia

Suffix	Meaning	Example
-algia	suffering, pain	neuralgia
-ase	enzyme	protease
-blast	cell that builds	osteoblast
-cide	causing death	pesticide
-clast	cell that destroys	osteoclast
-cyte	mature cell	erythrocyte
-ectomy	removal	thyroidectomy
-emia	blood	anemia
-gen	get or produce	antigen
-genesis	produce	glucogenesis
-gram	tracing or mark	cardiogram
-graph	instrument	cardiograph
-ia, iasis	disease of	cholelithiasis
-itis	inflammation of	hepatitis
-logy	study of	biology
-lysis	solution, breakdown	hydrolysis
-meter	instrument for measuring	calorimeter
-oid	like	lipoid
-oma	tumor, swelling	adenoma
-osis	disease of, state or condition	fluorosis
-pathy	suffering, disease	osteopathy
-phagia	swallowing, eating	hyperphagia
-phobia	fear of, antagonism	hydrophobia
-plasty	repair of	rhinoplasty
-rhea	flow, discharge	steatorrhea
-tomy	cut into	appendectomy

APPENDIX C

Food and Nutrition Board, National Academy of Sciences–National Research Council recommended daily dietary allowances,* revised 1974

*It is anticipated that the ninth revision will be available late in the spring of 1979. It may be obtained from the Food and Nutrition Board, National Academy of Sciences, 2100 Constitution Avenue, Washington, D. C. Preliminary reports indicate there will be no changes for the majority of nutrients and only minor ones for a few.

Designed for the maintenance of good nutrition of practically all healthy people in the United States*

								Fat-soluble vitamins			
	Age (years)	Weight (kg)	Weight (lb)	Height (cm)	Height (in)	Energy (kcal)†	Protein (g)	Vitamin A activity (RE)‡	Vitamin A activity (IU)	Vitamin D (IU)	Vitamin E activity‖ (IU)
Infants	0.0-0.5	6	14	60	24	kg × 117	kg × 2.2	420§	1400	400	4
	0.5-1.0	9	20	71	28	kg × 108	kg × 2.0	400	2000	400	5
Children	1-3	13	28	86	34	1300	23	400	2000	400	7
	4-6	20	44	110	44	1800	30	500	2500	400	9
	7-10	30	66	135	54	2400	36	700	3300	400	10
Males	11-14	44	97	158	63	2800	44	1000	5000	400	12
	15-18	61	134	172	69	3000	54	1000	5000	400	15
	19-22	67	147	172	69	3000	54	1000	5000	400	15
	23-50	70	154	172	69	2700	56	1000	5000	—	15
	51+	70	154	172	69	2400	56	1000	5000	—	15
Females	11-14	44	97	155	62	2400	44	800	4000	400	10
	15-18	54	119	162	65	2100	48	800	4000	400	11
	19-22	58	128	162	65	2100	46	800	4000	400	12
	23-50	58	128	162	65	2000	46	800	4000	—	12
	51+	58	128	162	65	1800	46	800	4000	—	12
Pregnant						+300	+30	1000	5000	400	15
Lactating						+500	+20	1200	6000	400	15

*The allowances are intended to provide for individual variations among most normal persons as they live in the United nutrients for which human requirements have been less well defined. See text for more detailed discussion of allowances and

†Kilojoules (KJ) = 4.2 × kcal.

‡Retinol equivalents.

§Assumed to be as retinol in milk during the first six months of life. All subsequent intakes are assumed to be one half as retinol and one fourth as β-carotene.

‖Total vitamin E activity, estimated to be 80% as α-tocopherol and 20% other tocopherols.

¶The folacin allowances refer to dietary sources as determined by *Lactobacillus casei* assay. Pure forms of folacin may be

** Although allowances are expressed as niacin, it is recognized that on the average 1 mg of niacin is derived from each

††This increased requirement cannot be met by ordinary diets; therefore, the use of supplemental iron is recommended.

Water-soluble vitamins							Minerals					
Ascorbic acid (mg)	Folacin¶ (μg)	Niacin** (mg)	Riboflavin (mg)	Thiamin (mg)	Vitamin B_6 (mg)	Vitamin B_{12} (μg)	Calcium (mg)	Phosphorus (mg)	Iodine (μg)	Iron (mg)	Magnesium (mg)	Zinc (mg)
35	50	5	0.4	0.3	0.3	0.3	360	240	35	10	60	3
35	50	8	0.6	0.5	0.4	0.3	540	400	45	15	70	5
40	100	9	0.8	0.7	0.6	1.0	800	800	60	15	150	10
40	200	12	1.1	0.9	0.9	1.5	800	800	80	10	200	10
40	300	16	1.2	1.2	1.2	2.0	800	800	110	10	250	10
45	400	18	1.5	1.4	1.6	3.0	1200	1200	130	18	350	15
45	400	20	1.8	1.5	1.8	3.0	1200	1200	150	18	400	15
45	400	20	1.8	1.5	2.0	3.0	800	800	140	10	350	15
45	400	18	1.6	1.4	2.0	3.0	800	800	130	10	350	15
45	400	16	1.5	1.2	2.0	3.0	800	800	110	10	350	15
45	400	16	1.3	1.2	1.6	3.0	1200	1200	115	18	300	15
45	400	14	1.4	1.1	2.0	3.0	1200	1200	115	18	300	15
45	400	14	1.4	1.1	2.0	3.0	800	800	100	18	300	15
45	400	13	1.2	1.0	2.0	3.0	800	800	100	18	300	15
45	400	12	1.1	1.0	2.0	3.0	800	800	80	10	300	15
60	800	+2	+0.3	+0.3	2.5	4.0	1200	1200	125	18+††	450	20
60	600	+4	+0.5	+0.3	2.5	4.0	1200	1200	150	18	450	25

States under usual environmental stresses. Diets should be based on a variety of common foods in order to provide other of nutrients not tabulated.

retinol and one half as β-carotene when calculated from international units. As retinol equivalents, three fourths are as

effective in doses less than one fourth of the RDA.
60 mg of dietary tryptophan.

APPENDIX D

United States recommended daily allowances (U.S. RDA)*

	Adults and children 4 or more years of age (For use in labeling conventional foods and also for "special dietary foods")	Infants	Children under 4 years of age (For use only with "special dietary foods")	Pregnant or lactating women (For use only with "special dietary foods")
*Nutrients which **must** be declared on the label (in the order below)*				
Protein†	45 g "high quality protein" 65 g "proteins in general"		—	—
Vitamin A	5000 IU	1500 IU	2500 IU	8000 IU
Vitamin C (or ascorbic acid)	60 mg	35 mg	40 mg	60 mg
Thiamin (or vitamin B_1)	1.5 mg	0.5 mg	0.7 mg	1.7 mg
Riboflavin (or vitamin B_2)	1.7 mg	0.6 mg	0.8 mg	2.0 mg
Niacin	20 mg	8 mg	9 mg	20 mg
Calcium	1.0 g	0.6 g	0.8 g	1.3 g
Iron	18 mg	15 mg	10 mg	18 mg
*Nutrients which **may** be declared on the label (in the order below)*				
Vitamin D	400 IU	400 IU	400 IU	400 IU
Vitamin E	30 IU	5 IU	10 IU	30 IU
Vitamin B_6	2.0 mg	0.4 mg	0.7 mg	2.5 mg
Folic acid (or folacin)	0.4 mg	0.1 mg	0.2 mg	0.8 mg
Vitamin B_{12}	6 μg	2 μg	3 μg	8 μg
Phosphorus	1.0 g	0.5 g	0.8 g	1.3 g
Iodine	150 μg	45 μg	70 μg	150 μg
Magnesium	400 mg	70 mg	200 mg	450 mg
Zinc‡	15 mg	5 mg	8 mg	15 mg
Copper‡	2 mg	0.5 mg	1 mg	2 mg
Biotin‡	0.3 mg	0.15 mg	0.15 mg	0.3 mg
Pantothenic acid‡	10 mg	3 mg	5 mg	10 mg

*"U.S. RDA" is a new term replacing "minimum daily requirement" (MDR). The U.S. RDA values chosen are derived from the highest value for each nutrient given in the NAS-NRC tables except for calcium and phosphorus.

†"High quality protein" is defined as having a protein efficiency ratio (PER) equal to or greater than that of casein; "proteins in general" are those with a PER less than that of casein. Total protein with a PER less than 20% that of casein are considered "not a significant source of protein" and would not be expressed on the label in terms of the U.S. RDA but only as amount per serving.

‡There are no NAS-NRC RDAs for biotin, pantothenic acid, zinc, and copper.

APPENDIX E

Canadian dietary standard

Recommended daily nutrient intakes—revised 1974 committee for revision of the

Age (yr)	Sex	Weight (kg)	Height (cm)	Energy[a] (kcal)	Protein (g)	Water-soluble vitamins: Thiamin (mg)	Niacin[e] (mg)	Riboflavin (mg)	Vit. B_6[f] (mg)	Folate[g] (μg)
0-6 mo	Both	6	—	kg × 117	kg × 2.2 (2.0)[d]	0.3	5	0.4	0.3	40
7-11 mo	Both	9	—	kg × 108	kg × 1.4	0.5	6	0.6	0.4	60
1-3	Both	13	90	1400	22	0.7	9	0.8	0.8	100
4-6	Both	19	110	1800	27	0.9	12	1.1	1.3	100
7-9	M	27	129	2200	33	1.1	14	1.3	1.6	100
	F	27	128	2000	33	1.0	13	1.2	1.4	100
10-12	M	36	144	2500	41	1.2	17	1.5	1.8	100
	F	38	145	2300	40	1.1	15	1.4	1.5	100
13-15	M	51	162	2800	52	1.4	19	1.7	2.0	200
	F	49	159	2200	43	1.1	15	1.4	1.5	200
16-18	M	64	172	3200	54	1.6	21	2.0	2.0	200
	F	54	161	2100	43	1.1	14	1.3	1.5	200
19-35	M	70	176	3000	56	1.5	20	1.8	2.0	200
	F	56	161	2100	41	1.1	14	1.3	1.5	200
36-50	M	70	176	2700	56	1.4	18	1.7	2.0	200
	F	56	161	1900	41	1.0	13	1.2	1.5	200
51+	M	70	176	2300[b]	56	1.4	18	1.7	2.0	200
	F	56	161	1800[b]	41	1.0	13	1.2	1.5	200
Pregnant				+300[c]	+20	+0.2	+2	+0.3	+0.5	+50
Lactating				+500	+24	+0.4	+7	+0.6	+0.6	+50

*Canadian Council on Nutrition: Dietary standards for Canada, Can. Bull. Nutr. **6**:1, 1964 (suppl. 1974).

[a]Recommendations assume characteristic activity pattern for each age group.

[b]Recommended energy allowance for age 66+ years reduced to 2000 for men and 1500 for women.

[c]Increased energy allowance recommended during second and third trimesters. An increase of 100 kcal per day is recommended during first

[d]Recommended protein allowance of 2.2 g/kg of body weight for infants age 0 to 2 mo and 2.0 g/kg of body weight for those age 3 to 5 mo.

[e]Approximately 1 mg of niacin is derived from each 60 mg of dietary tryptophan.

[f]Recommendations are based on the estimated average daily protein intake of Canadians.

[g]Recommendation given in terms of free folate.

[h]Considerably higher levels may be prudent for infants during the first week of life to guard against neonatal tyrosinemia.

[i]One μg retinol equivalent (1 μg RE) corresponds to a biological activity in humans equal to 1 μg of retinol (3.33 IU) and 6 μg of β-carotene

[j]One μg cholecalciferol is equivalent to 40 IU vitamin D activity.

[k]Most older children and adults receive enough vitamin D from irradiation but 2.5 μg daily is recommended. This recommended allowance periods.

[l]The intake of breast-fed infants may be less than the recommendation but is considered to be adequate.

[m]A recommended total intake of 15 mg daily during pregnancy and lactation assumes the presence of adequate stores of iron. If stores are

Canadian dietary standard, bureau of nutritional sciences, health and welfare Canada*

		Fat-soluble vitamins			Minerals					
Vit. B_{12} (μg)	Ascorbic acid (mg)	Vit. A (μg RE)[i]	Vit. D (μg choelcal-ciferol)[j]	Vit. E (mg α-to-copherol)	Ca (mg)	P (mg)	Mg (mg)	I (μg)	Fe (mg)	Zn (mg)
0.3	20[h]	400	10	3	500[l]	250[l]	50[l]	35[l]	7[l]	4[l]
0.3	20	400	10	3	500	400	50	50	7	5
0.9	20	400	10	4	500	500	75	70	8	5
1.5	20	500	5	5	500	500	100	90	9	6
1.5	30	700	2.5[k]	6	700	700	150	110	10	7
1.5	30	700	2.5[k]	6	700	700	150	100	10	7
3.0	30	800	2.5[k]	7	900	900	175	130	11	8
3.0	30	800	2.5[k]	7	1000	1000	200	120	11	9
3.0	30	1000	2.5[k]	9	1200	1200	250	140	13	10
3.0	30	800	2.5[k]	7	800	800	250	110	14	10
3.0	30	1000	2.5[k]	10	1000	1000	300	160	14	12
3.0	30	800	2.5[k]	6	700	700	250	110	14	11
3.0	30	1000	2.5[k]	9	800	800	300	150	10	10
3.0	30	800	2.5[k]	6	700	700	250	110	14	9
3.0	30	1000	2.5[k]	8	800	800	300	140	10	10
3.0	30	800	2.5[k]	6	700	700	250	100	14	9
3.0	30	1000	2.5[k]	8	800	800	300	140	10	10
3.0	30	800	2.5[k]	6	700	700	250	100	9	9
+1.0	+20	+100	+2.5[k]	+1	+500	+500	+25	+15	+1[m]	+3
+0.5	+30	+400	+2.5[k]	+2	+500	+500	+75	+25	+1[m]	+7

trimester.
Protein recommendation for infants, 0 to 11 mo, assumes consumption of breast milk or protein of equivalent quality.

(10 IU).

increases to 5.0 μg daily for pregnant and lactating women and for those who are confined indoors or otherwise deprived of sunlight for extended

suspected of being inadequate, additional iron as a supplement is recommended.

APPENDIX F

Desirable weights for height for adults

Desirable weights for men 25 years of age and over*†

Height with shoes on (1-inch heels)				
Feet	Inches	Small frame	Medium frame	Large frame
5	2	112-120	118-129	126-141
5	3	115-123	121-133	129-144
5	4	118-126	124-136	132-148
5	5	121-129	127-139	135-152
5	6	124-133	130-143	138-156
5	7	128-137	134-147	142-161
5	8	132-141	138-152	147-166
5	9	136-145	142-156	151-170
5	10	140-150	146-160	155-174
5	11	144-154	150-165	159-179
6	0	148-158	154-170	164-184
6	1	152-162	158-175	168-189
6	2	156-167	162-180	173-194
6	3	160-171	167-185	178-199
6	4	164-175	172-190	182-204

*Courtesy Metropolitan Life Insurance Co., How to control your weight, New York, 1960 supplement. Based on 1959 Build and blood pressure study.
†Weight in pounds, according to frame (in indoor clothing).

Desirable weights for women 25 years of age and over*†

Height with shoes on (2-inch heels)		Small frame	Medium frame	Large frame
Feet	Inches			
4	10	92-98	96-107	104-119
4	11	94-101	98-110	106-122
5	0	96-104	101-113	109-125
5	1	99-107	104-116	112-128
5	2	102-110	107-119	115-131
5	3	105-113	110-122	118-134
5	4	108-116	113-126	121-138
5	5	111-119	116-130	125-142
5	6	114-123	120-135	129-146
5	7	118-127	124-139	133-150
5	8	122-131	128-143	137-154
5	9	126-135	132-147	141-158
5	10	130-140	136-151	145-163
5	11	134-144	140-155	149-168
6	0	138-148	144-159	153-173

*Courtesy Metropolitan Life Insurance Co., How to control your weight, New York, 1960 supplement. Based on 1959 Build and blood pressure study.

†Weight in pounds, according to frame (in indoor clothing).

APPENDIX G

Table of food composition

Nutritive values of the edible part of foods*†

Foods, approximate measures, units, and weight in grams (edible part unless footnotes indicate otherwise)			Water (%)	Food energy (kcal)	Protein (g)	Fat (g)	Fatty acids		
							Saturated (total) (g)	Unsaturated	
								Oleic (g)	Linoleic (g)
DAIRY PRODUCTS (CHEESE, CREAM, IMITATION CREAM, MILK; RELATED PRODUCTS)									
Butter. See Fats, oils; related products									
Cheese									
Natural									
Blue	1 oz	28	42	100	6	8	5.3	1.9	0.2
Camembert (3 wedges per 4 oz container)	1 wedge	38	52	115	8	9	5.8	2.9	0.2
Cheddar									
Cut pieces	1 oz	28	37	115	7	9	6.1	2.1	0.2
	1 inch cube	17.2	37	70	4	6	3.7	1.3	0.1
Shredded	1 cup	113	37	455	28	37	24.2	8.5	0.7
Cottage (curd not pressed down)									
Creamed (cottage cheese, 4% fat)									
Large curd	1 cup	225	79	235	28	10	6.4	2.4	0.2
Small curd	1 cup	210	79	220	26	9	6.0	2.2	0.2
Low fat (2%)	1 cup	226	79	205	31	4	2.8	1.0	0.1
Low fat (1%)	1 cup	226	82	165	28	2	1.5	0.5	0.1
Uncreamed (cottage cheese dry curd, less than ½% fat)	1 cup	145	80	125	25	1	0.4	0.1	Trace
Cream	1 oz	28	54	100	2	10	6.2	2.4	0.2
Mozzarella, made with									
Whole milk	1 oz	28	48	90	6	7	4.4	1.7	0.2
Part skim milk	1 oz	28	49	80	8	5	3.1	1.2	0.1
Parmesan, grated									
Cup, not pressed down	1 cup	100	18	455	42	30	19.1	7.7	0.3
Tablespoon	1 tbsp	5	18	25	2	2	1.0	0.4	Trace
Ounce	1 oz	28	18	130	12	9	5.4	2.2	0.1
Provolone	1 oz	28	41	100	7	8	4.8	1.7	0.1
Ricotta, made with									
Whole milk	1 cup	246	72	1,790	28	32	20.4	7.1	0.7
Part skim milk	1 cup	246	74	340	28	19	12.1	4.7	0.5
Romano	1 oz	28	31	110	9	8	—	—	—

*From Nutritive value of foods, House and Garden Bulletin No. 72, Washington, D.C., 1977, U.S. Department of Agriculture, pp. 4 to 30.
†Dashes denote lack of reliable data for a constituent believed to be present in measurable amount.

NUTRIENTS IN INDICATED QUANTITY

Carbohydrate (g)	Calcium (mg)	Phosphorus (mg)	Iron (mg)	Potassium (mg)	Vitamin A value (IU)	Thiamin (mg)	Riboflavin (mg)	Niacin (mg)	Ascorbic acid (mg)
1	150	110	0.1	73	200	0.01	0.11	0.3	0
Trace	147	132	0.1	71	350	0.01	0.19	0.2	0
Trace	204	145	0.2	28	300	0.01	0.11	Trace	0
Trace	124	88	0.1	17	180	Trace	0.06	Trace	0
1	815	579	0.8	111	1,200	0.03	0.42	0.1	0
6	135	297	0.3	190	370	0.05	0.37	0.3	Trace
6	126	277	0.3	177	340	0.04	0.34	0.3	Trace
8	155	340	0.4	217	160	0.05	0.42	0.3	Trace
6	138	304	0.3	193	80	0.05	0.37	0.3	Trace
3	46	151	0.3	47	40	0.04	0.21	0.2	0
1	23	30	0.3	34	400	Trace	0.06	Trace	0
1	163	117	0.1	21	260	Trace	0.08	Trace	0
1	207	149	0.1	27	180	0.01	0.10	Trace	0
4	1,376	807	1.0	107	700	0.05	0.39	0.3	0
Trace	69	40	Trace	5	40	Trace	0.02	Trace	0
1	390	229	0.3	30	200	0.01	0.11	0.1	0
1	214	141	0.1	39	230	0.01	0.09	Trace	0
7	509	389	0.9	257	1,210	0.03	0.48	0.3	0
13	669	449	1.1	308	1,060	0.05	0.46	0.2	0
1	302	215	—	—	160	—	0.11	Trace	0

Continued.

Nutritive values of the edible part of food—cont'd

Foods, approximate measures, units, and weight in grams (edible part unless footnotes indicate otherwise)			Water (%)	Food energy (kcal)	Protein (g)	Fat (g)	Fatty acids		
							Saturated (total) (g)	Unsaturated	
								Oleic (g)	Linoleic (g)
Swiss	1 oz	28	37	105	8	8	5.0	1.7	0.2
Pasteurized process cheese									
American	1 oz	28	39	105	6	9	5.6	2.1	0.2
Swiss	1 oz	28	42	95	7	7	4.5	1.7	0.1
Pasteurized process cheese food, American	1 oz	28	43	95	6	7	4.4	1.7	0.1
Pasteurized process cheese spread, American	1 oz	28	48	82	5	6	3.8	1.5	0.1
Cream, sweet									
Half-and-half (cream and milk)	1 cup	242	81	315	7	28	17.3	7.0	0.6
	1 tbsp	15	81	20	Trace	2	1.1	0.4	Trace
Light, coffee, or table	1 cup	240	74	470	6	46	28.8	11.7	1.0
	1 tbsp	15	74	30	Trace	3	1.8	0.7	0.1
Whipping, unwhipped (volume about double when whipped)									
Light	1 cup	239	64	700	5	74	46.2	18.3	1.5
	1 tbsp	15	64	45	Trace	5	2.9	1.1	0.1
Heavy	1 cup	238	58	820	5	38	54.8	22.2	2.0
	1 tbsp	15	58	80	Trace	6	3.5	1.4	0.1
Whipped topping (pressurized)	1 cup	60	61	155	2	13	8.3	3.4	0.3
	1 tbsp	3	61	10	Trace	1	0.4	0.2	Trace
Cream, sour	1 cup	230	71	495	7	48	30.0	12.1	1.1
	1 tbsp	12	71	25	Trace	3	1.6	0.6	0.1
Cream products, imitation (made with vegetable fat)									
Sweet									
Creamers									
Liquid (frozen)	1 cup	245	77	335	2	24	22.8	0.3	Trace
	1 tbsp	15	77	20	Trace	1	1.4	Trace	0
Powdered	1 cup	94	2	515	5	33	30.6	0.9	Trace
	1 tsp	2	2	10	Trace	1	0.7	Trace	0
Whipped topping									
Frozen	1 cup	75	50	240	1	19	16.3	1.0	0.2
	1 tbsp	4	50	15	Trace	1	0.9	0.1	Trace
Powdered, made with whole milk	1 cup	80	67	150	3	10	8.5	0.6	0.1
	1 tbsp	4	67	10	Trace	Trace	0.4	Trace	Trace
Pressurized	1 cup	70	60	185	1	16	13.2	1.4	0.2
	1 tbsp	4	60	10	Trace	1	0.8	0.1	Trace
Sour dressing (imitation sour cream) made with nonfat dry milk	1 cup	235	75	415	8	39	31.2	4.4	1.1
	1 tbsp	12	75	20	Trace	2	1.6	0.2	0.1
Ice cream. See Milk desserts, frozen									
Ice milk. See Milk desserts, frozen									
Milk									
Fluid									
Whole (3.3% fat)	1 cup	244	88	150	8	8	5.1	2.1	0.2
Lowfat (2%)									
No milk solids added	1 cup	244	89	120	8	5	2.9	1.2	0.1

[1] Vitamin A value is largely from beta-carotene used for coloring. Riboflavin value for powdered imitation creamers apply to products with

[2] Applies to product without added vitamin A. With added vitamin A, value is 500 IU.

NUTRIENTS IN INDICATED QUANTITY

Carbohydrate (g)	Calcium (mg)	Phosphorus (mg)	Iron (mg)	Potassium (mg)	Vitamin A value (IU)	Thiamin (mg)	Riboflavin (mg)	Niacin (mg)	Ascorbic acid (mg)
1	272	171	Trace	31	240	0.01	0.10	Trace	0
Trace	174	211	0.1	46	340	0.01	0.10	Trace	0
1	219	216	0.2	61	230	Trace	0.08	Trace	0
2	163	130	0.2	79	260	0.01	0.13	Trace	0
2	159	202	0.1	69	220	0.01	0.12	Trace	0
10	254	230	0.2	314	260	0.08	0.36	0.2	2
1	16	14	Trace	19	20	0.01	0.02	Trace	Trace
9	231	192	0.1	292	1,730	0.08	0.36	0.01	2
1	14	12	Trace	18	110	Trace	0.02	Trace	Trace
7	166	146	0.1	231	2,690	0.06	0.30	0.1	1
Trace	10	9	Trace	15	170	Trace	0.02	Trace	Trace
7	154	149	0.1	179	3,500	0.05	0.26	0.1	1
Trace	10	9	Trace	11	220	Trace	0.02	Trace	Trace
7	61	54	Trace	88	550	0.02	0.04	Trace	0
Trace	3	3	Trace	4	30	Trace	Trace	Trace	0
10	268	195	0.1	331	1,820	0.08	0.34	0.2	2
1	14	10	Trace	17	90	Trace	0.02	Trace	Trace
28	23	157	0.1	467	[1]220	0	0	0	0
2	1	10	Trace	29	[1]10	0	0	0	0
52	21	397	0.1	763	[1]190	0	[1]0.16	0	0
1	Trace	8	Trace	16	[1]Trace	0	[1]Trace	0	0
17	5	6	0.1	14	[1]650	0	0	0	0
1	Trace	Trace	Trace	1	[1]30	0	0	0	0
13	72	69	Trace	121	[1]290	0.20	0.09	Trace	1
1	4	3	Trace	6	[1]10	Trace	Trace	Trace	Trace
11	4	13	Trace	13	[1]330	0	0	0	0
1	Trace	1	Trace	1	[1]20	0	0	0	0
11	266	205	0.1	380	[1]20	0.09	0.38	0.2	2
1	14	10	Trace	19	[1]Trace	0.01	0.02	Trace	Trace
11	291	228	0.1	370	[2]310	0.09	0.40	0.2	2
12	297	232	0.1	377	500	0.10	0.40	0.2	2

added riboflavin.

Continued.

Nutritive values of the edible part of food—cont'd

Foods, approximate measures, units, and weight in grams (edible part unless footnotes indicate otherwise)			Water (%)	Food energy (kcal)	Protein (g)	Fat (g)	Fatty acids: Saturated (total) (g)	Unsaturated: Oleic (g)	Unsaturated: Linoleic (g)
Milk solids added									
Label claim less than 10 g of protein/cup	1 cup	245	89	125	9	5	2.9	1.2	0.1
Label claim 10 or more grams of protein/cup (protein fortified)	1 cup	246	88	135	10	5	3.0	1.2	0.1
Lowfat (1%)									
No milk solids added	1 cup	244	90	100	8	3	1.6	0.7	0.1
Milk solids added									
Label claim less than 10 g of protein/cup	1 cup	245	90	105	9	2	1.5	0.6	0.1
Label claim 10 or more grams of protein/cup (protein fortified)	1 cup	246	89	120	10	3	1.8	0.7	0.1
Nonfat (skim)									
No milk solids added	1 cup	245	91	85	8	Trace	0.3	0.1	Trace
Milk solids added									
Label claim less than 10 g of protein/cup	1 cup	245	90	90	9	1	0.4	0.1	Trace
Label claim 10 or more grams of protein/cup (protein fortified)	1 cup	246	89	100	10	1	0.4	0.1	Trace
Buttermilk	1 cup	245	90	100	8	2	1.3	0.5	Trace
Canned									
Evaporated, unsweetened									
Whole milk	1 cup	252	74	340	17	19	11.6	5.3	0.4
Skim milk	1 cup	255	79	200	19	1	0.3	0.1	Trace
Sweetened, condensed	1 cup	306	27	980	24	27	16.8	6.7	0.7
Dried									
Buttermilk	1 cup	120	3	465	41	7	4.3	1.7	0.2
Nonfat instant									
Envelope, net wt, 3.2 oz[5]	1 envelope	91	4	325	32	1	0.4	0.1	Trace
Cup[7]	1 cup	68	4	245	24	Trace	0.3	0.1	Trace
Milk beverages									
Chocolate milk (commercial)									
Regular	1 cup	250	82	210	8	8	5.3	2.2	0.2
Lowfat (2%)	1 cup	250	84	180	8	5	3.1	1.3	0.1
Lowfat (1%)	1 cup	250	85	160	8	3	1.5	0.7	0.1
Eggnog (commercial)	1 cup	254	74	340	10	19	11.3	5.0	0.6

[3] Applies to product without vitamin A added.
[4] Applies to product with added vitamin A. Without added vitamin A, value is 20 IU.
[5] Yields 1 qt. of fluid milk when reconstituted according to package directions.
[6] Applies to product with added vitamin A.
[7] Weight applies to product with label claim of 1⅓ cups equal 3.2 oz.

NUTRIENTS IN INDICATED QUANTITY									
Carbohydrate (g)	Calcium (mg)	Phosphorus (mg)	Iron (mg)	Potassium (mg)	Vitamin A value (IU)	Thiamin (mg)	Riboflavin (mg)	Niacin (mg)	Ascorbic acid (mg)
12	313	245	0.1	397	500	0.10	0.42	0.2	2
14	352	276	0.1	447	500	0.11	0.48	0.2	3
12	300	235	0.1	381	500	0.10	0.41	0.2	2
12	313	245	0.1	397	500	0.10	0.42	0.2	2
14	349	273	0.1	444	500	0.11	0.47	0.2	3
12	302	247	0.1	406	500	0.09	0.37	0.2	2
12	316	255	0.1	418	500	0.10	0.43	0.2	2
14	352	275	0.1	446	500	0.11	0.48	0.2	3
12	285	219	0.1	371	[3]80	0.08	0.38	0.1	2
25	657	510	0.5	764	[3]610	0.12	0.80	0.5	5
29	738	497	0.7	845	[3]1,000	0.11	0.79	0.4	3
166	868	775	0.6	1,136	[3]1,000	0.28	1.27	0.6	8
59	1,421	1,119	0.4	1,910	[3]260	0.47	1.90	1.1	7
47	1,120	896	0.3	1,552	[6]2,160	0.38	1.59	0.8	5
35	837	670	0.2	1,160	[6]1,610	0.28	1.19	0.6	4
26	280	251	0.6	417	[3]300	0.09	0.41	0.3	2
26	284	254	0.6	422	500	0.10	0.42	0.3	2
26	287	257	0.6	426	500	0.10	0.40	0.2	2
34	330	278	0.5	420	890	0.09	0.48	0.3	4

Continued.

Nutritive values of the edible part of food—cont'd

Foods, approximate measures, units, and weight in grams (edible part unless footnotes indicate otherwise)			Water (%)	Food energy (kcal)	Protein (g)	Fat (g)	Fatty acids: Saturated (total) (g)	Fatty acids: Unsaturated: Oleic (g)	Fatty acids: Unsaturated: Linoleic (g)
Malted milk, home-prepared with 1 cup of whole milk and 2 to 3 heaping tsp of malted milk powder (about ¾ oz)									
Chocolate	1 cup of milk plus ¾ oz of powder	265	81	235	9	9	5.5	—	—
Natural	1 cup of milk plus ¾ oz of powder	265	81	235	11	10	6.0	—	—
Shakes, thick[8]									
Chocolate, container, net wt, 10.6 oz	1 container	300	72	355	9	8	5.0	2.0	0.2
Vanilla, container, net wt, 11 oz	1 container	313	74	350	12	9	5.9	2.4	0.2
Milk desserts, frozen									
Ice cream									
Regular (about 11% fat)									
Hardened	½ gal	1,064	61	2,155	38	115	71.3	28.8	2.6
	1 cup	133	61	270	5	14	8.9	3.6	0.3
	3 fl oz container	50	61	100	2	5	3.4	1.4	0.1
Soft serve (frozen custard)	1 cup	173	60	375	7	23	13.5	5.9	0.6
Rich (about 16% fat), hardened	½ gal	1,188	59	2,805	33	190	118.3	47.8	4.3
	1 cup	148	59	350	4	24	14.7	6.0	0.5
Ice milk									
Hardened (about 4.3% fat)	½ gal	1,048	69	1,470	41	45	28.1	11.3	1.0
	1 cup	131	69	185	5	6	3.5	1.4	0.1
Soft serve (about 2.6% fat)	1 cup	175	70	255	8	5	2.9	1.2	0.1
Sherbet (about 2% fat)	½ gal	1,542	66	2,160	17	31	19.0	7.7	0.7
	1 cup	193	66	270	2	4	2.4	1.0	0.1
Milk desserts, other									
Custard, baked	1 cup	265	77	305	14	15	6.8	5.4	0.7
Puddings									
From home recipe									
Starch base									
Chocolate	1 cup	260	66	385	8	12	7.6	3.3	0.3
Vanilla (blancmange)	1 cup	255	76	285	9	10	6.2	2.5	0.2
Tapioca cream	1 cup	165	72	220	8	8	4.1	2.5	0.5
From mix (chocolate) and milk									
Regular (cooked)	1 cup	260	70	320	9	8	4.3	2.6	0.2
Instant	1 cup	260	69	325	8	7	3.6	2.2	0.3
Yogurt									
With added milk solids									
Made with lowfat milk									
Fruit-flavored[9]	1 container, net wt, 8 oz	227	75	230	10	3	1.8	0.6	0.1

[8]Applies to products made from thick shake mixes and that do not contain added ice cream. Products made from milk shake mixes are higher

[9]Content of fat, vitamin A, and carbohydrate varies. Consult the label when precise values are needed for special diets.

NUTRIENTS IN INDICATED QUANTITY

Carbohydrate (g)	Calcium (mg)	Phosphorus (mg)	Iron (mg)	Potassium (mg)	Vitamin A value (IU)	Thiamin (mg)	Riboflavin (mg)	Niacin (mg)	Ascorbic acid (mg)
29	304	265	0.5	500	330	0.14	0.43	0.7	2
27	347	307	0.3	529	380	0.20	0.54	1.3	2
63	396	378	0.9	672	260	0.14	0.67	0.4	0
56	457	361	0.3	572	360	0.09	0.61	0.5	0
254	1,406	1,075	1.0	2,052	4,340	0.42	2.63	1.1	6
32	176	134	0.1	257	540	0.05	0.33	0.1	1
12	66	51	Trace	96	200	0.02	0.12	0.1	Trace
38	236	199	0.4	338	790	0.08	0.45	0.2	1
256	1,213	927	0.8	1,771	7,200	0.36	2.27	0.9	5
32	151	115	0.1	221	900	0.04	0.28	0.1	1
232	1,409	1,035	1.5	2,117	1,710	0.61	2.78	0.9	6
29	176	129	0.1	265	210	0.08	0.35	0.1	1
38	274	202	0.3	412	180	0.12	0.54	0.2	1
469	827	594	2.5	1,585	1,480	0.26	0.71	1.0	31
59	103	74	0.3	198	198	0.03	0.09	0.1	4
29	297	310	1.1	387	930	0.11	0.50	0.3	1
67	250	255	1.3	445	390	0.05	0.36	0.3	1
41	298	232	Trace	352	410	0.08	0.41	0.3	2
28	173	180	0.7	223	480	0.07	0.30	0.2	2
59	265	247	0.8	354	340	0.05	0.39	0.3	2
63	374	237	1.3	335	340	0.08	0.39	0.3	2
42	343	269	0.2	439	[10]120	0.08	0.40	0.2	1

in fat and usually contain added ice cream.

Continued.

Nutritive values of the edible part of food—cont'd

Foods, approximate measures, units, and weight in grams (edible part unless footnotes indicate otherwise)			Water (%)	Food energy (kcal)	Protein (g)	Fat (g)	Fatty acids: Saturated (total) (g)	Unsaturated: Oleic (g)	Unsaturated: Linoleic (g)
Yogurt—cont'd									
Plain	1 container, net wt, 8 oz	227	85	145	12	4	2.3	0.8	0.1
Made with nonfat milk	1 container, net wt, 8 oz	227	85	125	13	Trace	0.3	0.1	Trace
Without added milk solids									
Made with whole milk	1 container, net wt, 8 oz	227	88	140	8	7	4.8	1.7	0.1
EGGS									
Eggs, large (24 oz/dozen)									
Raw									
Whole, without shell	1 egg	50	75	80	6	6	1.7	2.0	0.6
White	1 white	33	88	15	3	Trace	0	0	0
Yolk	1 yolk	17	49	65	3	6	1.7	2.1	0.6
Cooked									
Fried in butter	1 egg	46	72	85	5	6	2.4	2.2	0.6
Hard-cooked, shell removed	1 egg	50	75	80	6	6	1.7	2.0	0.6
Poached	1 egg	50	74	80	6	6	1.7	2.0	0.6
Scrambled (milk added) in butter, also omlet	1 egg	64	76	95	6	7	2.8	2.3	0.6
FATS, OILS; RELATED PRODUCTS									
Butter									
Regular (1 brick or 4 sticks/lb)									
Stick (½ cup)	1 stick	113	16	815	1	92	57.3	23.1	2.1
Tablespoon (about ⅛ stick)	1 tbsp	14	16	100	Trace	12	7.2	2.9	0.3
Pat (1 inch square, ⅓ inch high; 90/lb)	1 pat	5	16	35	Trace	4	2.5	1.0	0.1
Whipped (6 sticks or two 8 oz containers/lb)									
Stick (½ cup)	1 stick	76	16	540	1	61	38.2	15.4	1.4
Tablespoon (about ⅛ stick)	1 tbsp	9	16	65	Trace	8	4.7	1.9	0.2
Pat (1¼ inch square, ⅓ inch high; 120/lb)	1 pat	4	16	25	Trace	3	1.9	0.8	0.1
Fats, cooking (vegetable shortenings)	1 cup	200	0	1,770	0	200	48.8	88.2	48.4
	1 tbsp	13	0	110	0	13	3.2	5.7	3.1
Lard	1 cup	205	0	1,850	0	205	81.0	83.8	20.5
	1 tbsp	13	0	115	0	13	5.1	5.3	1.3
Margarine									
Regular (1 brick or 4 sticks/lb)									
Stick (½ cup)	1 stick	113	16	815	1	92	16.7	42.9	24.9
Tablespoon (about ⅛ stick)	1 tbsp	14	16	100	Trace	12	2.1	5.3	3.1

[10] Applies to product made with milk containing no added vitamin A.
[11] Based on year-round average.
[12] Based on average vitamin A content of fortified margarine. Federal specifications for fortified margarine require a minimum of 15,000 IU of

NUTRIENTS IN INDICATED QUANTITY

Carbohydrate (g)	Calcium (mg)	Phosphorus (mg)	Iron (mg)	Potassium (mg)	Vitamin A value (IU)	Thiamin (mg)	Riboflavin (mg)	Niacin (mg)	Ascorbic acid (mg)
16	415	326	0.2	531	[10]150	0.10	0.49	0.3	2
17	452	355	0.2	579	[10]20	0.11	0.53	0.3	2
11	274	215	0.1	351	280	0.07	0.32	0.2	1
1	28	90	1.0	65	260	0.04	0.15	Trace	0
Trace	4	4	Trace	45	0	Trace	0.09	Trace	0
Trace	26	86	0.9	15	310	0.04	0.07	Trace	0
1	26	80	0.9	58	290	0.03	0.13	Trace	0
1	28	90	1.0	65	260	0.04	0.14	Trace	0
1	28	90	1.0	65	260	0.04	0.13	Trace	0
1	47	97	0.9	85	310	0.04	0.16	Trace	0
Trace	27	26	0.2	29	[11]3,470	0.01	0.04	Trace	0
Trace	3	3	Trace	4	[11]430	Trace	Trace	Trace	0
Trace	1	1	Trace	1	[11]150	Trace	Trace	Trace	0
Trace	18	17	0.1	20	[11]2,310	Trace	0.03	Trace	0
Trace	2	2	Trace	2	[11]290	Trace	Trace	Trace	0
Trace	1	1	Trace	1	[11]120	0	Trace	Trace	0
0	0	0	0	0	—	0	0	0	0
0	0	0	0	0	—	0	0	0	0
0	0	0	0	0	0	0	0	0	0
0	0	0	0	0	0	0	0	0	0
Trace	27	26	0.2	29	[12]3,750	0.01	0.04	Trace	0
Trace	3	3	Trace	4	[12]470	Trace	Trace	Trace	0

Continued.

vitamin A/lb.

Nutritive values of the edible part of food—cont'd

Foods, approximate measures, units, and weight in grams (edible part unless footnotes indicate otherwise)			Water (%)	Food energy (kcal)	Protein (g)	Fat (g)	Fatty acids: Saturated (total) (g)	Fatty acids: Unsaturated: Oleic (g)	Fatty acids: Unsaturated: Linoleic (g)
Margarine—cont'd									
Pat (1 inch square, ⅓ inch high; 90/lb)	1 pat	5	16	35	Trace	4	0.7	1.9	1.1
Soft, two 8 oz containers/lb	1 container	227	16	1,635	1	184	32.5	71.5	65.4
	1 tbsp	14	16	100	Trace	12	2.0	4.5	4.1
Whipped (6 sticks/lb)									
Stick (½ cup)	1 stick	76	16	545	Trace	61	11.2	28 7	16.7
Tablespoon (about ⅛ stick	1 tbsp	9	16	70	Trace	8	1.4	3.6	2.1
Oils, salad or cooking									
Corn	1 cup	218	0	1,925	0	218	27.7	53.6	125.1
	1 tbsp	14	0	120	0	14	1.7	3.3	7.8
Olive	1 cup	216	0	1,910	0	216	30.7	154.4	17.7
	1 tbsp	14	0	200	0	14	1.9	9.7	1.1
Peanut	1 cup	216	0	1,910	0	216	37.4	98.5	67.0
	1 tbsp	14	0	120	0	14	2.3	6.2	4.2
Safflower	1 cup	218	0	1,925	0	218	20.5	25.9	159.8
	1 tbsp	14	0	120	0	14	1.3	1.6	10.0
Soybean oil, hydrogenated (partially hardened)	1 cup	218	0	1,925	0	218	31.8	93.1	75.6
	1 tbsp	14	0	120	0	14	2.0	5.8	4.7
Soybean-cottonseed oil blend hydrogenated	1 cup	218	0	1,925	0	218	38.2	63.0	99.6
	1 tbsp	14	0	120	0	14	2.4	3.9	6.2
Salad dressings									
Commercial									
Blue cheese									
Regular	1 tbsp	15	32	75	1	8	1.6	1.7	3.8
Low calorie (5 Cal/tsp)	1 tbsp	16	84	10	Trace	1	0.5	0.3	Trace
French									
Regular	1 tbsp	16	39	65	Trace	6	1.1	1.3	3.2
Low calorie (5 Cal/tsp)	1 tbsp	16	77	15	Trace	1	0.1	0.1	0.4
Italian									
Regular	1 tbsp	15	28	85	Trace	9	1.6	1.9	4.7
Low calorie (2 Cal/tsp)	1 tbsp	15	90	10	Trace	1	0.1	0.1	0.4
Mayonnaise	1 tbsp	14	15	100	Trace	11	2.0	2.4	5.6
Mayonnaise type									
Regular	1 tbsp	15	41	65	Trace	6	1.1	1.4	3.2
Low calorie (8 Cal/tsp)	1 tbsp	16	81	20	Trace	2	0.4	0.4	1.0
Tartar sauce, regular	1 tbsp	14	34	75	Trace	8	1.5	1.8	4.1
Thousand island									
Regular	1 tbsp	16	32	80	Trace	8	1.4	1.7	4.0
Low calorie (10 Cal/tsp)	1 tbsp	15	68	25	Trace	2	0.4	0.4	1.0
From home recipe									
Cooked type[13]	1 tbsp	16	68	25	1	2	0.5	0.6	0.3

[13]Fatty acid values apply to product made with regular-type margarine.

NUTRIENTS IN INDICATED QUANTITY

Carbohydrate (g)	Calcium (mg)	Phosphorus (mg)	Iron (mg)	Potassium (mg)	Vitamin A value (IU)	Thiamin (mg)	Riboflavin (mg)	Niacin (mg)	Ascorbic acid (mg)
Trace	1	1	Trace	1	[12]170	Trace	Trace	Trace	0
Trace	53	52	0.4	59	[12]7,500	0.01	0.08	0.1	0
Trace	3	3	Trace	4	[12]470	Trace	Trace	Trace	0
Trace	18	17	0.1	20	[12]2,500	Trace	0.03	Trace	0
Trace	2	2	Trace	2	[12]310	Trace	Trace	Trace	0
0	0	0	0	0	—	0	0	0	0
0	0	0	0	0	—	0	0	0	0
0	0	0	0	0	—	0	0	0	0
0	0	0	0	0	—	0	0	0	0
0	0	0	0	0	—	0	0	0	0
0	0	0	0	0	—	0	0	0	0
0	0	0	0	0	—	0	0	0	0
0	0	0	0	0	—	0	0	0	0
0	0	0	0	0	—	0	0	0	0
0	0		0	0	—	0	0	0	0
0	0	0	0	0	—	0	0	0	0
0	0	0	0	0	—	0	0	0	0
1	12	11	Trace	6	30	Trace	0.02	Trace	Trace
1	10	8	Trace	5	30	Trace	0.01	Trace	Trace
3	2	2	0.1	13	—	—	—	—	—
2	2	2	0 1	13	—	—	—	—	—
1	2	1	Trace	2	Trace	Trace	Trace	Trace	—
Trace	Trace	1	Trace	2	Trace	Trace	Trace	Trace	—
Trace	3	4	0.1	5	40	Trace	0.01	Trace	—
2	2	4	Trace	1	30	Trace	Trace	Trace	—
2	3	4	Trace	1	40	Trace	Trace	Trace	—
1	3	4	0.1	11	30	Trace	Trace	Trace	Trace
2	2	3	0.1	18	50	Trace	Trace	Trace	Trace
2	2	3	0.1	17	50	Trace	Trace	Trace	Trace
2	14	15	0.1	19	80	0.01	0.03	Trace	Trace

Continued.

Nutritive values of the edible part of food—cont'd

Foods, approximate measures, units, and weight in grams (edible part unless footnotes indicate otherwise)			Water (%)	Food energy (kcal)	Protein (g)	Fat (g)	Fatty acids: Saturated (total) (g)	Fatty acids: Unsaturated Oleic (g)	Fatty acids: Unsaturated Linoleic (g)
FISH, SHELLFISH, MEAT, POULTRY; RELATED PRODUCTS									
Fish and shellfish									
Bluefish, baked with butter or margarine	3 oz	85	68	135	22	4	—	—	—
Clams									
Raw, meat only	3 oz	85	82	65	11	1	—	—	—
Canned, solids and liquid	3 oz	85	86	45	7	1	0.2	Trace	Trace
Crabmeat (white or king), canned, not pressed down	1 cup	135	77	135	24	3	0.6	0.4	0.1
Fish sticks, breaded, cooked, frozen (stick, 4 by 1 by ½ inch)	1 stick or 1 oz	28	66	50	5	3	—	—	—
Haddock, breaded, fried[14]	3 oz	85	66	140	17	5	1.4	2.2	1.2
Ocean perch, breaded, fried[14]	1 fillet	85	59	195	16	11	2.7	4.4	2.3
Oysters, raw, meat only (13-19 medium selects)	1 cup	240	85	160	20	4	1.3	0.2	0.1
Salmon, pink, canned, solids and liquid	3 oz	85	71	120	17	5	0.9	0.8	0.1
Sardines, Atlantic, canned in oil, drained solids	3 oz	85	62	175	20	9	3.0	2.5	0.5
Scallops, frozen, breaded, fried, reheated	6 scallops	90	60	175	16	8	—	—	—
Shad, baked with butter or margarine, bacon	3 oz	85	64	170	20	10	—	—	—
Shrimp									
Canned meat	3 oz	85	70	100	21	1	0.1	0.1	Trace
French fried[16]	3 oz	85	57	190	17	9	2.3	3.7	2.0
Tuna, canned in oil, drained solids	3 oz	85	61	170	24	7	1.7	1.7	0.7
Tuna salad[17]	1 cup	205	70	350	30	22	4.3	6.3	6.7
Meat and meat products									
Bacon (20 slices/lb, raw), broiled or fried, crisp	2 slices	15	8	85	4	8	2.5	3.7	0.7
Beef,[18] cooked									
Cuts braised, simmered or pot roasted									
Lean and fat (piece, 2½ by 2½ by ¾ inch)	3 oz	85	53	245	23	16	6.8	6.5	0.4
Lean only from above item	2.5 oz	72	62	140	22	5	2.1	1.8	0.2
Ground beef, broiled									
Lean with 10% fat	3 oz or patty 3 by ⅝ inch	85	60	185	23	10	4.0	3.9	0.3
Lean with 21% fat	2.9 oz or patty 3 by ⅝ inch	82	54	235	20	17	7.0	6.7	0.4

[14]Dipped in egg, milk or water, and breadcrumbs; fried in vegetable shortening.
[15]If bones are discarded, value for calcium will be greatly reduced.
[16]Dipped in egg, breadcrumbs, and flour or batter.
[17]Prepared with tuna, celery, salad dressing (mayonnaise type), pickle, onion, and egg.
[18]Outer layer of fat on the cut was removed to within approximately ½ inch of the lean. Deposits of fat within the cut were not removed.

NUTRIENTS IN INDICATED QUANTITY									
Carbohydrate (g)	Calcium (mg)	Phosphorus (mg)	Iron (mg)	Potassium (mg)	Vitamin A value (IU)	Thiamin (mg)	Riboflavin (mg)	Niacin (mg)	Ascorbic acid (mg)
0	25	244	0.6	—	40	0.09	0.08	1.6	—
2	59	138	5.2	154	90	0.08	0.15	1.1	8
2	47	116	3.5	119	—	0.01	0.09	0.9	—
1	61	246	1.1	149	—	0.11	0.11	2.6	—
2	3	47	0.1	—	0	0.01	0.02	0.5	—
5	34	210	1.0	296	—	0.30	0.06	2.7	2
6	28	192	1.1	242	—	0.10	0.10	1.6	—
8	226	343	13.2	290	740	0.34	0.43	6.0	—
0	[15]167	243	0.7	307	60	0.03	0.16	6.8	—
0	372	424	2.5	502	190	0.02	0.17	4.6	—
9	—	—	—	—	—	—	—	—	—
0	20	266	0.5	320	30	0.11	0.22	7.3	—
1	98	224	2.6	104	50	0.01	0.03	1.5	—
9	61	162	1.7	195	—	0.03	0.07	2.3	
0	7	199	1.6	—	70	0.04	0.10	10.1	—
7	41	291	2.7	—	590	0.08	0.23	10.3	2
Trace	2	34	0.5	35	0	0.08	0.05	0.8	—
0	10	114	2.9	184	30	0.04	0.18	3.6	—
0	10	108	2.7	176	10	0.04	0.17	3.3	—
0	10	196	3.0	261	20	0.08	0.20	5.1	—
0	9	159	2.6	221	30	0.07	0.17	4.4	—

Continued.

Nutritive values of the edible part of food—cont'd

Foods, approximate measures, units, and weight in grams (edible part unless footnotes indicate otherwise)			Water (%)	Food energy (kcal)	Protein (g)	Fat (g)	Fatty acids: Saturated (total) (g)	Fatty acids: Unsaturated: Oleic (g)	Fatty acids: Unsaturated: Linoleic (g)
Roast, oven cooked, no liquid added									
Relatively fat, such as rib									
Lean and fat (2 pieces, 4⅛ by 2¼ by ¼ inch)	3 oz	85	40	375	17	33	14.0	13.6	0.8
Lean only from above item	1.8 oz	51	57	125	14	7	3.0	2.5	0.3
Relatively lean, such as heel of round									
Lean and fat (2 pieces, 4⅛ by 2¼ by ¼ inch)	3 oz	85	62	165	25	7	2.8	2.7	0.2
Lean only from above item	2.8 oz	78	65	125	24	3	1.2	1.0	0.1
Steak									
Relatively fat sirloin, broiled									
Lean and fat (piece, 2½ by 2½ by ¾ inch)	3 oz	85	44	330	20	27	11.3	11.1	0.6
Lean only from above item	2.0 oz	56	59	115	18	4	1.8	1.6	0.2
Relatively lean round, braised									
Lean and fat (piece, 4⅛ by 2¼ by ½ inch)	3 oz	85	55	220	24	13	5.5	5.2	0.4
Lean only from above item	2.4 oz	68	61	130	21	4	1.7	1.5	0.2
Beef, canned									
Corned beef	3 oz	85	59	185	22	10	4.9	4.5	0.2
Corned beef hash	1 cup	220	67	400	19	25	11.9	10.9	0.5
Beef, dried, chipped	2½ oz jar	71	48	145	24	4	2.1	2.0	0.1
Beef and vegetable stew	1 cup	245	82	220	16	11	4.9	4.5	0.2
Beef potpie (home recipe), baked[19] (piece, ⅓ of 9-inch diam. pie)	1 piece	210	55	515	21	30	7.9	12.8	6.7
Chili con carne with beans, canned	1 cup	255	72	340	19	16	7.5	6.8	0.3
Chop suey with beef and pork (home recipe)	1 cup	250	75	300	26	17	8.5	6.2	0.7
Heart, beef, lean, braised	3 oz	85	61	160	27	5	1.5	1.1	0.6
Lamb, cooked									
Chop, rib (cut 3/lb with bone), broiled									
Lean and fat	3.1 oz	89	43	360	18	32	14.8	12.1	1.2
Lean only from above item	2 oz	57	60	120	16	6	2.5	2.1	0.2
Leg, roasted									
Lean and fat (2 pieces, 4⅛ by 2¼ by ¼ inch)	3 oz	85	54	235	22	16	7.3	6.0	0.6

[19]Crust made with vegetable shortening and enriched flour.

NUTRIENTS IN INDICATED QUANTITY									
Carbohydrate (g)	Calcium (mg)	Phosphorus (mg)	Iron (mg)	Potassium (mg)	Vitamin A value (IU)	Thiamin (mg)	Riboflavin (mg)	Niacin (mg)	Ascorbic acid (mg)
0	8	158	2.2	189	70	0.05	0.13	3.1	—
0	6	131	1.8	161	10	0.04	0.11	2.6	—
0	11	208	3.2	279	10	0.06	0.19	4.5	—
0	10	199	3.0	268	Trace	0.06	0.18	4.3	—
0	9	162	2.5	220	50	0.05	0.15	4.0	—
0	7	146	2.2	202	10	0.05	0.14	3.6	—
0	10	213	3.0	272	20	0.07	0.19	4.8	—
0	9	182	2.5	238	10	0.05	0.16	4.1	—
0	17	90	3.7	—	—	0.01	0.20	2.9	—
24	29	147	4.4	440	—	0.02	0.20	4.6	—
0	14	287	3.6	142	—	0.05	0.23	2.7	0
15	29	184	2.9	613	2,400	0.15	0.17	4.7	17
39	29	149	3.8	334	1,720	0.30	0.30	5.5	6
31	82	321	4.3	594	150	0.08	0.18	3.3	—
13	60	248	4.8	425	600	0.28	0.38	5.0	33
1	5	154	5.0	197	20	0.21	1.04	6.5	1
0	8	139	1.0	200	—	0.11	0.19	4.1	—
0	6	121	1.1	174	—	0.09	0.15	3.4	—
0	9	177	1.4	241	—	0.13	0.23	4.7	—

Continued.

Nutritive values of the edible part of food—cont'd

Foods, approximate measures, units, and weight in grams (edible part unless footnotes indicate otherwise)			Water (%)	Food energy (kcal)	Protein (g)	Fat (g)	Fatty acids: Saturated (total) (g)	Fatty acids: Unsaturated: Oleic (g)	Fatty acids: Unsaturated: Linoleic (g)
Leg, roasted—cont'd									
Lean only from above item	2.5 oz	71	62	130	20	5	2.1	1.8	0.2
Shoulder, roasted									
Lean and fat (3 pieces, 2½ by 2½ by ¼ inch)	3 oz	85	50	285	18	23	10.8	8.8	0.9
Lean only from above item	2.3 oz	64	61	130	17	6	3.6	2.3	0.2
Liver, beef, fried[20] (slice, 6½ by 2⅜ by ⅜ inch)	3 oz	85	56	195	22	9	2.5	3.5	0.9
Pork, cured, cooked									
Ham, light cure, lean and fat roasted (2 pieces, 4⅛ by 2¼ by ¼ inch)[22]	3 oz	85	54	245	18	19	6.8	7.9	1.7
Luncheon meat									
Boiled ham, slice (8/8 oz pkg)	1 oz	28	59	65	5	5	1.7	2.0	0.4
Canned, spiced or unspiced									
Slice, approx. 3 by 2 by ½ inch	1 slice	60	55	175	9	15	5.4	6.7	1.0
Pork, fresh,[18] cooked									
Chop, loin (cut 3/lb with bone), broiled									
Lean and fat	2.7 oz	78	42	305	19	25	8.9	10.4	2.2
Lean only from above item	2 oz	56	53	150	17	9	3.1	3.6	0.8
Roast, oven cooked, no liquid added									
Lean and fat (piece, 2½ by 2½ by ¾ inch)	3 oz	85	46	310	21	24	8.7	10.2	2.2
Lean only from above item	2.4 oz	68	55	175	20	10	3.5	4.1	0.8
Shoulder cut, simmered									
Lean and fat (3 pieces, 2½ by 2½ by ¼ inch)	3 oz	85	46	320	20	26	9.3	10.9	2.3
Lean only from above item	2.2 oz	63	60	135	18	6	2.2	2.6	0.6
Sausages (see also Luncheon meat)									
Bologna, slice (8/8 oz pkg)	1 slice	28	56	85	3	8	3.0	3.4	0.5
Braunschweiger, slice (6/6 oz pkg)	1 slice	28	53	90	4	8	2.6	3.4	0.8

[20] Regular-type margarine used.
[21] Value varies widely.
[22] About one fourth of the outer layer of fat on the cut was removed. Deposits of fat within the cut were not removed.

NUTRIENTS IN INDICATED QUANTITY

Carbohydrate (g)	Calcium (mg)	Phosphorus (mg)	Iron (mg)	Potassium (mg)	Vitamin A value (IU)	Thiamin (mg)	Riboflavin (mg)	Niacin (mg)	Ascorbic acid (mg)
0	9	169	1.4	227	—	0.12	0.21	4.4	—
0	9	146	1.0	206	—	0.11	0.20	4.0	—
0	8	140	1.0	193	—	0.10	0.18	3.7	—
5	9	405	7.5	323	[21]45,390	0.22	3.56	14.0	23
0	8	146	2.2	199	0	0.40	0.15	3.1	—
0	3	47	0.8	—	0	0.12	0.04	0.7	—
1	5	65	1.3	133	0	0.19	0.13	1.8	—
0	9	209	2.7	216	0	0.75	0.22	4.5	—
0	7	181	2.2	192	0	0.63	0.18	3.8	—
0	9	218	2.7	233	0	0.78	0.22	4.8	—
0	9	211	2.6	224	0	0.73	0.21	4.4	—
0	9	118	2.6	158	0	0.46	0.21	4.1	—
0	8	111	2.3	146	0	0.42	0.19	3.7	—
Trace	2	36	0.5	65	—	0.05	0.06	0.7	—
1	3	69	1.7	—	1,850	0.05	0.41	2.3	—

Continued.

Nutritive values of the edible part of food—cont'd

Foods, approximate measures, units, and weight in grams (edible part unless footnotes indicate otherwise)			Water (%)	Food energy (kcal)	Protein (g)	Fat (g)	Fatty acids: Saturated (total) (g)	Fatty acids: Unsaturated: Oleic (g)	Fatty acids: Unsaturated: Linoleic (g)
Sausages—cont'd									
Brown and serve (10 or 11/8 oz pkg), browned	1 link	17	40	70	3	6	2.3	2.8	0.7
Deviled ham, canned	1 tbsp	13	51	45	2	4	1.5	1.8	0.4
Frankfurter (8/1 lb pkg), cooked (reheated)	1 frankfurter	56	57	170	7	15	5.6	6.5	1.2
Meat, potted (beef, chicken, turkey), canned	1 tbsp	13	61	30	2	2	—	—	—
Pork link (16/1 lb pkg), cooked	1 link	13	35	60	2	6	2.1	2.4	0.5
Salami									
Dry type, slice (12/4 oz pkg)	1 slice	10	30	45	2	4	1.6	1.6	0.1
Cooked type, slice (8/8 oz pkg)	1 slice	28	51	90	5	7	3.1	3.0	0.2
Vienna sausage (7/4 oz can)	1 sausage	16	63	40	2	3	1.2	1.4	0.2
Veal, medium fat, cooked, bone removed									
Cutlet (4⅛ by 2¼ by ½ inch), braised or broiled	3 oz	85	60	185	23	9	4.0	3.4	0.4
Rib (2 pieces, 4⅛ by 2¼ by ¼ inch), roasted	3 oz	85	55	230	23	14	6.1	5.1	0.6
Poultry and poultry products									
Chicken, cooked									
Breast, fried,[23] bones removed, ½ breast (3.3 oz with bones)	2.8 oz	79	58	160	26	5	1.4	1.8	1.1
Drumstick, fried,[23] bones removed (2 oz with bones)	1.3 oz	38	55	90	12	4	1.1	1.3	0.9
Half broiler, broiled, bones removed (10.4 oz with bones)	6.2	176	71	240	42	7	2.2	2.5	1.3
Chicken, canned, boneless	3 oz	85	65	170	18	10	3.2	3.8	2.0
Chicken a la king, cooked (home recipe)	1 cup	245	68	470	27	34	12.7	14.3	3.3
Chicken and noodles, cooked (home recipe)	1 cup	240	71	365	22	18	5.9	7.1	3.5
Chicken chow mein									
Canned	1 cup	250	89	95	7	Trace	—	—	—
From home recipe	1 cup	250	78	255	31	10	2.4	3.4	3.1
Chicken potpie (home recipe), baked,[19] (piece ⅓ of 9-inch diam. pie)	1 piece	232	57	545	23	31	11.3	10.9	5.6
Turkey, roasted, flesh without skin									
Dark meat (piece, 2½ by 1⅝ by ¼ inch)	4 pieces	85	61	175	26	7	2.1	1.5	1.5

[23] Vegetable shortening used.

NUTRIENTS IN INDICATED QUANTITY

Carbohydrate (g)	Calcium (mg)	Phosphorus (mg)	Iron (mg)	Potassium (mg)	Vitamin A value (IU)	Thiamin (mg)	Riboflavin (mg)	Niacin (mg)	Ascorbic acid (mg)
Trace	—	—	—	—	—	—	—	—	—
0	1	12	0.3	—	0	0.02	0.01	0.2	—
1	3	57	0.8	—	—	0.08	0.11	1.4	—
0	—	—	—	—	—	Trace	0.03	0.2	—
Trace	1	21	0.3	35	0	0.10	0.04	0.5	—
Trace	1	28	0.4	—	—	0.04	0.03	0.5	—
Trace	3	57	0.7	—	—	0.07	0.07	1.2	—
Trace	1	24	0.3	—	—	0.01	0.02	0.4	—
0	9	196	2.7	258	—	0.06	0.21	4.6	—
0	10	211	2.9	259	—	0.11	0.26	6.6	—
1	9	218	1.3	—	70	0.04	0.17	11.6	—
Trace	6	89	0.9	—	50	0.03	0.15	2.7	—
0	16	355	3.0	483	160	0.09	0.34	15.5	—
0	18	210	1.3	117	200	0.03	0.11	3.7	3
12	127	358	2.5	404	1,130	0.10	0.42	5.4	12
26	26	247	2.2	149	430	0.05	0.17	4.3	Trace
18	45	85	1.3	418	150	0.05	0.10	1.0	13
10	58	293	2.5	473	280	0.08	0.23	4.3	10
42	70	232	3.0	343	3,090	0.34	0.31	5.5	5
0	—	—	2.0	338	—	0.03	0.20	3.6	—

Continued.

Nutritive values of the edible part of food—cont'd

Foods, approximate measures, units, and weight in grams (edible part unless footnotes indicate otherwise)			Water (%)	Food energy (kcal)	Protein (g)	Fat (g)	Fatty acids		
							Saturated (total) (g)	Unsaturated	
								Oleic (g)	Linoleic (g)
Turkey, roasted, flesh without skin—cont'd									
Light meat (piece, 4 by 2 by ¼ inch)	2 pieces	85	62	150	28	3	0.9	0.6	0.7
Light and dark meat									
Chopped or diced	1 cup	140	61	265	44	9	2.5	1.7	1.8
Pieces (1 slice white meat, 4 by 2 by ¼ inch with 2 slices dark meat, 2½ by 1⅝ by ¼ inch)	3 pieces	85	61	160	27	5	1.5	1.0	1.1
FRUITS AND FRUIT PRODUCTS									
Apples, raw, unpeeled, without cores									
2¾-inch diam. (about 3/lb with cores)	1 apple	138	84	80	Trace	1	—	—	—
3¼-inch diam (about 2/lb with cores)	1 apple	212	84	125	Trace	1	—	—	—
Apple juice, bottled or canned[24]	1 cup	248	88	120	Trace	Trace	—	—	—
Applesauce, canned									
Sweetened	1 cup	255	76	230	1	Trace	—	—	—
Unsweetened	1 cup	244	89	100	Trace	Trace	—	—	—
Apricots									
Raw, without pits (about 12/lb with pits)	3 apricots	107	85	55	1	Trace	—	—	—
Canned in heavy syrup (halves and syrup)	1 cup	258	77	220	2	Trace	—	—	—
Dried									
Uncooked (28 large or 37 medium halves/cup)	1 cup	130	25	340	7	1	—	—	—
Cooked, unsweetened, fruit and liquid	1 cup	250	76	215	4	1	—	—	—
Apricot nectar, canned	1 cup	251	85	145	1	Trace	—	—	—
Avocados, raw, whole, without skins and seeds									
California, mid- and late-winter (with skin and seed, 3⅛-inch diam.; wt, 10 oz)	1 avocado	216	74	370	5	37	5.5	22.0	3.7
Florida, late summer and fall (with skin and seed, 3⅝-inch diam.; wt, 1 lb)	1 avocado	304	78	390	4	33	6.7	15.7	5.3
Banana without peel (about 2.6/lb with peel)	1 banana	119	76	100	1	Trace	—	—	—
Banana flakes	1 tbsp	6	3	20	Trace	Trace	—	—	—

[24] Also applies to pasteurized apple cider.
[25] Applies to product without added ascorbic acid. For value of product with added ascorbic acid, refer to label.
[26] Based on product with label claim of 45% of U.S. RDA in 6 fl oz.

NUTRIENTS IN INDICATED QUANTITY

Carbohydrate (g)	Calcium (mg)	Phosphorus (mg)	Iron (mg)	Potassium (mg)	Vitamin A value (IU)	Thiamin (mg)	Riboflavin (mg)	Niacin (mg)	Ascorbic acid (mg)
0	—	—	1.0	349	—	0.04	0.12	9.4	—
0	11	351	2.5	514	—	0.07	0.25	10.8	—
0	7	213	1.5	312	—	0.04	0.15	6.5	—
20	10	14	0.4	152	120	0.04	0.03	0.1	6
31	15	21	0.6	233	190	0.06	0.04	0.2	8
30	15	22	1.5	250	—	0.02	0.05	0.2	[25]2
61	10	13	1.3	166	100	0.05	0.03	0.1	[25]3
26	10	12	1.2	190	100	0.05	0.02	0.1	[25]2
14	18	25	0.5	301	2,890	0.03	0.04	0.6	11
57	28	39	0.8	604	4,490	0.05	0.05	1.0	10
86	87	140	7.2	1,273	14,170	0.01	0.21	4.3	16
54	55	88	4.5	795	7,500	0.01	0.13	2.5	8
37	23	30	0.5	379	2,380	0.03	0.03	0.5	[26]36
13	22	91	1.3	1,303	630	0.24	0.43	3.5	30
27	30	128	1.8	1,836	880	0.33	0.61	4.9	43
26	10	31	0.8	440	230	0.06	0.07	0.8	12
5	2	6	0.2	92	50	0.01	0.01	0.2	Trace

Continued.

Nutritive values of the edible part of food—cont'd

Foods, approximate measures, units, and weight in grams (edible part unless footnotes indicate otherwise)			Water (%)	Food energy (kcal)	Protein (g)	Fat (g)	Fatty acids: Saturated (total) (g)	Unsaturated: Oleic (g)	Unsaturated: Linoleic (g)
Blackberries, raw	1 cup	144	85	85	2	1	—	—	—
Blueberries, raw	1 cup	145	83	90	1	1	—	—	—
Cantaloup. See Muskmelons									
Cherries									
Sour (tart), red, pitted, canned, water pack	1 cup	244	88	105	2	Trace	—	—	—
Sweet, raw, without pits and stems	10	68	80	45	1	Trace	—	—	—
Cranberry juice cocktail, bottled, sweetened	1 cup	253	83	165	Trace	Trace	—	—	—
Cranberry sauce, sweetened, canned, strained	1 cup	277	62	405	Trace	1	—	—	—
Dates									
Whole, without pits	10	80	23	220	2	Trace	—	—	—
Chopped	1 cup	178	23	490	4	1	—	—	—
Fruit cocktail, canned, in heavy syrup	1 cup	255	80	195	1	Trace	—	—	—
Grapefruit									
Raw, medium, 3¾-inch diam. (about 1 lb 1 oz)									
Pink or red	½ with peel[28]	241	89	50	1	Trace	—	—	—
White	½ with peel[28]	241	89	45	1	Trace	—	—	—
Canned, sections with syrup	1 cup	254	81	180	2	Trace	—	—	—
Grapefruit juice									
Raw, pink, red, or white	1 cup	246	90	95	1	Trace	—	—	—
Canned, white									
Unsweetened	1 cup	247	89	100	1	Trace	—	—	—
Sweetened	1 cup	250	86	135	1	Trace	—	—	—
Frozen, concentrate, unsweetened									
Undiluted, 6 fl oz can	1 can	207	62	300	4	1	—	—	—
Diluted with 3 parts water by volume	1 cup	247	89	100	1	Trace	—	—	—
Dehydrated crystals, prepared with water (1 lb yields about 1 gal)	1 cup	247	90	100	1	Trace	—	—	—
Grapes, European type (adherent skin), raw									
Thompson Seedless	10 grapes	50	81	35	Trace	Trace	—	—	—
Tokay and Emperor, seeded types	10 grapes[30]	60	81	40	Trace	Trace	—	—	—
Grape juice									
Canned or bottled	1 cup	253	83	165	1	Trace	—	—	—
Frozen concentrate, sweetened									
Undiluted, 6 fl oz can	1 can	216	53	395	1	Trace	—	—	—
Diluted with 3 parts water by volume	1 cup	250	86	135	1	Trace	—	—	—

[27] Based on product with label claim of 100% of U.S. RDA in 6 fl oz.

[28] Weight includes peel and membranes between sections. Without these parts, the weight of the edible portion is 123 g for pink or red and

[29] For white-fleshed varieties, value is about 20 IU per cup; for red-fleshed varieties, 1,080 IU.

[30] Weight includes seeds. Without seeds, weight of the edible portion is 57 g.

[31] Applies to product without added ascorbic acid. With added ascorbic acid, based on claim that 6 fl oz of reconstituted juice contain 45% or 50%

NUTRIENTS IN INDICATED QUANTITY

Carbohydrate (g)	Calcium (mg)	Phosphorus (mg)	Iron (mg)	Potassium (mg)	Vitamin A value (IU)	Thiamin (mg)	Riboflavin (mg)	Niacin (mg)	Ascorbic acid (mg)
19	46	27	1.3	245	290	0.04	0.06	0.6	30
22	22	19	1.5	117	150	0.04	0.09	0.7	20
26	37	32	0.7	317	1,660	0.07	0.05	0.5	12
12	15	13	0.3	129	70	0.03	0.04	0.3	7
42	13	8	0.08	25	Trace	0.03	0.03	0.1	[27]81
104	17	11	0.6	83	60	0.03	0.03	0.1	6
58	47	50	2.4	518	40	0.07	0.08	1.8	0
130	105	112	5.3	1,153	90	0.16	0.18	3.9	0
50	23	31	1.0	411	360	0.05	0.03	1.0	5
13	20	20	0.5	166	540	0.05	0.02	0.2	44
12	19	19	0.5	159	10	0.05	0.02	0.2	44
45	33	36	0.8	343	30	0.08	0.05	0.5	76
23	22	37	0.5	399	([29])	0.10	0.05	0.5	93
24	20	35	1.0	400	20	0.07	0.05	0.5	84
32	20	35	1.0	405	30	0.08	0.05	0.5	78
72	70	124	0.8	1,250	60	0.29	0.12	1.4	286
24	25	42	0.2	420	20	0.10	0.04	0.5	96
24	22	40	0.2	412	20	0.10	0.05	0.5	91
9	6	10	0.2	87	50	0.03	0.02	0.2	2
10	7	11	0.2	99	60	0.03	0.03	0.2	2
42	28	30	0.8	293	—	0.10	0.05	0.5	[25]Trace
100	22	32	0.9	255	40	0.13	0.22	1.5	[31]32
33	8	10	0.3	85	10	0.05	0.08	0.5	[31]10

Continued.

118 g for white.

of the U.S. RDA, value in milligrams is 108 or 120 for a 6 fl oz can, 36 or 40 for 1 cup of diluted juice.

Nutritive values of the edible part of food—cont'd

Foods, approximate measures, units, and weight in grams (edible part unless footnotes indicate otherwise)			Water (%)	Food energy (kcal)	Protein (g)	Fat (g)	Fatty acids: Saturated (total) (g)	Fatty acids: Unsaturated: Oleic (g)	Fatty acids: Unsaturated: Linoleic (g)
Grape drink, canned	1 cup	250	86	135	Trace	Trace	—	—	—
Lemon, raw, size 165, without peel and seeds (about 4/lb with peels and seeds)	1 lemon	74	90	20	1	Trace	—	—	—
Lemon juice									
Raw	1 cup	244	91	60	1	Trace	—	—	—
Canned, or bottled, unsweetened	1 cup	244	92	55	1	Trace	—	—	—
Frozen, single strength, unsweetened, 6 fl oz can	1 can	183	92	40	1	Trace	—	—	—
Lemonade concentrate, frozen									
Undiluted, 6 fl oz can	1 can	219	49	425	Trace	Trace	—	—	—
Diluted with 4⅓ parts water by volume	1 cup	248	89	105	Trace	Trace	—	—	—
Limeade concentrate, frozen									
Undiluted, 6 fl oz can	1 can	218	50	410	Trace	Trace	—	—	—
Diluted with 4⅓ parts water by volume	1 cup	247	89	100	Trace	Trace	—	—	—
Lime juice									
Raw	1 cup	246	90	65	1	Trace	—	—	—
Canned, unsweetened	1 cup	246	90	65	1	Trace	—	—	—
Muskmelons, raw, with rind, without seed cavity									
Cantaloup, orange-fleshed (with rind and seed cavity, 5-inch diam., 2⅓ lb)	½ melon with rind[33]	477	91	80	2	Trace	—	—	—
Honeydew (with rind and seed cavity, 6½-inch diam., 5¼ lb)	1/10 melon with rind[33]	226	91	50	1	Trace	—	—	—
Oranges, all commercial varieties, raw									
Whole, 2⅝-inch diam., without peel and seeds (about 2½/lb with peel and seeds)	1 orange	131	86	65	1	Trace	—	—	—
Sections without membranes	1 cup	180	86	90	2	Trace	—	—	—
Orange juice									
Raw, all varieties	1 cup	248	88	110	2	Trace	—	—	—
Canned, unsweetened	1 cup	249	87	120	2	Trace	—	—	—
Frozen concentrate									
Undiluted, 6 fl oz can	1 can	213	55	360	5	Trace	—	—	—
Diluted with 3 parts water by volume	1 cup	249	87	120	2	Trace	—	—	—
Dehydrated crystals, prepared with water (1 lb yields about 1 gal)	1 cup	248	88	115	1	Trace	—	—	—

[32]For products with added thiamin and riboflavin but without added ascorbic acid, values in milligrams would be 0.60 for thiamin, 0.80 for
[33]Weight includes rind. Without rind, the weight of the edible portion is 272 g for cantaloup and 149 g for honeydew.

NUTRIENTS IN INDICATED QUANTITY

Carbohydrate (g)	Calcium (mg)	Phosphorus (mg)	Iron (mg)	Potassium (mg)	Vitamin A value (IU)	Thiamin (mg)	Riboflavin (mg)	Niacin (mg)	Ascorbic acid (mg)
35	8	10	0.3	88	—	[32]0.03	[32]0.03	0.3	([32])
6	19	12	0.4	102	10	0.03	0.01	0.1	39
20	17	24	0.5	344	50	0.07	0.02	0.2	112
19	17	24	0.5	344	50	0.07	0.02	0.2	102
13	13	16	0.5	258	40	0.05	0.02	0.2	81
112	9	13	0.4	153	40	0.05	0.06	0.7	66
28	2	3	0.1	40	10	0.01	0.02	0.2	17
108	11	13	0.2	129	Trace	0.02	0.02	0.2	26
27	3	3	Trace	32	Trace	Trace	Trace	Trace	6
22	22	27	0.5	256	20	0.05	0.02	0.2	79
22	22	27	0.5	256	20	0.05	0.02	0.2	52
20	38	44	1.1	682	9,240	0.11	0.08	1.6	90
11	21	24	0.6	374	60	0.06	0.04	0.9	34
16	54	26	0.5	263	260	0.13	0.05	0.5	66
22	74	36	0.7	360	360	0.18	0.07	0.7	90
26	27	42	0.5	496	500	0.22	0.07	1.0	124
28	25	45	1.0	496	500	0.17	0.05	0.7	100
87	75	126	0.9	1,500	1,620	0.68	0.11	2.8	360
29	25	42	0.2	503	540	0.23	0.03	0.9	120
27	25	40	0.5	518	500	0.20	0.07	1.0	109

riboflavin, and trace for ascorbic acid. For products with only ascorbic acid added, value varies with the brand. Consult the label.

Continued.

Nutritive values of the edible part of food—cont'd

Foods, approximate measures, units, and weight in grams (edible part unless footnotes indicate otherwise)			Water (%)	Food energy (kcal)	Protein (g)	Fat (g)	Fatty acids: Saturated (total) (g)	Unsaturated: Oleic (g)	Unsaturated: Linoleic (g)
Orange and grapefruit juice									
Frozen concentrate									
Undiluted, 6 fl oz can	1 can	210	59	330	4	1	—	—	—
Diluted with 3 parts water by volume	1 cup	248	88	110	1	Trace	—	—	—
Papayas, raw, ½-inch cubes	1 cup	140	89	55	1	Trace	—	—	—
Peaches									
Raw									
Whole, 2½-inch diam., peeled, pitted (about 4/lb with peels and pits)	1 peach	100	89	40	1	Trace	—	—	—
Sliced	1 cup	170	89	65	1	Trace	—	—	—
Canned, yellow-fleshed, solids and liquid (halves or slices)									
Syrup pack	1 cup	256	79	200	1	Trace	—	—	—
Water pack	1 cup	244	91	75	1	Trace	—	—	—
Dried									
Uncooked	1 cup	160	25	420	5	1	—	—	—
Cooked, unsweetened, halves and juice	1 cup	250	77	205	3	1	—	—	—
Frozen, sliced, sweetened									
10 oz container	1	284	77	250	1	Trace	—	—	—
Cup	1 cup	250	77	220	1	Trace	—	—	—
Pears									
Raw, with skin, cored									
Bartlett, 2½-inch diam. (about 2½/lb with cores and stems)	1 pear	164	83	100	1	1	—	—	—
Bosc, 2½-inch diam. (about 3/lb with cores and stems)	1 pear	141	83	85	1	1	—	—	—
D'Anjou, 3-inch diam. (about 2/lb with cores and stems)	1 pear	200	83	120	1	1	—	—	—
Canned, solids and liquid, syrup pack, heavy (halves or slices)	1 cup	255	80	195	1	1	—	—	—
Pineapple									
Raw, diced	1 cup	155	85	80	1	Trace	—	—	—
Canned, heavy syrup pack, solids and liquid									
Crushed, chunks, tidbits	1 cup	255	80	190	1	Trace	—	—	—
Slices and liquid									
Large	1 slice; 2¼ tbsp liquid	105	80	80	Trace	Trace	—	—	—
Medium	1 slice; 1¼ tbsp liquid	58	80	45	Trace	Trace	—	—	—
Pineapple juice, unsweetened, canned	1 cup	250	86	140	1	Trace	—	—	—

[34]Represents yellow-fleshed varieties. For white-fleshed varieties, value is 50 IU for 1 peach, 90 IU for 1 cup of slices.

[35]Value represents products with added ascorbic acid. For products without added ascorbic acid, value in milligrams is 166 for a 10 oz

NUTRIENTS IN INDICATED QUANTITY

Carbohydrate (g)	Calcium (mg)	Phosphorus (mg)	Iron (mg)	Potassium (mg)	Vitamin A value (IU)	Thiamin (mg)	Riboflavin (mg)	Niacin (mg)	Ascorbic acid (mg)
78	61	99	0.8	1,308	800	0.48	0.06	2.3	302
26	20	32	0.2	439	270	0.15	0.02	0.7	102
14	28	22	0.4	328	2,450	0.06	0.06	0.4	78
10	9	19	0.5	202	[34]1,330	0.02	0.05	1.0	7
16	15	32	0.9	343	[34]2,260	0.03	0.09	1.7	12
51	10	31	0.8	333	1,100	0.03	0.05	1.5	8
20	10	32	0.7	334	1,100	0.02	0.07	1.5	7
109	77	187	9.6	1,520	6,240	0.02	0.30	8.5	29
54	38	93	4.8	743	3,050	0.01	0.15	3.8	5
64	11	37	1.4	352	1,850	0.03	0.11	2.0	[35]116
57	10	33	1.3	310	1,630	0.03	0.10	1.8	[35]103
25	13	18	0.5	213	30	0.03	0.07	0.2	7
22	11	16	0.4	83	30	0.03	0.06	0.1	6
31	16	22	0.6	260	40	0.04	0.08	0.2	8
50	13	18	0.5	214	10	0.03	0.05	0.3	3
21	26	12	0.8	226	110	0.14	0.05	0.3	26
49	28	13	0.8	245	130	0.20	0.05	0.5	18
20	12	5	0.3	101	50	0.08	0.02	0.2	7
11	6	3	0.2	56	30	0.05	0.01	0.1	4
34	38	23	0.8	373	130	0.13	0.05	0.5	[27]80

Continued.

container, 103 for 1 cup.

Nutritive values of the edible part of food—cont'd

Foods, approximate measures, units, and weight in grams (edible part unless footnotes indicate otherwise)			Water (%)	Food energy (kcal)	Protein (g)	Fat (g)	Fatty acids		
							Saturated (total) (g)	Unsaturated	
								Oleic (g)	Linoleic (g)
Plums									
Raw, without pits									
Japanese and hybrid (2⅛-inch diam., about 6½/lb with pits)	1 plum	66	87	30	Trace	Trace	—	—	—
Prune-type (1½-inch diam., about 15/lb with pits)	1 plum	28	79	20	Trace	Trace	—	—	—
Canned, heavy syrup pack (Italian prunes), with pits and liquid									
Cup	1 cup[36]	272	77	215	1	Trace	—	—	—
Portion	3 plums; 2¾ tbsp liquid[36]	140	77	110	1	Trace	—	—	—
Prunes, dried, "softenized," with pits									
Uncooked	4 extra large or 5 large prunes[36]	49	28	110	1	Trace	—	—	—
Cooked, unsweetened, all sizes, fruit and liquid	1 cup[36]	250	66	255	2	1	—	—	—
Prune juice, canned or bottled	1 cup	256	80	195	1	Trace	—	—	—
Raisins, seedless									
Cup, not pressed down	1 cup	145	18	420	4	Trace	—	—	—
Packet, ½ oz (1½ tbsp)	1	14	18	40	Trace	Trace	—	—	—
Raspberries, red									
Raw, capped, whole	1 cup	123	84	70	1	1	—	—	—
Frozen, sweetened, 10 oz container	1	284	74	280	2	1	—	—	—
Rhubarb, cooked, added sugar									
From raw	1 cup	270	63	380	1	Trace	—	—	—
From frozen, sweetened	1 cup	270	63	385	1	1	—	—	—
Strawberries									
Raw, whole berries, capped	1 cup	149	90	55	1	1	—	—	—
Frozen, sweetened									
Sliced, 10 oz container	1 container	284	71	310	1	1	—	—	—
Whole, 1 lb container (about 1¾ cups)	1 container	454	76	415	2	1	—	—	—
Tangerine, raw, 2⅜-inch diam., size 176, without peel (about 4/lb with peels and seeds)	1 tangerine	86	87	40	1	Trace	—	—	—
Tangerine juice, canned, sweetened	1 cup	249	87	125	1	Trace	—	—	—
Watermelon, raw, 4 by 8-inch wedge with rind and seeds (1/16 of 32⅔ lb melon, 10 by 16 inch)	1 wedge with rind and seeds[37]	926	93	110	2	1	—	—	—

[36] Weight includes pits. After removal of the pits, the weight of the edible portion is 258 g for 1 cup, 133 g for 1 portion, 43 g for uncooked

[37] Weight includes rind and seeds. Without rind and seeds, weight of the edible portion is 426 g.

NUTRIENTS IN INDICATED QUANTITY

Carbohydrate (g)	Calcium (mg)	Phosphorus (mg)	Iron (mg)	Potassium (mg)	Vitamin A value (IU)	Thiamin (mg)	Riboflavin (mg)	Niacin (mg)	Ascorbic acid (mg)
8	8	12	0.3	112	160	0.02	0.02	0.3	4
6	3	5	0.1	48	80	0.01	0.01	0.1	1
56	23	26	2.3	367	3,130	0.05	0.05	1.0	5
29	12	13	1.2	189	1,610	0.03	0.03	0.5	3
29	22	34	1.7	298	690	0.04	0.07	0.7	1
67	51	79	3.8	695	1,590	0.07	0.15	1.5	2
49	36	51	1.8	602	—	0.03	0.03	1.0	5
112	90	146	5.1	1,106	30	0.16	0.12	0.7	1
11	9	14	0.5	107	Trace	0.02	0.01	0.1	Trace
17	27	27	1.1	207	160	0.04	0.11	1.1	31
70	37	48	1.7	284	260	0.06	0.17	1.7	60
97	211	41	1.6	548	220	0.05	0.14	0.8	16
98	211	32	1.9	475	190	0.05	0.11	0.5	16
13	31	31	1.5	244	90	0.04	0.10	0.9	88
79	40	48	2.0	318	90	0.06	0.17	1.4	151
107	59	73	2.7	472	140	0.09	0.27	2.3	249
10	34	15	0.3	108	360	0.05	0.02	0.1	27
30	44	35	0.5	440	1,040	0.15	0.05	0.2	54
27	30	43	2.1	426	2,510	0.13	0.13	0.9	30

prunes, and 213 g for cooked prunes.

Continued.

Nutritive values of the edible part of food—cont'd

Foods, approximate measures, units, and weight in grams (edible part unless footnotes indicate otherwise)			Water (%)	Food energy (kcal)	Protein (g)	Fat (g)	Fatty acids: Saturated (total) (g)	Fatty acids: Unsaturated: Oleic (g)	Fatty acids: Unsaturated: Linoleic (g)
GRAIN PRODUCTS									
Bagel, 3-inch diam.									
Egg	1 bagel	55	32	165	6	2	0.5	0.9	0.8
Water	1 bagel	55	29	165	6	1	0.2	0.4	0.6
Barley, pearled, light, uncooked	1 cup	200	11	700	16	2	0.3	0.2	0.8
Biscuits, baking powder, 2-inch diam. (enriched flour, vegetable shortening)									
From home recipe	1 biscuit	28	27	105	2	5	1.2	2.0	1.2
From mix	1 biscuit	28	29	90	2	3	0.6	1.1	0.7
Bread crumbs (enriched)[38]									
Dry, grated	1 cup	100	7	390	13	5	1.0	1.6	1.4
Soft. See White bread									
Breads									
Boston brown bread, canned, slice, 3¼ by ½ inch[38]	1 slice	45	45	95	2	1	0.1	0.2	0.2
Cracked-wheat bread (¾ enriched wheat flour, ¼ cracked wheat)[38]									
Loaf, 1 lb	1 loaf	454	35	1,195	39	10	2.2	3.0	3.9
Slice (18/loaf)	1 slice	25	35	65	2	1	0.1	0.2	0.2
French or vienna bread, enriched[38]									
Loaf, 1 lb	1 loaf	454	31	1,315	41	14	3.2	4.7	4.6
Slice									
French (5 by 2½ by 1 inch)	1 slice	35	31	100	3	1	0.2	0.4	0.4
Vienna (4¾ by 4 by ½ inch)	1 slice	25	31	75	2	1	0.2	0.3	0.3
Italian bread, enriched									
Loaf, 1 lb	1 loaf	454	32	1,250	41	4	0.6	0.3	1.5
Slice, (4½ by 3¼ by ¾ inch)	1 slice	30	32	85	3	Trace	Trace	Trace	0.1
Raisin bread, enriched[38]									
Loaf, 1 lb	1 loaf	454	35	1,190	30	13	3.0	4.7	3.9
Slice (18/loaf)	1 slice	25	35	65	2	1	0.2	0.3	0.2
Rye bread									
American, light ⅔ enriched wheat flour, ⅓ rye flour)									
Loaf, 1 lb	1 loaf	454	36	1,100	41	5	0.7	0.5	2.2
Slice (4¾ by 3¾ by 7/16 inch)	1 slice	25	36	60	2	Trace	Trace	Trace	0.1
Pumpernickel (⅔ rye flour, ⅓ enriched wheat flour)									
Loaf, 1 lb	1 loaf	454	34	1,115	41	5	0.7	0.5	2.4
Slice (5 by 4 by ⅜ inch)	1 slice	32	34	80	3	Trace	0.1	Trace	0.2

[38] Made with vegetable shortening.

[39] Applies to product made with white cornmeal. With yellow cornmeal, value is 30 IU.

NUTRIENTS IN INDICATED QUANTITY

Carbohydrate (g)	Calcium (mg)	Phosphorus (mg)	Iron (mg)	Potassium (mg)	Vitamin A value (IU)	Thiamin (mg)	Riboflavin (mg)	Niacin (mg)	Ascorbic acid (mg)
28	9	43	1.2	41	30	0.14	0.10	1.2	0
30	8	41	1.2	42	0	0.15	0.11	1.4	0
158	32	378	4.0	320	0	0.24	0.10	6.2	0
13	34	49	0.4	33	Trace	0.08	0.08	0.7	Trace
15	19	65	0.6	32	Trace	0.09	0.08	0.8	Trace
73	122	141	3.6	152	Trace	0.35	0.35	4.8	Trace
21	41	72	0.9	131	[39]0	0.06	0.04	0.7	0
236	399	581	9.5	608	Trace	1.52	1.13	14.4	Trace
13	22	32	0.5	34	Trace	0.08	0.06	0.8	Trace
251	195	386	10.0	408	Trace	1.80	1.10	15.0	Trace
19	15	30	0.8	32	Trace	0.14	0.08	1.2	Trace
14	11	21	0.6	23	Trace	0.10	0.06	0.8	Trace
256	77	349	10.0	336	0	1.80	1.10	15.0	0
17	5	23	0.7	22	0	0.12	0.07	1.0	0
243	322	395	10.0	1,057	Trace	1.70	1.07	10.7	Trace
13	18	22	0.6	58	Trace	0.09	0.06	0.6	Trace
236	340	667	9.1	658	0	1.35	0.98	12.9	0
13	19	37	0.5	36	0	0.07	0.05	0.7	0
241	381	1,039	11.8	2,059	0	1.30	0.93	8.5	0
17	27	73	0.8	145	0	0.09	0.07	0.6	0

Continued.

Nutritive values of the edible part of food—cont'd

Foods, approximate measures, units, and weight in grams (edible part unless footnotes indicate otherwise)			Water (%)	Food energy (kcal)	Protein (g)	Fat (g)	Fatty acids: Saturated (total) (g)	Fatty acids: Unsaturated: Oleic (g)	Fatty acids: Unsaturated: Linoleic (g)
White bread, enriched[38]									
Soft-crumb type									
Loaf, 1 lb	1 loaf	454	36	1,225	39	15	3.4	5.3	4.6
Slice (18/loaf)	1 slice	25	36	70	2	1	0.2	0.3	0.3
Slice, toasted	1 slice	22	25	70	2	1	0.2	0.3	0.3
Slice (22/loaf)	1 slice	20	36	55	2	1	0.2	0.2	0.2
Slice, toasted	1 slice	17	25	55	2	1	0.2	0.2	0.2
Loaf, 1½ lb	1 loaf	680	36	1,835	59	22	5.2	7.9	6.9
Slice (24/loaf)	1 slice	28	36	75	2	1	0.2	0.3	0.3
Slice, toasted	1 slice	24	25	75	2	1	0.2	0.3	0.3
Slice (28/loaf)	1 slice	24	36	65	2	1	0.2	0.3	0.2
Slice, toasted	1 slice	21	25	65	2	1	0.2	0.3	0.2
Cubes	1 cup	30	36	80	3	1	0.2	0.3	0.3
Crumbs	1 cup	45	36	120	4	1	0.3	0.5	0.5
Firm-crumb type									
Loaf, 1 lb	1 loaf	454	35	1,245	41	17	3.9	5.9	5.2
Slice (20/loaf)	1 slice	23	35	65	2	1	0.2	0.3	0.3
Slice, toasted	1 slice	20	24	65	2	1	0.2	0.3	0.3
Loaf, 2 lb	1 loaf	907	35	2,495	82	34	7.7	11.8	10.4
Slice (34/loaf)	1 slice	27	35	75	2	1	0.2	0.3	0.3
Slice, toasted	1 slice	23	24	75	2	1	0.2	0.3	0.3
Whole wheat bread									
Soft-crumb type[38]									
Loaf, 1 lb	1 loaf	454	36	1,095	41	12	2.2	2.9	4.2
Slice (16/loaf)	1 slice	28	36	65	3	1	0.1	0.2	0.2
Slice, toasted	1 slice	24	24	65	3	1	0.1	0.2	0.2
Firm-crumb type[38]									
Loaf, 1 lb	1 loaf	454	36	1,100	48	14	2.5	3.3	4.9
Slice (18/loaf)	1 slice	25	36	60	3	1	0.1	0.2	0.3
Slice, toasted	1 slice	21	24	60	3	1	0.1	0.2	0.3
Breakfast cereals									
Hot type, cooked									
Corn (hominy) grits, degermed									
Enriched	1 cup	245	87	125	3	Trace	Trace	Trace	0.1
Unenriched	1 cup	245	87	125	3	Trace	Trace	Trace	0.1
Farina, quick-cooking, enriched	1 cup	245	89	105	3	Trace	Trace	Trace	0.1
Oatmeal or rolled oats	1 cup	240	87	130	5	2	0.4	0.8	0.9
Wheat, rolled	1 cup	240	80	180	5	1	—	—	—
Wheat, whole-meal	1 cup	245	88	110	4	1	—	—	—
Ready-to-eat									
Bran flakes (40% bran), added sugar, salt, iron, vitamins	1 cup	35	3	105	4	1	—	—	—
Bran flakes with raisins, added sugar, salt, iron, vitamins	1 cup	50	7	145	4	1	—	—	—
Corn flakes									
Plain, added sugar, salt, iron, vitamins	1 cup	25	4	95	2	Trace	—	—	—

[40] Applies to white varieties. For yellow varieties, value is 150 IU.

[41] Applies to products that do not contain disodium phosphate. If disodium phosphate is an ingredient, value is 162 mg.

[42] Value may range from less than 1 mg to about 8 mg depending on the brand. Consult the label.

[43] Value varies with the brand. Consult the label.

NUTRIENTS IN INDICATED QUANTITY

Carbohydrate (g)	Calcium (mg)	Phosphorus (mg)	Iron (mg)	Potassium (mg)	Vitamin A value (IU)	Thiamin (mg)	Riboflavin (mg)	Niacin (mg)	Ascorbic acid (mg)
229	381	440	11.3	476	Trace	1.80	1.10	15.0	Trace
13	21	24	0.6	26	Trace	0.10	0.06	0.8	Trace
13	21	24	0.6	26	Trace	0.08	0.06	0.8	Trace
10	17	19	0.5	21	Trace	0.08	0.05	0.7	Trace
10	17	19	0.5	21	Trace	0.06	0.05	0.7	Trace
343	571	660	17.0	714	Trace	2.70	1.65	22.5	Trace
14	24	27	0.7	29	Trace	0.11	0.07	0.9	Trace
14	24	27	0.7	29	Trace	0.09	0.07	0.9	Trace
12	20	23	0.6	25	Trace	0.10	0.06	0.8	Trace
12	20	23	0.6	25	Trace	0.08	0.06	0.8	Trace
15	25	29	0.8	32	Trace	0.12	0.07	1.0	Trace
23	38	44	1.1	47	Trace	0.18	0.11	1.5	Trace
228	435	463	11.3	549	Trace	1.80	1.10	15.0	Trace
12	22	23	0.6	28	Trace	0.09	0.06	0.8	Trace
12	22	23	0.6	28	Trace	0.07	0.06	0.8	Trace
455	871	925	22.7	1,097	Trace	3.60	2.20	30.0	Trace
14	26	28	0.7	33	Trace	0.11	0.06	0.9	Trace
14	26	28	0.7	33	Trace	0.09	0.06	0.9	Trace
224	381	1,152	13.6	1,161	Trace	1.37	0.45	12.7	Trace
14	24	71	0.8	72	Trace	0.09	0.03	0.8	Trace
14	24	71	0.8	72	Trace	0.07	0.03	0.8	Trace
216	449	1,034	13.6	1,238	Trace	1.17	0.54	12.7	Trace
12	25	57	0.8	68	Trace	0.06	0.03	0.7	Trace
12	25	57	0.8	68	Trace	0.05	0.03	0.7	Trace
27	2	25	0.7	27	[40]Trace	0.10	0.07	1.0	0
27	2	25	0.2	27	[40]Trace	0.05	0.02	0.5	0
22	147	[41]113	([42])	25	0	0.12	0.07	1.0	0
23	22	137	1 4	146	0	0.19	0.05	0.2	0
41	19	182	1.7	202	0	0.17	0.07	2.2	0
23	17	127	1.2	118	0	0.15	0.05	1.5	0
28	19	125	12.4	137	1,650	0.41	0.49	4.1	12
40	28	146	17.7	154	2,350	0.58	0.71	5.8	18
21	([43])	9	0.6	30	1,180	0.29	0.35	2.9	9

Continued.

Nutritive values of the edible part of food—cont'd

Foods, approximate measures, units, and weight in grams (edible part unless footnotes indicate otherwise)			Water (%)	Food energy (kcal)	Protein (g)	Fat (g)	Fatty acids: Saturated (total) (g)	Fatty acids: Unsaturated: Oleic (g)	Fatty acids: Unsaturated: Linoleic (g)
Corn flakes—cont'd									
Sugar-coated, added salt, iron, vitamins	1 cup	40	2	155	2	Trace	—	—	—
Corn, puffed, plain, added sugar, salt, iron, vitamins	1 cup	20	4	80	2	1	—	—	—
Corn, shredded, added sugar, salt, iron, thiamin, niacin	1 cup	25	3	95	2	Trace	—	—	—
Oats, puffed, added sugar, salt, minerals, vitamins	1 cup	25	3	100	3	1	—	—	—
Rice, puffed									
Plain, added iron, thiamin, niacin	1 cup	15	4	60	1	Trace	—	—	—
Presweetened, added salt, iron, vitamins	1 cup	28	3	115	1	0	—	—	—
Wheat flakes, added sugar, salt, iron, vitamins	1 cup	30	4	105	3	Trace	—	—	—
Wheat puffed									
Plain, added iron, thiamin, niacin	1 cup	15	3	55	2	Trace	—	—	—
Presweetened, added salt, iron, vitamins	1 cup	38	3	140	3	Trace	—	—	—
Wheat, shredded, plain (oblong biscuit or ½ cup spoon-size biscuits)	1 biscuit	25	7	90	2	1	—	—	—
Wheat germ, without salt and sugar, toasted	1 tbsp	6	4	25	2	1	—	—	—
Buckwheat flour, light, sifted	1 cup	98	12	340	6	1	0.2	0.4	0.4
Bulgur, canned, seasoned	1 cup	135	56	245	8	4	—	—	—
Cake icings. See Sugars and sweets									
Cakes made from cake mixes with enriched flour[46]									
Angel food									
Whole cake (9¾-inch diam. tube cake)	1 cake	635	34	1,645	36	1	—	—	—
Piece, 1/12 of cake	1 piece	53	34	135	3	Trace	—	—	—
Coffeecake									
Whole cake (7¾ by 5⅝ by 1¼ inch)	1 cake	430	30	1,385	27	41	11.7	16.3	8.8
Piece, 1/6 of cake	1 piece	72	30	230	5	7	2.0	2.7	1.5
Cupcakes, made with egg, milk, 2½-inch diam.									
Without icing	1 cupcake	25	26	90	1	3	0.8	1.2	0.7
With chocolate icing	1 cupcake	36	22	130	2	5	2.0	1.6	0.6

[44] Value varies with the brand. Consult the label.

[45] Applies to product with added ascorbic acid. Without added ascorbic acid, value is trace.

[46] Excepting angel food cake, cakes were made from mixes containing vegetable shortening; icings, with butter.

NUTRIENTS IN INDICATED QUANTITY

Carbohydrate (g)	Calcium (mg)	Phosphorus (mg)	Iron (mg)	Potassium (mg)	Vitamin A value (IU)	Thiamin (mg)	Riboflavin (mg)	Niacin (mg)	Ascorbic acid (mg)
37	1	10	1.0	27	1,880	0.46	0.56	4.6	14
16	4	18	2.3	—	940	0.23	0.28	2.3	7
22	1	10	0.6	—	0	0.11	0.05	0.5	0
19	44	102	2.9	—	1,180	0.29	0.35	2.9	9
13	3	14	0.3	15	0	0.07	0.01	0.7	0
26	3	14	[44]1.1	43	1,250	0.38	0.43	5.0	[45]15
24	12	83	([43])	81	1,410	0.35	0.42	3.5	11
12	4	48	0.6	51	0	0.08	0.03	1.2	0
33	7	52	[44]1.6	63	1,680	0.50	0.57	6.7	[45]20
20	11	97	0.9	87	0	0.06	0.03	1.1	0
3	3	70	0.5	57	10	0.11	0.05	0.3	1
78	11	86	1.0	314	0	0.08	0.04	0.4	0
44	27	263	1.9	151	0	0.08	0.05	4.1	0
377	603	756	2.5	381	0	0.37	0.97	3.6	0
32	50	63	0.2	32	0	0.03	0.08	0.3	0
225	262	748	6.9	469	690	0.82	0.91	7.7	1
38	44	125	1.2	78	120	0.14	0.15	1.3	Trace
14	40	59	0.3	21	40	0.05	0.05	0.4	Trace
21	47	71	0.4	42	60	0.05	0.06	0.4	Trace

Continued.

Nutritive values of the edible part of food—cont'd

Foods, approximate measures, units, and weight in grams (edible part unless footnotes indicate otherwise)			Water (%)	Food energy (kcal)	Protein (g)	Fat (g)	Fatty acids: Saturated (total) (g)	Unsaturated: Oleic (g)	Unsaturated: Linoleic (g)
Devil's food with chocolate icing									
Whole, 2 layer cake (8- or 9-inch diam.)	1 cake	1,107	24	3,755	49	136	50.0	44.9	17.0
Piece, 1/16 of cake	1 piece	69	24	235	3	8	3.1	2.8	1.1
Cupcake, 2½-inch diam.	1 cupcake	35	24	120	2	4	1.6	1.4	0.5
Gingerbread									
Whole cake (8-inch square)	1 cake	570	37	1,575	18	39	9.7	16.6	10.0
Piece, 1/9 of cake	1 piece	63	37	175	2	4	1.1	1.8	1.1
White, 2 layer with chocolate icing									
Whole cake (8- or 9-inch diam.)	1 cake	1,140	21	4,000	44	122	48.2	46.4	20.0
Piece, 1/16 of cake	1 piece	71	21	250	3	8	3.0	2.9	1.2
Yellow, 2 layer with chocolate icing									
Whole cake (8- or 9-inch diam.)	1 cake	1,108	26	3,735	45	125	47.8	47.8	20.3
Piece, 1/16 of cake	1 piece	69	26	235	3	8	3.0	3.0	1.3
Cakes made from home recipes using enriched flour[47]									
Boston cream pie with custard filling									
Whole cake (8-inch diam.)	1 cake	825	35	2,490	41	78	23.0	30.1	15.2
Piece, 1/12 of cake	1 piece	69	35	210	3	6	1.9	2.5	1.3
Fruitcake, dark									
Loaf, 1 lb (7½ by 2 by 1½ inch)	1 loaf	454	18	1,720	22	69	14.4	33.5	14.8
Slice, 1/30 of loaf	1 slice	15	18	55	1	2	0.5	1.1	0.5
Plain, sheet cake									
Without icing									
Whole cake (9-inch square)	1 cake	777	25	2,830	35	108	29.5	44.4	23.9
Piece, 1/9 of cake	1 piece	86	25	315	4	12	3.3	4.9	2.6
With uncooked white icing									
Whole cake (9-inch square)	1 cake	1,096	21	4,020	37	129	42.2	49.5	24.4
Piece, 1/9 of cake	1 piece	121	21	445	4	14	4.7	5.5	2.7
Pound[49]									
Loaf, 8½ by 3½ by 3¼ inches	1 loaf	565	16	2,725	31	170	42.9	73.1	39.6
Slice, 1/17 of loaf	1 slice	33	16	160	2	10	2.5	4.3	2.3
Spongecake									
Whole cake (9¾-inch diam. tube cake)	1 cake	790	32	2,345	60	45	13.1	15.8	5.7
Piece, 1/12 of cake	1 piece	66	32	195	5	4	1.1	1.3	0.5
Cookies made with enriched flour[50,51]									

[47] Excepting spongecake, vegetable shortening used for cake portion; butter, for icing. If butter or margarine used for cake portion, vitamin A

[48] Applies to product made with a sodium aluminum-sulfate type baking powder. With a low-sodium type baking powder containing potassium,

[49] Equal weights of flour, sugar, eggs, and vegetable shortening.

[50] Products are commercial unless otherwise specified.

[51] Made with enriched flour and vegetable shortening except for macaroons which do not contain flour or shortening.

NUTRIENTS IN INDICATED QUANTITY

Carbohydrate (g)	Calcium (mg)	Phosphorus (mg)	Iron (mg)	Potassium (mg)	Vitamin A value (IU)	Thiamin (mg)	Riboflavin (mg)	Niacin (mg)	Ascorbic acid (mg)
645	653	1,162	16.6	1,439	1,660	1.06	1.65	10.1	1
40	41	72	1.0	90	100	0.07	0.10	0.6	Trace
20	21	37	0.5	46	50	0.03	0.05	0.3	Trace
291	513	570	8.6	1,562	Trace	0.84	1.00	7.4	Trace
32	57	63	0.9	173	Trace	0.09	0.11	0.8	Trace
716	1,129	2,041	11.4	1,322	680	1.50	1.77	12.5	2
45	70	127	0.7	82	40	0.09	0.11	0.8	Trace
638	1,008	2,017	12.2	1,208	1,550	1.24	1.67	10.6	2
40	63	126	0.8	75	100	0.08	0.10	0.7	Trace
412	553	833	8.2	[48]734	1,730	1.04	1.27	9.6	2
34	46	70	0.7	[48]61	140	0.09	0.11	0.8	Trace
271	327	513	11.8	2,250	540	0.72	0.73	4.9	2
9	11	17	0.4	74	20	0.02	0.02	0.2	Trace
434	497	793	8.5	[48]614	1,320	1.21	1.40	10.2	2
48	55	88	0.9	[48]68	150	0.13	0.15	1.1	Trace
694	548	822	8.2	[48]669	2,190	1.22	1.47	10.2	2
77	61	91	0.8	[48]74	240	0.14	0.16	1.1	Trace
273	107	418	7.9	345	1,410	0.90	0.99	7.3	0
16	6	24	0.5	20	80	0.05	0.06	0.4	0
427	237	885	13.4	687	3,560	1.10	1.64	7.4	Trace
36	20	74	1.1	57	300	0.09	0.14	0.6	Trace

values would be higher.

value would be about twice the amount shown.

Continued.

Nutritive values of the edible part of food—cont'd

Foods, approximate measures, units, and weight in grams (edible part unless footnotes indicate otherwise)			Water (%)	Food energy (kcal)	Protein (g)	Fat (g)	Fatty acids: Saturated (total) (g)	Fatty acids: Unsaturated: Oleic (g)	Fatty acids: Unsaturated: Linoleic (g)
Brownies with nuts									
Home-prepared, 1¾ by 1¾ by ⅞ inch									
From home recipe	1 brownie	20	10	95	1	6	1.5	3.0	1.2
From commercial recipe	1 brownie	20	11	85	1	4	0.9	1.4	1.3
Frozen, with chocolate icing,[52] 1½ by 1¾ by ⅞ inch	1 brownie	25	13	105	1	5	2.0	2.2	0.7
Chocolate chip									
Commercial, 2¼-inch diam., ⅜ inch thick	4 cookies	42	3	200	2	9	2.8	2.9	2.2
From home recipe, 2⅓-inch diam.	4 cookies	40	3	205	2	12	3.5	4.5	2.9
Fig bars, square (1⅝ by 1⅝ by ⅜ inch) or rectangular (1½ by 1¾ by ½ inch)	4 cookies	56	14	200	2	3	0.8	1.2	0.7
Gingersnaps, 2-inch diam., ¼ inch thick	4 cookies	28	3	90	2	2	0.7	1.0	0.6
Macaroons, 2¾-inch diam., ¼ inch thick	2 cookies	38	4	180	2	9	—	—	—
Oatmeal with raisins, 2⅝-inch diam., ¼ inch thick	4 cookies	52	3	235	3	8	2.0	3.3	2.0
Plain, prepared from commercial chilled dough, 2½-inch diam., ¼ inch thick	4 cookies	48	5	240	2	12	3.0	5.2	2.9
Sandwich type (chocolate or vanilla), 1¾-inch diam., ⅜ inch thick	4 cookies	40	2	200	2	9	2.2	3.9	2.2
Vanilla wafers, 1¾-inch diam., ¼-inch thick	10 cookies	40	3	185	2	6	—	—	—
Cornmeal									
Whole-ground, unbolted, dry form	1 cup	122	12	435	11	5	0.5	1.0	2.5
Bolted (nearly whole-grain), dry form	1 cup	122	12	440	11	4	0.5	0.9	2.1
Degermed, enriched									
Dry form	1 cup	138	12	500	11	2	0.2	0.4	0.9
Cooked	1 cup	240	88	120	3	Trace	Trace	0.1	0.2
Degermed, unenriched									
Dry form	1 cup	138	12	500	11	2	0.2	0.4	0.9
Cooked	1 cup	240	88	120	3	Trace	Trace	0.1	0.2
Crackers[38]									
Graham, plain, 2½-inch square	2 crackers	14	6	55	1	1	0.3	0.5	0.3
Rye wafers, whole-grain, 1⅞ by 3½ inches	2 wafers	13	6	45	2	Trace	—	—	—
Saltines, made with enriched flour	4 crackers or 1 packet	11	4	50	1	1	0.3	0.5	0.4

[52] Icing made with butter.

[53] Applies to yellow varieties; white varieties contain only a trace.

NUTRIENTS IN INDICATED QUANTITY

Carbohydrate (g)	Calcium (mg)	Phosphorus (mg)	Iron (mg)	Potassium (mg)	Vitamin A value (IU)	Thiamin (mg)	Riboflavin (mg)	Niacin (mg)	Ascorbic acid (mg)
10	8	30	0.4	38	40	0.04	0.03	0.2	Trace
13	9	27	0.4	34	20	0.03	0.02	0.2	Trace
15	10	31	0.4	44	50	0.03	0.03	0.2	Trace
29	16	48	1.0	56	50	0.10	0.17	0.9	Trace
24	14	40	0.8	47	40	0.06	0.06	0.5	Trace
42	44	34	1.0	111	60	0.04	0.14	0.9	Trace
22	20	13	0.7	129	20	0.08	0.06	0.7	0
25	10	32	0.3	176	0	0.02	0.06	0.2	0
38	11	53	1.4	192	30	0.15	0.10	1.0	Trace
31	17	35	0.6	23	30	0.10	0.08	0.9	0
28	10	96	0.7	15	0	0.06	0.10	0.7	0
30	16	25	0.6	29	50	0.10	0.09	0.8	0
90	24	312	2.9	346	[53]620	0.46	0.13	2.4	0
91	21	272	2.2	303	[53]590	0.37	0.10	2.3	0
108	8	137	4.0	166	[53]610	0.61	0.36	4.8	0
26	2	34	1.0	38	[53]140	0.14	0.10	1.2	0
108	8	137	1.5	166	[53]610	0.19	0.07	1.4	0
26	2	34	0.5	38	[53]140	0.05	0.02	0.2	0
10	6	21	0.5	55	0	0.02	0.08	0.5	0
10	7	50	0.5	78	0	0.04	0.03	0.2	0
8	2	10	0.5	13	0	0.05	0.05	0.4	0

Continued.

Nutritive values of the edible part of food—cont'd

Foods, approximate measures, units, and weight in grams (edible part unless footnotes indicate otherwise)			Water (%)	Food energy (kcal)	Protein (g)	Fat (g)	Fatty acids: Saturated (total) (g)	Fatty acids: Unsaturated: Oleic (g)	Fatty acids: Unsaturated: Linoleic (g)
Danish pastry (enriched flour), plain without fruit or nuts[54]									
Packaged ring, 12 oz	1 ring	340	22	1,435	25	80	24.3	31.7	16.5
Round piece, about 4¼-inch diam. by 1 inch	1 pastry	65	22	275	5	15	4.7	6.1	3.2
Ounce	1 oz	28	22	120	2	7	2.0	2.7	1.4
Doughnuts, made with enriched flour[38]									
Cake type, plain, 2½-inch diam., 1 inch high	1 doughnut	25	24	100	1	5	1.2	2.0	1.1
Yeast-leavened, glazed, 3¾-inch diam., 1¼ inch high	1 doughnut	50	26	205	3	11	3.3	5.8	3.3
Macaroni, enriched, cooked (cut lengths, elbows, shells)									
Firm stage (hot)	1 cup	130	64	190	7	1	—	—	—
Tender stage									
Cold macaroni	1 cup	105	73	115	4	Trace	—	—	—
Hot macaroni	1 cup	140	73	155	5	1	—	—	—
Macaroni (enriched) and cheese									
Canned[55]	1 cup	240	80	230	9	10	4.2	3.1	1.4
From home recipe (served hot)[56]	1 cup	200	58	430	17	22	8.9	8.8	2.9
Muffins made with enriched flour[38]									
From home recipe									
Blueberry, 2⅜-inch diam., 1½ inch high	1 muffin	40	39	110	3	4	1.1	1.4	0.7
Bran	1 muffin	40	35	105	3	4	1.2	1.4	0.8
Corn (enriched degermed cornmeal and flour), 2⅜-inch diam., 1½ inch high	1 muffin	40	33	125	3	4	1.2	1.6	0.9
Plain, 3-inch diam., 1½ inches high	1 muffin	40	38	120	3	4	1.0	1.7	1.0
From mix, egg, milk									
Corn, 2⅜-inch diam., 1½ inch high[58]	1 muffin	40	30	130	3	4	1.2	1.7	0.9
Noodles (egg noodles), enriched, cooked	1 cup	160	71	200	7	2	—	—	—
Noodles, chow mein, canned	1 cup	45	1	220	6	11	—	—	—
Pancakes (4-inch diam.)[38]									
Buckwheat, made from mix (with buckwheat and enriched flours), egg and milk added	1 cake	27	58	55	2	2	0.8	0.9	0.4

[54]Contains vegetable shortening and butter.
[55]Made with corn oil.
[56]Made with regular margarine.
[57]Applies to product made with yellow cornmeal.
[58]Made with enriched degermed cornmeal and enriched flour.

NUTRIENTS IN INDICATED QUANTITY

Carbohydrate (g)	Calcium (mg)	Phosphorus (mg)	Iron (mg)	Potassium (mg)	Vitamin A value (IU)	Thiamin (mg)	Riboflavin (mg)	Niacin (mg)	Ascorbic acid (mg)
155	170	371	6.1	381	1,050	0.97	1.01	8.6	Trace
30	33	71	1.2	73	200	0.18	0.19	1.7	Trace
13	14	31	0.5	32	90	0.08	0.08	0.7	Trace
13	10	48	0.4	23	20	0.05	0.05	0.4	Trace
22	16	33	0.6	34	25	0.10	0.10	0.8	0
39	14	85	1.4	103	0	0.23	0.13	1.8	0
24	8	53	0.9	64	0	0.15	0.08	1.2	0
32	11	70	1.3	85	0	0.20	0.11	1.5	0
26	199	182	1.0	139	260	0.12	0.24	1.0	Trace
40	362	322	1.8	240	860	0.20	0.40	1.8	Trace
17	34	53	0.6	46	90	0.09	0.10	0.7	Trace
17	57	162	1.5	172	90	0.07	0.10	1.7	Trace
19	42	68	0.7	54	[57]120	0.10	0.10	0.7	Trace
17	42	60	0.6	50	40	0.09	0.12	0.9	Trace
20	96	152	0.6	44	[57]100	0.08	0.09	0.7	Trace
37	16	94	1.4	70	110	0.22	0.13	1.9	0
26	—	—	—	—	—	—	—	—	—
6	59	91	0.4	66	60	0.04	0.05	0.2	Trace

Continued.

Nutritive values of the edible part of food—cont'd

Foods, approximate measures, units, and weight in grams (edible part unless footnotes indicate otherwise)			Water (%)	Food energy (kcal)	Protein (g)	Fat (g)	Fatty acids: Saturated (total) (g)	Fatty acids: Unsaturated: Oleic (g)	Fatty acids: Unsaturated: Linoleic (g)
Pancakes—cont'd									
Plain									
Made from home recipe using enriched flour	1 cake	27	50	60	2	2	0.5	0.8	0.5
Made from mix with enriched flour, egg and milk added	1 cake	27	51	60	2	2	0.7	0.7	0.3
Pies, piecrust made with enriched flour, vegetable shortening (9-inch diam.)									
Apple									
Whole	1 pie	945	48	2,420	21	105	27.0	44.5	25.2
Sector, 1/7 of pie	1 sector	135	48	345	3	15	3.9	6.4	3.6
Banana cream									
Whole	1 pie	910	54	2,010	41	85	26.7	33.2	16.2
Sector, 1/7 of pie	1 sector	130	54	285	6	12	3.8	4.7	2.3
Blueberry									
Whole	1 pie	945	51	2,285	23	102	24.8	43.7	25.1
Sector, 1/7 of pie	1 sector	135	51	325	3	15	3.5	6.2	3.6
Cherry									
Whole	1 pie	945	47	2,465	25	107	28.2	45.0	25.3
Sector, 1/7 of pie	1 sector	135	47	350	4	15	4.0	6.4	3.6
Custard									
Whole	1 pie	910	58	1,985	56	101	33.9	38.5	17.5
Sector, 1/7 of pie	1 sector	130	58	285	8	14	4.8	5.5	2.5
Lemon meringue									
Whole	1 pie	840	47	2,140	31	86	26.1	33.8	16.4
Sector, 1/7 of pie	1 sector	120	47	305	4	12	3.7	4.8	2.3
Mince									
Whole	1 pie	945	43	2,560	24	109	28.0	45.9	25.2
Sector, 1/7 of pie	1 sector	135	43	365	3	16	4.0	6.6	3.6
Peach									
Whole	1 pie	945	48	2,410	24	101	24.8	43.7	25.1
Sector, 1/7 of pie	1 sector	135	48	345	3	14	3.5	6.2	3.6
Pecan									
Whole	1 pie	825	20	3,450	42	189	27.8	101.0	44.2
Sector, 1/7 of pie	1 sector	118	20	495	6	27	4.0	14.4	6.3
Pumpkin									
Whole	1 pie	910	59	1,920	36	102	37.4	37.5	16.6
Sector, 1/7 of pie	1 sector	130	59	275	5	15	5.4	5.4	2.4
Piecrust (home recipe) made with enriched flour and vegetable shortening, baked, 9-inch diam.	1 pie shell	180	15	900	11	60	14.8	26.1	14.9
Piecrust mix for 2-crust pie with enriched flour and vegetable shortening, 10 oz pkg prepared and baked, 9-inch diam.	1 mix	320	19	1,485	20	93	22.7	39.7	23.4
Pizza (cheese) baked, 4¾-inch sector; ⅛ of 12-inch diam. pie[19]	1 sector	60	45	145	6	4	1.7	1.5	0.6
Popcorn, popped									
Plain, large kernel	1 cup	6	4	25	1	Trace	Trace	0.1	0.2
With oil (coconut) and salt added, large kernel	1 cup	9	3	40	1	2	1.5	0.2	0.2

NUTRIENTS IN INDICATED QUANTITY

Carbohydrate (g)	Calcium (mg)	Phosphorus (mg)	Iron (mg)	Potassium (mg)	Vitamin A value (IU)	Thiamin (mg)	Riboflavin (mg)	Niacin (mg)	Ascorbic acid (mg)
9	27	38	0.4	33	30	0.06	0.07	0.5	Trace
9	58	70	0.3	42	70	0.04	0.06	0.2	Trace
360	76	208	6.6	756	280	1.06	0.79	9.3	9
51	11	30	0.9	108	40	0.15	0.11	1.3	2
279	601	746	7.3	1,847	2,280	0.77	1.51	7.0	9
40	86	107	1.0	264	330	0.11	0.22	1.0	1
330	104	217	9.5	614	280	1.03	0.80	10.0	28
47	15	31	1.4	88	40	0.15	0.11	1.4	4
363	132	236	6.6	992	4,160	1.09	0.84	9.8	Trace
52	19	34	0.9	142	590	0.16	0.12	1.4	Trace
213	874	1,028	8.2	1,247	2,090	0.79	1.92	5.6	0
30	125	147	1.2	178	300	0.11	0.27	0.8	0
317	118	412	6.7	420	1,430	0.61	0.84	5.2	25
45	17	59	1.0	60	200	0.09	0.12	0.7	4
389	265	359	13.3	1,682	20	0.96	0.86	9.8	9
56	38	51	1.9	240	Trace	0.14	0.12	1.4	1
361	95	274	8.5	1,408	6,900	1.04	0.97	14.0	28
52	14	39	1.2	201	990	0.15	0.14	2.0	4
423	388	850	25.6	1,015	1,320	1.80	0.95	6.9	Trace
61	55	122	3.7	145	190	0.26	0.14	1.0	Trace
223	464	628	7.3	1,456	22,480	0.78	1.27	7.0	Trace
32	66	90	1.0	208	3,210	0.11	0.18	1.0	Trace
79	25	90	3.1	89	0	0.47	0.40	5.0	0
141	131	272	6.1	179	0	1.07	0.79	9.9	0
22	86	89	1.1	67	230	0.16	0.18	1.6	4
5	1	17	0.2	—	—	—	0.01	0.1	0
5	1	19	0.2	—	—	—	0.01	0.2	0

Continued.

Nutritive values of the edible part of food—cont'd

Foods, approximate measures, units, and weight in grams (edible part unless footnotes indicate otherwise)			Water (%)	Food energy (kcal)	Protein (g)	Fat (g)	Fatty acids: Saturated (total) (g)	Fatty acids: Unsaturated: Oleic (g)	Fatty acids: Unsaturated: Linoleic (g)
Popcorn, popped—cont'd									
Sugar coated	1 cup	35	4	135	2	1	0.5	0.2	0.4
Pretzels, made with enriched flour									
Dutch, twisted, 2¾ by 2⅝ inches	1 pretzel	16	5	60	2	1	—	—	—
Thin, twisted, 3¼ by 2¼ by ¼ inch	10 pretzels	60	5	235	6	3	—	—	—
Stick, 2¼ inches long	10 pretzels	3	5	10	Trace	Trace	—	—	—
Rice, white, enriched									
Instant, ready-to-serve, hot	1 cup	165	73	180	4	Trace	Trace	Trace	Trace
Long grain									
Raw	1 cup	185	12	670	12	1	0.2	0.2	0.2
Cooked, served hot	1 cup	205	73	225	4	Trace	0.1	0.1	0.1
Parboiled									
Raw	1 cup	185	10	685	14	1	0.2	0.1	0.2
Cooked, served hot	1 cup	175	73	185	4	Trace	0.1	0.1	0.1
Rolls, enriched[38]									
Commercial									
Brown-and-serve (12/12 oz pkg), browned	1 roll	26	27	85	2	2	0.4	0.7	0.5
Cloverleaf or pan, 2½-inches diam., 2 inches high	1 roll	28	31	85	2	2	0.4	0.6	0.4
Frankfurter and hamburger (8/11½ oz pkg.)	1 roll	40	31	120	3	2	0.5	0.8	0.6
Hard, 3¾-inch diam., 2 inches high	1 roll	50	25	155	5	2	0.4	0.6	0.5
Hoagie or submarine, 11½ by 3 by 2½ inches	1 roll	135	31	390	12	4	0.9	1.4	1.4
From home recipe									
Cloverleaf, 2½-inch diam., 2 inches high	1 roll	35	26	120	3	3	0.8	1.1	0.7
Spaghetti, enriched, cooked									
Firm stage, "al dente," served hot	1 cup	130	64	190	7	1	—	—	—
Tender stage, served hot	1 cup	140	73	155	5	1	—	—	—
Spaghetti (enriched) in tomato sauce with cheese									
From home recipe	1 cup	250	77	260	9	9	2.0	5.4	0.7
Canned	1 cup	250	80	190	6	2	0.5	0.3	0.4
Spaghetti (enriched) with meat balls and tomato sauce									
From home recipe	1 cup	248	70	330	19	12	3.3	6.3	0.9
Canned	1 cup	250	78	260	12	10	2.2	3.3	3.9
Toaster pastries	1 pastry	50	12	200	3	6	—	—	—
Waffles, made with enriched flour, 7-inch diam.[38]									
From home recipe	1 waffle	75	41	210	7	7	2.3	2.8	1.4
From mix, egg and milk added	1 waffle	75	42	205	7	8	2.8	2.9	1.2

[59] Product may or may not be enriched with riboflavin. Consult the label.
[60] Value varies with the brand. Consult the label.

NUTRIENTS IN INDICATED QUANTITY

Carbohydrate (g)	Calcium (mg)	Phosphorus (mg)	Iron (mg)	Potassium (mg)	Vitamin A value (IU)	Thiamin (mg)	Riboflavin (mg)	Niacin (mg)	Ascorbic acid (mg)
30	2	47	0.5	—	—	—	0.02	0.4	0
12	4	21	0.2	21	0	0.05	0.04	0.7	0
46	13	79	0.9	78	0	0.20	0.15	2.5	0
2	1	4	Trace	4	0	0.01	0.01	0.1	0
40	5	31	1.3	—	0	0.21	([59])	1.7	0
149	44	174	5.4	170	0	0.81	0.06	6.5	0
50	21	57	1.8	57	0	0.23	0.02	2.1	0
150	111	370	5.4	278	0	0.81	0.07	6.5	0
41	33	100	1.4	75	0	0.19	0.02	2.1	0
14	20	23	0.5	25	Trace	0.10	0.06	0.9	Trace
15	21	24	0.5	27	Trace	0.11	0.07	0.9	Trace
21	30	34	0.8	38	Trace	0.16	0.10	1.3	Trace
30	24	46	1.2	49	Trace	0.20	0.12	1.7	Trace
75	58	115	3.0	122	Trace	0.54	0.32	4.5	Trace
20	16	36	0.7	41	30	0.12	0.12	1.2	Trace
39	14	85	1.4	103	0	0.23	0.13	1.8	0
32	11	70	1.3	85	0	0.20	0.11	1.5	0
37	80	135	2.3	408	1,080	0.25	0.18	2.3	13
39	40	88	2.8	303	930	0.35	0.28	4.5	10
39	124	236	3.7	665	1,590	0.25	0.30	4.0	22
29	53	113	3.3	245	1,000	0.15	0.18	2.3	5
36	[60]54	[60]67	1.9	[60]74	500	0.16	0.17	2.1	([60])
28	85	130	1.3	109	250	0.17	0.23	1.4	Trace
27	179	257	1.0	146	170	0.14	0.22	0.9	Trace

Continued.

Nutritive values of the edible part of food—cont'd

Foods, approximate measures, units, and weight in grams (edible part unless footnotes indicate otherwise)			Water (%)	Food energy (kcal)	Protein (g)	Fat (g)	Fatty acids: Saturated (total) (g)	Fatty acids: Unsaturated: Oleic (g)	Fatty acids: Unsaturated: Linoleic (g)
Wheat flours									
All-purpose or family flour, enriched									
Sifted, spooned	1 cup	115	12	420	12	1	0.2	0.1	0.5
Unsifted, spooned	1 cup	125	12	455	13	1	0.2	0.1	0.5
Cake or pastry flour, enriched, sifted, spooned	1 cup	96	12	350	7	1	0.1	0.1	0.3
Self-rising, enriched, unsifted, spooned	1 cup	125	12	440	12	1	0.2	0.1	0.5
Whole-wheat, from hard wheats, stirred	1 cup	120	12	400	16	2	0.4	0.2	1.0
LEGUMES (DRY), NUTS, SEEDS; RELATED PRODUCTS									
Almonds, shelled									
Chopped (about 130 almonds)	1 cup	130	5	775	24	70	5.6	47.7	12.8
Slivered, not pressed down (about 115 almonds)	1 cup	115	5	690	21	62	5.0	42.2	11.3
Beans, dry									
Common varieties as Great Northern, navy, and others									
Cooked, drained									
Great Northern	1 cup	180	69	210	14	1	—	—	—
Pea (navy)	1 cup	190	69	225	15	1	—	—	—
Canned, solids and liquid									
White with—									
Frankfurters (sliced)	1 cup	255	71	365	19	18	—	—	—
Pork and tomato sauce	1 cup	255	71	310	16	7	2.4	2.8	0.6
Pork and sweet sauce	1 cup	255	66	385	16	12	4.3	5.0	1.1
Red kidney	1 cup	255	76	230	15	1	—	—	—
Lima, cooked, drained	1 cup	190	64	260	16	1	—	—	—
Blackeye peas, dry, cooked (with residual cooking liquid)	1 cup	250	80	190	13	1	—	—	—
Brazil nuts, shelled (6-8 large kernels)	1 oz	28	5	185	4	19	4.8	6.2	7.1
Cashew nuts, roasted in oil	1 cup	140	5	785	24	64	12.9	36.8	10.2
Coconut meat, fresh									
Piece, about 2 by 2 by ½ inch	1 piece	45	51	155	2	16	14.0	0.9	0.3
Shredded or grated, not pressed down	1 cup	80	51	275	3	28	24.8	1.6	0.5
Filberts (hazelnuts), chopped (about 80 kernels)	1 cup	115	6	730	14	72	5.1	55.2	7.3
Lentils, whole, cooked	1 cup	200	72	210	16	Trace	—	—	—
Peanuts, roasted in oil, salted (whole, halves, chopped)	1 cup	144	2	840	37	72	13.7	33.0	20.7

NUTRIENTS IN INDICATED QUANTITY

Carbohydrate (g)	Calcium (mg)	Phosphorus (mg)	Iron (mg)	Potassium (mg)	Vitamin A value (IU)	Thiamin (mg)	Riboflavin (mg)	Niacin (mg)	Ascorbic acid (mg)
88	18	100	3.3	109	0	0.74	0.46	6.1	0
95	20	109	3.6	119	0	0.80	0.50	6.6	0
76	16	70	2.8	91	0	0.61	0.38	5.1	0
93	331	583	3.6	—	0	0.80	0.50	6.6	0
85	49	446	4.0	444	0	0.66	0.14	5.2	0
25	304	655	6.1	1,005	0	0.31	1.20	4.6	Trace
22	269	580	5.4	889	0	0.28	1.06	4.0	Trace
38	90	266	4.9	749	0	0.25	0.13	1.3	0
40	95	281	5.1	790	0	0.27	0.13	1.3	0
32	94	303	4.8	688	330	0.18	0.15	3.3	Trace
48	138	235	4.6	536	330	0.20	0.08	1.5	5
54	161	291	5.9	—	—	0.15	0.10	1.3	—
42	74	278	4.6	673	10	0.13	0.10	1.5	—
49	55	293	5.9	1,163	—	0.25	0.11	1.3	—
35	43	238	3.3	573	30	0.40	0.10	1.0	—
3	53	196	1.0	203	Trace	0.27	0.03	0.5	—
41	53	522	5.3	650	140	0.60	0.35	2.5	—
4	6	43	.8	115	0	0.02	0.01	0.2	1
8	10	76	1.4	205	0	0.04	0.02	0.4	2
19	240	388	3.9	810	—	0.53	—	1.0	Trace
39	50	238	4.2	498	40	0.14	0.12	1.2	0
27	107	577	3.0	971	—	0.46	0.19	24.8	0

Continued.

Nutritive values of the edible part of food—cont'd

Foods, approximate measures, units, and weight in grams (edible part unless footnotes indicate otherwise)			Water (%)	Food energy (kcal)	Protein (g)	Fat (g)	Fatty acids: Saturated (total) (g)	Fatty acids: Unsaturated: Oleic (g)	Fatty acids: Unsaturated: Linoleic (g)
Peanut butter	1 tbsp	16	2	95	4	8	1.5	3.7	2.3
Peas, split, dry, cooked	1 cup	200	70	230	16	1	—	—	—
Pecans, chopped or pieces (about 120 large halves)	1 cup	118	3	810	11	84	7.2	50.5	20.0
Pumpkin and squash kernels, dry, hulled	1 cup	140	4	775	41	65	11.8	23.5	27.5
Sunflower seeds, dry, hulled	1 cup	145	5	810	35	69	8.2	13.7	43.2
Walnuts									
Black									
Chopped or broken kernels	1 cup	125	3	785	26	74	6.3	13.3	45.7
Ground (finely)	1 cup	80	3	500	16	47	4.0	8.5	29.2
Persian or English, chopped (about 60 halves)	1 cup	120	4	780	18	77	8.4	11.8	42.2
SUGARS AND SWEETS									
Cake icings									
Boiled, white									
Plain	1 cup	94	18	295	1	0	0	0	0
With coconut	1 cup	166	15	605	3	13	11.0	0.9	Trace
Uncooked									
Chocolate made with milk and butter	1 cup	275	14	1,035	9	38	23.4	11.7	1.0
Creamy fudge from mix and water	1 cup	245	15	830	7	16	5.1	6.7	3.1
White	1 cup	319	11	1,200	2	21	12.7	5.1	0.5
Candy									
Caramels, plain or chocolate	1 oz	28	8	115	1	3	1.6	1.1	0.1
Chocolate									
Milk, plain	1 oz	28	1	145	2	9	5.5	3.0	0.3
Semisweet, small pieces (60/oz)	1 cup or 6 oz pkg	170	1	860	7	61	36.2	19.8	1.7
Chocolate-coated peanuts	1 oz	28	1	160	5	12	4.0	4.7	2.1
Fondant, uncoated (mints, candy corn, other)	1 oz	28	8	105	Trace	1	0.1	0.3	0.1
Fudge, chocolate, plain	1 oz	28	8	115	1	3	1.3	1.4	0.6
Gum drops	1 oz	28	12	100	Trace	Trace	—	—	—
Hard	1 oz	28	1	110	0	Trace	—	—	—
Marshmallows	1 oz	28	17	90	1	Trace	—	—	—
Chocolate-flavored beverage powders (about 4 heaping tsp/oz)									
With nonfat dry milk	1 oz	28	2	100	5	1	0.5	0.3	Trace
Without milk	1 oz	28	1	100	1	1	0.4	0.2	Trace
Honey, strained or extracted	1 tbsp	21	17	65	Trace	0	0	0	0
Jams and preserves	1 tbsp	20	29	55	Trace	Trace	—	—	—
	1 packet	14	29	40	Trace	Trace	—	—	—
Jellies	1 tbsp	18	29	50	Trace	Trace	—	—	—
	1 packet	14	29	40	Trace	Trace	—	—	—
Syrups									
Chocolate-flavored syrup or topping									
Thin type	1 fl oz or 2 tbsp	38	32	90	1	1	0.5	0.3	Trace

NUTRIENTS IN INDICATED QUANTITY

Carbohydrate (g)	Calcium (mg)	Phosphorus (mg)	Iron (mg)	Potassium (mg)	Vitamin A value (IU)	Thiamin (mg)	Riboflavin (mg)	Niacin (mg)	Ascorbic acid (mg)
3	9	61	.3	100	—	0.02	0.02	2.4	0
42	22	178	3.4	592	80	0.30	0.18	1.8	—
17	86	341	2.8	712	150	1.01	0.15	1.1	2
21	71	1,602	15.7	1,386	100	0.34	0.27	3.4	—
29	174	1,214	10.3	1,334	70	2.84	0.33	7.8	—
19	Trace	713	7.5	575	380	0.28	0.14	0.9	—
12	Trace	456	4.8	368	240	0.18	0.09	0.6	—
19	119	456	3.7	540	40	0.40	0.16	1.1	2
75	2	2	Trace	17	0	Trace	0.03	Trace	0
124	10	50	0.8	277	0	0.02	0.07	0.3	0
185	165	305	3.3	536	580	0.06	0.28	0.6	1
183	96	218	2.7	238	Trace	0.05	0.20	0.7	Trace
260	48	38	Trace	57	860	Trace	0.06	Trace	Trace
22	42	35	0.4	54	Trace	0.01	0.05	0.1	Trace
16	65	65	0.3	109	80	0.02	0.10	0.1	Trace
97	51	255	4.4	553	30	0.02	0.14	0.9	0
11	33	84	0.4	143	Trace	0.10	0.05	2.1	Trace
25	4	2	0.3	1	0	Trace	Trace	Trace	0
21	22	24	0.3	42	Trace	0.01	0.03	0.1	Trace
25	2	Trace	0.1	1	0	0	Trace	Trace	0
28	6	2	0.5	1	0	0	0	0	0
23	5	2	0.5	2	0	0	Trace	Trace	0
20	167	155	0.5	227	10	0.04	0.21	0.2	1
25	9	48	0.6	142	—	0.01	0.03	0.1	0
17	1	1	0.1	11	0	Trace	0.01	0.1	Trace
14	4	2	0.2	18	Trace	Trace	0.01	Trace	Trace
10	3	1	0.1	12	Trace	Trace	Trace	Trace	Trace
13	4	1	0.3	14	Trace	Trace	0.01	Trace	1
10	3	1	0.2	11	Trace	Trace	Trace	Trace	1
24	6	35	0.6	106	Trace	0.01	0.03	0.2	0

Continued.

Nutritive values of the edible part of food—cont'd

Foods, approximate measures, units, and weight in grams (edible part unless footnotes indicate otherwise)			Water (%)	Food energy (kcal)	Protein (g)	Fat (g)	Fatty acids: Saturated (total) (g)	Fatty acids: Unsaturated: Oleic (g)	Fatty acids: Unsaturated: Linoleic (g)
Syrups—cont'd									
Fudge type	1 fl oz or 2 tbsp	38	25	125	2	5	3.1	1.6	0.1
Molasses, cane									
Light (first extraction)	1 tbsp	20	24	50	—	—	—	—	—
Blackstrap (third extraction)	1 tbsp	20	24	45	—	—	—	—	—
Sorghum	1 tbsp	21	23	55	—	—	—	—	—
Table blends, chiefly corn, light and dark	1 tbsp	21	24	60	0	0	0	0	0
Sugars									
Brown, pressed down	1 cup	220	2	820	0	0	0	0	0
White									
Granulated	1 cup	200	1	770	0	0	0	0	0
	1 tbsp	12	1	45	0	0	0	0	0
	1 packet	6	1	23	0	0	0	0	0
Powdered, sifted, spooned into cup	1 cup	100	1	385	0	0	0	0	0
VEGETABLE AND VEGETABLE PRODUCTS									
Asparagus, green									
Cooked, drained									
Cuts and tips, 1½- to 2-inch lengths									
From raw	1 cup	145	94	30	3	Trace	—	—	—
From frozen	1 cup	180	93	40	6	Trace	—	—	—
Spears, ½-inch diam. at base									
From raw	4 spears	60	94	10	1	Trace	—	—	—
From frozen	4 spears	60	92	15	2	Trace	—	—	—
Canned, spears, ½-inch diam. at base	4 spears	80	93	15	2	Trace	—	—	—
Beans									
Lima, immature seeds, frozen, cooked, drained									
Thick-seeded types (Fordhooks)	1 cup	170	74	170	10	Trace	—	—	—
Thin-seeded types (baby limas)	1 cup	180	69	210	13	Trace	—	—	—
Snap									
Green									
Cooked, drained									
From raw (cuts and French style)	1 cup	125	92	30	2	Trace	—	—	—
From frozen									
Cuts	1 cup	135	92	35	2	Trace	—	—	—
French style	1 cup	130	92	35	2	Trace	—	—	—
Canned, drained solids (cuts)	1 cup	135	92	30	2	Trace	—	—	—
Yellow or wax									
Cooked, drained									
From raw (cuts and French style)	1 cup	125	93	30	2	Trace	—	—	—
From frozen (cuts)	1 cup	135	92	35	2	Trace	—	—	—
Canned, drained solids (cuts)	1 cup	135	92	30	2	Trace	—	—	—

NUTRIENTS IN INDICATED QUANTITY

Carbohydrate (g)	Calcium (mg)	Phosphorus (mg)	Iron (mg)	Potassium (mg)	Vitamin A value (IU)	Thiamin (mg)	Riboflavin (mg)	Niacin (mg)	Ascorbic acid (mg)
20	48	60	0.5	107	60	0.02	0.08	0.2	Trace
13	33	9	0.9	183	—	0.01	0.01	Trace	—
11	137	17	3.2	585	—	0.02	0.04	0.4	—
14	35	5	2.6	—	—	—	0.02	Trace	—
15	9	3	0.8	1	0	0	0	0	0
212	187	42	7.5	757	0	0.02	0.07	0.4	0
199	0	0	0.2	6	0	0	0	0	0
12	0	0	Trace	Trace	0	0	0	0	0
6	0	0	Trace	Trace	0	0	0	0	0
100	0	0	0.1	3	0	0	0	0	0
5	30	73	0.9	265	1,310	0.23	0.26	2.0	38
6	40	115	2.2	396	1,530	0.25	0.23	1.8	41
2	13	30	0.4	110	540	0.10	0.11	0.8	16
2	13	30	0.7	143	470	0.10	0.08	0.7	16
3	15	42	1.5	133	640	0.05	0.08	0.6	12
32	34	153	2.9	724	390	0.12	0.09	1.7	29
40	63	227	4.7	709	400	0.16	0.09	2.2	22
7	63	46	0.8	189	680	0.09	0.11	0.6	15
8	54	43	0.9	205	780	0.09	0.12	0.5	7
8	49	39	1.2	177	690	0.08	0.10	0.4	9
7	61	34	2.0	128	630	0.04	0.07	0.4	5
6	63	46	0.8	189	290	0.09	0.11	0.6	16
8	47	42	0.9	221	140	0.09	0.11	0.5	8
7	61	34	2.0	128	140	0.04	0.07	0.4	7

Continued.

Nutritive values of the edible part of food—cont'd

Foods, approximate measures, units, and weight in grams (edible part unless footnotes indicate otherwise)			Water (%)	Food energy (kcal)	Protein (g)	Fat (g)	Fatty acids: Saturated (total) (g)	Fatty acids: Unsaturated: Oleic (g)	Fatty acids: Unsaturated: Linoleic (g)
Beans, mature. See Beans, dry and Blackeye peas, dry									
Bean sprouts (mung)									
Raw	1 cup	105	89	35	4	Trace	—	—	—
Cooked, drained	1 cup	125	91	35	4	Trace	—	—	—
Beets									
Cooked, drained, peeled									
Whole beets, 2-inch diam.	2	100	91	30	1	Trace	—	—	—
Diced or sliced	1 cup	170	91	55	2	Trace	—	—	—
Canned, drained solids									
Whole beets, small	1 cup	160	89	60	2	Trace	—	—	—
Diced or sliced	1 cup	170	89	65	2	Trace	—	—	—
Beet greens, leaves and stems, cooked, drained	1 cup	145	94	25	2	Trace	—	—	—
Blackeye peas, immature seeds, cooked and drained									
From raw	1 cup	165	72	180	13	1	—	—	—
From frozen	1 cup	170	66	220	15	1	—	—	—
Broccoli, cooked, drained									
From raw									
Stalk, medium size	1	180	91	45	6	1	—	—	—
Stalks cut into ½-inch pieces	1 cup	155	91	40	5	Trace	—	—	—
From frozen									
Stalk, 4½ to 5 inches long	1	30	91	10	1	Trace	—	—	—
Chopped	1 cup	185	92	50	5	1	—	—	—
Brussels sprouts, cooked, drained									
From raw, 7-8 sprouts (1¼- to 1½-inch diam.)	1 cup	155	88	55	7	1	—	—	—
From frozen	1 cup	155	89	50	5	Trace	—	—	—
Cabbage									
Common varieties									
Raw									
Coarsely shredded or sliced	1 cup	70	92	15	1	Trace	—	—	—
Finely shredded or chopped	1 cup	90	92	20	1	Trace	—	—	—
Cooked, drained	1 cup	145	94	30	2	Trace	—	—	—
Red, raw, coarsely shredded or sliced	1 cup	70	90	20	1	Trace	—	—	—
Savoy, raw, coarsely shredded or sliced	1 cup	70	92	15	2	Trace	—	—	—
Cabbage, celery (also called pe-tsai or wongbok), raw, 1-inch pieces	1 cup	75	95	10	1	Trace	—	—	—
Cabbage, white mustard (also called bokchoy or pakchoy), cooked, drained	1 cup	170	95	25	2	Trace	—	—	—
Carrots									
Raw, without crowns and tips, scraped									

NUTRIENTS IN INDICATED QUANTITY

Carbohydrate (g)	Calcium (mg)	Phosphorus (mg)	Iron (mg)	Potassium (mg)	Vitamin A value (IU)	Thiamin (mg)	Riboflavin (mg)	Niacin (mg)	Ascorbic acid (mg)
7	20	67	1.4	234	20	0.14	0.14	0.8	20
7	21	60	1.1	195	30	0.11	0.13	0.9	8
7	14	23	0.5	208	20	0.03	0.04	0.3	6
12	24	39	0.9	354	30	0.05	0.07	0.5	10
14	30	29	1.1	267	30	0.02	0.05	0.2	5
15	32	31	1.2	284	30	0.02	0.05	0.2	5
5	144	36	2.8	481	7.400	0.10	0.22	0.4	22
30	40	241	3.5	625	580	0.50	0.18	2.3	28
40	43	286	4.8	573	290	0.68	0.19	2.4	15
8	158	112	1.4	481	4,500	0.16	0.36	1.4	162
7	136	96	1.2	414	3,880	0.14	0.31	1.2	140
1	12	17	0.2	66	570	0.02	0.03	0.2	22
9	100	104	1.3	392	4,810	0.11	0.22	0.9	105
10	50	112	1.7	423	810	0.12	0.22	1.2	135
10	33	95	1.2	457	880	0.12	0.16	0.9	126
4	34	20	0.3	163	90	0.04	0.04	0.02	33
5	44	26	0.4	210	120	0.05	0.05	0.3	42
6	64	29	0.4	236	190	0.06	0.06	0.4	48
5	29	25	0.6	188	30	0.06	0.04	0.3	43
3	47	38	0.6	188	140	0.04	0.06	0.2	39
2	32	30	0.5	190	110	0.04	0.03	0.5	19
4	252	56	1.0	364	5,270	0.07	0.14	1.2	26

Continued.

Nutritive values of the edible part of food—cont'd

Foods, approximate measures, units, and weight in grams (edible part unless footnotes indicate otherwise)			Water (%)	Food energy (kcal)	Protein (g)	Fat (g)	Fatty acids: Saturated (total) (g)	Fatty acids: Unsaturated: Oleic (g)	Fatty acids: Unsaturated: Linoleic (g)
Carrots—cont'd									
Whole, 7½ by 1⅛ inches, or strips, 2½ to 3 inches long	1 carrot or 18 strips	72	88	30	1	Trace	—	—	—
Grated	1 cup	110	88	45	1	Trace	—	—	—
Cooked (crosswise cuts), drained	1 cup	155	91	50	1	Trace	—	—	—
Canned									
Sliced, drained solids	1 cup	155	91	45	1	Trace	—	—	—
Strained or junior (baby food)	1 oz (1¾ to 2 tbsp)	28	92	10	Trace	Trace	—	—	—
Cauliflower									
Raw, chopped	1 cup	115	91	31	3	Trace	—	—	—
Cooked, drained									
From raw (flower buds)	1 cup	125	93	30	3	Trace	—	—	—
From frozen (flowerets)	1 cup	180	94	30	3	Trace	—	—	—
Celery, Pascal type, raw									
Stalk, large outer, 8 by 1½ inches, at root end	1	40	94	5	Trace	Trace	—	—	—
Pieces, diced	1 cup	120	94	20	1	Trace	—	—	—
Collards, cooked, drained									
From raw (leaves without stems)	1 cup	190	90	65	7	1	—	—	—
From frozen (chopped)	1 cup	170	90	50	5	1	—	—	—
Corn, sweet									
Cooked, drained									
From raw, ear 5 by 1¾ inches	1 ear[61]	140	74	70	2	1	—	—	—
From frozen									
Ear, 5 inch long	1 ear[61]	229	73	120	4	1	—	—	—
Kernels	1 cup	165	77	130	5	1	—	—	—
Canned									
Cream style	1 cup	256	76	210	5	2	—	—	—
Whole kernel									
Vacuum pack	1 cup	210	76	175	5	1	—	—	—
Wet pack, drained solids	1 cup	165	76	140	4	1	—	—	—
Cowpeas. See Blackeye peas									
Cucumber slices, ⅛ inch thick (large, 2⅛-inches diam.; small, 1¾-inches diam.)									
With peel	6 large or 8 small slices	28	95	5	Trace	Trace	—	—	—
Without peel	6½ large or 9 small pieces	28	96	5	Trace	Trace	—	—	—
Dandelion greens, cooked, drained	1 cup	105	90	35	2	1	—	—	—
Endive, curly (including escarole), raw, small pieces	1 cup	50	93	10	1	Trace	—	—	—
Kale, cooked, drained									
From raw (leaves without stems and midribs)	1 cup	110	88	45	5	1	—	—	—

NUTRIENTS IN INDICATED QUANTITY									
Carbohydrate (g)	Calcium (mg)	Phosphorus (mg)	Iron (mg)	Potassium (mg)	Vitamin A value (IU)	Thiamin (mg)	Riboflavin (mg)	Niacin (mg)	Ascorbic acid (mg)
7	27	26	0.5	246	7,930	0.04	0.04	0.4	6
11	41	40	0.8	375	12,100	0.07	0.06	0.7	9
11	51	48	0.9	344	16,280	0.08	0.08	0.8	9
10	47	34	1.1	186	23,250	0.03	0.05	0.6	3
2	7	6	0.1	51	3,690	0.01	0.01	0.1	1
6	29	64	1.3	339	70	0.13	0.12	0.8	90
5	26	53	0.9	258	80	0.11	0.10	0.8	69
6	31	68	0.9	373	50	0.07	0.09	0.7	74
2	16	11	0.1	136	110	0.01	0.01	0.1	4
5	47	34	0.4	409	320	0.04	0.04	0.4	11
10	357	99	1.5	498	14,820	0.21	0.38	2.3	144
10	299	87	1.7	401	11,560	0.10	0.24	1.0	56
16	2	69	0.5	151	[62]310	0.09	0.08	1.1	7
27	4	121	1.0	291	[62]440	0.18	0.10	2.1	9
31	5	120	1.3	304	[62]580	0.15	0.10	2.5	8
51	8	143	1.5	248	[62]840	0.08	0.13	2.6	13
43	6	153	1.1	204	[62]740	0.06	0.13	2.3	11
33	8	81	0.8	160	[62]580	0.05	0.08	1.5	7
1	7	8	0.3	45	70	0.01	0.01	0.1	3
1	5	5	0.1	45	Trace	0.01	0.01	0.1	3
7	147	44	1.9	244	12,290	0.14	0.17	—	19
2	41	27	0.9	147	1,650	0.04	0.07	0.3	5
7	206	64	1.8	243	9,130	0.11	0.20	1.8	102

Continued.

Nutritive values of the edible part of food—cont'd

Foods, approximate measures, units, and weight in grams (edible part unless footnotes indicate otherwise)			Water (%)	Food energy (kcal)	Protein (g)	Fat (g)	Fatty acids		
							Saturated (total) (g)	Unsaturated	
								Oleic (g)	Linoleic (g)
Kale, cooked, drained—cont'd									
From frozen (leaf style)	1 cup	130	91	40	4	1	—	—	—
Lettuce, raw									
Butterhead, as Boston types									
Head, 5-inch diam.	1 head[63]	220	95	25	2	Trace	—	—	—
Leaves	1 outer or 2 inner or 3 heart leaves	15	95	Trace	Trace	Trace	—	—	—
Crisphead, as Iceberg									
Head, 6-inch diam.	1 head[64]	567	96	70	5	1	—	—	—
Wedge, ¼ of head	1 wedge	135	96	20	1	Trace	—	—	—
Pieces, chopped or shredded	1 cup	55	96	5	Trace	Trace	—	—	—
Looseleaf (bunching varieties including romaine or cos), chopped or shredded pieces	1 cup	55	94	10	1	Trace	—	—	—
Mushrooms, raw, sliced or chopped	1 cup	70	90	20	2	Trace	—	—	—
Mustard greens, without stems and midribs, cooked, drained	1 cup	140	93	30	3	1	—	—	—
Okra pods, 3 by ⅝ inch, cooked	10 pods	106	91	30	2	Trace	—	—	—
Onions									
Mature									
Raw									
Chopped	1 cup	170	89	65	3	Trace	—	—	—
Sliced	1 cup	115	89	45	2	Trace	—	—	—
Cooked (whole or sliced), drained	1 cup	210	92	60	3	Trace	—	—	—
Young green, bulb (⅜-inch diam.) and white portion of top	6 onions	30	88	15	Trace	Trace	—	—	—
Parsley, raw, chopped	1 tbsp	4	85	Trace	Trace	Trace	—	—	—
Parsnips, cooked (diced or 2-inch lengths)	1 cup	155	82	100	2	1	—	—	—
Peas, green									
Canned									
Whole, drained solids	1 cup	170	77	150	8	1	—	—	—
Strained (baby food)	1 oz (1¾ to 2 tbsp)	28	86	15	1	Trace	—	—	—
Frozen, cooked, drained	1 cup	160	82	110	8	Trace	—	—	—
Peppers, hot, red, without seeds, dried (ground chili powder, added seasonings)	1 tsp	2	9	5	Trace	Trace	—	—	—
Peppers, sweet (about 5/lb, whole), stem and seeds removed									
Raw	1 pod	74	93	15	1	Trace	—	—	—
Cooked, boiled, drained	1 pod	73	95	15	1	Trace	—	—	—

[63]Weight includes refuse of outer leaves and core. Without these parts, weight is 163 g.

[64]Weight includes core. Without core, weight is 539 g.

[65]Value based on white-fleshed varieties. For yellow-fleshed varieties, value in International Units is 70 for chopped raw onions, 50 for sliced

NUTRIENTS IN INDICATED QUANTITY

Carbohydrate (g)	Calcium (mg)	Phosphorus (mg)	Iron (mg)	Potassium (mg)	Vitamin A value (IU)	Thiamin (mg)	Riboflavin (mg)	Niacin (mg)	Ascorbic acid (mg)
7	157	62	1.3	251	10,660	0.08	0.20	0.9	49
44	57	42	3.3	430	1,580	0.10	0.10	0.5	13
Trace	5	4	0.3	40	150	0.01	0.01	Trace	1
16	108	118	2.7	943	1,780	0.32	0.32	1.6	32
4	27	30	0.7	236	450	0.08	0.08	0.4	8
2	11	12	0.3	96	180	0.03	0.03	0.2	3
2	37	14	0.8	145	1,050	0.03	0.04	0.2	10
3	4	81	0.6	290	Trace	0.07	0.32	2.9	2
6	193	45	2.5	308	8,120	0.11	0.20	0.8	67
6	98	43	0.5	184	520	0.14	0.19	1.0	21
15	46	61	0.9	267	[65]Trace	0.05	0.07	0.3	17
10	31	41	0.6	181	[65]Trace	0.03	0.05	0.2	12
14	50	61	0.8	231	[65]Trace	0.06	0.06	0.4	15
3	12	12	0.2	69	Trace	0.02	0.01	0.1	8
Trace	7	2	0.2	25	300	Trace	0.01	Trace	6
23	70	96	0.9	587	50	0.11	0.12	0.2	16
29	44	129	3.2	163	1,170	0.15	0.10	1.4	14
3	3	18	0.3	28	140	0.02	0.03	0.3	3
19	30	138	3.0	216	960	0.43	0.14	2.7	21
1	5	4	0.3	20	1,300	Trace	0.02	0.2	Trace
4	7	16	0.5	157	310	0.06	0.06	0.4	94
3	7	12	0.4	109	310	0.05	0.05	0.4	70

Continued.

raw onions, and 80 for cooked onions.

Nutritive values of the edible part of food—cont'd

Foods, approximate measures, units, and weight in grams (edible part unless footnotes indicate otherwise)			Water (%)	Food energy (kcal)	Protein (g)	Fat (g)	Fatty acids: Saturated (total) (g)	Fatty acids: Unsaturated: Oleic (g)	Fatty acids: Unsaturated: Linoleic (g)
Potatoes, cooked									
Baked, peeled after baking (about 2/lb, raw)	1 potato	156	75	145	4	Trace	—	—	—
Boiled (about 3/lb, raw)									
Peeled after boiling	1 potato	137	80	105	3	Trace	—	—	—
Peeled before boiling	1 potato	135	83	90	3	Trace	—	—	—
French-fried, strip, 2 to 3½ inches long									
Prepared from raw	10 strips	50	45	135	2	7	1.7	1.2	3.3
Frozen, oven heated	10 strips	50	53	110	2	4	1.1	0.8	2.1
Hashed brown, prepared from frozen	1 cup	155	56	345	3	18	4.6	3.2	9.0
Mashed, prepared from—									
Raw									
Milk added	1 cup	210	83	135	4	2	0.7	0.4	Trace
Milk and butter added	1 cup	210	80	195	4	9	5.6	2.3	0.2
Dehydrated flakes (without milk), water, milk, butter, and salt added	1 cup	210	79	195	4	7	3.6	2.1	0.2
Potato chips, 1¾ by 2½ inches oval cross section	10 chips	20	2	115	1	8	2.1	1.4	4.0
Potato salad, made with cooked salad dressing	1 cup	250	76	250	7	7	2.0	2.7	1.3
Pumpkin, canned	1 cup	245	90	80	2	1	—	—	—
Radishes, raw (prepackaged) stem ends, rootlets cut off	4 radishes	18	95	5	Trace	Trace	—	—	—
Sauerkraut, canned, solids and liquid	1 cup	235	93	40	2	Trace	—	—	—
Souther peas. See Blackeye peas									
Spinach									
Raw, chopped	1 cup	55	91	15	2	Trace	—	—	—
Cooked, drained									
From raw	1 cup	180	92	40	5	1	—	—	—
From frozen									
Chopped	1 cup	205	92	45	6	1	—	—	—
Leaf	1 cup	190	92	45	6	1	—	—	—
Canned, drained solids	1 cup	205	91	50	6	1	—	—	—
Squash, cooked									
Summer (all varieties), diced, drained	1 cup	210	96	30	2	Trace	—	—	—
Winter (all varieties), baked, mashed	1 cup	205	81	130	4	1	—	—	—
Sweet potatoes									
Cooked (raw, 5 by 2 inches; about 2½/lb)									
Baked in skin, peeled	1 potato	114	64	160	2	1	—	—	—
Boiled in skin, peeled	1 potato	151	71	170	3	1	—	—	—
Candied, 2½ by 2-inch piece	1 piece	105	60	175	1	3	2.0	0.8	0.1
Canned									
Solid pack (mashed)	1 cup	255	72	275	5	1	—	—	—
Vacuum pack, piece 2¾ by 1 inch	1 piece	40	72	45	1	Trace	—	—	—

NUTRIENTS IN INDICATED QUANTITY

Carbohydrate (g)	Calcium (mg)	Phosphorus (mg)	Iron (mg)	Potassium (mg)	Vitamin A value (IU)	Thiamin (mg)	Riboflavin (mg)	Niacin (mg)	Ascorbic acid (mg)
33	14	101	1.1	782	Trace	0.15	0.07	2.7	31
23	10	72	0.8	556	Trace	0.12	0.05	2.0	22
20	8	57	0.7	385	Trace	0.12	0.05	1.6	22
18	18	56	0.7	427	Trace	0.07	0.04	1.6	11
17	5	43	0.9	326	Trace	0.07	0.01	1.3	11
45	28	78	1.9	439	Trace	0.11	0.03	1.6	12
27	50	103	0.8	548	40	0.17	0.11	2.1	21
26	50	101	0.8	525	360	0.17	0.11	2.1	19
30	65	99	0.6	601	270	0.08	0.08	1.9	11
10	8	28	0.4	226	Trace	0.04	0.01	1.0	3
41	80	160	1.5	798	350	0.20	0.18	2.8	28
19	61	64	1.0	588	15,680	0.07	0.12	1.5	12
1	5	6	0.2	58	Trace	0.01	0.01	0.1	5
9	85	42	1.2	329	120	0.07	0.09	0.5	33
2	51	28	1.7	259	4,460	0.06	0.11	0.3	28
6	167	68	4.0	583	14,580	0.13	0.25	0.9	50
8	232	90	4.3	683	16,200	0.14	0.31	0.8	39
7	200	84	4.8	688	15,390	0.15	0.27	1.0	53
7	242	53	5.3	513	16,400	0.04	0.25	0.6	29
7	53	53	0.8	296	820	0.11	0.17	1.7	21
32	57	98	1.6	945	8,610	0.10	0.27	1.4	27
37	46	66	1.0	342	9,230	0.10	0.08	0.8	25
40	48	71	1.1	367	11,940	0.14	0.09	0.9	26
36	39	45	0.9	200	6,620	0.06	0.04	0.4	11
63	64	105	2.0	510	19,890	0.13	0.10	1.5	36
10	10	16	0.3	80	3,120	0.02	0.02	0.2	6

Continued.

Nutritive values of the edible part of food—cont'd

Foods, approximate measures, units, and weight in grams (edible part unless footnotes indicate otherwise)			Water (%)	Food energy (kcal)	Protein (g)	Fat (g)	Fatty acids		
							Saturated (total) (g)	Unsaturated	
								Oleic (g)	Linoleic (g)
Tomatoes									
Raw, 2 3/5-inch diam. (3/12 oz pkg)	1 tomato[66]	135	94	25	1	Trace	—	—	—
Canned, solids and liquid	1 cup	241	94	50	2	Trace	—	—	—
Tomato catsup	1 cup	273	69	290	5	1	—	—	—
	1 tbsp	15	69	15	Trace	Trace	—	—	—
Tomato juice, canned									
Cup	1 cup	243	94	45	2	Trace	—	—	—
Glass (6 fl oz)	1 glass	182	94	35	2	Trace	—	—	—
Turnips, cooked, diced	1 cup	155	94	35	1	Trace	—	—	—
Turnip greens, cooked, drained									
From raw (leaves and stems)	1 cup	145	94	30	3	Trace	—	—	—
From frozen (chopped)	1 cup	165	93	40	4	Trace	—	—	—
Vegetables, mixed, frozen, cooked	1 cup	182	83	115	6	1	—	—	—
MISCELLANEOUS ITEMS									
Baking powders for home use									
Sodium aluminum sulfate									
With monocalcium phosphate monohydrate	1 tsp	3.0	2	5	Trace	Trace	0	0	0
With monocalcium phosphate monohydrate, calcium sulfate	1 tsp	2.9	1	5	Trace	Trace	0	0	0
Straight phosphate	1 tsp	3.8	2	5	Trace	Trace	0	0	0
Low sodium	1 tsp	4.3	2	5	Trace	Trace	0	0	0
Barbecue sauce	1 cup	250	81	230	4	17	2.2	4.3	10.0
Beverages, alcoholic									
Beer	12 fl oz	360	92	150	1	0	0	0	0
Gin, rum, vodka, whisky									
80-proof	1½ fl oz jigger	42	67	95	—	—	0	0	0
86-proof	1½ fl oz jigger	42	64	105	—	—	0	0	0
90-proof	1½ fl oz jigger	42	62	110	—	—	0	0	0
Wines									
Dessert	3½ fl oz glass	103	77	140	Trace	0	0	0	0
Table	3½ fl oz glass	102	86	85	Trace	0	0	0	0
Beverages, carbonated, sweetened, nonalcoholic									
Carbonated water	12 fl oz	366	92	115	0	0	0	0	0
Cola type	12 fl oz	369	90	145	0	0	0	0	0
Fruit-flavored sodas and Tom Collins mixer	12 fl oz	372	88	170	0	0	0.	0	0
Ginger ale	12 fl oz	366	92	115	0	0	0	0	0
Root beer	12 fl oz	370	90	150	0	0	0	0	0
Chili powder. See Peppers, hot, red									
Chocolate									
Bitter or baking	1 oz	28	2	145	3	15	8.9	4.9	0.4

[66] Weight includes cores and stem ends. Without these parts, weight is 123 g.
[67] Based on year-round average. For tomatoes marketed from November through May, value is about 12 mg; from June through October, 32 mg.
[68] Applies to product without calcium salts added. Value for products with calcium salts added may be as much as 63 mg for whole tomatoes,

NUTRIENTS IN INDICATED QUANTITY

Carbohydrate (g)	Calcium (mg)	Phosphorus (mg)	Iron (mg)	Potassium (mg)	Vitamin A value (IU)	Thiamin (mg)	Riboflavin (mg)	Niacin (mg)	Ascorbic acid (mg)
6	16	33	0.6	300	1,110	0.07	0.05	0.9	[67]28
10	[68]14	46	1.2	523	2,170	0.12	0.07	1.7	41
69	60	137	2.2	991	3,820	0.25	0.19	4.4	41
4	3	8	0.1	54	210	0.01	0.01	0.2	2
10	17	44	2.2	552	1,940	0.12	0.07	1.9	39
8	13	33	1.6	413	1,460	0.09	0.05	1.5	29
8	54	37	0.6	291	Trace	0.06	0.08	0.5	34
5	252	49	1.5	—	8,270	0.15	0.33	0.7	68
6	195	64	2.6	246	11,390	0.08	0.15	0.7	31
24	46	115	2.4	348	9,010	0.22	0.13	2.0	15

Carbohydrate (g)	Calcium (mg)	Phosphorus (mg)	Iron (mg)	Potassium (mg)	Vitamin A value (IU)	Thiamin (mg)	Riboflavin (mg)	Niacin (mg)	Ascorbic acid (mg)
1	58	87	—	5	0	0	0	0	0
1	183	45	—	—	0	0	0	0	0
1	239	359	—	6	0	0	0	0	0
2	207	314	—	471	0	0	0	0	0
20	53	50	2.0	435	900	0.03	0.03	0.8	13
14	18	108	Trace	90	—	0.01	0.11	2.2	—
Trace	—	—	—	1	—	—	—	—	—
Trace	—	—	—	1	—	—	—	—	—
Trace	—	—	—	1	—	—	—	—	—
8	8	—	—	77	—	0.01	0.02	0.2	—
4	9	10	0.4	94	—	Trace	0.01	0.1	—
29	—	—	—	—	0	0	0	0	0
37	—	—	—	—	0	0	0	0	0
45	—	—	—	—	0	0	0	0	0
29	—	—	—	0	0	0	0	0	0
39	—	—	—	0	0	0	0	0	0
8	22	109	1.9	235	20	0.01	0.07	0.4	0

Continued.

241 mg for cut forms.

Nutritive values of the edible part of food—cont'd

Foods, approximate measures, units, and weight in grams (edible part unless footnotes indicate otherwise)			Water (%)	Food energy (kcal)	Protein (g)	Fat (g)	Fatty acids		
							Saturated (total) (g)	Unsaturated	
								Oleic (g)	Linoleic (g)
Chocolate—cont'd									
Semisweet, see Candy, chocolate									
Gelatin, dry	1,7 g envelope	7	13	25	6	Trace	0	0	0
Gelatin dessert prepared with gelatin dessert powder and water	1 cup	240	84	140	4	0	0	0	0
Mustard, prepared, yellow	1 tsp or individual serving pouch or cup	5	80	5	Trace	Trace	—	—	—
Olives, pickled, canned									
Green	4 medium or 3 extra large or 2 giant[69]	16	78	15	Trace	2	0.2	1.2	0.1
Ripe, Mission	3 small or 2 large[69]	10	73	15	Trace	2	0.2	1.2	0.1
Pickles, cucumber									
Dill, medium, whole, 3¾ inches long, 1¼-inch diam.	1 pickle	65	93	5	Trace	Trace	—	—	—
Fresh-pack, slices 1½-inch diam., ¼ inches thick	2 slices	15	79	10	Trace	Trace	—	—	—
Sweet, gherkin, small, whole, about 2½ inches long, ¾-inch diam.	1 pickle	15	61	20	Trace	Trace	—	—	—
Relish, finely chopped, sweet	1 tbsp	15	63	20	Trace	Trace	—	—	—
Popcorn									
Popsicle, 3 fl oz size	1	95	80	70	0	0	0	0	0
Soups									
Canned, condensed									
Prepared with equal volume of milk									
Cream of chicken	1 cup	245	85	180	7	10	4.2	3.6	1.3
Cream of mushroom	1 cup	245	83	215	7	14	5.4	2.9	4.6
Tomato	1 cup	250	84	175	7	7	3.4	1.7	1.0
Prepared with equal volume of water									
Bean with pork	1 cup	250	84	170	8	6	1.2	1.8	2.4
Beef broth, bouillon, consomme	1 cup	240	96	30	5	0	0	0	0
Beef noodle	1 cup	240	93	65	4	3	0.6	0.7	0.8
Clam chowder, Manhattan type (with tomatoes, without milk)	1 cup	245	92	80	2	3	0.5	0.4	1.3
Cream of chicken	1 cup	240	92	95	3	6	1.6	2.3	1.1
Cream of mushroom	1 cup	240	90	135	2	10	2.6	1.7	4.5
Minestrone	1 cup	245	90	105	5	3	0.7	0.9	1.3
Split pea	1 cup	245	85	145	9	3	1.1	1.2	0.4
Tomato	1 cup	245	91	90	2	3	0.5	0.5	1.0

[69] Weight includes pits. Without pits, weight is 13 g for green olives, 9 g for ripe olives.

NUTRIENTS IN INDICATED QUANTITY									
Carbohydrate (g)	Calcium (mg)	Phosphorus (mg)	Iron (mg)	Potassium (mg)	Vitamin A value (IU)	Thiamin (mg)	Riboflavin (mg)	Niacin (mg)	Ascorbic acid (mg)
0	—	—	—	—	—	—	—	—	—
34	—	—	—	—	—	—	—	—	—
Trace	4	4	0.1	7	—	—	—	—	—
Trace	8	2	0.2	7	40	—	—	—	—
Trace	9	1	0.1	2	10	Trace	Trace	—	—
1	17	14	0.7	130	70	Trace	0.01	Trace	4
3	5	4	0.3	—	20	Trace	Trace	Trace	1
5	2	2	0.2	—	10	Trace	Trace	Trace	1
5	3	2	0.1	—	—	—	—	—	—
18	0	—	Trace	—	0	0	0	0	0
15	172	169	0.5	260	610	0.05	0.27	0.7	2
16	191	152	0.5	279	250	0.05	0.34	0.7	1
23	168	155	0.8	418	1,200	0.10	0.25	1.3	15
22	63	128	2.3	395	650	0.13	0.08	1.0	3
3	Trace	31	0.5	130	Trace	Trace	0.02	1.2	—
7	7	48	1.0	77	50	0.05	0.07	1.0	Trace
12	34	47	1.0	184	880	0.02	0.02	1.0	—
8	24	34	0.5	79	410	0.02	0.05	0.5	Trace
10	41	50	0.5	98	70	0.02	0.12	0.7	Trace
14	37	59	1.0	314	2,350	0.07	0.05	1.0	—
21	29	149	1.5	270	440	0.25	0.15	1.5	1
16	15	34	0.7	230	1,000	0.05	0.05	1.2	12

Continued.

Nutritive values of the edible part of food—cont'd

Foods, approximate measures, units, and weight in grams (edible part unless footnotes indicate otherwise)			Water (%)	Food energy (kcal)	Protein (g)	Fat (g)	Fatty acids: Saturated (total) (g)	Fatty acids: Unsaturated: Oleic (g)	Fatty acids: Unsaturated: Linoleic (g)
Soups—cont'd									
Vegetable beef	1 cup	245	92	80	5	2	—	—	—
Vegetarian	1 cup	245	92	80	2	2	—	—	—
Dehydrated									
Bouillon cube, ½ inch	1 cube	4	4	5	1	Trace	—	—	—
Mixes									
Unprepared									
Onion	1½ oz pkg	43	3	150	6	5	1.1	2.3	1.0
Prepared with water									
Chicken noodle	1 cup	240	95	55	2	1	—	—	—
Onion	1 cup	240	96	35	1	1	—	—	—
Tomato vegetable with noodles	1 cup	240	93	65	1	1	—	—	—
Vinegar, cider	1 tbsp	15	94	Trace	Trace	0	0	0	0
White sauce, medium, with enriched flour	1 cup	250	73	405	10	31	19.3	7.8	0.8
Yeast									
Baker's, dry, active	1 pkg	7	5	20	3	Trace	—	—	—
Brewer's, dry	1 tbsp	8	5	25	3	Trace	—	—	—

[70] Value may vary from 6 to 60 mg.

NUTRIENTS IN INDICATED QUANTITY

Carbohydrate (g)	Calcium (mg)	Phosphorus (mg)	Iron (mg)	Potassium (mg)	Vitamin A value (IU)	Thiamin (mg)	Riboflavin (mg)	Niacin (mg)	Ascorbic acid (mg)
10	12	49	0.7	162	2,700	0.05	0.05	1.0	—
13	20	39	1.0	172	2,940	0.05	0.05	1.0	—
Trace	—	—	—	4	—	—	—	—	—
23	42	49	0.6	238	30	0.05	0.03	0.3	6
8	7	19	0.2	19	50	0.07	0.05	0.5	Trace
6	10	12	0.2	58	Trace	Trace	Trace	Trace	2
12	7	19	0.2	29	480	0.05	0.02	0.5	5
1	1	1	0.1	15	—	—	—	—	—
22	288	233	0.5	348	1,150	0.12	0.43	0.7	2
3	3	90	1.1	140	Trace	0.16	0.38	2.6	Trace
3	[70]17	140	1.4	152	Trace	1.25	0.34	3.0	Trace

APPENDIX H

Pyridoxine, vitamin B_{12}, pantothenic acid, folic acid, biotin, magnesium, and zinc content of some representative foods

Food and serving size	B_6 (μg)	B_{12} (μg)	Pantothenic acid (μg)	Folic acid (μg)	Biotin (mg)	Magnesium (mg)	Zinc (mg)
Apple, 1 medium	45	0	150	3	2	8	0
Banana, 1 medium	480	0	450	40	6	46	0.3
Beef chuck, braised, 3 oz	297	1.53	340	3	3	20	2.1
Beef, ground, 3 oz	85	1.56	510	3	3	23	2.6
Bread, white, 1 slice	9	0	92	4	0	6	0.3
Bread, whole wheat, 1 slice	41	0	184	9	0	10	0.6
Broccoli, ½ cup	107	0	315	14	1	13	0.1
Carrots, raw, 1 small	75	0	150	8	2	9	0.3
Cheese, cheddar, 1 oz	22	0.28	140	2	1	10	0.3
Chicken, fried, 3 oz	340	0.36	765	5	9	16	3.9
Cookies, assorted, 2	20	0	160	4	2	6	0.7
Cottage cheese, creamed, ½ cup	46	1.14	228	31	2	9	1.6
Egg, hard cooked, 1	49	1.10	1,100	16	13	7	0.8
Grapefruit, ½ medium	30	0	300	2	3	9	0.1
Halibut, broiled, 3 oz	289	0.85	255	14	7	20	0.8
Lettuce, head, ½ cup chunks	22	0	74	74	1	4	0
Milk, whole, 1 cup	98	0.98	984	22	5	37	1.0
Orange juice, ½ cup	36	0	240	5	0	14	0.1
Peanut butter, 2 tbsp	92	0	476	4	11	49	0.6
Pear, ¼ cup	110	0	255	13	2	18	0.8
Pizza with cheese, 2 slices	100	0.48	600	6	2	54	2.2
Potato, baked, 1 medium	200	0	400	12	2	22	0.2
Raisins, 2 tbsp	67	0	28	3	1	9	0.1
Rice, white, enriched ½ cup	30	0	150	1	4	5	0.1
Sweet potato, baked, 1 medium	238	0	980	27	3	17	1.0
Tuna, canned, ⅓ can	258	1.32	180	1	2	16	0.2
Wheat flakes, 1 cup	81	0	140	5	0	27	0.7

APPENDIX I

Diabetic exchange lists

Milk (12 g carbohydrate, 8 g protein, 0 fat, 80 kcal)

1 cup nonfat milk
1 cup yougurt
1 cup buttermilk
1 cup 2% milk (omit 1 fat exchange)
1 cup whole milk (omit 2 fat exchanges)

Vegetables (5 g carbohydrate, 2 g protein, 0 fat, 25 kcal)

½ cup asparagus
½ cup cabbage
½ cup carrots
½ cup celery
½ cup eggplant
½ cup green pepper
½ cup mushrooms
½ cup onions
½ cup rhubarb
½ cup string beans
½ cup tomatoes
½ cup turnips

Fruit (10 g carbohydrate, 0 fat, 40 kcal)

1 apple
1 tangerine
1 orange
1 fig
1 nectarine
½ banana
½ grapefruit
½ mango
2 tbsp raisins
½ cup berries
½ cup grapefruit juice
½ cup pineapple
½ cup applesauce
½ cup orange juice

Bread (15 g carbohydrate, 2 g protein, 0 fat, 70 kcal)

1 slice white bread
1 slice whole wheat bread
1 slice pumpernickel bread
1 slice raisin bread
½ hamburger bun
½ English muffin
1 tortilla
1 biscuit
5 crackers
8 french-fried potatoes
⅓ cup corn
⅓ cup lima beans
½ cup green peas
½ cup potatoes

Meat, 1 oz (7 g protein, 3 g fat, 55 kcal)

Low fat	1 oz beef, lamb, pork, veal, poultry, fish, ¼ cup cottage cheese
Medium fat	Omit ½ fat exchange
High fat	Omit 1 fat exchange
	1 oz cheddar cheese
	1 frankfurter

Fat exchange (5 g fat, 55 kcal)

1 tsp margarine, oil, butter, mayonnaise
1 tbsp heavy cream, cream cheese
1 strip bacon
6 walnuts
20 peanuts
5 olives

APPENDIX J

Food sources of nutrients in relation to United States recommended dietary allowances*

Nutrient	Sources: Excellent (75% U.S. RDA)	Good (50% U.S. RDA)	Significant (25% U.S. RDA)	Fair (10% U.S. RDA)
Ascorbic acid	Orange Strawberries Cauliflower Broccoli Br. sprouts Green pepper Tomato Grapefruit Honeydew melon Mustard greens	Cabbage Spinach Tangerine Asparagus	Banana Blueberries Lima beans Raspberries Green peas Radishes Sauerkraut	Apple Peach Corn
Vitamin A	Liver Carrot Pumpkin Sweet potatoes Spinach Winter squash Turnip greens Mustard greens Beet greens	Apricots Watermelon Broccoli	Honeydew melon Peaches Prunes Tomato Nectarines	Asparagus Green beans Br. sprouts Cheddar cheese Green peas Tomato juice
Thiamin	Pork	Dried peas Macaroni	Green peas Ham Peanuts	Orange Watermelon Dried beans Noodles Spaghetti Lamb liver

*Based on average serving size as follows:
Meat—3 oz, edible portion
Fruit—3 to 4 oz
Vegetables—3 to 4 oz
Cereals—1 oz
Milk—8 oz

Nutrient	Sources: Excellent (75% U.S. RDA)	Good (50% U.S. RDA)	Significant (25% U.S. RDA)	Fair (10% U.S. RDA)
Thiamin—cont'd				Rice
				Cashew nuts
Riboflavin	Liver		Macaroni	Avocado
			Cottage cheese	Tangerine
			Buttermilk	Prunes
			Milk	Asparagus
			Yogurt	Broccoli
				Mushrooms
				Ice cream
				Beef
				Salmon
				Turkey
Vitamin B_6		Soybeans	Lima beans	Cauliflower
		Beef liver	Pork	Green pepper
		Tuna	Beef	Potatoes
			Veal	Spinach
			Halibut	Raisins
			Salmon	Perch
			Chicken	
			Bananas	
			Avocado	
Vitamin B_{12}	Beef liver		Veal	
	Clams		Cheese	
	Salmon		Scallops	
	Trappist cheese		Swordfish	
	Lamb			
	Eggs			
Magnesium	Molasses	Beet greens	Spinach	Raisins
	Peanuts		Lima beans	Sweet potatoes
			Green peas	Br. sprouts
				Cod
Iron	Calves and pork liver	Beef liver	Asparagus	Banana
	Clams		Ham	Beans
			Veal	Br. sprouts
			Beef	Cod
			Chicken	Green peas
			Macaroni	Noodles
			Prunes	Rice
			Raisins	Cashew nuts
			Spinach	Peanuts
Calcium			Turnip greens	Prunes
			Swiss cheese	Broccoli
			Buttermilk	Beet greens
			Milk	Cottage cheese
			Yogurt	Ice cream
			Salmon	Haddock
				Scallops

APPENDIX K

Selected sources of reliable nutrition information

American Dental Association
222 E. Superior Street
Chicago, Ill. 60611

American Dietetic Association
Publications Department
430 N. Michigan Avenue
Chicago, Ill. 60611

American Home Economics Association
Division of Public Affairs
2010 Massachusetts Avenue, NW
Washington, D.C. 20036

American Institute of Baking
400 E. Ontario Street
Chicago, Ill. 60611

American Institute of Nutrition
9650 Rockville Pike
Bethesda, Md. 20014

American Meat Institute
59 E. Van Buren Street
P.O. Box 3556
Washington, D.C. 20007

American Medical Association
Council on Foods and Nutrition
Order Department
535 N. Dearborn Street
Chicago, Ill. 60610

American Public Health Association
1015 18th Street, NW
Washington, D.C. 20036

American School Food Service
P.O. Box 10095
Denver, Colo. 80210

Cereal Institute
135 S. LaSalle Street
Chicago, Ill. 60603

Children's Bureau
U.S. Department of Health, Education, and Welfare
Washington, D.C. 20203

Food and Agriculture Organization (FAO) of the U.N.
c/o American Public Health Association
1740 Broadway
New York, N.Y. 10019

Food and Drug Administration (FDA)
Parklane Building
5600 Fishers Lane
Rockville, Md. 20852

Food and Nutrition Board
National Academy of Sciences
2101 Constitution Avenue
Washington, D.C. 20418

National Dairy Council
6300 N. River Road
Rosemont, Ill. 60018

National Foundation—March of Dimes
Health Information Department
P.O. Box 2000
White Plains, N.Y. 10602

National Livestock and Meat Board
444 N. Michigan Avenue
Chicago, Ill. 60611

National Nutrition Consortium
2121 P Street
Suite 216
Washington, D.C. 20037

Nutrition Foundation, Inc.
888 17th Street, NW
Washington, D.C. 20016

Nutrition Today Society
101 Ridgly Avenue
P.O. Box 773
Annapolis, Md. 21404

Society for Nutrition Education
National Nutrition Education
Clearing House
2140 Shattuck Avenue
Suite 1110
Berkeley, Calif. 94704

Superintendent of Documents
U.S. Government Printing Office
Washington, D.C. 20402

U.S. Department of Agriculture

Cooperative Extension Service
Home Economics
Washington, D.C. 20250

Nutrition Program
Consumer and Food Economics Division
Agricultural Research Service
Hyattsville, Md. 20782

Office of Communication
Washington, D.C. 20250

School Lunch Program
Information Division
Food and Nutrition Service
Washington, D.C. 20250

(Your local Cooperative Extension Service)

World Health Organization (WHO)
Distribution and Sales Service
1211 Geneva 27, Switzerland

APPENDIX L

Formulas of vitamins and amino acids

FAT-SOLUBLE VITAMINS

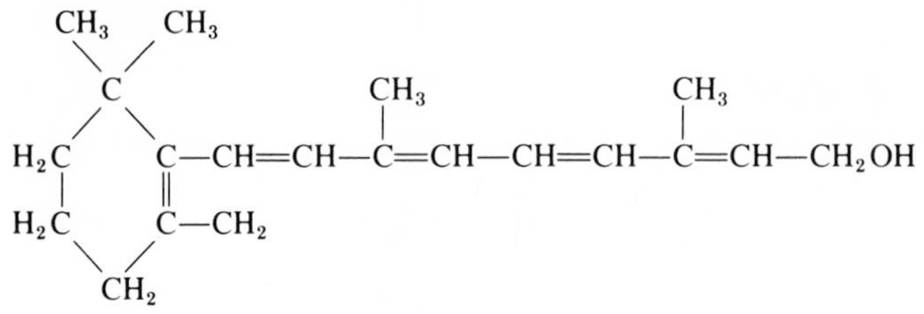

```
       CH3    CH3
         \    /
           C                    CH3                        CH3
         /   \                   |                          |
     H2C       C—CH═CH—CH—C═CH—CH═CH—C═CH—CH2OH
      |        ‖
     H2C       C—CH3
         \    /
          CH2
```

Retinol (vitamin A)

```
                                    CH3               CH3   CH3
                     H2     H        |                 |     |
                     C   CH3C————CH—CH═CH—CH—CH—CH3
                   /   \  |  /  \
               H2C       C       CH2
     H   H2     |        |        |
     C   C     H2C       C———————CH2
   /   \ ‖         \   / |
H2C      C           C   H
 |       |           ‖
H—C      C           CH
 /  \   / \\        /
HO    C      C
      H2
```

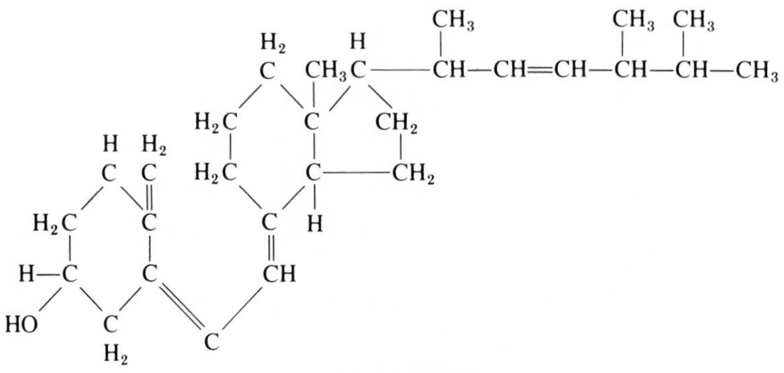

Cholecalciferol (vitamin D)

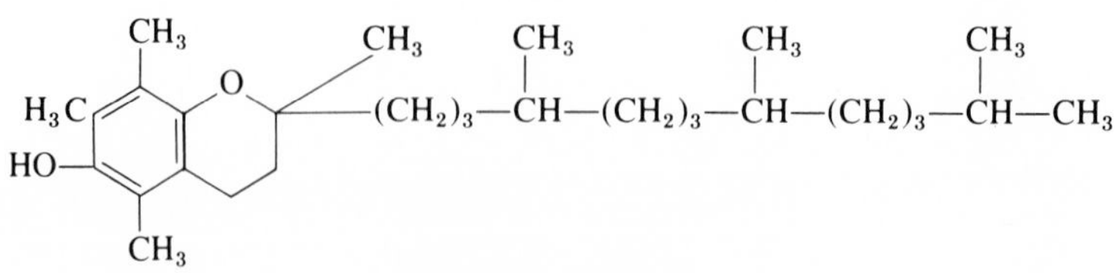

```
        CH3                 CH3      CH3            CH3            CH3
                          /           |              |              |
 H3C                 O  /——(CH2)3—CH—(CH2)3—CH—(CH2)3—CH—CH3
 HO—
        CH3
```

Tocopherol (vitamin E)

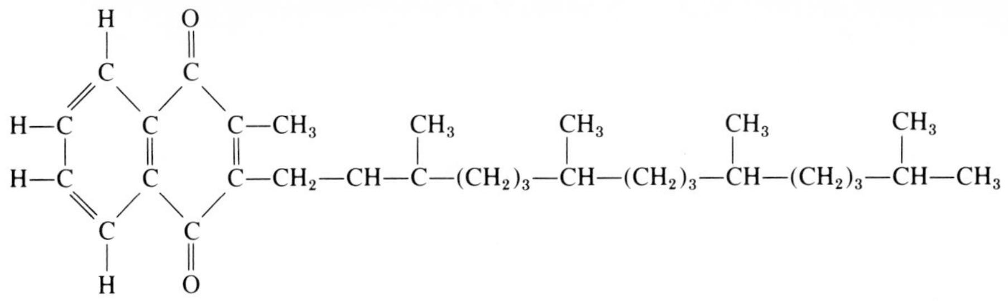

Phylloquinone (vitamin K)

WATER-SOLUBLE VITAMINS

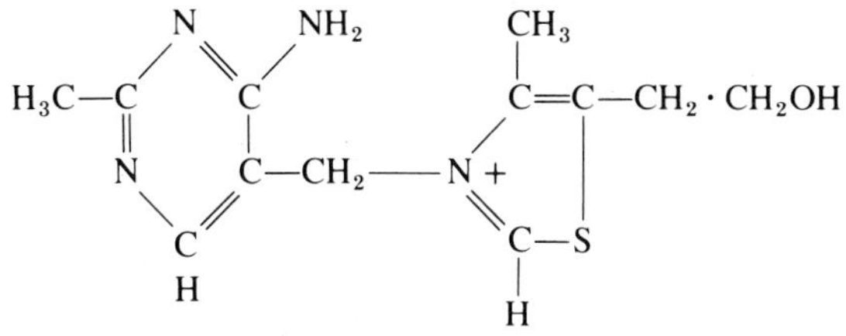

Thiamin (vitamin B_1)

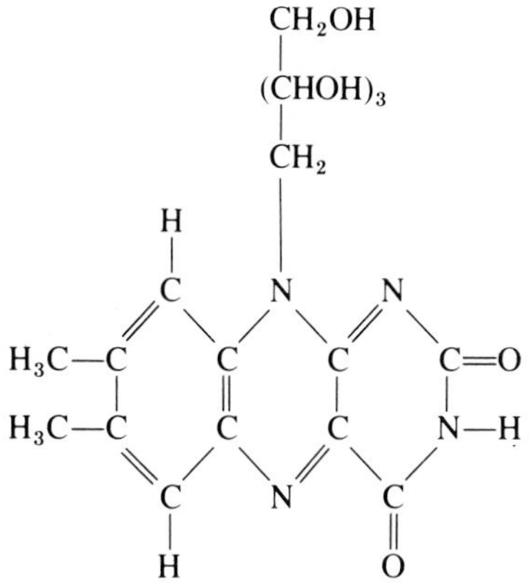

Niacin (nicotinic acid)

Riboflavin (vitamin B_2)

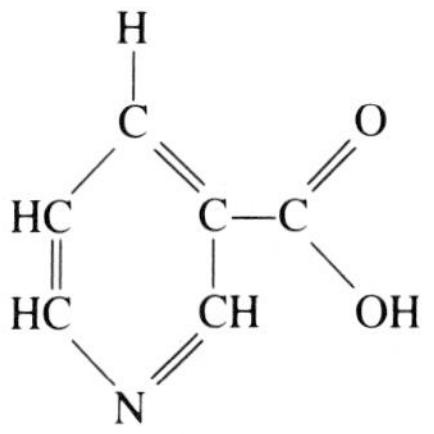

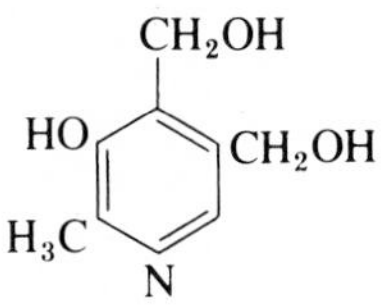

Pyridoxine (vitamin B_6)

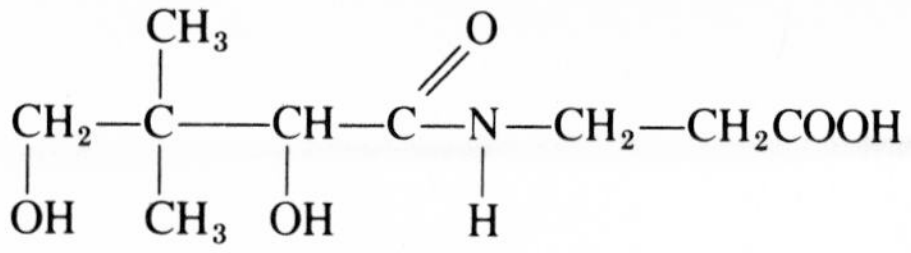

CH₃ O CH₂—C—CH—C—N—CH₂—CH₂COOH OH CH₃ OH H

Pantothenic acid

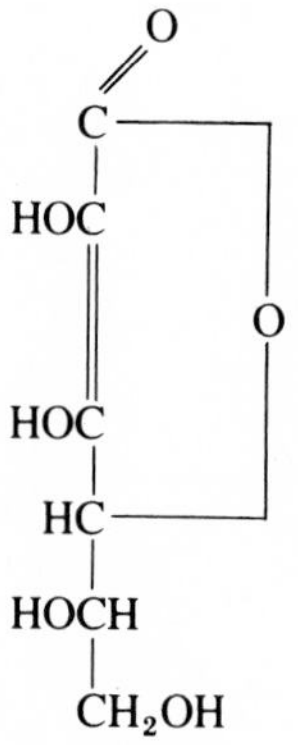

O C HOC O HOC HC HOCH CH₂OH

Ascorbic acid (vitamin C)

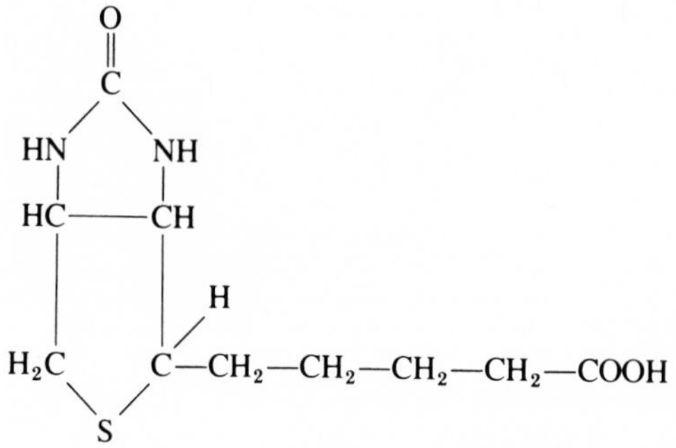

O C HN NH HC CH H H₂C C—CH₂—CH₂—CH₂—CH₂—COOH S

Biotin

H H O H H N N HOOC—C—N—C— —N—C— NH₂ N N CH₂ H OH HOOC—CH₂

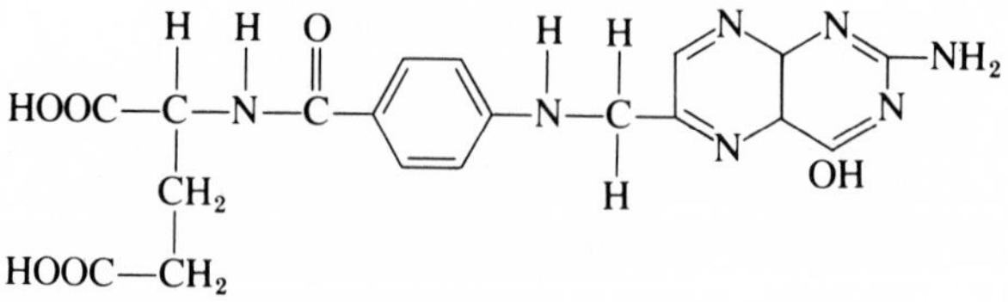

Folacin

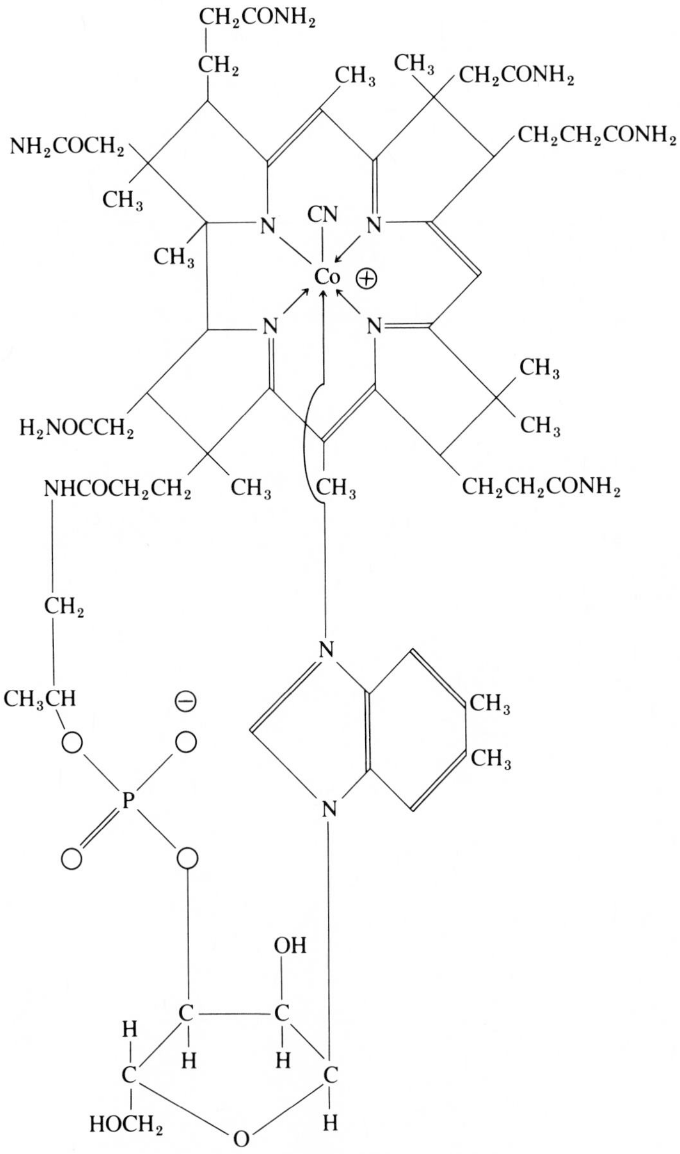

CH_2CONH_2
CH_2
CH_3 CH_3 CH_2CONH_2
NH_2COCH_2 $CH_2CH_2CONH_2$
CH_3
N CN N
CH_3
Co $\oplus$
N N
CH_3
H_2NOCCH_2 CH_3
$NHCOCH_2CH_2$ CH_3 CH_3 $CH_2CH_2CONH_2$
CH_2
N
CH_3CH $\ominus$ CH_3
O O CH_3
P N
O O
OH
C C
H H H
C C
$HOCH_2$ O H

Vitamin B_{12}

ESSENTIAL AMINO ACIDS

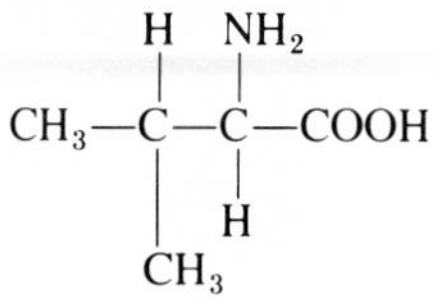

```
         H   NH2
         |   |
CH3 —C — C —COOH
         |   |
         |   H
        CH3
```

Valine

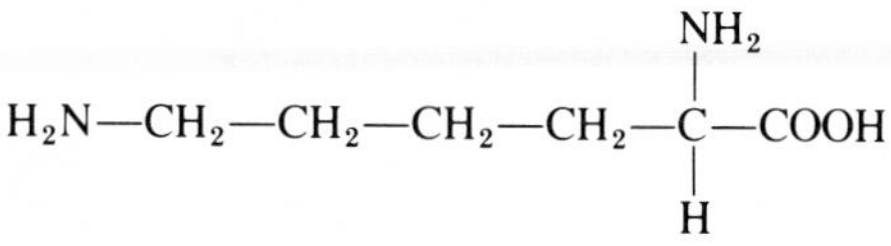

```
                                         NH2
                                         |
H2N—CH2—CH2—CH2—CH2—C—COOH
                                         |
                                         H
```

Lysine

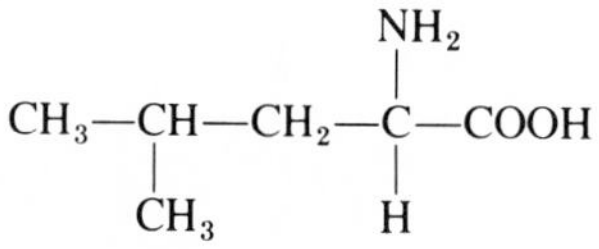

```
                      NH2
                      |
CH3—CH—CH2—C—COOH
        |             |
       CH3            H
```

Leucine

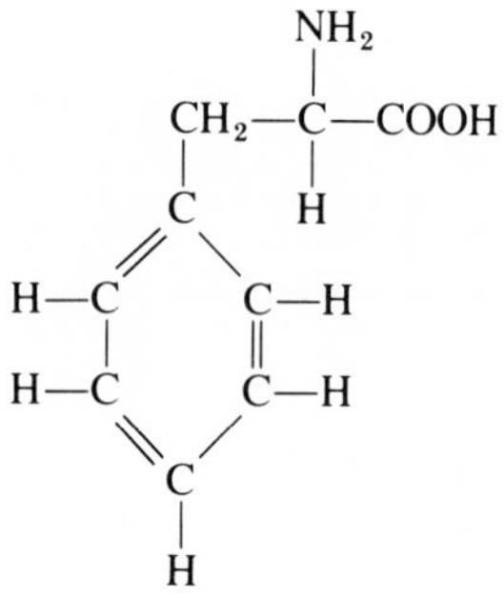

```
          NH2
          |
CH2—C—COOH
 |        |
 C        H
// \
H—C      C—H
  |      ||
H—C      C—H
   \\   /
     C
     |
     H
```

Phenylalanine

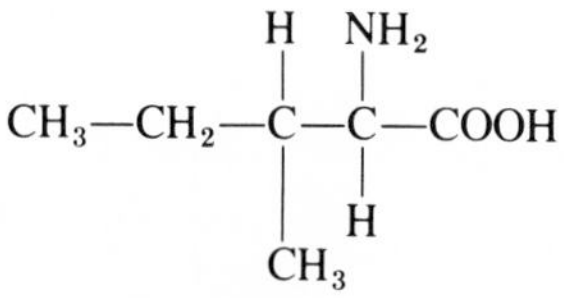

```
                H    NH2
                |    |
CH3—CH2—C—C—COOH
                |    |
                |    H
               CH3
```

Isoleucine

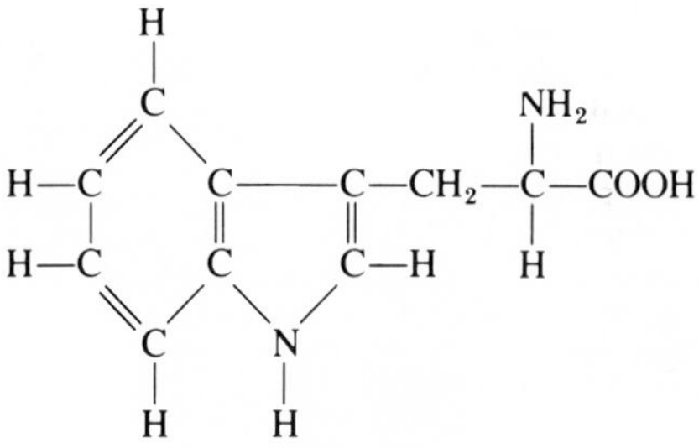

```
      H
      |
      C                                NH2
   //   \                              |
H—C        C———C—CH2—C—COOH
  |        ||      ||           |
H—C        C       C—H         H
   \\    /   \   /
      C        N
      |        |
      H        H
```

Tryptophan

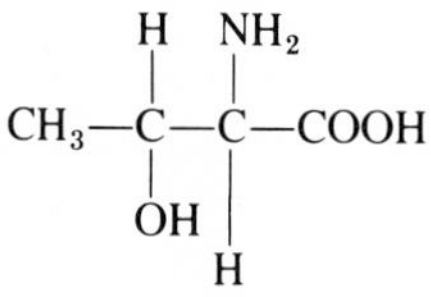

```
         H   NH2
         |   |
CH3—C—C—COOH
         |   |
        OH   |
             H
```

Threonine

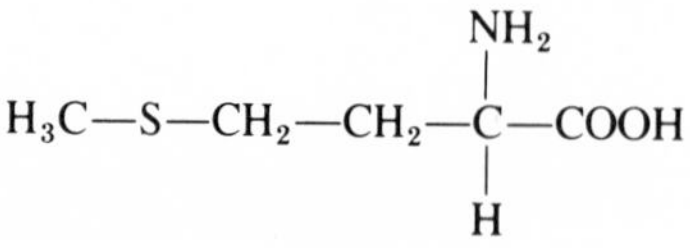

```
                                   NH2
                                   |
H3C—S—CH2—CH2—C—COOH
                                   |
                                   H
```

Methionine

```
H
C=====C—CH2—CH—COOH
|        |          |
N        NH         NH2
  \\    /
    C
    H
```

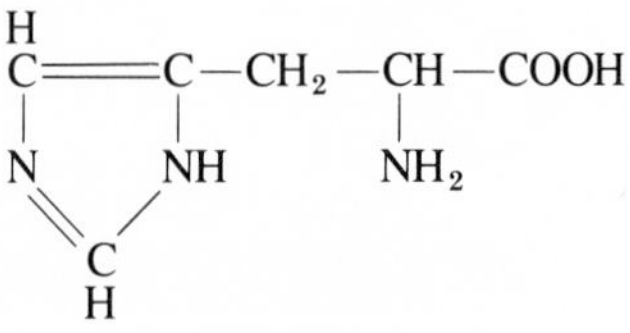

Histidine

Index

C

D

G

J

K

L

M

O

Q

R

S

T

W